H. Yasui (Editor-in-Chief), H. Kado · M. Masuda (Editors)

Cardiovascular Surgery for Congenital Heart Disease

Hisataka Yasui (Editor-in-Chief)
Hideaki Kado · Munetaka Masuda (Editors)

Cardiovascular Surgery for Congenital Heart Disease

Springer

Hisataka Yasui, M.D.
Professor Emeritus, Kyushu University
President, Hamanomachi General Hospital
Fukuoka, Japan

Hideaki Kado, M.D.
Clinical Professor, Kyushu University
Vice President, Fukuoka Children's Hospital
Fukuoka, Japan

Munetaka Masuda, M.D.
Professor and Chairman
Department of Surgery, Yokohama City University
Yokohama, Japan

ISBN: 978-4-431-56321-1 Springer Tokyo Berlin Heidelberg New York

DOI 10.1007/978-4-431-99470-1

Springer is a part of Springer Science+Business Media
springer.com

Softcover re-print of the Hardcover 1st edition 2009

This English translation is based on the Japanese edition

Originally published in Japan in 2003 by MEDICAL VIEW Co., Ltd.

Typesetting: SNP Best-set Typesetter Ltd., Hong Kong

Printed on acid-free paper

Foreword

Surgery for congenital heart disease has been an area of scientific endeavor where many innovative techniques and procedures have been contributed by international surgeons, including a large number from Japan. The publication of *Cardiovascular Surgery for Congenital Heart Disease* in English is an opportunity for many of these techniques to gain a wider audience.

Cardiovascular Surgery for Congenital Heart Disease is an excellent textbook of techniques in pediatric cardiothoracic surgery. The artwork is clear and valuable for trainees in cardiovascular surgery and for practicing pediatric cardiovascular surgeons who wish to have increased information on several variations in surgical techniques that have been pioneered by Japanese surgeons.

Several important modifications are very nicely described in the text, including the Yamaguchi modification of annular enlarging procedures and creative techniques for many operations to avoid the need for homograft material, which is not readily available in Japan or other Asian countries. Some of these unique technical procedures include the very nice illustrations of Yasui's operation for interrupted aortic arch and the Darling series of operations for total anomalous pulmonary venous return. Other creative approaches to unusual coronary anatomy are demonstrated in the chapter on Transposition with VSD. A particularly useful section is on Kawashima's operation for Transposition with VSD, which gives a very nice clear diagrammatic illustration of this creative operation. Other excellent illustrations include the modifications of Jatene's rerouting operation for Taussig-Bing anomaly and transposition VSD with arch obstruction.

There is an excellent series of illustrations of the Sano modification of the Norwood operation for hypoplastic left heart syndrome demonstrating clearly how the operation can be done without the use of artificial material or homograft material. Another excellent chapter includes the various techniques for repair of anomalous origin of the left coronary artery from the pulmonary artery with the unique spiral technique to elongate the origin of the coronary prior to reimplantation, and a nice description of the elongation technique for the unusual situation of anterior descending coronary from the pulmonary artery.

I believe *Cardiovascular Surgery for Congenital Heart Disease* is an excellent addition to the literature and is an important addition to the library of any international pediatric cardiothoracic surgeon practicing in the field. Dr. Yasui and his colleagues are to be commended on pursuing publication of this text in English so that it can achieve the wider audience that it deserves.

Thomas L. Spray, M.D.
President, 2008 and 2009, The American Association for Thoracic Surgery
Head and Chief, Division of Cardiothoracic Surgery
The Children's Hospital Philadelphia
Professor of Surgery (Tenure)
University of Pennsylvania
Philadelphia, USA

Foreword

Preface to the English Edition

Two years ago a Japanese surgeon who practices in the United States contacted me inquiring about the possibility of translating and publishing our book, *Cardiovascular Surgery for Congenital Heart Disease*, because his colleagues so admired the book. We never imagined publishing our surgical textbook in English, because much of what we know in Japan was learned from surgeons in the United States and Europe. When I went to Toronto in 1972 to be trained by Dr. Wilfred G. Bigelow, it was supposed that cardiac surgery in Japan was more than 10 years behind that in North America. It is a great pleasure that more than 40 years later, I can publish this surgical book in English and contribute to the world's surgical community.

Surgery that was initiated by pioneers with novel ideas and techniques has been refined with multiple modifications over the years by successors. The majority of this book is an accumulation of my experience and that of other alumni of Kyushu University Cardiovascular Surgery, whose ideas, techniques, and procedures have evolved over the past 40 years. Because the illustrations herein were drawn from the surgeon's view, I believe they will be efficient and helpful references for paramedical personnel such as nurses, perfusionists, and medical students as well as for cardiac surgeons.

Access to the homograft is very limited in Japan; therefore, many surgical techniques that use only autologous tissue or utilize nonhomograft material have been invented and utilized here. These kinds of modifications which are characteristic of and unique to our practice in Japan may not be applicable or necessarily considered in the United States, as homografts are easily available there. These modifications, however, may become useful resources to surgeons in Asia, Africa, South America, and some parts of Europe where the homograft is not readily available. In addition, a new chapter on cardiac transplantation was added, and several original chapters were revised on this occasion.

For the support and encouragement resulting in the publishing of this English edition, I wish to express my great appreciation to Dr. Thomas L. Spray at the University of Pennsylvania School of Medicine, who kindly wrote the Foreword for this book. I thank Drs. Michiaki Imamura and Robert D.B. Jaquiss at the University of Arkansas for Medical Sciences, who initiated this publishing project and translated the entire book. I gratefully acknowledge also the Kyushu University Cardiovascular Surgery Alumni Association for their participation in supporting this publication.

Hisataka Yasui, M.D.
Professor Emeritus, Kyushu University
President, Hamanomachi General Hospital
Fukuoka, Japan
6 March 2009

Preface to the Japanese Edition

The dawn of pediatric cardiac surgery occurred in the 1960s, at a time when many adorable children with congenital heart disease, who deeply believed doctors could rescue them, were dying as a consequence of our limited knowledge and resources. Doctors were unable to do much to save them. However, over the last half-century many significant advancements in technique and surgical inventions have been achieved in the field of congenital heart disease. These include a more precise understanding of the morphology of congenital heart anomalies with conduction system anatomy, remarkable improvement of neonatal cardiopulmonary bypass from a better understanding of fetal and neonatal circulation, introduction of cardioplegia, and the advancement of mechanical ventilation. A survey in 2000 by The Japanese Association for Thoracic Surgery showed the overall mortality rate of pediatric heart surgery to be less than 5%, although neonatal open heart surgery still has a high mortality rate of 32%.

When Fukuoka Children's Hospital was opened in Japan in 1980, neonatal open heart surgery was thought not to be practical and surgery was either postponed until the baby attained a weight of more than 5 kg or deep hypothermic circulatory arrest was used for challenging complex open heart procedures in small babies. We were unavoidably involved in neonatal open heart surgery and the management of complex congenital heart disease with little experience and only a limited understanding. In attempting to solve the difficult problems involved in surgical procedures in congenital heart disease, much knowledge was obtained from articles published in the world. Many imitations were tried, usually in vain. Inspired by the findings from the report of neonate hemodynamics by Abraham M. Rudolph and his colleagues, however, we moved forward and initiated moderate hypothermic high-flow cardiopulmonary bypass and were able to resolve many problems.

My initial experience included many operations for complex congenital heart disease. I spent many nights contemplating and reflecting on how to treat patients with complicated problems, combining observations in the operating room during visits to other countries with information available in journals. I have many colleagues to thank for their useful suggestions during these early years. In order to obtain a better understanding of complex congenital heart disease and improve surgical techniques as we sought to move ahead in our field, an association of peers called Genkai was formed in 1985 (Genkai had an appropriate double meaning for our purposes in Fukuoka. It is the name of the sea at Fukuoka, and also denote the sense of limitation, which we keenly felt at that time). Annual meetings were started with founding members Drs. Yasuharu Imai, Yasuaki Naito, Kennichi Kosuga, Shigeyuki Takeuchi, Michio Yokota, Masahiro Yamaguchi, and Hisataka Yasui. Many junior and senior colleagues were involved in these meetings and they have contributed greatly to the advancements of pediatric and congenital heart surgery in Japan.

Over the years, cardiac surgery has evolved based on our predecessors' knowledge, techniques, and clinical decisions. Those who succeeded them have been applying previously acquired knowledge, and honing their skills with some modification based on close examination of daily practice. Cardiac surgery is one of the supreme arts in medicine. Treatment results can be improved with subtle modification, and small advances in surgical techniques. This book is intended to present all surgical procedures, highlighting key steps, offering tips, and cautioning against pitfalls. At the time of retirement from cardiac surgery, my desire is to share these

30 years' experience as others have shared theirs with me in this specialized field. The authors are my close colleagues who are currently chief surgeons of cardiac surgery and have achieved excellent results in their practices.

It is my hope that this book will contribute to improving surgical treatment, with the goal of ultimately improving the quality of life for small children.

Hisataka Yasui, M.D.
Professor and Chairman
Department of Cardiovascular Surgery
Kyushu University School of Medicine
Fukuoka, Japan
1 January 2003

Contents

Contributors

Editor-in-Chief
Hisataka Yasui, M.D.
Professor Emeritus, Kyushu University
President, Hamanomachi General Hospital, Fukuoka, Japan

Editors
Hideaki Kado, M.D.
Clinical Professor, Kyushu University
Vice President, Fukuoka Children's Hospital, Fukuoka, Japan

Munetaka Masuda, M.D.
Professor and Chairman
Department of Surgery, Yokohama City University, Yokohama, Japan

Authors
Toshihide Asou, M.D.
Clinical Professor, Yokohama City University
Chief, Department of Cardiovascular Surgery
Kanagawa Children's Medical Center, Yokohama, Japan

Kouji Fukae, M.D.
Chief, Department of Pediatric Cardiac Surgery
Kumamoto City Hospital, Kumamoto, Japan

Michiaki Imamura, M.D., Ph.D.
Associate Professor of Surgery, University of Arkansas for Medical Sciences
Pediatric and Congenital Cardiothoracic Surgery
Arkansas Children's Hospital, Little Rock, AR, USA

Yutaka Imoto, M.D.
Chief, Department of Cardiovascular Surgery
Kyushu Koseinenkin Hospital, Kitakyushu, Japan

Robert D.B. Jaquiss, M.D.
Professor of Surgery, University of Arkansas for Medical Sciences
Pediatric and Congenital Cardiothoracic Surgery
Arkansas Children's Hospital, Little Rock, AR, USA

Hideaki Kado, M.D.
Clinical Professor, Kyushu University
Vice President, Fukuoka Children's Hospital, Fukuoka, Japan

Kazuhiro Kurisu, M.D.
Chief, Department of Cardiovascular Surgery
Kitakyushu Municipal Medical Center, Kitakyushu, Japan

Munetaka Masuda, M.D.
Professor and Chairman
Department of Surgery, Yokohama City University, Yokohama, Japan

Toshihide Nakano, M.D.
Chief, Department of Pediatric Cardiac Surgery
Fukuoka Children's Hospital, Fukuoka, Japan

Akira Sese, M.D.
Vice President
Kyushu Koseinenkin Hospital, Kitakyushu, Japan

Yuichi Shiokawa, M.D.
Assistant Professor, Department of Cardiovascular Surgery
Kyushu University Hospital, Fukuoka, Japan

Shigehiko Tokunaga, M.D.
Assistant Professor, Department of Cardiovascular Surgery
Kyushu University Hospital, Fukuoka, Japan

Yasutaka Ueno
Chief, Department of Cardiovascular Surgery
Shimonoseki City Central Hospital, Shimonoseki, Japan

Hisataka Yasui, M.D.
Professor Emeritus, Kyushu University
President, Hamanomachi General Hospital, Fukuoka, Japan

Kunihiro Yonenaga, M.D. (Deceased)
Chief, Department of Cardiovascular Surgery
Kumamoto City Hospital, Kumamoto, Japan

English Translation

Michiaki Imamura, M.D., Ph.D.
Associate Professor of Surgery, University of Arkansas for Medical Sciences
Pediatric and Congenital Cardiothoracic Surgery
Arkansas Children's Hospital, Little Rock, AR, USA

Robert D.B. Jaquiss, M.D.
Professor of Surgery, University of Arkansas for Medical Sciences
Pediatric and Congenital Cardiothoracic Surgery
Arkansas Children's Hospital, Little Rock, AR, USA

I. General Considerations

I-1. Cardiopulmonary Bypass and Myocardial Protection

In the past two decades, there have been enormous advances in pediatric and congenital heart surgery as a consequence of improvements in cardiopulmonary bypass (CPB) and cardioplegic protection. Especially in very small babies, the relatively large priming volume of the CPB circuit affects the vulnerable capillary endothelial integrity. This vascular insult is more serious in small children than in adults. Several techniques and drugs have been tried to reduce these adverse effects. Attention has been directed to reducing the volume from the cardiopulmonary circuit and washing out the priming solution [1,2]. Several methods of filtration, such as dilutional ultrafiltration (DUF) and modified ultrafiltration (MUF), are widely utilized to remove the harmful substances from the patient's body [3]. In the clinical setting, the safety of CPB is very important. In small babies, especially, smooth cannulation, precise technique, and greater experience are required.

In considering cardioplegic myocardial protection, it should be emphasized that the myocardium in small children is very susceptible to edema. It is necessary to modify the composition of the cardioplegic solution and to avoid excessive pressure during infusion [4]. Cardiopulmonary bypass and inadequate myocardial protection may cause multiple organ failure, including heart failure and other organ dysfunction, and may worsen postoperative outcome.

Prime Composition of the Bypass Circuit and Filtration of the Priming Solution

Many different-sized pump circuits are available, and circuit selection is based on the body weight of the patient (Table I-1-1). In neonates and small infants, it is important to have a prime composition that is similar to that of blood as well as to decrease the priming volume as much as possible. As shown in Table I-1-2, in neonates and small infants the priming volume is decreased to 270–300 ml, and the hematocrit and total protein are kept at about 30% and 4 g/dl, respectively. To achieve this composition, red blood cells and albumin are used. Bank blood may have citrate/phosphate dextrose and other vasoactive substances such as bradykinin. These vasoactive substances can induce adverse affects in the body after bypass. To remove these substances, the priming solution is washed and filtered.

To wash the priming solution of CPB, a hemofiltration solution is used because this type of fluid does not need further modulation. Initially, red blood cells and albumin solution are placed in the reservoir. Then, 300–500 ml of washing solution is gradually added into the circuit. The priming solution is circulated in the circuit, and filtration is instituted. After filtration, other components of the priming solution are added to the priming solution to obtain the final concentration. Washing of the priming solution can prevent hypotension soon after initiation of CPB, and it is more important than DUF, especially in short pump time cases.

Management During Bypass: Flow and Temperature

In neonates, normal cardiac output is about 350 ml/kg/min shortly after birth. It progressively falls to about 150 ml/kg/min by about 6 weeks of life, which is still a much higher output than that of an adult (80 ml/kg/min) [5,6]. Inadequate pump flow has been noted to cause maldistribution of blood flow [7], resulting in metabolic acidosis during cardiopulmonary bypass. Therefore, a rather high flow rate, 2.5–3.5 l/min/m^2, is utilized in neonates and young infants [8]. Poirier et al. [9] and Karl et al. [10] reported excellent surgical results using this high-flow cardiopulmonary bypass strategy. In our institution, high pump flow bypass was introduced in the early 1980s. Before the mid-1980s, a pulsatile flow pump was used to improve peripheral circulation and venous drainage [8]. Subsequently, a nonpulsatile pump has been used with the addition of a vasodilator.

In a relatively short case such as ventricular septal defect (VSD) closure, mild hypothermia of greater than 32°C can be used. In a patient with cyanotic heart disease, a higher flow is used to compensate for flow through aortopulmonary collateral vessels, which otherwise might cause a "steal" phenomenon. Even at a rectal temperature of 28°C, a flow of more than 3.0–3.5 l/min/m^2 is necessary. To improve visualization of the surgical field by decreasing the blood return to the intracardiac cavity, the flow may need to be reduced temporarily. When this reduced flow is required for a longer period, the patient should be cooled further.

Although deep hypothermic circulatory arrest is still used in the United States and in European countries for complex congenital heart surgery in neonates and small infants, in

Japan this modality has been used infrequently and only during surgical procedures requiring aortic arch reconstruction. A safe duration of circulatory arrest is believed to be less than 40–60 min at a rectal temperature of 18°C. However, subtle neurodevelopmental injury has been identified in long-term follow-up studies of patients who had even shorter duration of deep hypothermic circulatory arrest. Therefore, the safe limits of circulatory arrest time remain uncertain.

In lesions requiring aortic arch reconstruction such as interrupted aortic arch or hypoplastic left heart syndrome, with the use of regional cerebral perfusion through the brachiocephalic artery combined with descending aortic perfusion [11,12], surgery may be performed without any circulatory arrest to either the lower body or the brain. Even the Norwood procedure can be performed under moderate hypothermia with total body high-flow bypass, which may markedly improve surgical results for hypoplastic left heart syndrome [12,13].

During bypass, the peripheral vasculature undergoes vasoconstriction, and maldistribution of flow may occur. It is believed that this happens as a result of vascular response to the changed flow and temperature under artificial perfusion; this causes hypoperfusion of some parts of the body, producing metabolic acidosis. This vasoconstriction burdens the susceptible systemic ventricle during the early postoperative period as an excessive afterload. To avoid this vasoconstriction, chlorpromazine is used during surgery as a vasodilator. With a vasodilatory strategy during bypass, a higher bypass flow and adequate urine output are maintained, and stable postoperative hemodynamics can be easily obtained. To maintain a mean systemic pressure of 40–50 mmHg during bypass, 1–2 mg chlorpromazine is administered every 10–20 min. In general, a total dose will be 2 mg/kg; in neonates, 3–4 mg/kg can be used [14].

Table I-1-1. Circuit size and priming volume

Circuit	Patient weight (kg)	Priming volume (ml)	Oxygenator	Arterial tube size (in.)	Venous tube size (in.)
SS	<10	270	Dideco D-901	3/16	1/4
S	10–25	500	Dideco D-902	1/4	5/16
M	25–40	640	Dideco D-905	1/4	3/8
L	>40	900	Dideco D-905	3/8	1/2

Table I-1-2. Composition of priming solution (SS circuit)

Packed red blood cell	200 ml
15% Mannitol	10 ml
8.4% Sodium bicarbonate	15 ml
25% Albumin	50 ml
Heparin	5 mg
Ascorbic acid	250 mg
Antibiotic	
Total volume	275 ml

Dilutional Ultrafiltration (DUF)

It is known that several inflammatory mediators are released soon after initiation of bypass. These potentially injurious vasoactive substances should be removed from the circulation during the operation, because their concentration becomes elevated with prolonged bypass [15]. During bypass, as supplemental fluid is intermittently added to the circuit, an equivalent volume is removed through filtration (Fig. I-1-1). This added washing solution should be the same

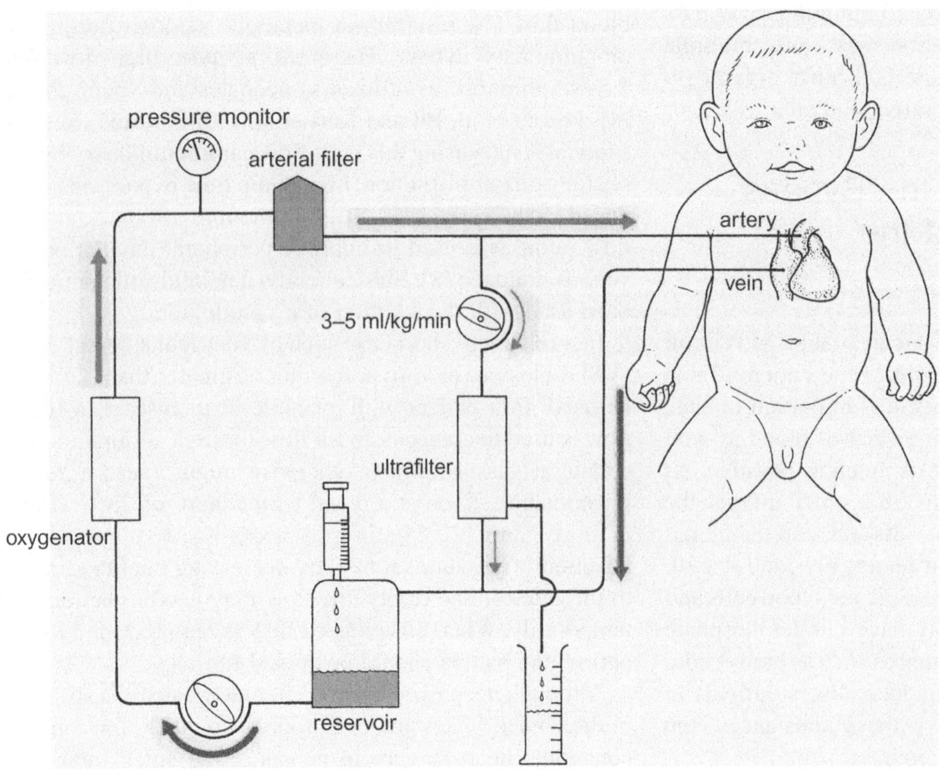

Fig. I-1-1. Dilutional ultrafiltration (DUF) circuit. During bypass, the pump in the filtration circuit is run at a rate of 3–5 ml/kg/min. Crystalloid solution of an amount equivalent to the filtrate is added to the reservoir

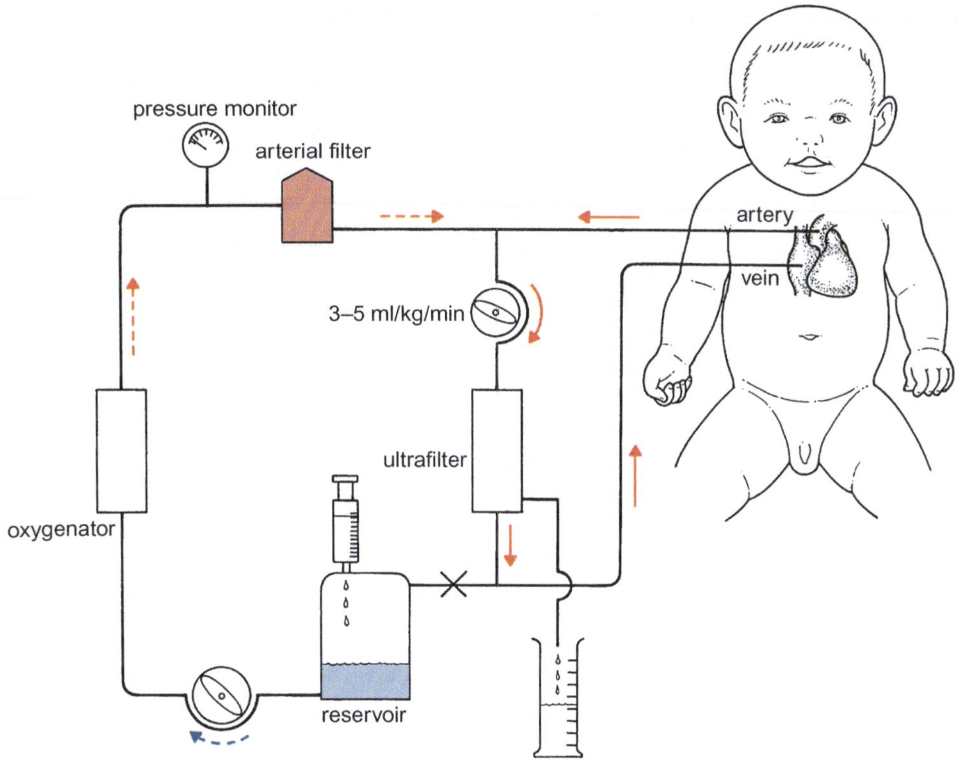

Fig. I-1-2. Modified ultrafiltration (MUF) circuit. After bypass is discontinued, filtration is started with a flow rate of 3–5 ml/kg/min drained from the arterial cannula and returned to the venous cannula. To compensate for decreases in central venous and left atrial pressures, blood in the reservoir is gradually returned. The blood in the reservoir is replaced with crystalloid solution. Ultimately, the oxygenator, the arterial filter, and the arterial tubing are filled with crystalloid solution to displace all sanguinary fluid into the filtration system

as the priming washing solution. In neonates and small infants, 1000–2000 ml of volume is exchanged during and after aortic cross-clamping. The flow rate of the filtration pump is 3–5 ml/kg/min.

Modified Ultrafiltration (MUF)

The superiority of MUF over DUF for removing inflammatory mediators is still controversial. Several studies, however, have clearly demonstrated that MUF removes total body free water, reduces myocardial edema, and improves cardiac contractility. Elevation of hematocrit and hemodynamic stability with improved blood pressure are usually observed. Better hemostasis with decreased transfusion has also been reported. After separation from bypass, MUF is instituted with a flow rate of 3–5 ml/kg/min by draining from the aortic cannula and returning an equivalent volume to the venous cannula (Fig. I-1-2).

Because a negative pressure at the site of the aortic cannula may cause air migration into the aortic cannula, care is taken to avoid producing excessively negative pressure at the aortic root. In hemodynamically unstable patients, MUF is started with a low flow rate. We do not use any special cannulae for MUF. The bypass cannulae during surgery are continuously used for MUF. The benefits of this maneuver are smooth transition from the bypass to MUF and rapid reinstitution of the bypass if necessary. As free water is removed from the patient, the central venous and left atrial pressures may decrease. Therefore, the blood from the reservoir is returned to the patient intermittently. The speed of the filtration is adjusted with the resistance at the drainage site of the filter as with DUF. When the level of the reservoir is low, crystalloid solution is added. It takes 10–15 min to finish the filtration. Usually hematocrit increases about 6%. In patients using a SS circuit, hematocrit rises about 10%–15%. Total protein increases from 4 to 7 g/dl.

Although some surgical teams worry about prolonging the operating time by using MUF, we spend this time placing chest tubes and pacing wires. Even in coagulopathic or bleeding patients, an increase in hematocrit above 50% at the end of MUF can be achieved. Platelets and fresh-frozen plasma are administered during or after MUF, if required, and may produce some hemodilution.

Cardiopulmonary Bypass without Transfusion

Nontransfusion bypass can avoid transfusion-related inflammatory response and infection. Adverse effects on several organs, particularly the lungs, may decrease, and postoperative recovery may be facilitated. Nontransfusion surgery should be performed very cautiously, because excessive hemodilution during bypass may cause neurological injury.

During nontransfusion bypass, care should be taken to (1) minimize hemodilution by decreasing the priming volume, (2) minimize bypass time, and (3) maintain higher bypass flow and Po_2 in the arterial blood. The priming volume can be reduced to less than 300 ml by shortening of the tubing and miniaturization of the oxygenator and filter. With a separate type of oxygenator and reservoir, the priming volume may be reduced to less than 200 ml. Although the lowest "safe" hematocrit is not known, because of the influence of bypass duration and the temperature of the patient, we believe a hematocrit less than 18% should be avoided. When the bypass time is longer than expected, transfusion should be considered at an earlier stage. As a simple approximation of oxygen delivery during CPB, mixed venous oxygen saturation (SvO_2) can be used. A $SvO_2 \geq 70\%$ is considered safe. If SvO_2 decreases toward this limit, pump flow should be increased. During rewarming, the SvO_2 may decrease as a result of increased oxygen consumption, so close attention is important during this phase.

During the period between separation from CPB and completely returning the blood from the bypass circuit, the patient is in a very vulnerable condition because hematocrit is low. High arterial oxygen saturation with 100% oxygen ventilation and high cardiac output with inotropic support should be maintained. During ventilation, it is especially important to avoid atelectasis. If the SvO_2 is inadequate under low flow conditions, separation from bypass is considered unsafe. To rapidly increase the low hematocrit, MUF is very effective, and can raise the hematocrit by 5%–8% within 10–15 min after separation from bypass without volume loading the heart. Compared to simply returning the blood from the bypass circuit, this maneuver is much safer and faster. In older children or patients with polycythemia caused by cyanotic heart disease, perioperative blood conservation and autotransfusion is utilized; this step can help to raise the hematocrit rapidly after separation from bypass [16].

Myocardial Protection

We use a multidose cardioplegic solution with topical cooling. The composition of the albumin-added crystalloid cardioplegia is shown in Table I-1-3. A simple gravity circuit with a filter is used to infuse the cardioplegic solution through a needle with side holes that has been placed in the root of the ascending aorta. Cooled cardioplegic solution is infused from a height of 100 cm, but the presence of the filter caused the actual pressure of infusion to be more likely less than 50 cmH_2O. The cardioplegic infusion pressure should not exceed 60 cmH_2O, as the coronary arteries in neonates may lack autoregulation [4]. Infusion using gravity can avoid excessive pressure and is the safest system. The infusion volume is 10 ml/kg as an initial dose, and 5 ml/kg in subsequent doses, re-administered every 20–30 min. For topical cooling, ice slush from Ringer's solution is used.

Table I-1-3. Composition of cardioplegic solution

5% Glucose	250 ml
Normal saline	250 ml
Sodium bicarbonate	5 ml
8.5% Calcium gluconate	1.5 ml
Potassium chloride	10 mEq
Lidocaine	50 mg
25% Albumin	20 ml
Regular insulin	2.5 unit
Na^+	90 mEq/l
K^+	20 mEq/l
Cl^-	100 mEq/l
Ca^{++}	0.4 mmol/l

When an aortotomy is required, retrograde cardioplegic administration is useful [17]. The initial dose is given antegrade through the aortic root. After right atriotomy, a retrograde cannula is inserted into the coronary sinus. After balloon inflation with 1 ml saline, the catheter is pulled back slowly until resistance is noticed. This cannula is connected to the cardioplegia circuit, and cardioplegic solution is injected with 50 cmH_2O pressure gravity. The seal at the coronary sinus and confirmation of delivery by blood dripping from the coronary artery orifices are checked. The volume of the cardioplegic solution and the interval of injections are the same as with antegrade cardioplegia. Because of lower injection pressure, a longer time is required to deliver the solution retrograde. This longer infusion time is not a problem, however, because the surgical procedure does not need to be interrupted during retrograde cardioplegia injection. When the balloon cannot be secured or the identification of the coronary sinus is not possible, occasionally direct coronary ostial antegrade cardioplegia is used. In neonates, a small feeding tube is used to perfuse the orifices selectively.

The manner of reperfusion after aortic declamping is important in myocardial recovery and attenuation of reperfusion injury. The perfusion pressure is kept low in the initial 10–15 min after declamping, and the heart is kept unloaded to facilitate recovery from the ischemic insult caused by aortic cross-clamping. After electrolytes are corrected, the preload to the heart is gradually increased.

Cardiopulmonary Bypass: Surgical Aspects

Selection of Cannulae

Selection of appropriate-sized cannulae is very important in pediatric CPB. To improve venous drainage, the largest cannula that fits the vessel should be chosen. When the correct cannula is chosen, inappropriate positioning of the venous cannula should be suspected if venous drainage is inadequate. We have evaluated the properties of our circuit and venous cannulae (Fig. I-1-3). The results may differ from the data supplied by the manufacturers, because these property changes are influenced by the size and length of the bypass tubing. Several kinds of arterial and venous can-

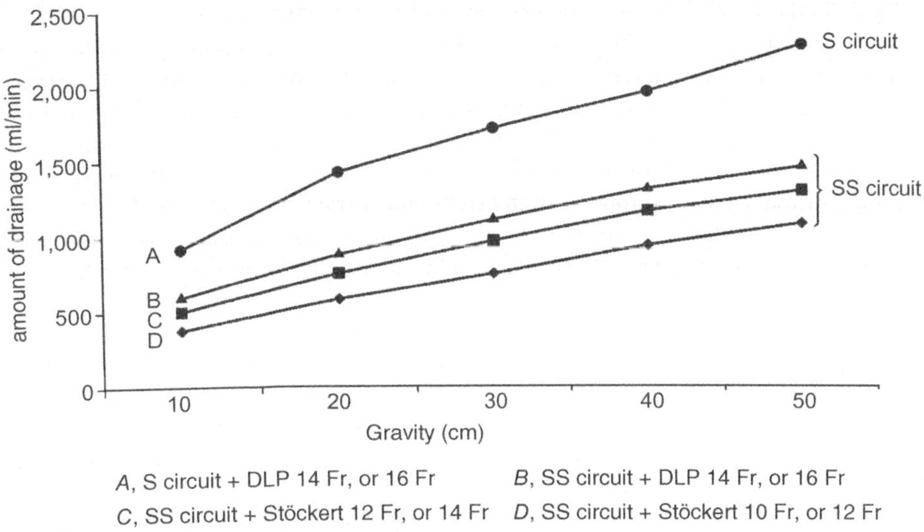

Fig. I-1-3. Venous cannula properties. Venous drainage according to the gravity using (S) and (SS) circuits with different kinds of venous cannulae

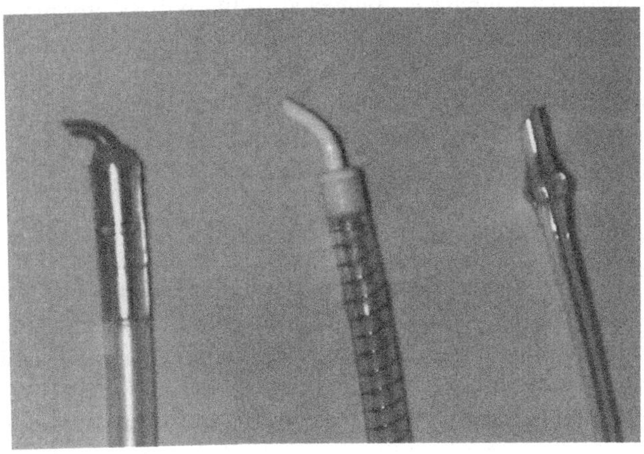

Fig. I-1-4. Arterial cannulae. From *left to right*: JMS, 2.1 mm; Stöckert, 2.0 mm; Research Medical, 8 Fr.

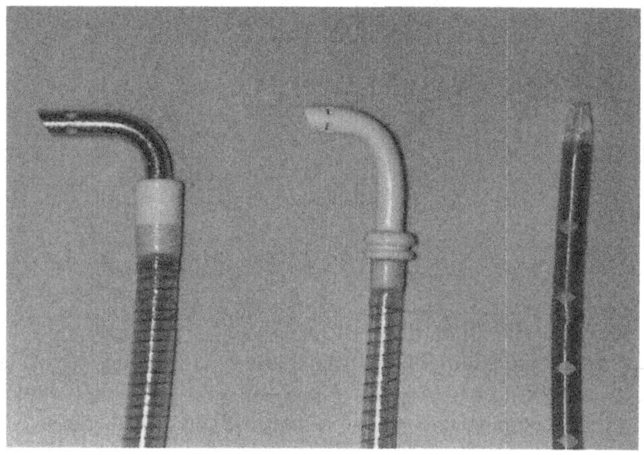

Fig. I-1-5. Venous cannulae. From *left to right*: DLP, 12 Fr.; Stöckert, 12 Fr.; Kuraray, 12 Fr.

nulae are available from different manufactures (Figs. I-1-4, I-1-5). The arterial cannula should be resistant to kinking, thin walled, light, and easy to insert. Cannulae by JMS (Japan Medical Supply, Hiroshima, Japan) were produced to obtain excellent flow characteristics [18]. When intracardiac surgery or surgical procedure on the SVC, such as a Glenn shunt, is required, a right-angled venous cannula from DLP or Stöckert is used for venous drainage. The bypass tubing can be retracted superiorly and inferiorly and tucked to the drapes to facilitate visualization of the operating field, because the tubing portions of these cannulae are flexible and resistant to kinking.

Cannulation

Cannulation is the most important surgical procedure in the establishment of CPB. Vessel damage or stenosis at the cannulation site can easily occur, because in neonates the vessels are small and the tissues are fragile. Hemodynamic instability may occur by compression of the heart, so extra care is necessary during cannulation.

Arterial Cannulation

The ascending aorta proximal to the base of the brachiocephalic artery is usually used for arterial cannulation. In neonates when the surgical procedure is on the ascending aorta, such as in the arterial switch operation, the aortic cannula is inserted into the aortic arch distal to the base of the brachiocephalic artery.

To improve visualization and stabilization of the ascending aorta, the adventitia of the ascending aorta is held with a mosquito clamp and pulled caudally. This maneuver is useful especially in minimal access surgery with a short skin incision. A single purse-string suture is placed in patients weighing less than 15 kg; in larger patients, two sutures are placed. A longitudinal or longitudinally oval-shaped purse-string suture is preferable in a small patient to avoid iatrogenic stenosis (Fig. I-1-6). The stitch is started from the cephalic side of the ascending aorta caudally. As the length of these stitches depends on the size of the cannula, the cannula is brought inside the surgeon's field of vision. This technique is also used for the purse-string suture for the venous cannula.

The other end of the stitch is placed parallel to the first suture. The suture is placed through the media of the aortic wall, and care is taken to avoid placing the stitch inside the aortic lumen. When bleeding occurs, hemostasis is obtained with compression, and then cannulation is completed. Cannulation is generally performed by securing a three-point fixation (Fig. I-1-7). The first assistant holds the clamp, which is securing the proximal ascending aorta caudally, with the left hand, and the forceps, which is securing the aortic adventitia 1–2 mm lateral to the left-side purse-string suture, with the right hand. The surgeon holds the adventitia lateral to the right-side purse-string suture, with a left hand and the forceps. The adventitia between the purse-string suture is carefully incised. With tension held by the two pairs of forceps, a knife is advanced into the aortic lumen with care not to damage the posterior wall of the aortic wall. After the knife is removed from the aorta, bleeding is controlled by approximation of the two forceps. At the time of inserting the aortic cannula, these two forceps are pulled to create tension on the aortic wall, and can help cannulation even in small children with low blood pressure. When a sufficient length of adventitia is incised, and enough tension at the aortic wall is present, the cannula can be inserted easily. After blood return into the aortic cannula has been confirmed, the cannula is connected to the bypass circuit. The aortic cannula is secured at the cephalic end of the skin incision edge using a heavy silk suture. When the left side of the ascending aorta is the main surgical focus, such as in supracristal VSD closure, the aortic cannula is secured on the right side of the skin incision.

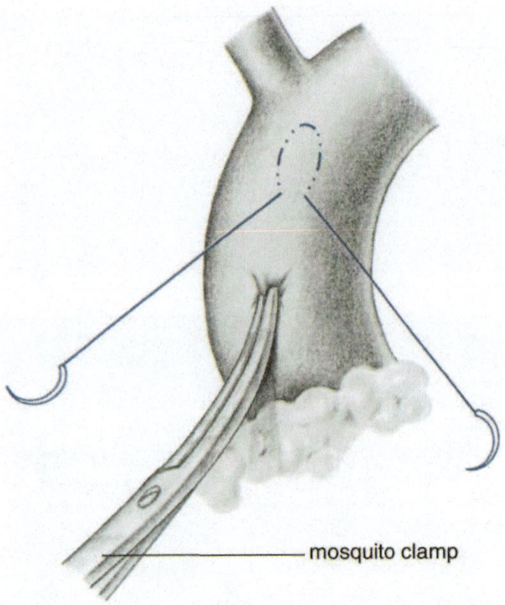

Fig. I-1-6. Ascending aortic cannulation: purse-string suture. The aortic adventitia is held with a mosquito clamp and pulled caudally, and the rectangular or oblong purse-string suture is placed

Venous Cannulation

Generally, venous cannulae are inserted directly into both cavae. During venous cannulation, excessive manipulation to the heart and bleeding may cause hemodynamic instability. In neonates, delicate handling is required for SVC cannulation. In these patients, therefore, purse-string sutures are

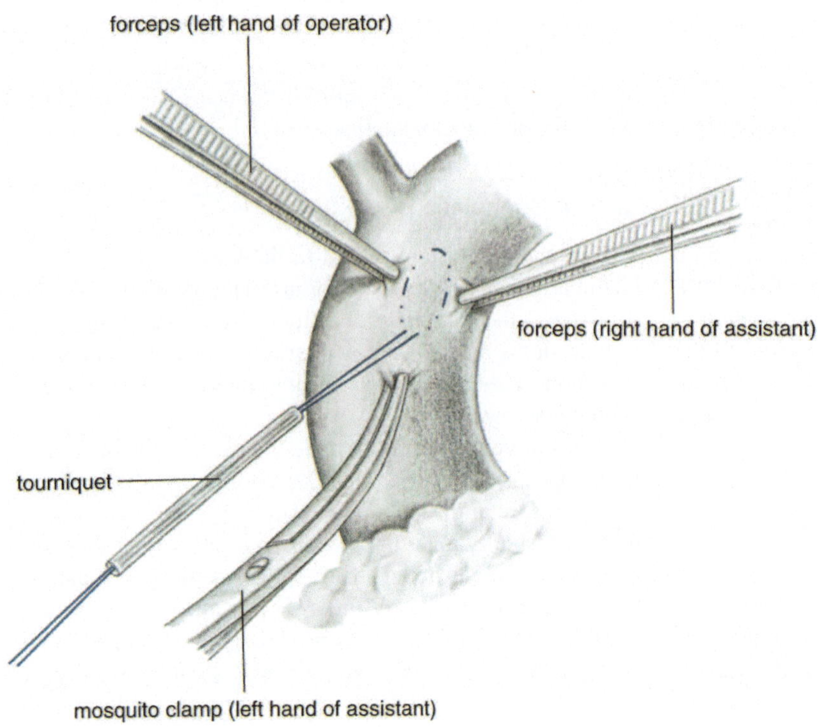

Fig. I-1-7. Ascending aortic cannulation: cannula insertion. The surgeon and the assistant hold the aortic adventitia 1–2 mm lateral to the proposed cannulation site

placed in the SVC and IVC. Then, the IVC cannula is inserted, and bypass is initiated with a single venous cannula. The SVC cannula is then inserted under stable conditions.

To insert the cannula directly into the SVC, the length of the SVC may be inadequate. The pericardial reflection is dissected to visualize the distal part of the SVC. During this dissection, care is taken not to damage the phrenic nerve situated lateral to the SVC. For surgery, such as total cavo-pulmonary connection or the Glenn procedure, because the SVC cannulation site needs to be very high, the junction with the innominate vein is also dissected. To facilitate dissection of the SVC, the right lobe of the thymus is partially excised. For the purse-string suture, a 4-0 or 5-0 monofilament suture is used in an older child and in an infant, respectively. In neonates or small infants, to avoid iatrogenic SVC stenosis, a narrow purse-string suture is placed. One arm of a double-armed suture is started 2–3 mm above the SVC-RA junction and advanced superiorly. Similar to the aortic purse-string suture, the cannula is brought in the viewing field of the operator to decide the length of the purse-string suture. Next, the other arm of the suture is placed parallel to the first suture (Fig. I-1-8). For opening the SVC, three points are secured as with aortic cannulation. The assistant holds the SVC distal to the purse-string suture site with the right hand. Opposite sides of the purse-string suture are held by the left hands of the surgeon and the assistant (Fig. I-1-9). With a no. 11 knife positioned vertically, the SVC incision is started from the caudal end of the purse-string suture and advanced superiorly. Forceps holding the side of the purse-string suture are pulled toward the surgeon and assistant to avoid damage to the posterior wall of the SVC. This maneuver can increase the width of the purse-string suture and avoid injury to the purse-string sutures. If the superior ends are kept slightly wider to obtain a large hole in the SVC, the incision can be extended to the end of the purse-string sutures. The incision is opened with three-point tension and the cannula is inserted. The cannula is usually held with the fingers. In neonates, the cannula is occasionally held with a hemostat clamp. When the cannulation is difficult for reason of a small incision, the incision is enlarged by gentle spreading of the tips of a mosquito clamp. After cannula insertion, the purse-string suture is snugged with a tourniquet. After blood return is checked, the cannula is connected to the circuit. At the time of connecting the tube and the cannula, the cannula is held steady by the assistant to avoid its dislodgement from the insertion site.

Because cannulation of the IVC is easier and less complicated than that of the SVC, IVC cannulation is performed first. For cannulation of the IVC, dissection around the IVC is not usually necessary. When direct cannulation of the IVC is required, the IVC is dissected at the junction of the IVC and diaphragm with care to protect the phrenic nerve. To improve visualization of the IVC, the pericardial edge of the diaphragm site is sutured to the skin edge (Figs. I-1-10, I-1-11).

To facilitate placement of purse-string sutures for IVC cannulation, the right atrial wall is retracted with two peanut retractors (gauze balls held in the end of a mosquito clamp) (see Fig. I-1-10). The suture is started from the junction of the diaphragm and IVC and brought superiorly. The other arm is placed parallel to the first stitch, and both sutures are put through the tourniquet. The incision to the IVC and cannulation procedure are similar to SVC cannulation, using three-point fixation in conjunction with an assistant (see Fig. I-1-11). An incision using a no. 11 knife is started from the diaphragmatic end and advanced cephalad. The tip of the

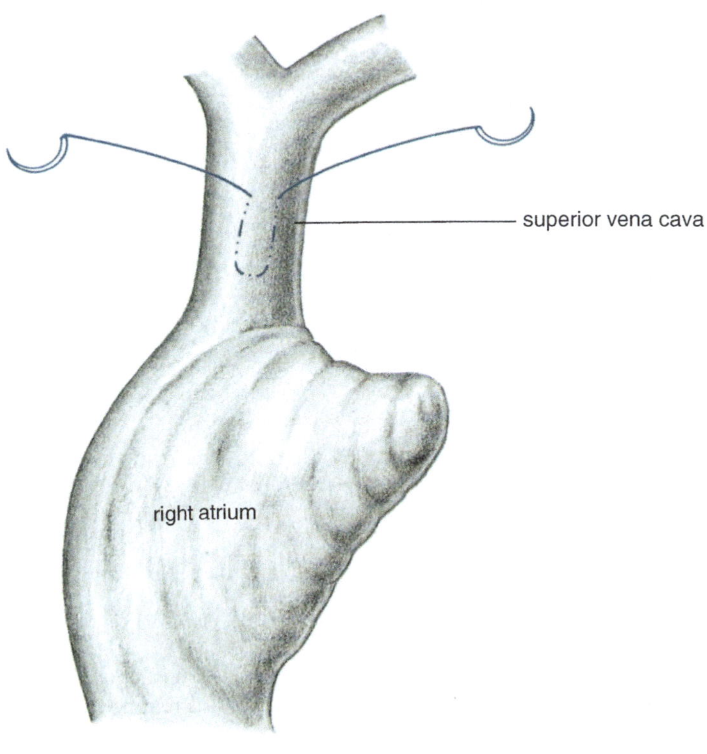

Fig. I-1-8. Superior vena cava (SVC) cannulation: purse-string suture. A narrow rectangular purse-string suture is placed. The cephalic ends of the sutures are kept wide open to be able to extend the incision as much as possible

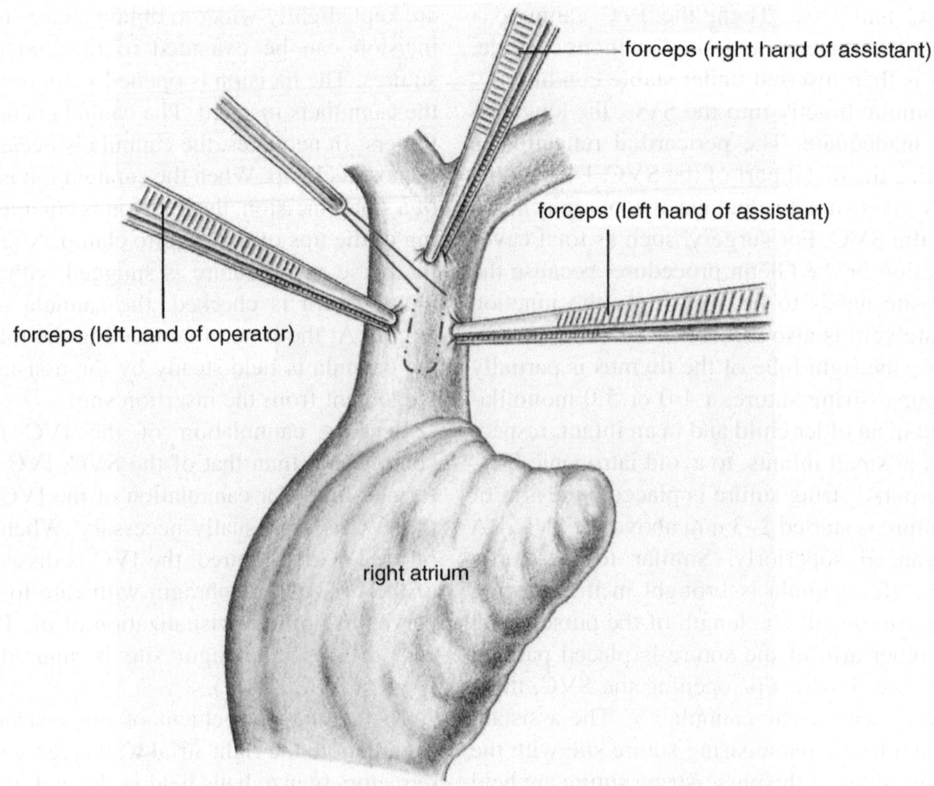

Fig. I-1-9. SVC cannulation: cannula insertion. The assistant holds the SVC distal to the purse-string suture site with the right hand. Each side of the purse-string suture is held by the left hands of the surgeon and assistant

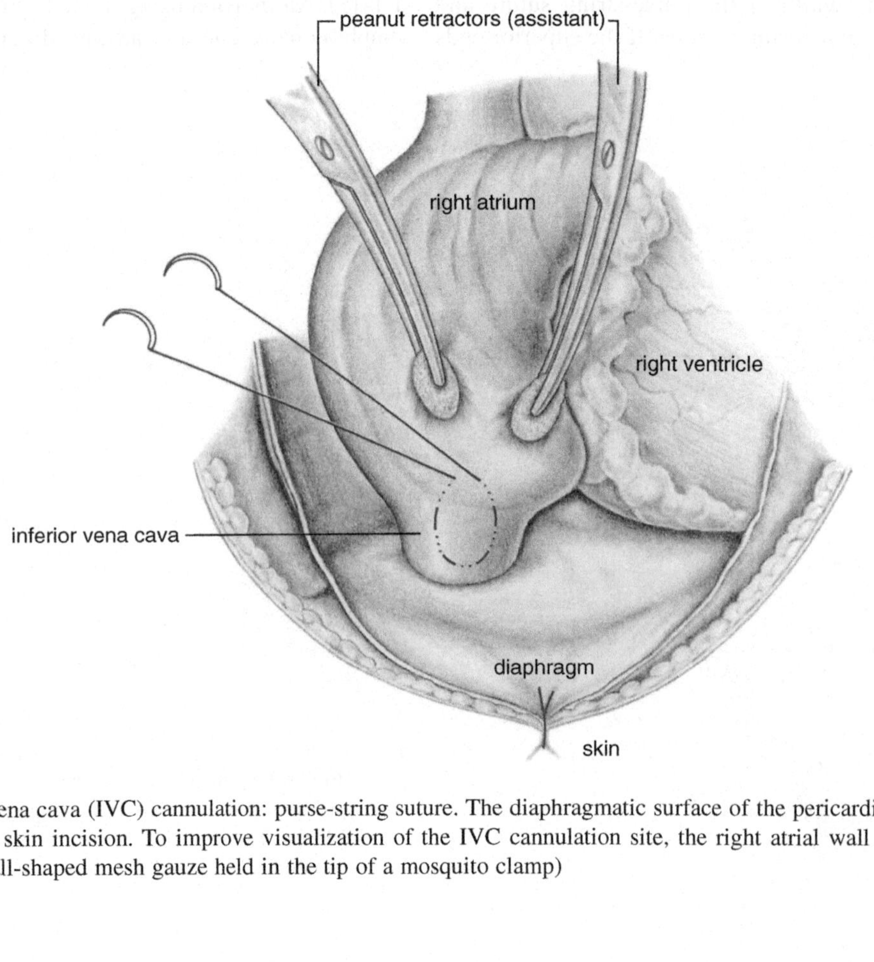

Fig. I-1-10. Inferior vena cava (IVC) cannulation: purse-string suture. The diaphragmatic surface of the pericardium is retracted to the inferior margin of the skin incision. To improve visualization of the IVC cannulation site, the right atrial wall is retracted with two "peanut" retractors (ball-shaped mesh gauze held in the tip of a mosquito clamp)

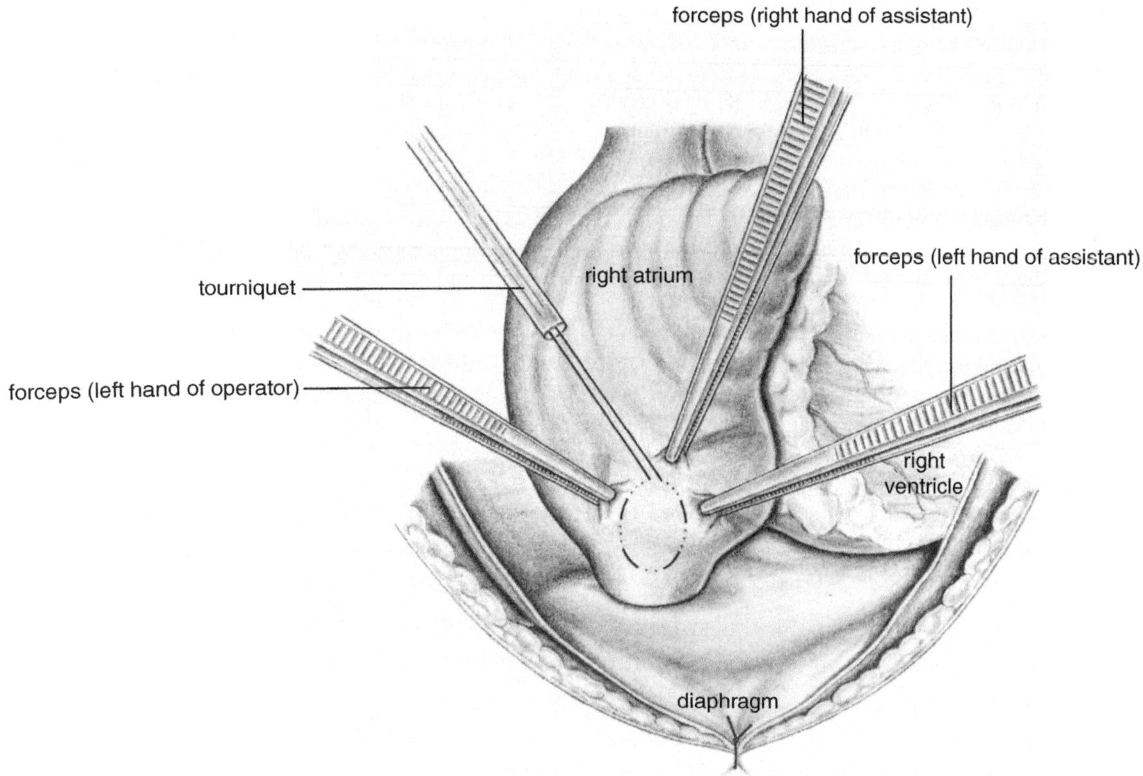

Fig. I-1-11. IVC cannulation: cannula insertion. Cannulation is performed in a fashion similar to SVC cannulation, using three-point fixation

cannula is placed into the right atrium (RA) body first and is turned counterclockwise and positioned into the IVC. If the tip of the cannula is trapped in the Eustachian valve or other intracardiac structure, the cannula is pulled back, turned, and directed toward the IVC. In most situations, inappropriate location of the IVC cannula tip causes inadequate venous drainage. Smooth cannula insertion into the IVC, without resistance, is important. When a ball-tip cannula is used, particularly deep cannulation, implying cannula tip placement in a hepatic vein, may cause inadequate venous drainage. To prevent this occurrence, the surgeon must pay particular attention to the length of the cannula and the depth of insertion. The surgeon should also ask for confirmation of the adequacy of venous drainage.

Another pitfall of IVC cannulation is cutting the purse-string suture with caval incision placement. If this happens, the cannula is kept in place and a new purse-string suture is placed to control the bleeding during surgery. If this purse-string suture is too wide, another narrow purse-string suture is placed during CPB or at the time of decannulation, and the previous too-wide suture is removed.

Reinforcement After Decannulation

After finishing the bypass, purse-string sutures are tied and hemostasis is obtained. Even if hemostasis is adequate, unexpected heavy bleeding may occasionally occur if the tied cannulation suture loosens or breaks as a consequence of coughing during the postoperative course, especially in older children. To prevent this disastrous occurrence, supplemental reinforcement sutures are additionally placed at all cannulation sites.

References

1. Fukumura F, Kado H, Imoto Y, et al (2004) Usefulness of low-priming-volume cardiopulmonary bypass circuits and dilutional ultrafiltration in neonatal open-heart surgery. J Artif Organs 7:9–12
2. Shimpo H, Shimamoto A, Sawamura Y, et al (2001) Ultrafiltration of the priming blood before cardiopulmonary bypass attenuates inflammatory response and improves postoperative clinical course in pediatric patients. Shock 16:s51–s54
3. Millar AB, Armstrong L, van der Linden J, et al (1993) Cytokine production and hemofiltration in children undergoing cardiopulmonary bypass. Ann Thorac Surg 56:1499–1502
4. Ishiyama N, Morita S, Nishida T, et al (2006) Different responses in adult and neonatal hearts to changes in coronary perfusion pressure. Pediatr Cardiol 27:13–18
5. Klopfenstein HS, Rudolph AM (1978) Postnatal changes in the circulation and responses to volume loading in sheep. Circ Res 42:839–845
6. Heymann MA (1989) Fetal and neonatal circulations. In: Adams F, Emmanouilides GC, Riemenschneider TA (eds) Heart disease in infants, children and adolescents, 4th edn. Williams & Wilkins, Baltimore, p 30
7. Galletti PM, Brecher GA (1962) Hemodynamic aspect of total heart-lung bypass, in Principle and technique of extracorporeal circulation. Grune & Stratton, New York, p 194–212

8. Yasui H, Yonenaga K, Kado H, et al (1989) Open-heart surgery in infants using pulsatile high-flow cardiopulmonary bypass. J Cardiovasc Surg 30:661–668
9. Poirier NC, Drummond-Webb JJ, Hisamochi K, et al (2000) Modified Norwood procedure with a high-flow cardiopulmonary bypass strategy results in low mortality without late arch obstruction. J Thorac Cardiovasc Surg 120:875–884
10. Karl TR, Hall S, Ford G, et al (2004) Arterial switch with full-flow cardiopulmonary bypass and limited circulatory arrest: neurodevelopmental outcome. J Thorac Cardiovasc Surg 127:213–222
11. Imoto Y (2000) Cannulation of the distal descending thoracic aorta: Reply to the Editor. Ann Thorac Surg 70:2187
12. Imoto Y, Kado H, Shiokawa Y, et al (2001) Experience with the Norwood procedure without circulatory arrest. J Thorac Cardiovasc Surg 122:879–882
13. Nakano T, Kado H, Shiokawa Y, et al (2004) The low resistance strategy for the perioperative management of the Norwood procedure. Ann Thorac Surg 77:908–912
14. Imoto Y, Kado H, Masuda M, et al (2002) Effects of chlorpromazine as a systemic vasodilator during cardiopulmonary bypass in neonates. Jpn J Thorac Cardiovasc Surg 50:241–245
15. Daggett CW, Lodge AJ, Scaborough JE, et al (1998) Modified ultrafiltration versus conventional ultrafiltration: a randomized prospective study in neonatal piglets. J Thorac Cardiovasc Surg 115:336–341
16. Murayama H, Maeda M, Miyahara K, et al (2003) The current role of preoperative and intraoperative autologous blood donation in pediatric open-heart surgery. Jpn J Thorac Cardiovasc Surg 51:91–97
17. Yonenaga K, Yasui H, Kado H, et al (1990) Myocardial protection by retrograde cardioplegia in arterial switch operation. Ann Thorac Surg 50:238–242
18. Asou T, Yasui H, Kado H, et al (1997) The use of a newly developed pediatric arterial perfusion cannula for neonates. Cardiol Young 7:71–73

I-2. Postoperative Management for Pediatric Cardiac Surgery

In neonates and infants during the perioperative period, special attention and care are required as the patient is small, the anatomy is complex, cardiac as well as pulmonary and renal systems are immature, and the functional reserve of these organ systems is limited.

Hemodynamic Management

Heart Rate and Electrocardiogram

The normal expectation for a neonate or infant is a postoperative heart rate between 130 and 150 bpm. If the rate exceeds 180 bpm, the cause of this phenomenon is investigated. The type of this tachycardia is explored whether it is ventricular, or supraventricular. When supraventricular tachycardia is identified, causes of tachycardia such as awaking, fever, and pain should be treated. Supraventricular tachycardia after Fontan surgery is often resistant to pharmacological treatment and may require hypothermia. Ventricular tachycardia requires emergent treatment such as cardiopulmonary resuscitation or cardioversion. Acute severe bradycardia may cause cardiorespiratory decompensation, manifested by hypoxia and low cardiac output syndrome. In neonates, heart rates lower than 80 bpm may lead to cardiac arrest if appropriate treatment is not instituted rapidly by atrial pacing, which is the treatment of choice, except in cases of severe bradycardia, which require cardiopulmonary resuscitation. If pacing does not achieve the desired effect, β-agonists such as isoproterenol or epinephrine are administered (Fig. I-2-1).

Blood Pressure

So long as at least 1 ml/kg/h of urine output is obtained, low blood pressure with adequate cardiac output in low systemic vascular resistance is probably desirable. In neonates, a systemic systolic pressure of 60 mmHg is adequate. When the left ventricular function is impaired, such as early after an arterial switch operation or total anomalous pulmonary venous return repair, systolic pressures of 55–60 mmHg are acceptable. When the peripheral perfusion is not adequate despite high arterial blood pressure, circulatory collapse may result from excessive afterload. The target systemic systolic pressure is 70–80 and 80–90 mmHg in toddlers and in school-age children, respectively.

Central Venous Pressure

So long as the central venous pressure (CVP) is lower than 10 mmHg, the trend of the pressure change is more important than the absolute value. After cavopulmonary connection, the target CVP is under 15 mmHg.

Left Atrial Pressure (LAP) and Pulmonary Arterial Pressure

Because atrial pressure reflects the ventricular end diastolic pressure, LAP is a useful measure of left ventricular function. Pulmonary artery pressure monitoring is useful to detect and identify a pulmonary hypertensive crisis, which is a rare but severe complication in pediatric cardiac surgery.

Respiratory Management

First, chest wall movement and breathing sounds are evaluated. A mucous plug in the airway and endotracheal tube position may be detected by diminished breath sounds or chest wall motion. Respiratory function deteriorates, typically declining in the first 6–12 h after cardiopulmonary bypass, and thereafter gradually recovers. Respiratory efficiency, as measured by respiratory index, declines most after surgery for total anomalous pulmonary venous return or transposition of the great arteries, less after unrestrictive ventricular septal defect (VSD) repair, and does not change after atrial septal defect (ASD) repair (Fig. I-2-2). Respiratory index was calculated using the following equation: respiratory index = $AaDo_2/Pao_2$ ($AaDo_2$ = alveolar—arterial oxygen tension difference). In patients with decreased pulmonary blood flow preoperatively, such as tetralogy of Fallot, deterioration of oxygen respiratory index is rare. It seems likely that preoperative pulmonary hypertension or pulmonary overcirculation may contribute to postoperative pulmonary dysfunction, as may longer cardiopulmonary bypass time.

Ventilator and Ventilator Settings

In neonates and infants, a ventilator that permits time-cycled/pressure control should be used. On arrival to the intensive care unit (ICU), the ventilator is set with the

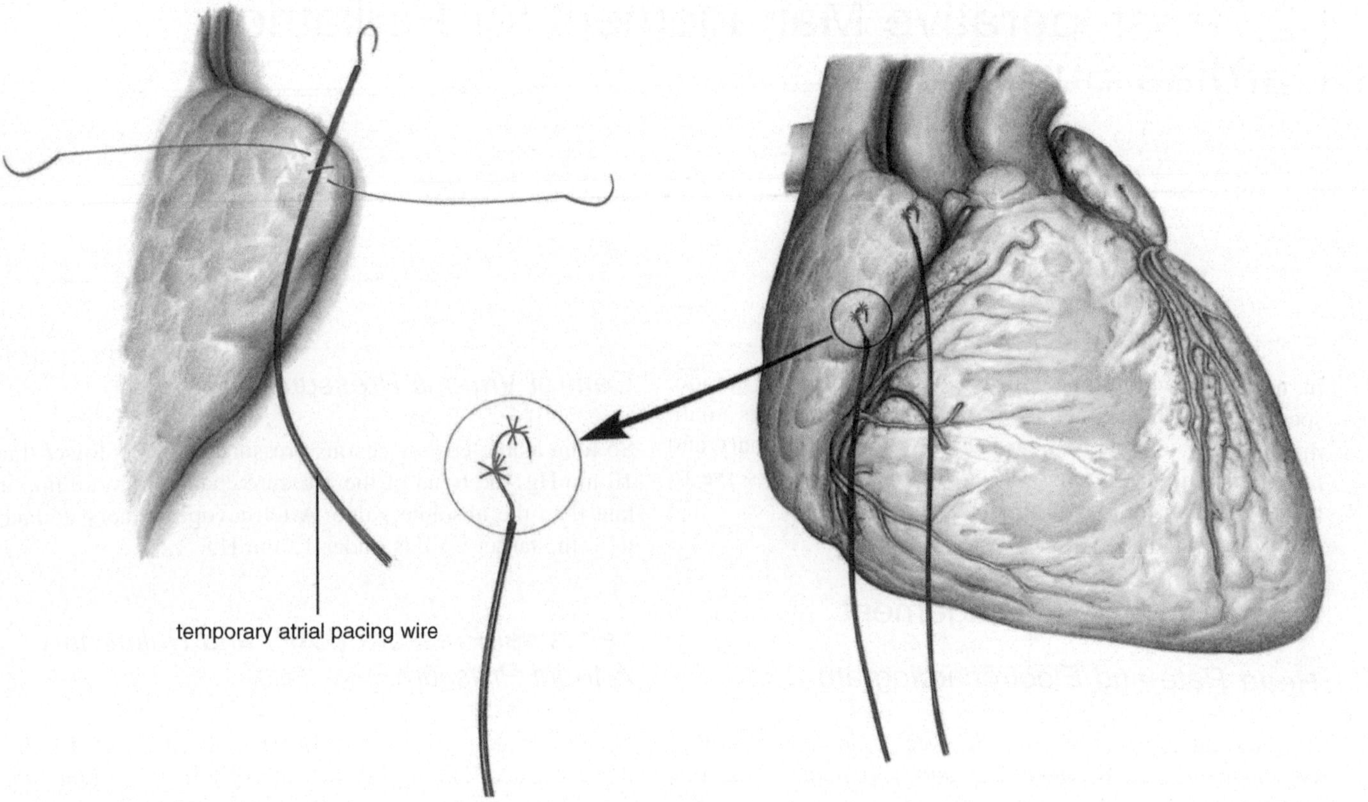

Fig. I-2-1. Temporary pacing wire placement. Two pairs of pacing wires are sutured with a fine monofilament suture to the right atrium and right ventricle

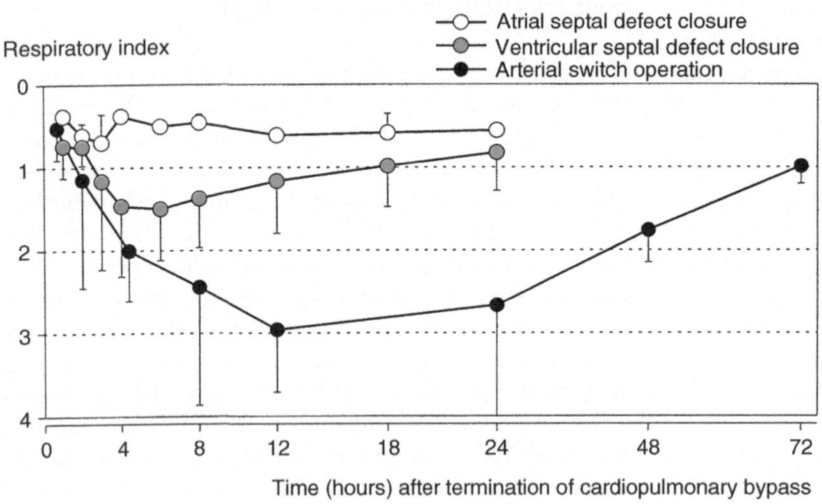

Fig. I-2-2. Postoperative time course of respiratory index. Deterioration of oxygenation is mild after ventricular septal defect (VSD) closure and severe after arterial switch operation. After an arterial switch operation, recovery to normal is prolonged

following parameters: inspiratory time of 0.6 s, peak inspiratory pressure of 15–20 cmH_2O, positive end-expiratory pressure (PEEP) of 2 cmH_2O, and respiratory rate of 15–25 breaths/min. Fractional concentration of oxygen (Fio_2) is lowered from 100% to less than 70% as soon as possible. To avoid barotrauma and oxygen toxicity, the minimum required inspiratory pressure, respiratory rate, and oxygen concentration should be used. In neonates after biventricular repair, oxygen tension in arterial blood (Pao_2) of 70–100 mmHg is acceptable. Carbon dioxide tension in arterial blood ($Paco_2$) is kept between 35 and 40 mmHg after biventricular repair in young infants. In neonates with single ventricle physiology, especially in the presence of atrioventricular valve regurgitation and a morphological right ventricle, Pao_2 may be kept around 35 mmHg to prevent excessive pulmonary blood flow after Blalock–Taussig shunt operation. In unusual cases, Pao_2 of 30 mmHg may be acceptable, early after surgery. It is important to keep the hematocrit higher than 45% in the early postoperative phase. By increasing blood viscosity, acute drops in pulmonary vascular resistance can be prevented. Other means to avoid acute increase in pulmonary blood flow related to falls in pulmonary resistance include (1) FiO_2 is decreased to 21% (room air) (occasionally nitrogen is added into the inspiratory gas and FiO_2 is decreased to 18%–20%); (2) intrathoracic pressure is increased by increasing PEEP to a maximum of 5 cmH_2O; (3) hypoventilation is instituted with muscle relaxant and lower respiratory rate to permit $PaCO_2$ values of up to 60 mmHg; (4) pulmonary vasodilators are discontinued; and (5) systemic vasodilators are used to favorably change the ratio of systemic to pulmonary flow.

Even with the aforementioned interventions, cardiac arrest may still be a concern as a result of pulmonary overcirculation, and additional surgery such as a patent ductus arteriosus (PDA) ligation or shunt banding may be required.

Endotracheal Tube Suction

Endotracheal tube suctioning may trigger acute deterioration in hemodynamics during the early, unstable postoperative period. Because excessive bagging with an ambu-bag can cause barotrauma and pneumothorax, manual ventilation should be performed with great care in watching chest wall movement. Before and during suctioning, the FiO_2 is increased by 10% or 20%. Bilateral breath sounds should be confirmed before and after suctioning.

Other Issues

In the presence of atelectasis, position changes may be instituted soon after surgery. Frequent suction and physiotherapy with vibration and percussion are often effective. A pneumothorax during mechanical ventilation should be treated with a chest tube as soon as possible. In the case of a tension pneumothorax, emergent intervention is required. Occasionally there is no time to obtain a chest X-ray to confirm this diagnosis, and a chest tube should be inserted based only on physical examination.

Weaning the Ventilator and Extubation Criteria

Guidelines for weaning from the ventilator and extubation are as follows: (1) stable hemodynamic conditions, (2) no excessive bleeding, (3) awake patient with spontaneous movement (in school-age child, response to the verbal interaction), (4) PaO_2 of about 100 mmHg (except for single ventricle physiology) with less than 60% FiO_2, (5) tidal volume of more than 7 ml/kg with spontaneous breathing, (6) forced or crying vital capacity of greater than 15 ml/kg, and (7) negative inspiratory force of −20 cmH_2O pressure.

Early Extubation

The merits of early extubation include (1) avoidance of accidental extubation or occlusion of an endotracheal tube by a mucous plug, (2) no need for excessive sedation, (3) increase in cardiac output, and (4) shorter ICU stay. With the recent introduction of propofol for anesthesia, early extubation (2–3 h after surgery) has become possible. After introduction of an early extubation protocol, the dose of fentanyl was decreased from 50–60 to 20–25 μg/kg with the help of propofol (patients older than 3 years) and sevoflurane during anesthesia. Except for neonates, the majority of patients are extubated 2–4 h after surgery. In patients who have cavopulmonary connection surgery, early extubation has the additional benefit of increasing cardiac output by lowering the intrathoracic pressure and central venous pressure by converting to negative pressure (spontaneous).

Fluid Therapy and Transfusion

In the intraoperative and perioperative period, major shifts occur between fluid compartments (intravascular, extracellular, intracellular), especially in neonates who are prone to the so-called capillary leak syndrome. Precise fluid management and adjustment are required, as organ reserve is especially limited in neonates and young infants.

Composition of Maintenance Intravenous Fluid

A 20% glucose solution is usually used as maintenance fluid. Calorie requirements for small children are shown in the following table.

Weight	Daily Caloric Requirement
<10 kg	100 kcal/kg
10–20 kg	1000 kcal + 50 kcal × (weight in kg − 10)
>20 kg	1500 kcal + 20 kcal × (weight in kg − 20)

For maintenance fluid, the potassium level is kept between 30 and 40 mEq/l, but potassium is not added until the level is checked after surgery and adequate urine output confirmed.

Main Fluid Infusion Volume

Daily fluid requirements are shown in the following table.

Weight	Daily Fluid Requirements
<10 kg	100 ml/kg
10–20 kg	1000 ml + 50 ml × (weight in kg − 10)
>20 kg	1500 ml + 20 ml × (weight in kg − 20)

Usually in the ICU, the maintenance fluid is started at the rate of 1 ml/kg/h, to account for the volume administered with infusions of various medications.

Transfusion

With stable hemodynamics in older infants and children, transfusion should be considered when the hematocrit becomes lower than 30%. If a "bloodless surgery" protocol is being employed, a lower transfusion target of 25% may be used. After open heart surgery in neonates, the target hematocrit is kept above 45%. After neonatal surgery for single ventricle physiology, such as the Norwood procedure, the hematocrit is maintained around 50%. After construction of a systemic-to-pulmonary shunt in single ventricle physiology, acute heart failure may occur as a result of pulmonary overcirculation. To avoid this, the hematocrit is kept high to increase the viscosity of the blood, which may reduce pulmonary high flow. To avoid graft-versus-host disease in small patients, cellular blood products are irradiated before transfusion. Blood products should be administered slowly to avoid hyperkalemia, because the potassium level of the blood product may be elevated after irradiation.

Electrolyte and Acid–Base Balance

Potassium Adjustment

After open heart surgery, hypokalemia is often observed, especially in patients receiving diuretics. This hypokalemia will increase susceptibility to arrhythmias during the early postoperative period. Potassium supplementation is used to keep a level above 3.5 mEq/l. During treatment with digoxin, careful attention should be paid because this medication increases the potential for hypokalemia-associated arrhythmia. To correct hypokalemia in infants, potassium is given at a rate of 0.5–1.0 mEq/h and 2 mEq/h at most. Hyperkalemia is treated when the potassium level is above 5.0 mEq/l. If the potassium level is above 6.5 mEq/l, the patient should be treated emergently, because this degree of hyperkalemia may cause a life-threatening arrhythmia. In this situation, calcium gluconate, sodium bicarbonate, and diuretics are administered to rapidly decrease the potassium level. In neonates receiving a highly concentrated glucose solution, insulin should be given very cautiously to avoid a precipitous drop of both glucose and potassium. In mild hyperkalemia, the initial approach is to change to a potassium-free solution, and acidosis is corrected. If oliguria and moderate hyperkalemia persist for more than 4 h, peritoneal dialysis is considered. If severe hyperkalemia (potassium more than 6.5 mEq/l) continues, peritoneal dialysis should be initiated immediately.

Sodium Adjustment

After open heart surgery, hyponatremia is usually secondary to fluid overload, which is treated with fluid restriction and diuretics. If the sodium level is lower than 125 mEq/l, supplemental sodium should be administered to prevent neurological symptoms. Hypernaturemia often occurs during treatment with sodium bicarbonate or hemoconcentration secondary to body fluid loss. If the sodium level exceeds 155 mEq/l, the risk of cerebral bleeding increases and treatment should be instituted. Initially, a 5% glucose solution and diuretics are administered. If this condition persists, peritoneal dialysis is utilized.

Calcium Adjustment

Hypocalcemia is often observed after open heart surgery in neonates and young infants, and this may lead to cardiac dysfunction and seizures. To prevent these occurrences, ionized calcium level is kept above 1.0 mmol/l by use of a calcium gluconate infusor. Calcium should only be administered through a central line.

Glucose Adjustment

Glucose levels tend to become unstable soon after open heart surgery in neonates. Levels should be checked every 2–3 h in the early postoperative period, because significant hypoglycemia may cause severe neurological injury and seizure. In severe hypoglycemia (glucose level lower than 50 mg/dl), a 50% glucose infusion should be started at the rate of 1 ml/kg/h. Hyperglycemia is usually much better tolerated postoperatively but should be treated if severe (glucose level higher than 350 mg/dl) by continuous infusion or bolus injection of insulin.

Acidosis and Alkalosis

Postoperative metabolic acidosis is most often caused by low cardiac output and poor systemic perfusion. The low cardiac output or poor perfusion should be corrected first, before correcting the metabolic acidosis. However, severe acidosis may compromise cardiac function and aggravate low cardiac output and poor perfusion. In this situation, metabolic acidosis should be treated with sodium bicarbonate. The usual approach is the half-correction of the metabolic acidosis. A dose of sodium bicarbonate (ml) is calculated as the product of the base excess (mmol/l) and the body weight (kg) divided by 6. Metabolic alkalosis early after surgery usually does not require treatment.

Medications

Catecholamines

Dopamine

Dopamine has vasodilative effects on the renal artery and no peripheral vasoconstriction effects in low doses, as well as a positive inotropic effect. Dopamine is used as the drug of first choice for mild cardiac dysfunction. During treatment with this drug, careful attention should be paid to the cardiac rhythm because of the proarrhythmic effect of dopamine. It is administered in a dose of 2–10 μg/kg/min.

Dobutamine

Dobutamine is used for patients who have mild to moderate cardiac dysfunction with increased susceptibility to arrhythmias and pulmonary hypertension, because this drug has properties of less proarrhythmic and pulmonary vasodilation. The dosage is the same as that of dopamine.

Isoproterenol

Isoproterenol increases heart rate and reduces pulmonary vascular resistance. Therefore, this drug is useful in patients with bradycardia or pulmonary hypertension. In children with bradycardia, atrial pacing is the treatment of choice. Because of its arrhythmogenic properties, currently this drug is not used frequently.

Norepinephrine

Norepinephrine is the treatment of choice to increase systemic vascular tone in the presence of significant vasodilation with good ventricular function, as in septic shock.

Epinephrine

Epinephrine has potent positive inotropic effects but causes significant peripheral and renal vasoconstriction at higher doses. In situations where the positive inotropic effects are desired without vasoconstriction, vasodilators such as nitroglycerin or chlorpromazine are often used simultaneously. We often use low-dose epinephrine infusion (0.01–0.05 μg/kg/min) after neonatal surgery with excellent results. At these doses, epinephrine improves cardiac output without increasing afterload. It causes coronary vasodilation and also bronchial dilation via β_2-adrenergic receptor stimulation.

Vasodilators

Afterload reduction is one of the mainstays of therapy for postoperative low cardiac output syndrome. There are a variety of vasodilators in clinical use, and the selection of these vasodilators is very important.

Chlorpromazine

Chlorpromazine is very useful after pediatric cardiac surgery because of its sedative properties and its effect on decreasing systemic vascular resistance at maintenance doses of 2–3 μg/kg/min. The initial starting dose is usually one-half or one-third of the final maintenance dose. The dose is gradually increased with titration to the systemic blood pressure. When high doses of epinephrine (more than 0.1 μg/kg/min) are required, chlorpromazine is very useful to counteract severe peripheral vasoconstriction. The main adverse effects are extrapyramidal symptoms of conjugate eye deviation and tremors, which may continue for 2–3 days after termination of this drug therapy.

Nitroglycerin

Nitroglycerin causes pulmonary and coronary vasodilation, and it is useful at doses of 1–3 μg/kg/min for patients at high risk of pulmonary hypertension and coronary artery spasm after surgery such as arterial switch operation.

Milrinone [1,2]

This phosphodiesterase inhibitor has positive inotropic and vasodilative effects. This drug is used during the postoperative period to treat low cardiac output syndrome. The drug is effective for the patient requiring afterload reduction, and is administered at a rate of 0.25–0.75 μg/kg/min. The drug may be used with a loading dose and continuous infusion, although the loading dose must be administrated cautiously to avoid hypotension and tachycardia.

Diuretics

Furosemide

To maintain and optimize postoperative fluid balance, furosemide may be used either as bolus dose of 1 mg/kg or by continuous infusion at a rate of 0.5–1.0 mg/kg/h. If necessary, the dose can be gradually increased. Care is taken to avoid electrolyte disturbance during diuretic therapy. After oral intake is started, an oral dose of furosemide 1–5 mg/kg/day divided into two to four doses may be initiated.

Carperitide (Alpha-Human Atrial Natriuretic Peptide) [3,4]

Atrial natriuretic peptide is naturally released by atrial myocytes in response to stretch. Carperitide, a synthetic analogue, is used as a diuretic and vasodilator during the postoperative period to decrease both pre- and afterload. It has potassium-sparing properties and therefore causes less electrolyte imbalance. The initial dose is 0.05 μg/kg/min, which is increased to 0.2 μg/kg/min depending on clinical response. The drug is tapered gradually before it is discontinued. The most common side effect of carperitide is hypotension.

Anticoagulation

If the patient requires anticoagulation after surgery, infractionated heparin is administered at 4 mg/kg/day (continuously, or as 1 mg/kg bolus doses every 6 h) after postoperative bleeding from chest tubes has decreased. Following placement of a modified Blalock–Taussig shunt, aspirin (1–2 mg/kg/day) is started after oral feeding is established. In patients with a mechanical valve replacement or Fontan-type surgery, anticoagulation is transitioned from heparin to coumadin once chest tubes are removed. The INR (international normalized ratio) is kept between 2.5 and 3.0 after valve replacement and between 1.5 and 2.0 after Fontan-type surgery.

Antibiotics

Intraoperatively, prophylactic antibiotics are administered, and these are continued for the first two postoperative days.

If infection is suspected, appropriate cultures are used to identify the organisms, and treatment is started.

Analgesics, Sedatives, and Muscle Relaxants

In the early postoperative period, patients are generally treated with analgesics, sedatives, and muscle relaxants to avoid hemodynamic and respiratory instability. For postoperative analgesia, bolus doses of morphine (0.1 mg/kg) or fentanyl (0.5–1 µg/kg) may be used. Alternatively, to provide a more consistent analgesic effect, a morphine continuous infusion (25–50 µg/kg/h) can be utilized. Sedation is achieved with benzodiazepines, by either bolus midazolam (0.05–0.1 mg/kg i.v.) or continuous infusion (0.05–0.2 mg/kg/h). In patients on an early extubation protocol, analgesia and sedatives are titrated at lower doses. After extubation, chloral hydrate, used orally or rectally, provides excellent sedation. In neonates and young infants with single ventricle physiology, muscle relaxants are often used in the acute setting to prevent abrupt hemodynamic instability by sudden awakening, which might increase cardiac and respiratory demand.

Antiarrhythmic Agents

Occasional premature atrial contractions are commonly seen in the postoperative period and do not require treatment. In patients with paroxysmal supraventricular tachycardia, an adenosine bolus (0.1–0.3 mg/kg) can be used. As adenosine may cause sudden sinus arrest, ventricular pacing via temporary pacing wires should be available. Adenosine is also useful to differentiate various subtypes of supraventricular arrhythmia. If supraventricular arrhythmia compromise severe hemodynamics, synchronized cardioversion (0.25–1 J/kg) should be carried out. Junctional ectopic tachycardia, a common postoperative arrhythmia, may cause severe hemodynamic instability; this is usually treated with a class III drug such as amiodarone.

In frequent or multifocal premature ventricular contraction, lidocaine or amiodarone is useful. However, when ventricular tachycardia causes hemodynamic instability, cardioversion should be rapidly instituted.

Other Treatment

Peritoneal Dialysis

In patients with preoperative cardiogenic shock, open heart surgery for single ventricle, or oliguria during the postoperative period, a peritoneal dialysis catheter is placed. In addition to optimizing management of acute renal failure and fluid status in these clinical situations, it also is used for removal of inflammatory mediators and can be used for temperature management [5].

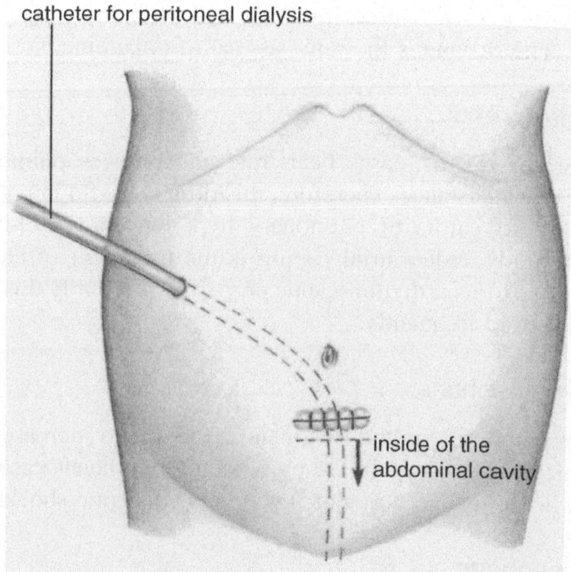

Fig. I-2-3. Peritoneal dialysis catheter placement: pelvis. A peritoneal dialysis catheter is inserted into the abdomen midway between the pubic symphysis and umbilicus. The tip of the catheter is placed toward the pouch of Douglas. A preperitoneal tunnel is created, and the catheter is brought through the skin in the right upper quadrant

Catheter Placement

Intrapelvic Placement

The intrapelvic site is the most standard site for placement of a peritoneal dialysis catheter. The catheter is inserted through the peritoneum beneath the umbilicus. The tip of the catheter is positioned in the pelvis. A subcutaneous tunnel is created, and the catheter exits the skin at the right upper abdominal quadrant (Fig. I-2-3). In children, this technique has the disadvantages of unstable positioning because of the shallow pelvis and easy occlusion of the catheter by the omentum.

Left Subdiaphragmatic Placement

Left subdiaphragmatic placement has been applied in neonates and young infants as it is a more stable location and there is less risk of omental occlusion of the catheter. An incision is made on the peritoneum at the transition between the diaphragm and peritoneum. The peritoneal dialysis catheter is positioned above the left lobe of the liver with the tip of the catheter reaching behind the spleen (Fig. I-2-4). In the neonate, the area behind the spleen is the lowest point in the peritoneum in the supine position, which enhances drainage.

Dialysis Protocol

Initially, isotonic dialysate solution is used. If further body fluid needs to be removed, hypertonic dialysate solution is used. Potassium is added to the dialysate solution in the presence of hypokalemia. The amount of inflow of the dialysate fluid is 10–15 ml/kg per cycle. Each cycle is 60 min, with 30 min dwelling and 30 min drainage.

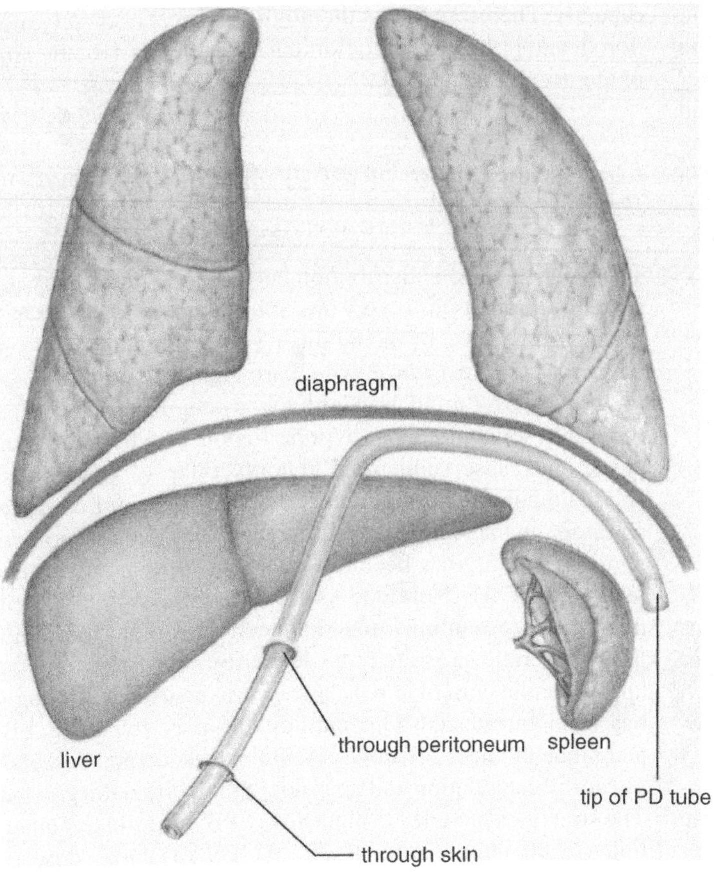

Fig. I-2-4. Peritoneal dialysis catheter placement: left subdiaphragmatic. A peritoneal dialysis (*PD*) catheter is inserted into the abdomen at the transition between the diaphragm and peritoneum. This catheter is placed above the left lobe of the liver with the tip of the catheter directed toward the spleen

Complications of Peritoneal Dialysis

Catheter Malfunction

Catheter entrapment by the omentum may occur, which may cause ineffective drainage. In this situation, milking of the dialysis catheter or pressure on the abdomen will not help. Omental entrapment may be prevented by leaving a small inflow drip during each cycle. If a dialysis catheter occlusion persists, replacement of the catheter should be considered.

Peritonitis

The appearance of the dialysis effluent is continuously examined. If the effluent becomes cloudy, a sample is sent for culture, Gram stain, and white blood cell count. Antibiotic medications may be added to the dialysis solution.

Hyperglycemia

In neonates and young infants, hyperglycemia commonly occurs as a consequence of systemic absorption of glucose from the dialysis fluid, although a higher glucose dialysate allows more effective fluid removal. After an adequate amount of fluid is removed from the body, a lower glucose concentration dialysis fluid should be used.

Respiratory Complication

In small children, peritoneal dialysis may increase the abdominal pressure and thus affect the respiratory status adversely. Therefore, especially in critically ill neonates, large volume instillation and quick drainage and rapid cycling should be avoided.

Prophylaxis for Pulmonary Hypertensive Crisis

In patients with increased pulmonary blood flow before surgery or preoperative pulmonary vein obstruction, a pulmonary hypertensive crisis can be triggered by various types of stimulation during the postoperative period [6]. In these conditions, pulmonary hypertension is more prone to occur because of decreased production of endothelial-derived relaxing factor and increased production of endothelial-derived vasoconstricting factor after open heart surgery. Hypoxia, hypercapnea, metabolic acidosis, decreased sedation, endotracheal suction, extubation, physiotherapy, and pain may all trigger a pulmonary hypertensive crisis. To prevent pulmonary hypertensive crises, minimization of these mentioned factors is ideal. Specific therapies that may prevent crises include (1) adequate sedation and muscle relaxation, (2) higher inspired oxygen concentration ($Fio_2 > 70\%$), (3) hyperventilation, (4) nitroglycerin infusion (2–3 μg/kg/min), and (5) prophylactic use of inhaled nitric oxide (5–10 ppm). When pulmonary hypertension occurs, treatment should be instituted rapidly. The condition is heralded by acute systemic hypotension, arterial desaturation, and high central venous pressure with no change or lowering left atrial pressure. Patients should be immediately ventilated using hand-bagging with 100% oxygen. Then, inhaled nitric oxide (10–20 ppm) is started. Electrolytes and acidosis are promptly corrected. When spontaneous movement and respiratory efforts are observed, sedatives and muscle relaxants are administered. Severe hypotension may require bolus dose catecholamine. If refractory bradycardia (heart rate less than 90 bpm) and severe hypotension (systolic blood pressure less than 40 mmHg) continue, cardiopulmonary resuscitation should be instituted promptly. Phosphodiesterase III inhibitors and human atrial natriuretic peptide are also effective for treatment of pulmonary hypertension.

Nitric Oxide [7–9]

Inhaled nitric oxide decreases pulmonary vascular resistance and improves right ventricular function and cardiac output. Inhaled nitric oxide has great benefit in smoothing the postoperative course in patients with pulmonary overcirculation before surgery such as complete atrioventricular septal defect, transposition of the great arteries with VSD, truncus arteriosus, and obstructed total anomalous pulmonary venous return. Recently, patients with right heart bypass (bidirectional cavopulmonary anastomosis or Fontan completion) also have been shown to benefit from inhaled nitric oxide treatment. In these patients, a lower pulmonary vascular resistance is advantageous to increase cardiac output (Fig. I-2-5). During the early postoperative period, inhaled nitric oxide may reverse the elevated pulmonary vascular resistance caused by cardiopulmonary bypass. As the injured pulmonary endothelium recovers with normal function, inhaled nitric oxide is gradually weaned. Inhaled nitric oxide is started at 20 ppm and weaned according to arterial blood gas and pulmonary artery pressure. The lowest maintenance dose is 2 ppm. One of the side effects of inhaled nitric oxide is the production of methemoglobin, which has fewer heme moieties to bind oxygen, thus reducing the oxygen carrying capacity. Therefore the methemoglobin level is closely monitored, and if the methemoglobin level exceeds 1%, the nitric oxide dose is decreased.

Low-Resistance Strategy After the Norwood Procedure [10]

The balance of flow distribution between the pulmonary and systemic circulations is very unstable soon after the Norwood procedure because of the lability of the pulmonary and systemic vascular resistance, which are changing continuously. Pulmonary overcirculation with low systemic cardiac output (or conversely pulmonary hypoperfusion with hypoxia) may ensue and cause sudden circulatory collapse. To maintain adequate pulmonary vascular resistance, a careful cardiorespiratory management is required, as this acute hemodynamic instability has been the cause for some poor surgical results after the Norwood procedure. Since 1998 in our institution, to minimize the changes in systemic to pulmonary flow ratio, a strategy to decrease both the pulmonary and systemic vascular resistance (low-resistance strategy) has been introduced. Our cardiopulmonary bypass (CPB) technique includes selective cerebral perfusion and descending aortic cannulation and does not require circulatory arrest. The strategies include (1) high-flow CPB, (2) mild hypothermia (rectal temperature of 30°–32°C), (3) large dose of vasodilator (chlorpromazine 5 mg/kg), and (4) removal of inflammatory cytokines with dilutional ultrafiltration and modified ultrafiltration. At the time of separation from bypass, the patient is ventilated with 100% oxygen and inhaled nitric oxide (20 ppm), and high-dose infusion of nitroglycerin (2–4 μg/kg/min) is instituted to decrease both pulmonary and systemic vascular resistances. To control pulmonary blood flow in patients having a right ventricle to pulmonary artery (RV-PA) conduit, clips are applied to this conduit to maintain Pa_{O_2} of 35–40 mmHg. Once the patient is transferred to the ICU, the management

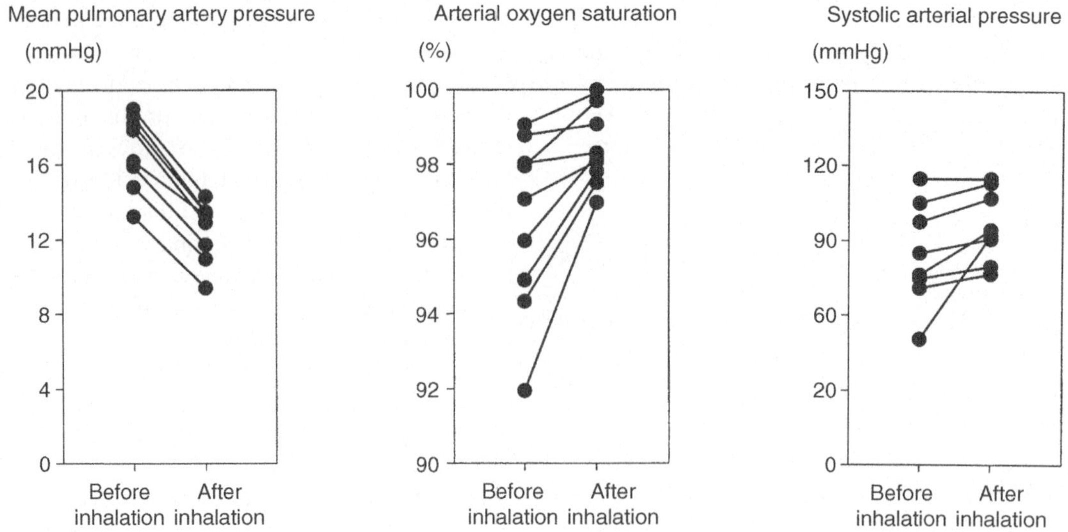

Fig. I-2-5. Effects of inhaled nitric oxide after the Fontan procedure. A decrease in the pulmonary artery pressure and increase in arterial oxygen saturation are observed after the initiation of inhaled nitric oxide

goal is to minimize acute change in vascular resistance. Therapies used include the continuation of inhaled nitric oxide (5–10 ppm), administration of analgesia, sedatives, muscle relaxants, and vasodilators such as chlorpromazine and nitroglycerin. Airway suctioning via the endotracheal tube is minimized in the first 24 h after surgery to prevent a pulmonary hypertensive crisis. Based on the gradual reduction of the pulmonary vascular resistance in an early postoperative period, FiO_2 and inhaled nitric oxide are gradually weaned. This management strategy allows for a more stable postoperative course after the Norwood procedure.

Delayed Sternal Closure

After open heart surgery to establish stable neonatal single ventricle physiology or extended times on CPB, hemodynamics may become unstable at the time of chest closure. Therefore, delayed sternal closure is often employed. At our institution, delayed sternal closure is used in all patients who have undergone the Norwood procedure. In a majority of these patients, struts are placed between the sternum, and the skin can be primarily closed. When the sternum needs to be widely open, a PTFE sheet is applied. To decrease the risk of infection, open sternotomy wounds should undergo the delayed closure by the third postoperative day. However, the timing of chest closure must be guided by the hemodynamic condition and resolution of chest wall edema.

Mechanical Circulatory Support After Open Heart Surgery

Historically, the intraaortic balloon pump (IABP) has been used in children for circulatory support only rarely because IABP-generated diastolic augmentation does not predictably present because of the very compliant aortic wall in children. Placement of the large IABP catheter is also difficult in the small vessels in children. Recently, extracorporeal membrane oxygenation (ECMO) with a heparin-coated circuit or left ventricular assist systems (LVAS) are being increasingly used in children. ECMO has an oxygenator in the circuit and, thus, an ability to support respiratory function. In the immediate postoperative period, ECMO is usually instituted using transthoracic cannulation of the ascending aorta and right atrium. Our team has used a centrifugal pump for both ECMO and LVAS.

Miscellaneous Issues

Temperature

In neonates and young infants, systemic vasodilation can be effectively achieved with warming extremities. This vasodilation using warm blankets is more effective than that achieved using vasodilator therapy. Younger and smaller patients are vulnerable to hypothermia, and careful attention should be paid to prevent this. Core temperature is kept between 36.0° and 37.0°C in infants using a radiant warmer. The core and peripheral temperatures are closely monitored because an increase in core temperature and an increasing difference between core and peripheral temperature are sensitive indicators of low cardiac syndrome. Topical warming must be accomplished with caution to avoid cutaneous burns. During the early postoperative period in small patients, hyperthermia is treated with ice bags applied to the head, the flanks, or the groins.

Drain Management

Suction on the mediastinal chest tubes is maintained between −10 and −13 cmH_2O. Frequent milking of the chest tubes is performed soon after surgery to optimize drainage of blood and prevent tube occlusion by blood clots. When the mediastinal chest tube output exceeds 3 ml/kg/h in older children and 4 ml/kg/h in neonates and infants, mediastinal re-exploration should be considered. Reliance on administration of coagulation factors and blood products should not be a substitute for timely re-exploration. If the drainage decreases abruptly, echocardiography should be considered to rule out the possibility of cardiac tamponade.

References

1. Hoffman TM, Wernovsky G, Atz AM, et al (2003) Efficacy and safety of milrinone in preventing low cardiac output syndrome in infants and children after corrective surgery for congenital heart disease. Circulation 107:996–1002
2. Chang AC, Atz AM, Wernovsky G, et al (1995) Milrinone: systemic and pulmonary hemodynamic effects in neonates after cardiac surgery. Crit Care Med 23:1907–1914
3. Hamawaki M, Tomino T, Sato H, et al (2000) Human atrial natriuretic peptide infusion for a neonate with congestive heart failure after total correction of total anomalous pulmonary venous connection. Jpn Circ J 64:708–710
4. Hiramatsu T, Imai Y, Takanashi Y, et al (1998) Hemodynamic effects of human atrial natriuretic peptide after modified Fontan procedure. Ann Thorac Surg 65:761–764
5. Riznik VM, Griswold WR, Peterson BM, et al (1991) Peritoneal dialysis for acute renal failure in children. Pediatr Nephrol 5:715–717
6. Raisher BD, Grant JW, Martin TC, et al (1992) Complete repair of total anomalous pulmonary venous connection in infancy. J Thorac Cardiovasc Surg 104:443–448
7. Curran RD, Mavroudis C, Backer CL, et al (1995) Inhaled nitric oxide for children with congenital heart disease and pulmonary hypertension. Ann Thorac Surg 60:1765–1771
8. Khambadkone S, Li J, de Leval MR, et al (2003) Basal pulmonary vascular resistance and nitric oxide responsiveness late after Fontan-type operation. Circulation 107:3204–3208
9. Miller OI, Tang SF, Keech A, et al (2000) Inhaled nitric oxide and prevention of pulmonary hypertension after congenital heart surgery: a randomized double-blind study. Lancet 356:1464–1469
10. Nakano T, Kado H, Shiokawa Y, et al (2004) The low resistance strategy for the perioperative management of the Norwood procedure. Ann Thorac Surg 77:908–912

II. Specific Defects and Procedure

II-1. Patent Ductus Arteriosus

Surgery is thought to be indicated for all patients with patent ductus arteriosus, even if there is only a small amount of shunt through the ductus. Long-term observation should be avoided due to the chance of infective endocarditis. The optimal timing for surgery is toddler age; however, some patients need surgery in the neonatal period. Early surgery is recommended for premature babies with patent ductus arteriosus, if the patient has failed indomethacin treatment or has renal failure [1,2]. Ductal closure is contraindicated if irreversible pulmonary vascular obstructive disease is demonstrated by lung biopsy or if the patient has a predominant right-to-left shunt.

The aortic arch, descending aorta, and the branching pattern of the aortic arch should be evaluated before surgery. The possibility of aneurysmal or calcific changes should be evaluated in adults. The use of cardiopulmonary bypass should be considered in adults if fragility of ductal tissue is suspected [3]. A pulse oxygen saturation monitor should be placed on the foot to check the blood flow to the descending aorta during surgery.

Duct Ligation via Left Thoracotomy

Via a left lateral or posterolateral thoracotomy, the chest is entered through the third or fourth intercostal space. The lung is retracted anteriorly, and the vessels and nerves are identified. It is mandatory to identify the aortic arch and the left subclavian artery. Palpation of a thrill at the duct site is useful. An incision is started in the parietal pleura overlying the descending aorta. This incision is advanced superiorly up to the left subclavian artery. During this dissection, the left superior intercostal vein is ligated and divided. To avoid chylothorax, the connective tissue at the base of the left subclavian artery is ligated and divided. Five to six 3-0 silk strings are placed in the edge of the pleura, and the pleura is retracted (Fig. II-1-1). This retraction elevates the operative field for better identification of the ductus arteriosus. The vagus and phrenic nerves are elevated with the pleura, and surgical manipulation is facilitated. An umbilical tape is placed around the descending aorta. With gentle traction on this tape, further dissection of the descending aorta from the connective tissue is advanced, especially behind the aorta. Care is taken not to damage the intercostal arteries from the descending aorta. Tapes are then placed around the left subclavian artery and the distal aortic arch. For taping around the distal aortic arch, the tape is placed around the descending aorta just distal to the left subclavian artery, and then this tape is put behind the left subclavian artery (Fig. II-1-2).

Dissection around the ductus then proceeds behind the ductus from above and below the ductus. During this dissection, the recurrent laryngeal nerve is carefully identified. The ductus wall is not dissected directly, but the connective tissues are dissected from the aortic wall at the junction of the descending aorta and ductus. Adequate space behind the ductus should be freed. When passing a right-angled clamp around the ductus, it is important that the tip of the clamp actually passes behind the descending aorta to avoid damage to the ductus or pulmonary artery. A heavy silk ligature is doubly folded on itself and passed around the ductus. This manipulation allows placement of two strings around the ductus in one movement (Fig. II-1-3). A vascular forceps is applied to the ductus temporarily, and the resultant changes in the arterial blood pressure, especially the elevation of the diastolic pressure and pulse oximeter reading, should be confirmed. At the time of ductus ligation, the assistant may clamp the aortic arch to decrease the pressure in the ductus as the surgeon ties the ligature. Ligation is accomplished first on the aortic side and then on the pulmonary side. Absence of a thrill confirms ductal closure. If the patient has severe pulmonary hypertension or significant right-to-left shunting is suspected, the duct is temporarily closed, and the hemodynamic conditions are followed closely for a short period. If severe hemodynamic changes or desaturation occur, the duct is left open.

If the duct is to be divided, because the ductal diameter is relatively large, typically two clamps are used. On the aortic end, the clamp is partially placed on the descending aorta to avoid clamping the ductal tissue. The two clamps must be placed for enough apart to allow sufficient length for safe division of the ductus, leaving adequate tissue for safe suture closure. In this regard, it is important to place the clamp on the pulmonary end of the ductus quite deeply (Fig. II-1-4). The assistant holds both clamps steady, and the duct is divided midway between clamps with a scalpel. For the pulmonary side, a double-armed 5-0 monofilament suture is used in an over-and-over fashion. For the aortic side, a double-layer closure is used with a deep running mattress suture and a second superficial over-and-over running suture (Fig. II-1-5). After suture closure, the clamps are released slowly. Needle hole bleeding is controlled by compressing the suture line with a sponge.

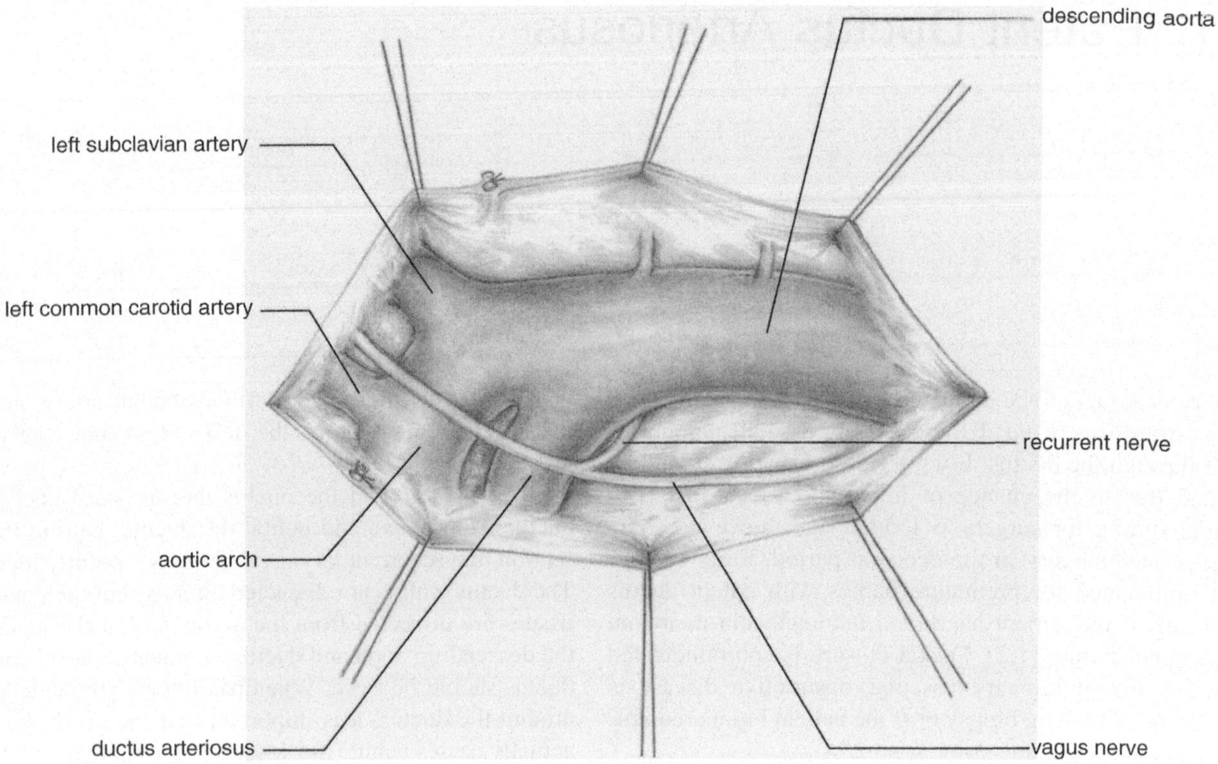

Fig. II-1-1. Surgical anatomy around the ductus arteriosus. The parietal pleura is opened and retracted with five or six silk sutures. The vagus nerve is pulled medially

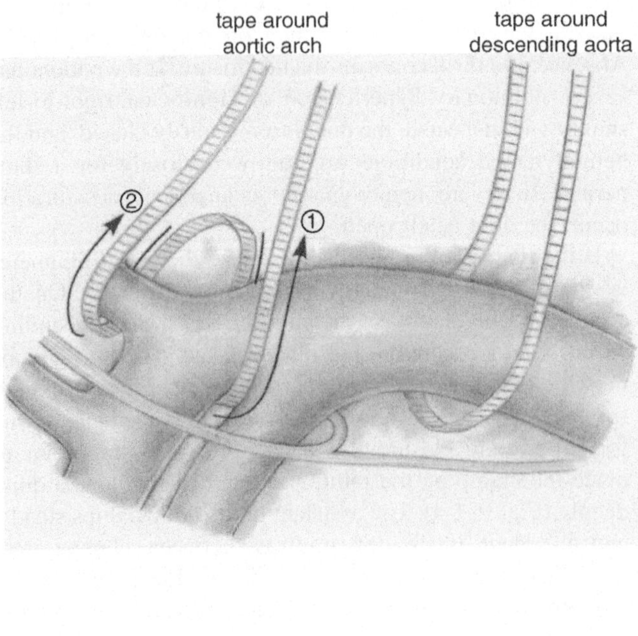

Fig. II-1-2. Placement of tape around the aortic arch. First, a tape is placed around the descending aorta just distal to the left subclavian artery ①, then around the left subclavian artery itself ②. The tape is thus placed around the aortic arch easily

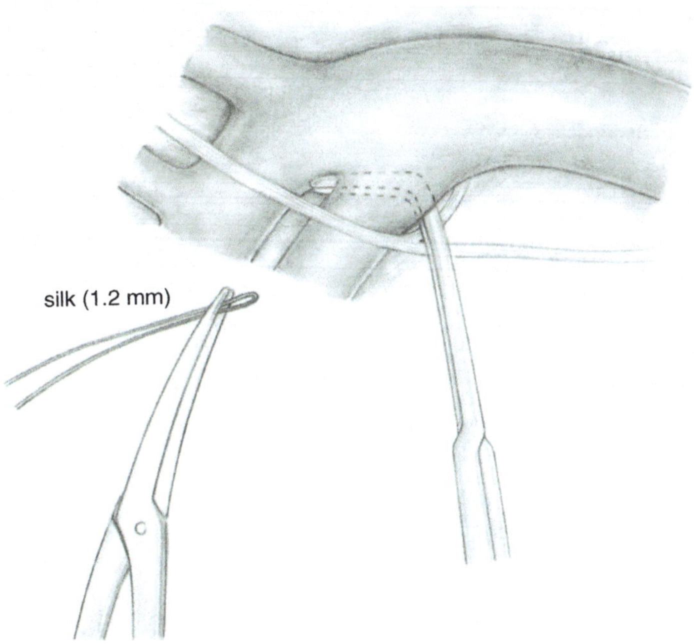

Fig. II-1-3. Placement of ductal ligatures. A heavy silk ligature is folded in half, and this fold is grasped with a right-angled clamp. After ligature passage, the tie is divided at the fold point. This procedure allows placement of two ties in one motion

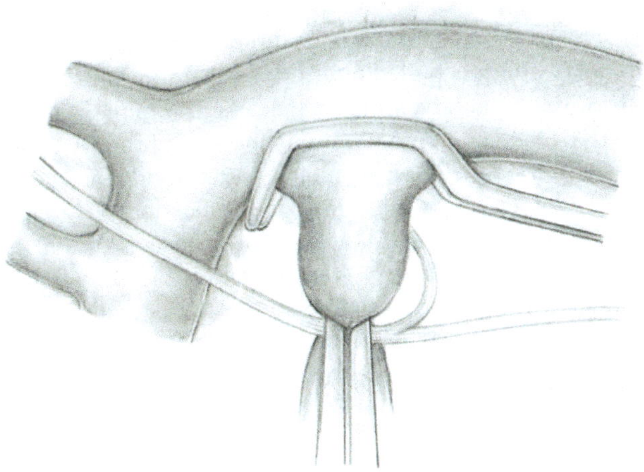

Fig. II-1-4. Technique of clamp placement. A C-shaped clamp is placed on the descending aorta, with care to avoid placing the clamp on ductal tissue. Attention must be paid posteriorly because there is a tendency to place the clamp in a too-shallow position, leaving the posterior clamp jaw on ductal rather than aortic tissue

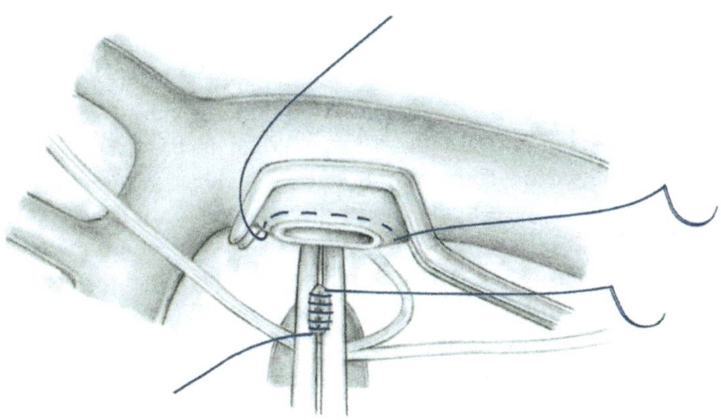

Fig. II-1-5. Division and closure of the ductus. After division of the ductus, divided ends are closed using a fine monofilament suture with mattress and then over-and-over running suture technique

If the duct is damaged and severe bleeding is encountered, immediate management is required. The injury site is compressed with a finger, and the bleeding is controlled. Immediately, the aorta is dissected above and below the damaged site, tapes are placed, and clamps are applied. Sutures are placed at the damaged site. The pulmonary site is treated similarly. If the pulmonary site is retracted into the pericardium, the pericardium is opened, and a clamp is placed on the left pulmonary artery to control bleeding. The injury to the pulmonary end is then repaired.

After ductal closure is complete, hemostasis and chylothorax are checked, and the opened pleura is closed. A drainage tube is placed regardless of the absence of bleeding.

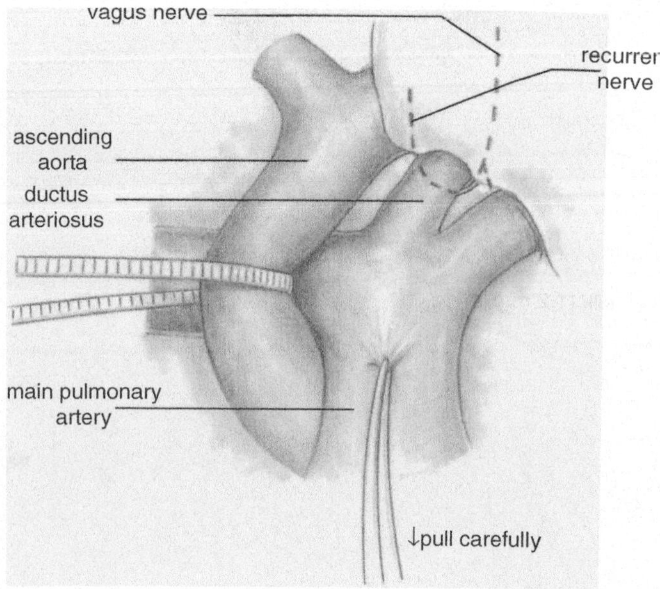

Fig. II-1-6. Dissection of the duct via median sternotomy. A mosquito clamp is placed on the anterior surface of the main pulmonary artery, and this clamp is pulled inferiorly to facilitate the visualization of the ductus. The location of the recurrent laryngeal nerve should be identified

Duct Ligation for the Premature Baby

Perioperative management is especially important for duct ligation in a premature baby. Because premature babies become hypothermic easily, an infant warmer is used to avoid hypothermia. Because of the significant stress involved in transportation, if feasible the surgery should be performed in the neonatal intensive care unit (NICU). Placement of an arterial monitoring line is often difficult; therefore, blood pressure is measured with a cuff. A posterolateral thoracotomy is utilized. Because the duct is short and blood pressure is low, a single string is enough to ligate the duct. As an alternative the duct may be simply closed with a surgical clip, which avoids the need for circumferential dissection of the ductus, which may be very hazardous in ultralow birth weight babies (<750 g). A chest tube is not placed [4]. A small catheter is left in the chest during chest closure. After chest closure the catheter is removed with suction to evacuate the air.

Duct Ligation via Median Sternotomy

A median sternotomy is rarely necessary for the simple duct ligation. However, this approach is used in children undergoing intracardiac repair of other anomalies and in adults.

For the patient undergoing intracardiac repair, it is important to control the ductal blood flow at the initiation of cardiopulmonary bypass. Therefore, dissection of the duct and placement of a ligature around the duct is completed before cardiopulmonary bypass. Adequate exposure is the key to dissection of the duct. A tape is placed around the ascending aorta, and the connective tissue behind the aorta is dissected. Dissection is then advanced leftward from the superior surface of the right pulmonary artery to the right side of the duct. The dissection of the superior surface of the left pulmonary artery is advanced toward the duct. After completion of preliminary dissection around the duct, a heavy silk ligature is placed around the duct with a right-angle clamp. To enhance visualization of the duct, the main pulmonary artery is pulled inferiorly with a mosquito clamp used to grasp the adventitia of the main pulmonary artery (Fig. II-1-6). It is important to remember the fragility of the duct and retract the main pulmonary artery with care. After initiation of cardiopulmonary bypass, the duct is doubly ligated. Care should be taken not to place tension on the ligated duct during surgery. In some cases, the duct should be divided to facilitate visualization of the operative field. In such cases, after double ligation, the duct is divided and a fine monofilament suture is placed in the aortic wall near the duct origin. The divided end of the pulmonary side duct is likewise reinforced.

The operative procedure for adult patients is completely different from that of children. Because of aneurysmal change and calcification of the duct, the usual procedure of ligation or division is very dangerous; therefore, the duct opening site is closed through the pulmonary arteriotomy directly or by using a patch [3,5]. To improve visualization of the operative field, a 6 or 8 Fr. Foley catheter is placed in the aorta through the main pulmonary artery and duct, the balloon is inflated, and blood flow through the duct is controlled temporarily (Fig. II-1-7). When the blood return from the duct obscures the operative field, cardiopulmonary bypass flow is reduced or, after hypothermia, circulatory arrest is utilized with the patient in Trendelenburg position. Purse-string suture placement or patch placement is chosen. The balloon is removed before tying the suture for the direct closure and finishing patch placement. In either approach, 4-0 polypropylene monofilament sutures are used for adults.

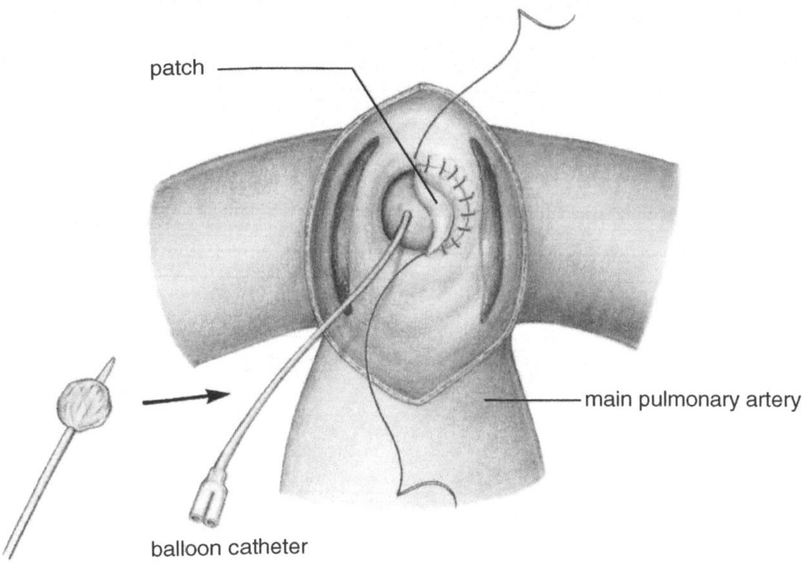

Fig. II-1-7. Patch closure of ductus arteriosus using a balloon. The ductus is temporarily closed using a balloon, which is placed into the descending aorta through the ductus and inflated to minimize back-bleeding from the aorta

References

1. Trus T, Winthrop AL, Pipe S, et al (1993) Optimal management of patent ductus arteriosus in the neonate weighing less than 800 g. J Pediatr Surg 28:1137–1139
2. Uchita S, Imai Y, Takanashi Y, et al (1998) Surgical management of patent ductus arteriosus in low body weight infants. Jpn J Thorac Cardiovasc Surg 46:1088–1092
3. Toda R, Moriyama Y, Yamashita M, et al (2000) Operation for adult patent ductus arteriosus using cardiopulmonary bypass. Ann Thorac Surg 70:1935–1937
4. Miles RH, DeLeon SY, Muraskas J, et al (1995) Safety of patent ductus arteriosus closure in premature infants without tube thoracostomy. Ann Thorac Surg 59:668–670
5. Drinkwater DC, Laks H, Perloff JK (1991) Surgical considerations. In: Perloff JK, Child JS (eds) Congenital heart disease in adults. Saunders, Philadelphia, pp 193–212

II-2. Aortopulmonary Window

The malformation called aortopulmonary window consists of a large defect between the ascending aorta and the main pulmonary artery. Because of the resultant large left-to-right shunt and pulmonary hypertension, the patient develops severe heart failure and respiratory distress as a neonate or infant, requiring early surgery. The surgical approach is patch placement for the orifice of the aortopulmonary window through the ascending aorta or main pulmonary artery. Residual shunt through a patch leak and stenosis of the ascending aorta are possible complications after surgery [1]. As an alternative, the aortopulmonary window may be divided and autologous tissue used for the reconstruction of the resulting defects in the aorta and pulmonary artery [2]. Native great arterial tissue is most often used for repair of the aortic wall in a neonate or young infant.

Operative Procedure

A median sternotomy is performed, and the pericardium is opened in an inverted T shape. The aortic arch and ascending aorta are dissected. A tape is placed around the ascending aorta distal to the window site. The superior and inferior vena cavae and bilateral branch pulmonary arteries are dissected, and tapes placed around them. Tourniquets are placed on the tapes on the branch pulmonary arteries (Fig. II-2-1). After dissection of the ascending aorta proximal to the window site, a tape is placed around the window site. If the window site has enough length, which is rare, ligation or division and oversewing after clamp placement are possible without cardiopulmonary bypass.

Cardiopulmonary bypass is initiated using aortic and bicaval cannulation. As bypass is initiated, the branch pulmonary arteries are occluded with the previously placed tourniquets. The aorta is cross-clamped, and cardioplegic solution is injected. After cardiac arrest, a right atriotomy is performed and a vent is inserted into the left atrium through the patent foramen ovale (PFO). In the absence of a PFO, a small stab wound is made in the foramen and a vent is inserted.

Autologous tissue is usually used for repair of the aortic wall. The window is incised as close as possible to the main pulmonary artery to leave a larger aortic flap. A short incision is placed in the anterior surface of the window connecting to the main pulmonary artery (Fig. II-2-2). This incision is extended longitudinally, close to the main pulmonary artery. After division of the window, the aortic side defect is closed primarily, because enough tissue is left for direct suture closure (Fig. II-2-3). The defect is closed longitudinally in two layers using fine absorbable monofilament suture. Usually the main pulmonary artery is dilated because of the left-to-right shunt and can also be closed primarily. The suture line is carefully oriented so as not to create stenosis at the origin of the right pulmonary artery (Fig. II-2-4). If right pulmonary artery stenosis seems likely, an autologous pericardial patch is used instead to close the defect.

In the patient with interrupted aortic arch (IAA), the right pulmonary artery often originates from the right side of the ascending aorta (Fig. II-2-5). As the aortopulmonary window is opened, and the right pulmonary artery is removed, a large defect is created in the ascending aorta. The anterior surface of the main pulmonary artery is incised to create a large aortic flap, which is then used to close this aortic defect [3]. In the patient with aortopulmonary window and interrupted aortic arch, the aortic arch is repaired first. Bypass is initiated with the arterial cannulae, one in a graft sewn to the brachiocephalic artery and the other placed in the descending aorta to perfuse the lower body. After cooling, the duct is divided and the descending aorta is directly anastomosed to the ascending aorta (cf. "Interrupted aortic arch"). After repair of the aortic arch, the window site is divided. The middle of the anterior surface of the main pulmonary artery is opened longitudinally. The window site and the orifice of the right pulmonary artery are identified. Then the incision is extended and the window site is divided (Fig. II-2-6). This pulmonary artery flap is used to close the defect in the aorta. A generous autologous pericardial patch is used to close the pulmonary artery defect. After trimming the patch, it is placed behind the ascending aorta, and the patch insertion is started at the distal right pulmonary artery from the right side of the ascending aorta. Then the suture line passes behind the ascending aorta, the patch and sutures are pulled to the left side of the ascending aorta, and patch insertion is completed (Fig. II-2-7).

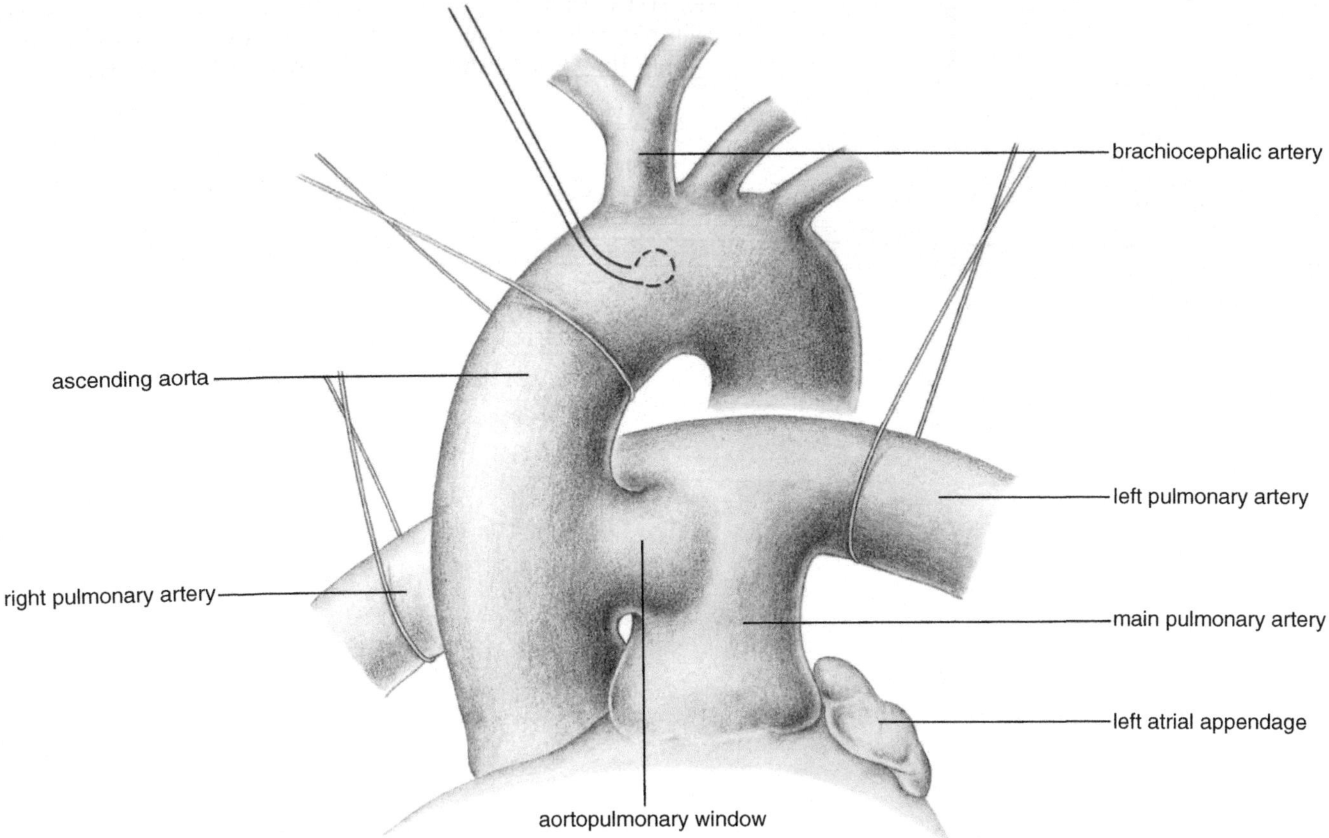

Fig. II-2-1. Aortopulmonary window. Tapes are applied to the ascending aorta and the branch pulmonary arteries. A purse-string suture is placed on the ascending aorta at the base of the brachiocephalic artery

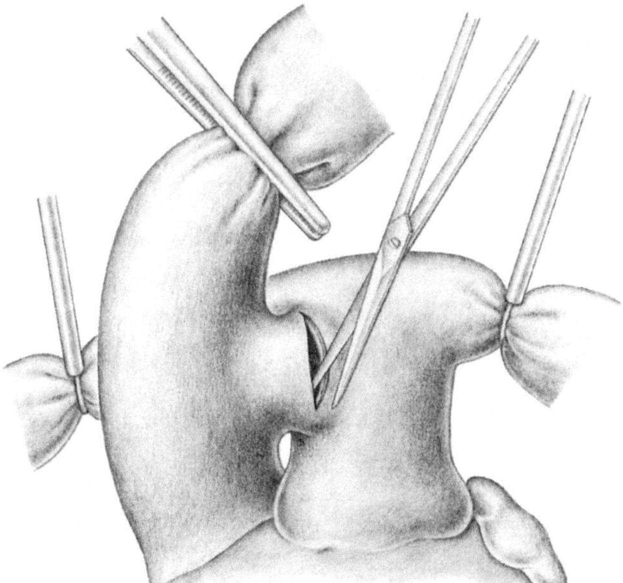

Fig. II-2-2. Division of the aortopulmonary window. The incision is placed as close as possible to the pulmonary artery

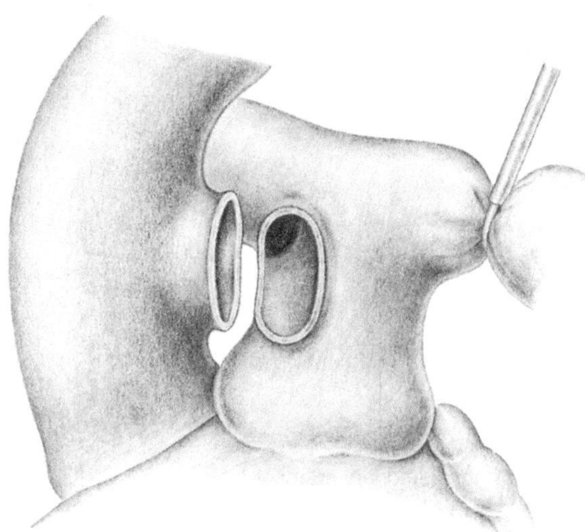

Fig. II-2-3. After division of aortopulmonary window. More tissue should be left on the aortic side, to maximize the possibility of primary closure

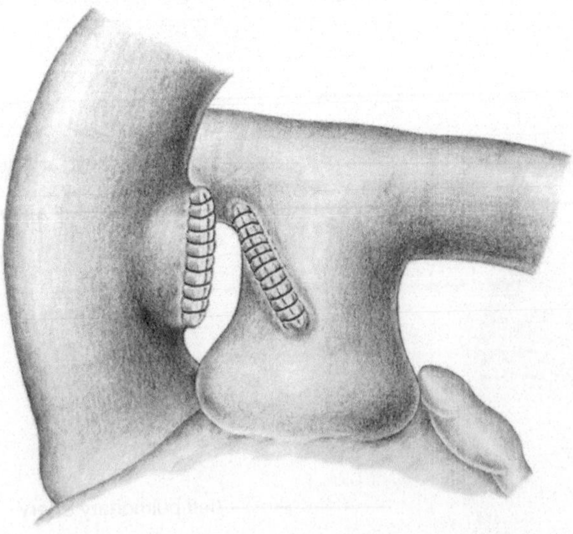

Fig. II-2-4. Closure of aorta and pulmonary artery. Because the main pulmonary artery is usually dilated, primary closure often does not cause stenosis. However, if stenosis seems likely, a patch closure is used

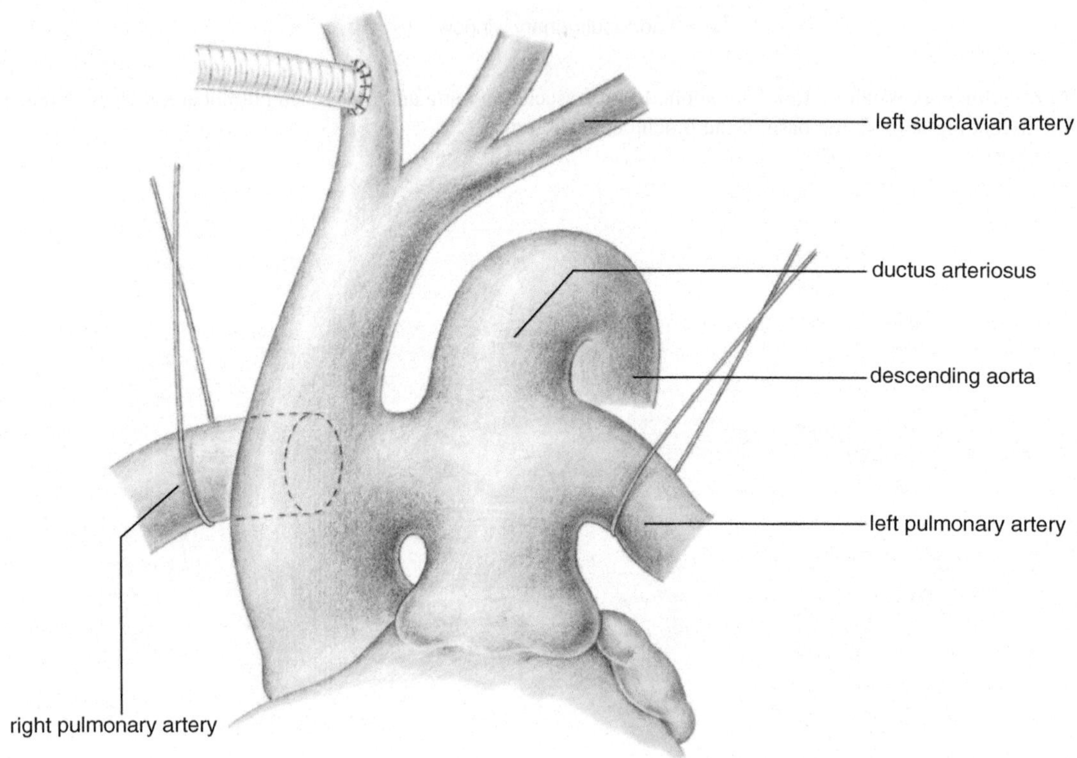

Fig. II-2-5. Combination of interrupted aortic arch (type A) and aortopulmonary window. A graft is anastomosed to the brachiocephalic artery for perfusion

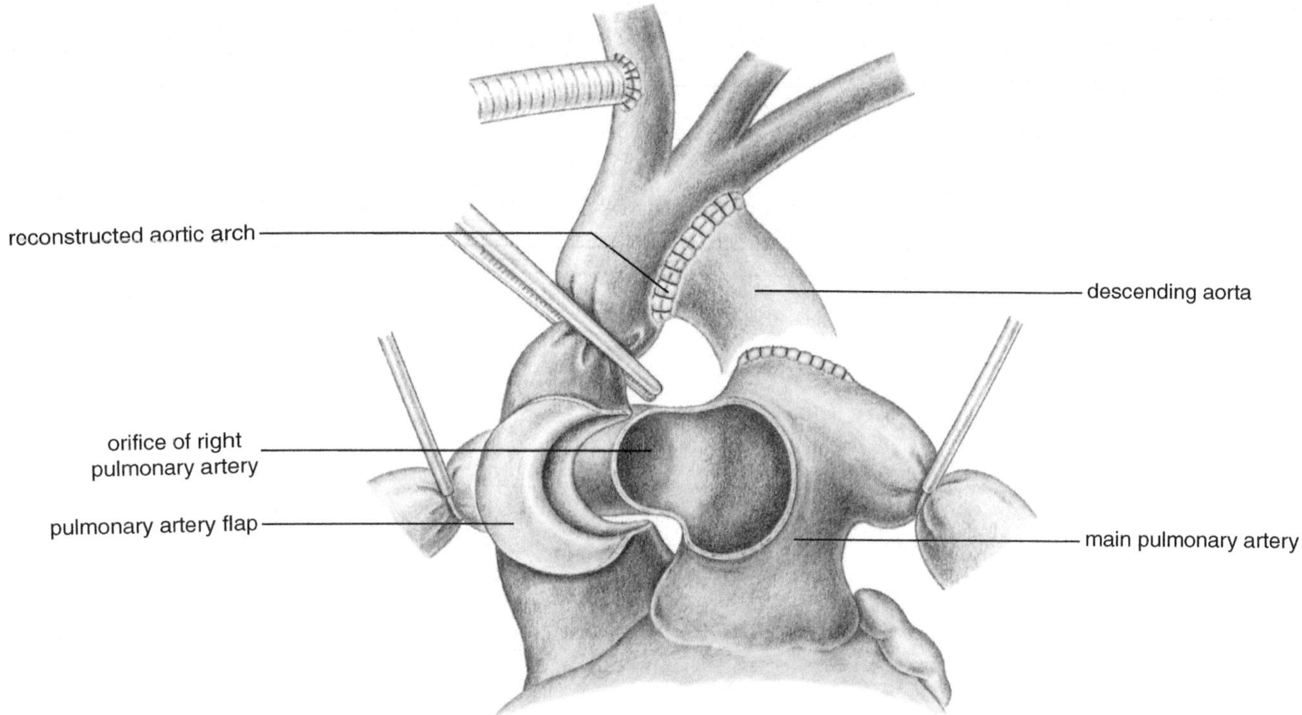

Fig. II-2-6. Division of the pulmonary artery from the ascending aorta. A large main pulmonary artery wall flap is preserved to repair the ascending aortic defect

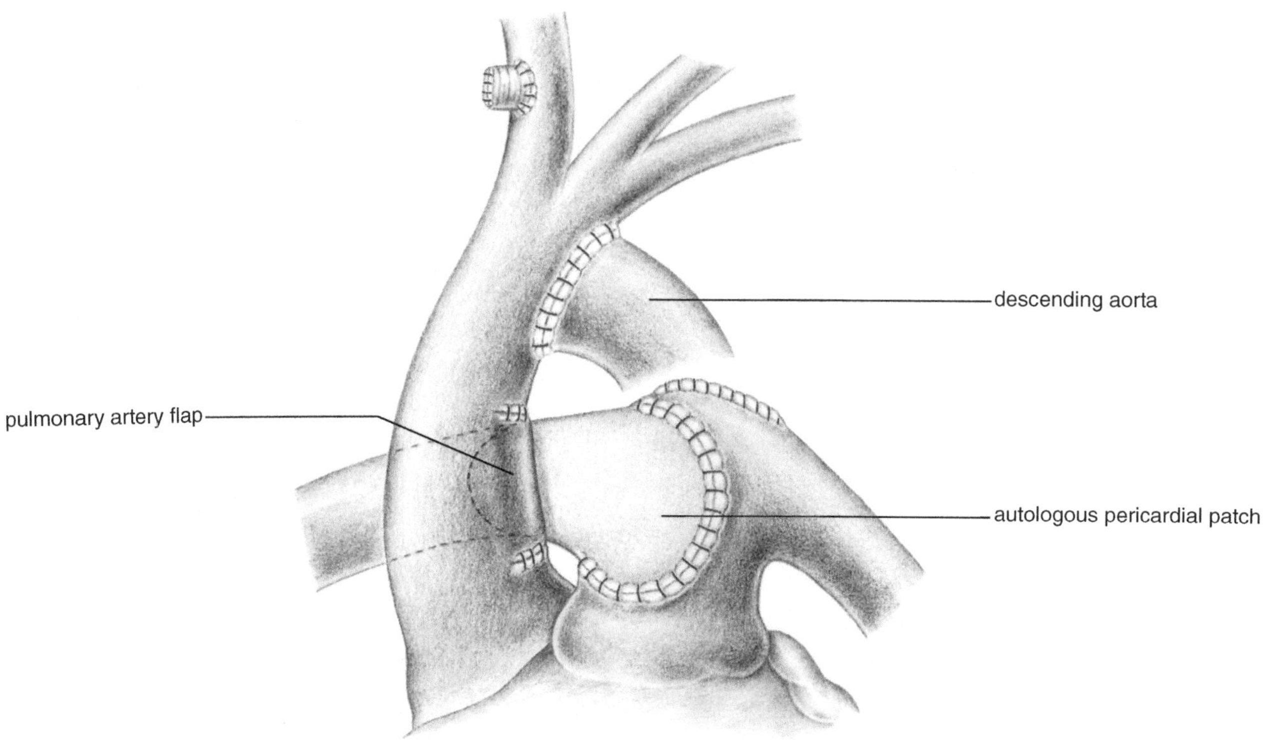

Fig. II-2-7. Completion of repair. The ascending aorta is repaired with the pulmonary artery flap. The defect in the main pulmonary artery and right pulmonary artery is repaired using an autologous pericardial patch

References

1. Uematsu M, Yamaguchi M, Ohashi H, et al (1994) Severe ascending aortic stenosis after one-stage repair of aortopulmonary window and interrupted aortic arch. Nippon Kyobu Geka Gakkai Zasshi 42:1247–1253
2. Prasad TR, Valiathan MS, Shyamakrishnan KG, et al (1989) Surgical management of aortopulmonary septal defect. Ann Thorac Surg 47:877–879
3. Sano T, Sese A, Ueno Y, et al (1995) Surgical treatment of interrupted aortic arch with aortopulmonary window. Nippon Kyobu Geka Gakkai Zasshi 43:300–305

II-3. Coarctation of the Aorta: Subclavian Flap Aortoplasty and Direct Anastomosis (Extended Aortic Arch Anastomosis)

Surgical Indication

There are two types of coarctation, divided depending on the location of coarctation: preductal (or infantile) and postductal (or adult) type (Fig. II-3-1) [1]. Not infrequently, hypoplasia of the aortic arch is present with the infantile form of this disease. In early infancy, patients with significant stenosis (a blood pressure gradient of more than 20–30 mmHg) are thought to have an indication for operation. If there is no coexisting intracardiac anomaly, only an aortoplasty is performed. If there is a significant intracardiac anomaly, either a single- or two-stage approach is chosen, based on institutional preference and experience. In patients associated with intracardiac anomaly, preoperative cardiac catheterization may be required to analyze it.

Subclavian Flap Aortoplasty (SFA) [2]

This procedure uses the left subclavian artery for repair of the coarctation. The benefit of this technique is the longitudinal suture line of the anastomosis, which allows potential for growth because only native tissue is used. Even if stenosis develops, it is usually amenable to relief by balloon angioplasty. The disadvantage of the technique is the sacrifice of blood supply to the left arm. In a neonate or small infant, however, this is usually not an issue because ischemia or functional deficit does not develop and limb growth is normal. Complications are bleeding and paraplegia. The risk factors for the development of paraplegia are (1) cross-clamp time of more than 40 min, (2) hyperthermia higher than 38°C during surgery, (3) hypotension during anastomosis, (4) mild stenosis and inadequate collateral vessels, and (5) aberrant right subclavian artery. Rectal temperature is monitored during surgery and is kept between 35° and 37°C using a blanket.

Thoracotomy: Dissection

A left thoracotomy is performed, and the chest is entered through the third or fourth intercostal space. The lung is retracted anteriorly (Fig. II-3-2). To avoid pulmonary hemorrhage, gentle ventilation is important. The superior intercostal vein is divided, and the pleura overlying the descending aorta is incised inferiorly and superiorly. Dissection of the aortic arch is advanced up to the left carotid artery, and a tape is placed around the aortic arch. The artery of Abbott, which arises from the distal arch behind the origin of the left subclavian artery, is only seen in the patient with coarctation of the aorta, and care is taken not to damage this artery. The descending aorta is mobilized 20 mm distal from the coarctation site, and a tape placed around the vessel. The duct is dissected so as to avoid damage to the recurrent laryngeal nerve. A heavy silk ligature is used to close the duct. The left subclavian artery is dissected completely. The branches of the left subclavian artery, including the vertebral artery, are doubly ligated and divided. Depending on the severity and length of the coarctation, the requirement of the subclavian artery is different. In all cases, the subclavian artery flap should be placed 10 mm beyond the coarctation site. When pulmonary artery banding is required, a loose band is placed before aortic reconstruction and is adjusted afterward.

Clamp and Division

To decrease lower extremity ischemia, the vessels are managed in the following order: (1) ligation of the left subclavian artery, (2) ligation of the duct, (3) clamping the distal aortic arch between the left subclavian artery and left carotid artery, and (4) clamp placement on the descending aorta. The descending aorta distal to the duct is opened longitudinally using a Potts knife scissors, and this incision is advanced proximally up to the distal subclavian artery (Fig. II-3-3). After opening up to the subclavian artery ligation site, the subclavian artery is divided. If the subclavian artery is divided before opening longitudinally, there is the risk of creating a spiral opening in this vessel. The membranous tissue at the coarctation site is resected carefully, because perforation or late aneurysm formation may occur if the resection is too deep.

Anastomosis

A mattress suture is placed between the bottom of the aortotomy of the descending aorta and the tip of the flap, and this suture is tied. Three to four stitches are advanced proximally. Stitches are placed on each side of the base of the flap (Fig. II-3-4). To avoid stenosis at the base of the

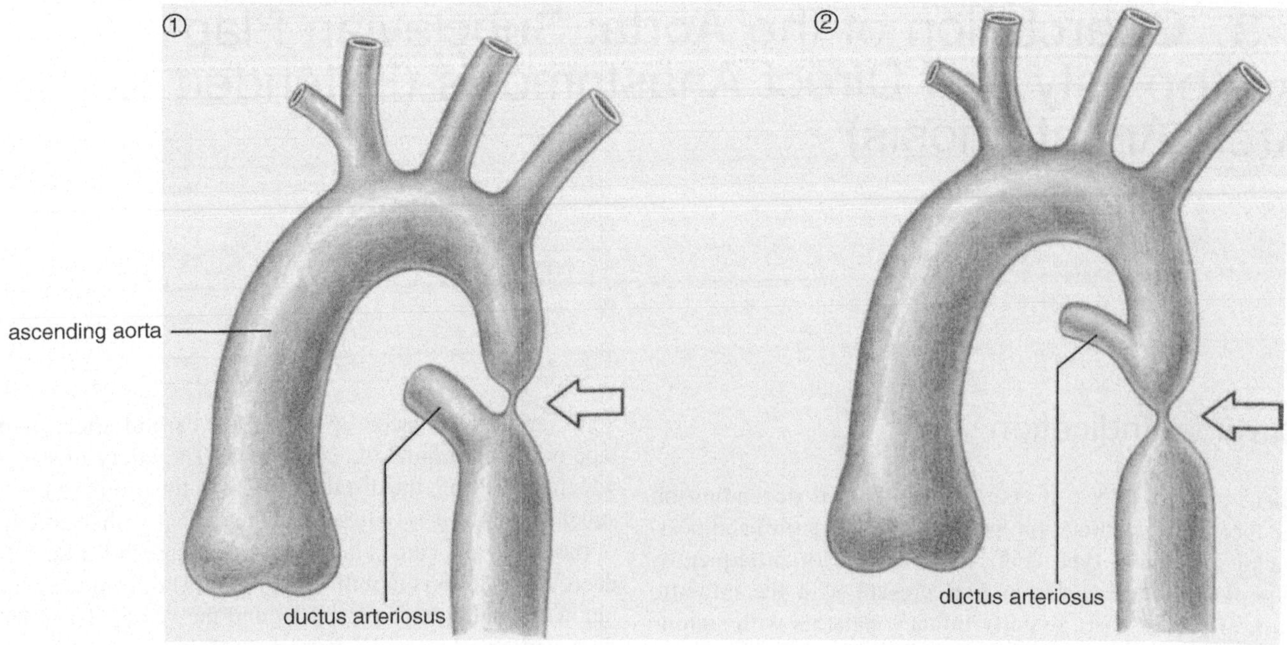

Fig. II-3-1. Type of coarctation of the aorta. Preductal type ①: the patient with this type of coarctation (*arrow*) develops symptoms in the neonatal or infantile period, and this type of coarctation is termed the infantile type. It is often associated with a variable degree of aortic arch hypoplasia. Postductal type ②: the patient with this type of coarctation with stenosis distal to the ductal insertion site (*arrow*) may not be identified until later childhood or adulthood, and this type of coarctation is often called the adult type

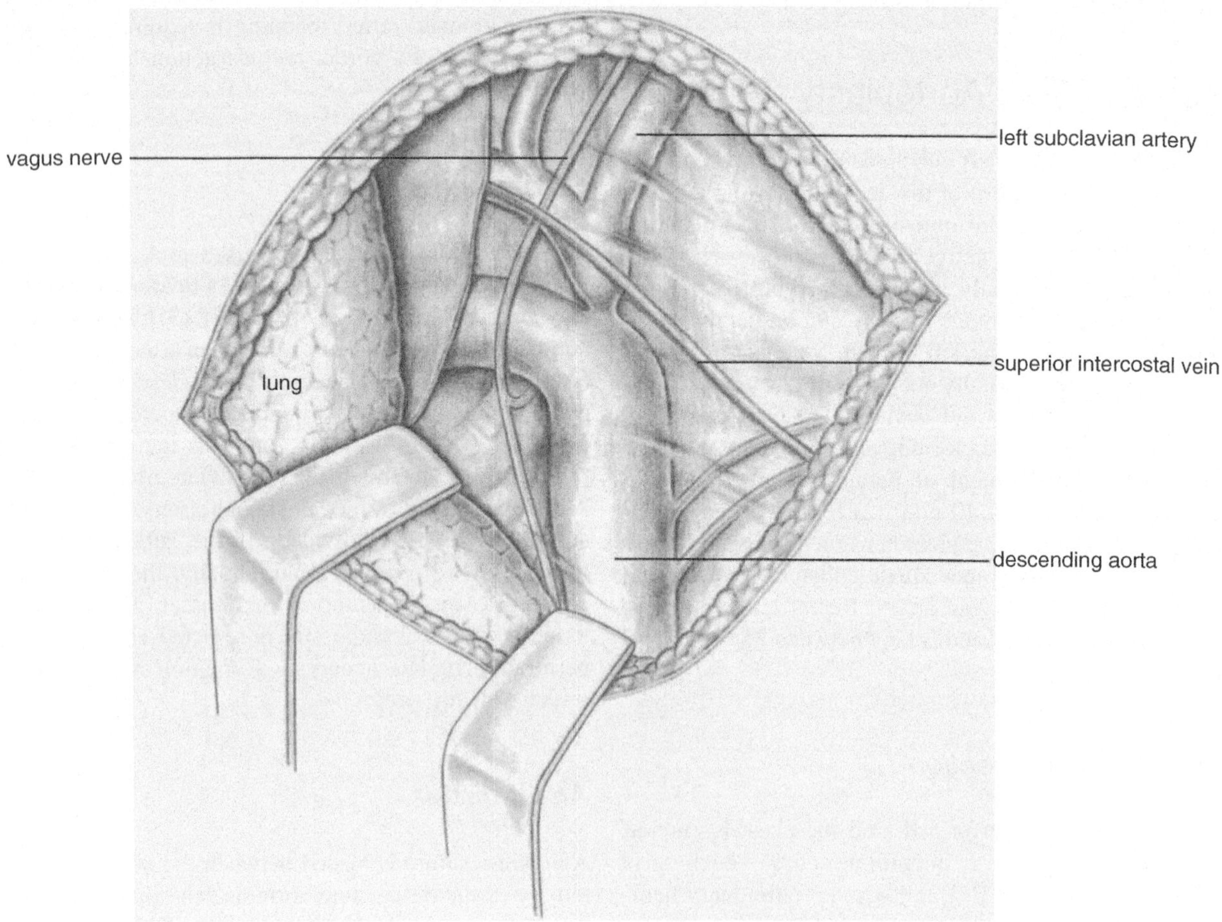

Fig. II-3-2. Subclavian flap aortoplasty: 1. The chest is entered via a left thoracotomy, and the lung is retracted inferiorly and anteriorly

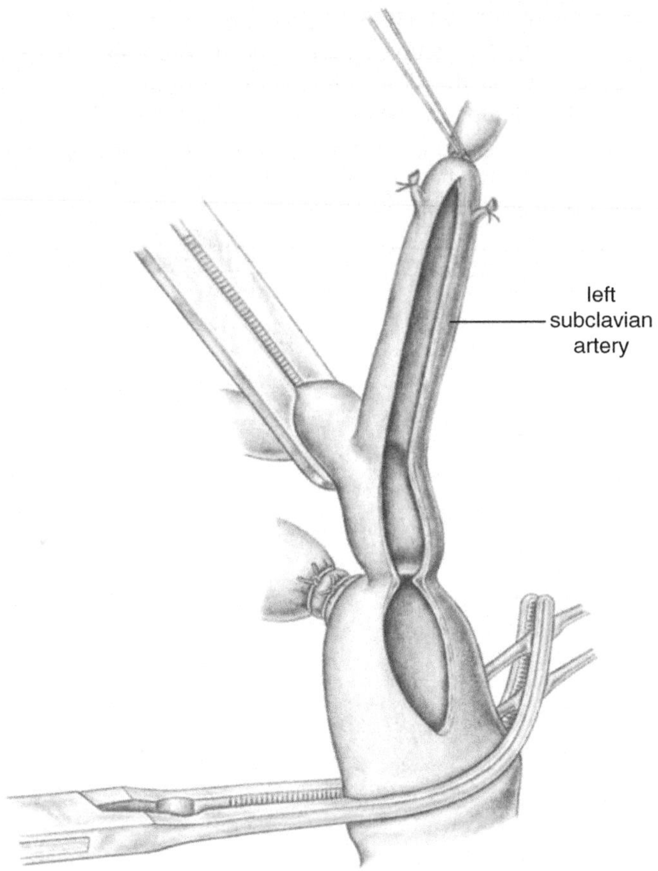

Fig. II-3-3. Subclavian flap aortoplasty: 2. A longitudinal incision is made from the descending aorta to the subclavian artery

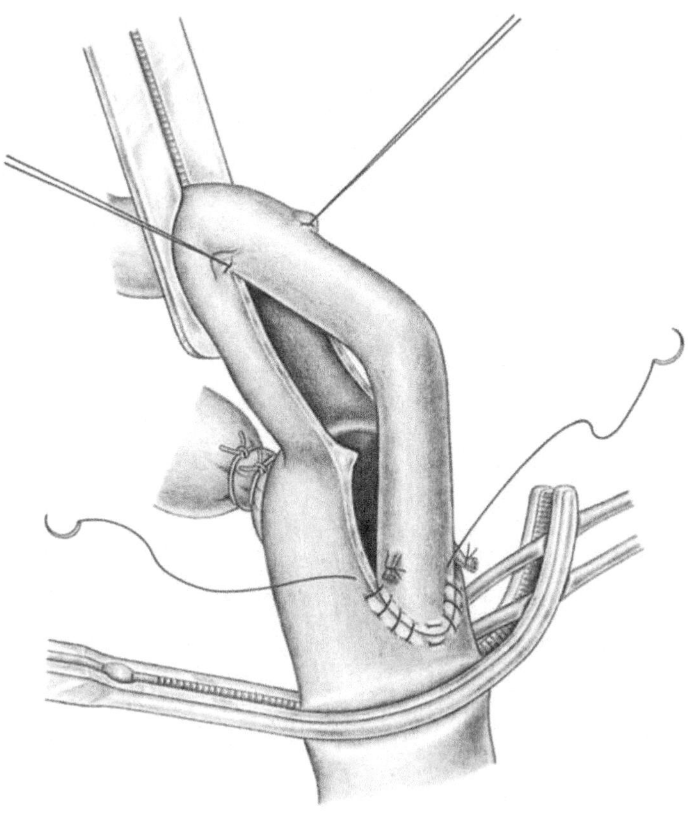

Fig. II-3-4. Subclavian flap aortoplasty: 3. Anastomosis of the flap is started distally

flap, sutures are placed in the flap 1–2 mm distal from the hinge point (Fig. II-3-5). Fine monofilament sutures are used to advance the anastomosis distally (Fig. II-3-6). These sutures are tied to the sutures begun at the distal end. Before finishing the anastomosis, the inside of the aorta is irrigated with saline. When the coarctation site is very small, a few interrupted stitches are placed at the coarctation site, which augments the vessel diameter (Fig. II-3-7). This procedure is performed before flap placement. The clamp on the descending aorta is released first, and then the clamp on the arch is removed. At the time of removal of a clamp, volume resuscitation and inotropic support are readied to treat hypotension involved with release of the clamp.

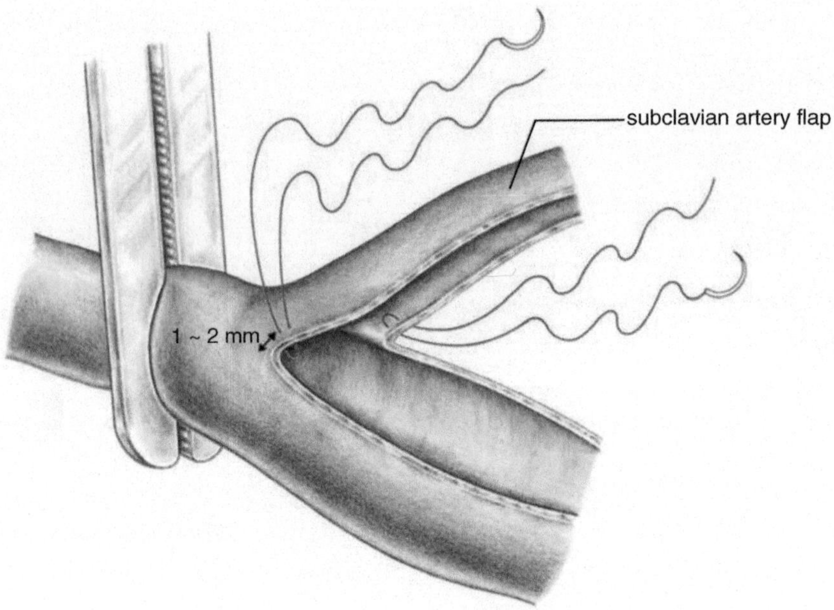

Fig. II-3-5. Subclavian flap aortoplasty: 4. Sutures are placed at the base of the flap. To avoid stenosis, the sutures are begun 1–2 mm distal to the hinge point in the base of the flap

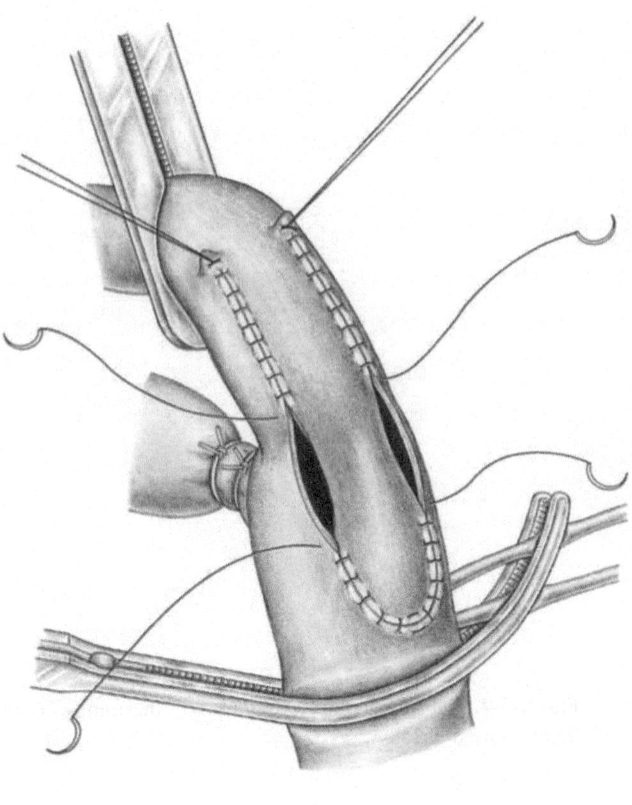

Fig. II-3-6. Subclavian flap aortoplasty: 5. Proximal and distal suture lines are joined

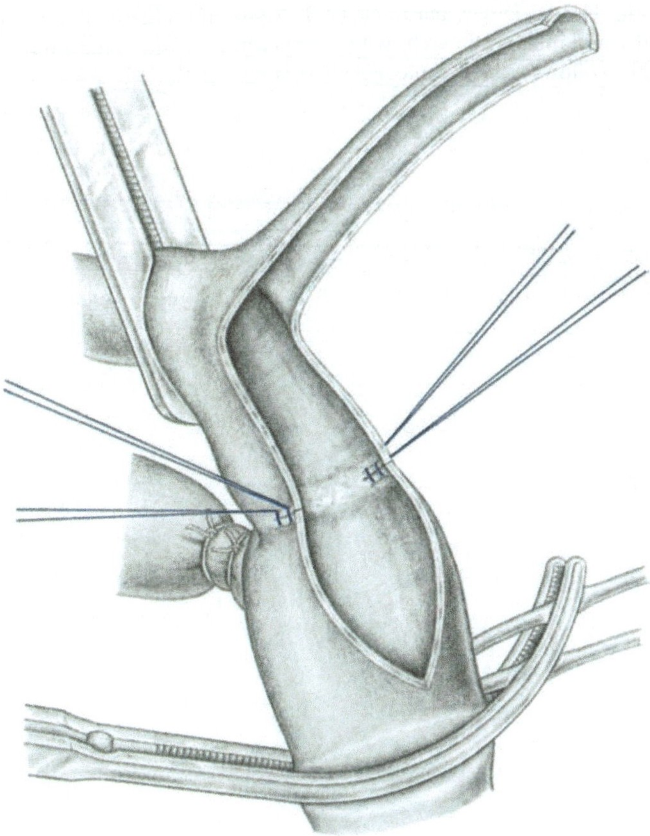

Fig. II-3-7. Subclavian flap aortoplasty: 6. If the coarctation site is especially narrow, a few interrupted sutures are used to fashion a transverse aortoplasty, which enlarges the coarctation site

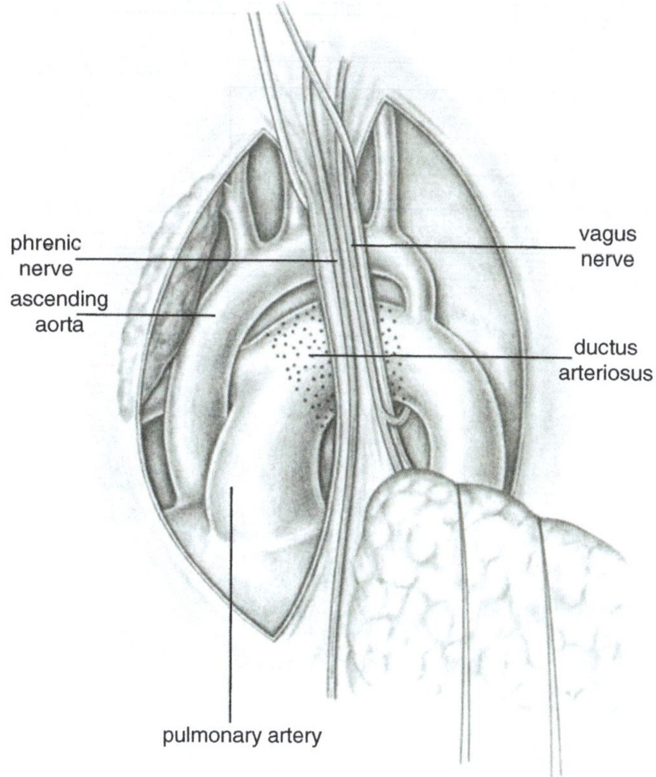

Fig. II-3-8. Direct anastomosis: 1. The *stippled area* shows ductal tissue. The pericardium is entered through an opening anterior to the phrenic nerve. The phrenic and vagus nerves are isolated together

Direct Anastomosis (Extended Aortic Arch Anastomosis)

In circumstances of severe aortic arch hypoplasia extending proximally, this procedure may require cardiopulmonary bypass, as discussed in Chapter II-4 for repair of interrupted aortic arch. In this chapter, the approach via left thoracotomy is described. Depending on the extent of aortotomy onto the arch this procedure is named differently. For limited proximal aortotomy, the terms coarctectomy and end-to-end anastomosis are used. When the term extended aortic arch anastomosis is employed, the implication is that the proximal aortotomy reaches close to the ascending aorta. In this chapter, extended aortic arch anastomosis is mentioned. In this surgery, there is potential for obstruction of blood flow into the brachiocephalic artery, and thus right radial or superficial temporal arterial blood pressure should be monitored. The mean arterial pressure needs to be kept above 30 mmHg.

Thoracotomy: Dissection

A thoracotomy through the third or fourth intercostal space is used as with subclavian flap aortoplasty. To improve visualization at the arch, the incision is often extended anteriorly. Dissection on the arch is advanced to the base of the brachiocephalic artery. To obtain better visualization, the left lobe of the thymus is resected. The pericardium is opened longitudinally anterior to the phrenic nerve. The ascending aorta, the main pulmonary artery, and the left carotid artery are dissected. The branches of the aortic arch are mobilized as distally as possible. To decrease tension at the anastomosis, the descending aorta is also mobilized as distally as possible. The intercostal arteries are isolated, but not ligated (Fig. II-3-8).

Aortic Clamp

The duct is doubly ligated at the pulmonary end. Clamps are placed on the proximal arch, left carotid artery, and left subclavian artery, with careful attention to the blood pressure in the right radial artery (Fig. II-3-9). Cerebral hemorrhage caused by acute hypertension at the time of aortic clamping has been reported, so acute hypertension should be avoided. Then the descending aorta is clamped, isolating the coarctation region.

Aortotomy and Anastomosis

The aorta is divided at the junction of the duct, and ductal tissue is completely resected from the descending aorta with inspection of the aortic lumen. Ductal tissue is fragile and swollen, appearing to have two layers. The border between the ductal tissue and normal aortic tissue is thus relatively easily distinguished. The dorsal part of the descending aorta is longitudinally incised to enlarge the anastomotic orifice. Fine monofilament absorbable running suture is used (Fig. II-3-10).

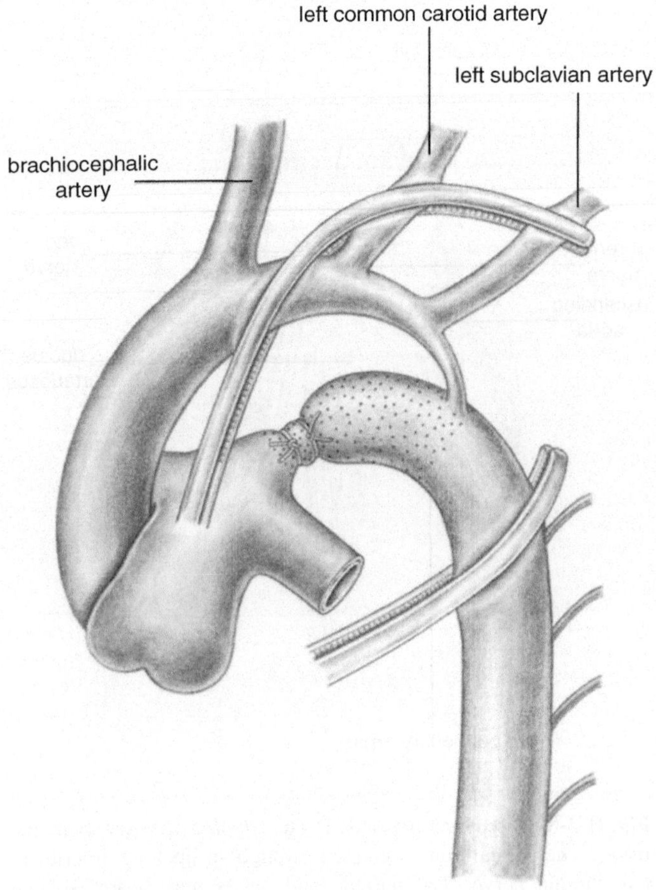

Fig. II-3-9. Direct anastomosis: 2. A vascular clamp is placed on the proximal aortic arch, with care taken to avoid compromise of blood flow in the brachiocephalic artery

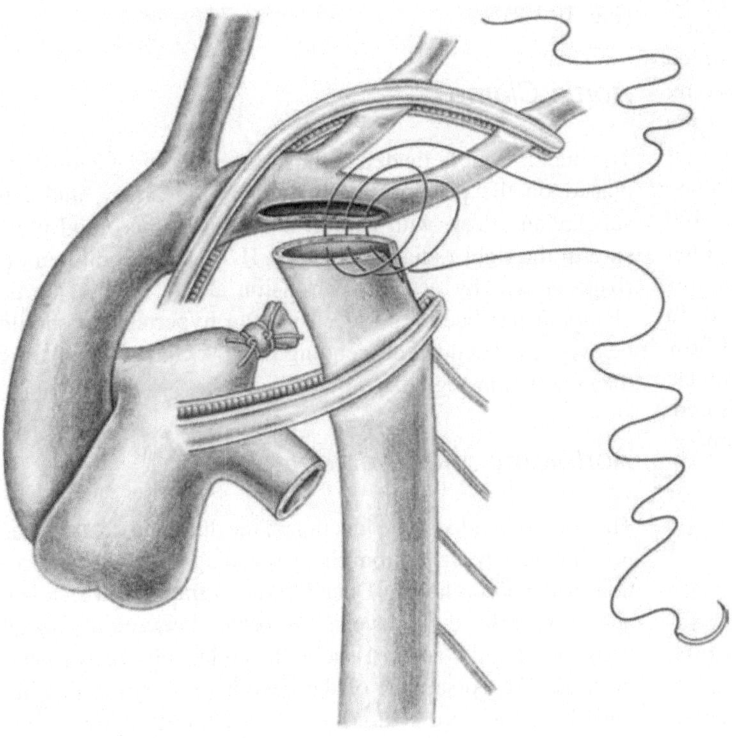

Fig. II-3-10. Direct anastomosis: 3. With a longitudinal incision at the posterior aspect of the descending aorta, the orifice is enlarged. An anastomosis is started using a running suture

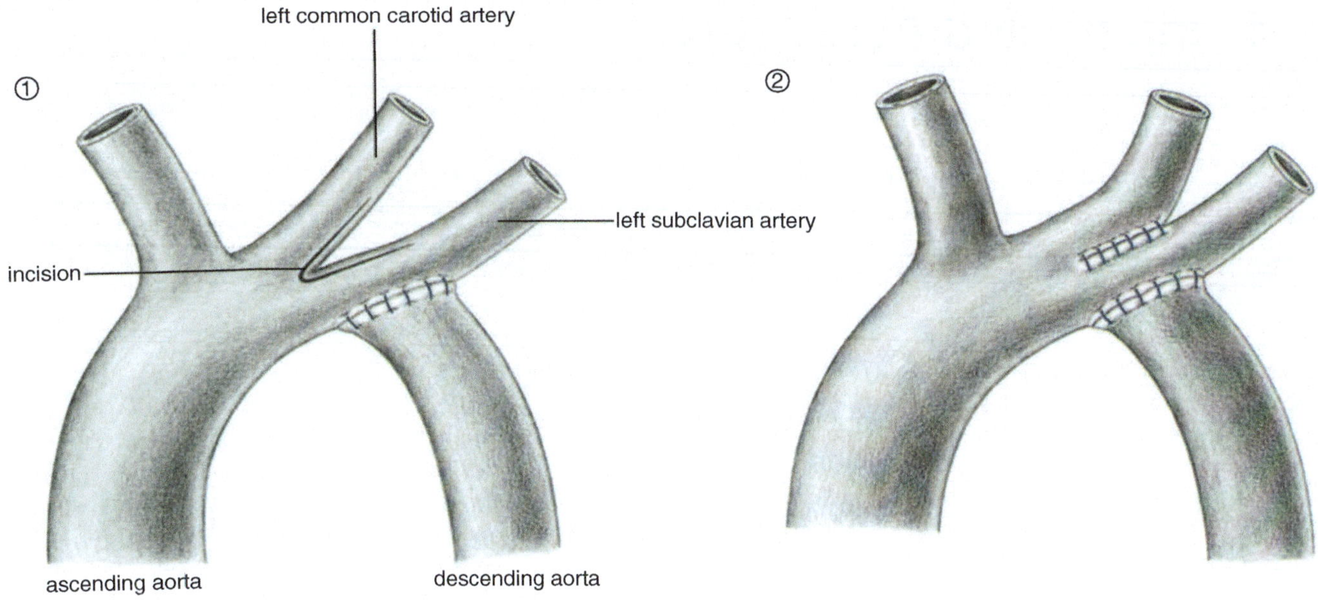

Fig. II-3-11. Direct anastomosis: 4. Technique for enlargement of hypoplastic aortic arch

For the patient with a hypoplastic aortic arch, the bases of left carotid and left subclavian arteries and distal aortic arch are longitudinally opened (Fig. II-3-11). The left carotid and left subclavian arteries are anastomosed in a side-to-side fashion, and the distal aortic arch is enlarged [3]. It may be wise to allow a period of distal reperfusion before completing later reconstruction.

References

1. Bonnett LM (1903) Sur la lesion site stenose congenitale de l'aorte dans la region de l'isthme. Rev Med Paris 23:108
2. Waldhausen JA, Nahrwold DL (1966) Repair of coarctation of the aorta with a subclavian flap. J Thorac Cardiovasc Surg 51:532–533
3. Yasui H, Kado H, Nakamura Y, et al (1983) Surgical treatment for neonatal and infant with coarctation of the aorta or interrupted aortic arch (in Japanese). Pediatr Cardiol Cardiac Surg Suppl: 182–183

II-4. Interrupted Aortic Arch

Because most patients with an interrupted aortic arch have coexisting intracardiac anomalies, this condition is called the interruption complex in Japan. For preoperative evaluation, it is vital to define any intracardiac anomalies and aortic arch anatomy. Intracardiac anomalies may include ventricular septal defect, truncus arteriosus, transposition of the great arteries, double outlet right ventricle, and aortopulmonary window. Because valvular, subvalvular, or supravalvular aortic stenosis is frequently observed, careful assessment of the entire left ventricular outflow tract is mandatory. Interrupted aortic arch is classified by the site of the interruption: type A (distal to the left subclavian artery), type B (between the left subclavian artery and left carotid artery), and type C (between the brachiocephalic artery and left carotid artery), as described by Celoria and Patton [1]. The incidence of type A is 42%, that of type B is 53%, and that of type C is 4% (Fig. II-4-1). Evaluation of the length of the missing aortic segment is important, because this influences the need for more extensive dissection and mobilization of the proximal and distal segments.

Historically, there have been two types of approach for interrupted aortic arch: a single-stage repair and a two-stage repair. The latter involves establishment of aortic continuity and pulmonary artery banding for the first stage, followed later by intracardiac repair with pulmonary artery debanding. The two-stage repair involves either a direct anastomosis (discussed in Chapter II-3: Coarctation of the Aorta) or a Blalock–Park procedure.

Blalock–Park Procedure

This procedure is used for type A interruption of the aortic arch. The left subclavian artery is divided and is anastomosed to the descending aorta.

Thoracotomy and Dissection

Thoracotomy and dissection are the same as subclavian flap aortoplasty (see p. 35).

Aortic Cross-Clamp

The left subclavian artery is extensively dissected and ligated. The duct is doubly ligated, and the descending aorta is clamped (Fig. II-4-2).

Division

The left subclavian artery is divided distally, and the inferior surface of the distal end of the artery is incised longitudinally for at least 1 cm. A longitudinal incision is placed in the dorsal surface of the descending aorta, also for at least 1 cm length. This incision should not include ductal tissue. To avoid involvement of ductal tissue in the anastomosis, the first incision is made far distal from the duct insertion site, and this incision is enlarged superiorly. The incision is stopped when the ductal tissue is reached. If a larger orifice is needed, the incision is extended inferiorly. It is essential to open the subclavian artery proximal to the origin of its first branch.

Anastomosis

An absorbable fine monofilament suture in a running technique is used for the anastomosis (Fig. II-4-3). At the end, the adventitia of the proximal descending aorta and the base of the left subclavian artery are approximated (Fig. II-4-4). This maneuver decreases the tension at the anastomosis suture line and may facilitate growth at the anastomosis site.

Aortic Arch Reconstruction in Single-Stage Repair

Single-stage repair includes arch reconstruction by direct anastomosis and intracardiac repair. Cardiopulmonary bypass techniques vary by institution [2–6]. Some use regional cerebral perfusion through the brachiocephalic artery and lower body circulatory arrest [3] or lower body perfusion through a graft anastomosed to the descending aorta [4]. Here we mention our current procedure of choice including descending aortic cannulation to allow perfusion of both the descending aorta and brachiocephalic artery, which completely avoids circulatory arrest [5,6].

The only modification of cardiopulmonary bypass circuit is a Y-connector at the arterial site (Fig. II-4-5). Because the relative distribution of blood flow to the upper and lower circulations depends on vascular resistance, it is desirable to monitor both upper and lower extremity blood pressure.

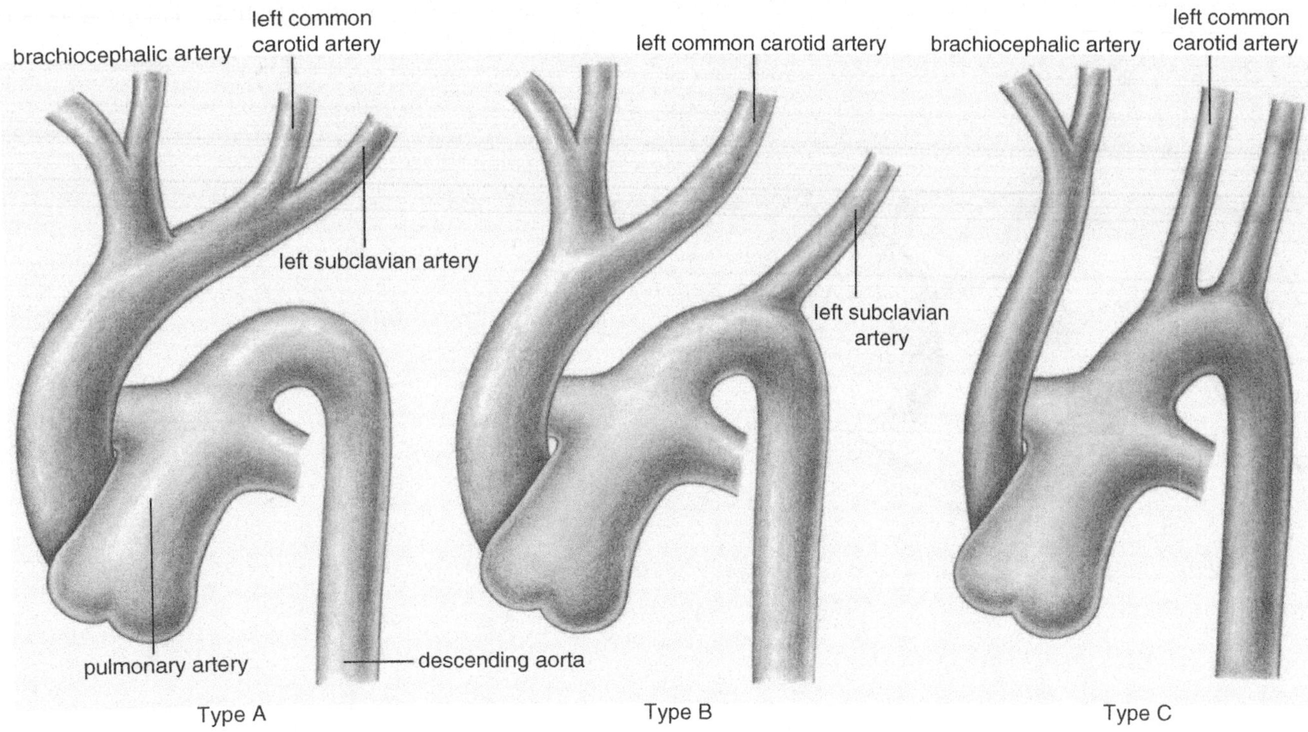

Fig. II-4-1. Classification of interrupted aortic arch by Celoria and Patton

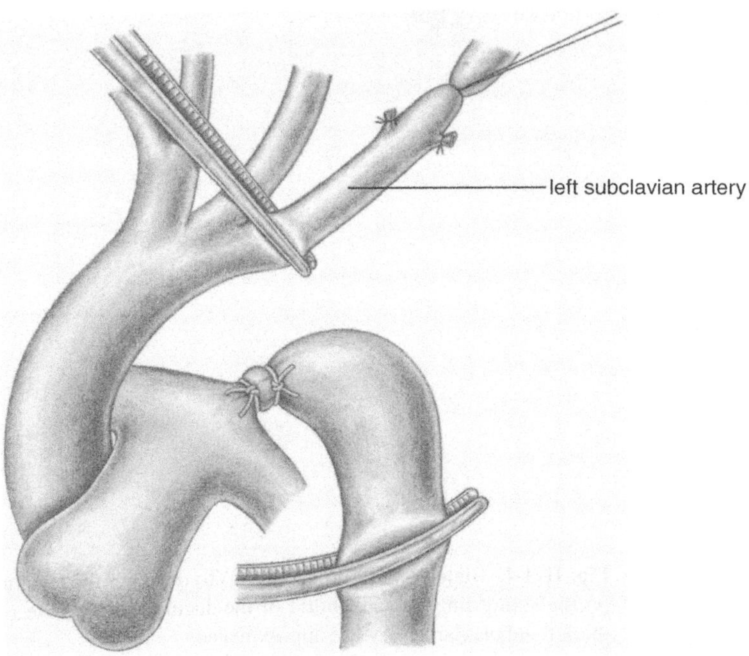

Fig. II-4-2. Blalock–Park procedure: 1. The left subclavian artery is ligated and divided distally

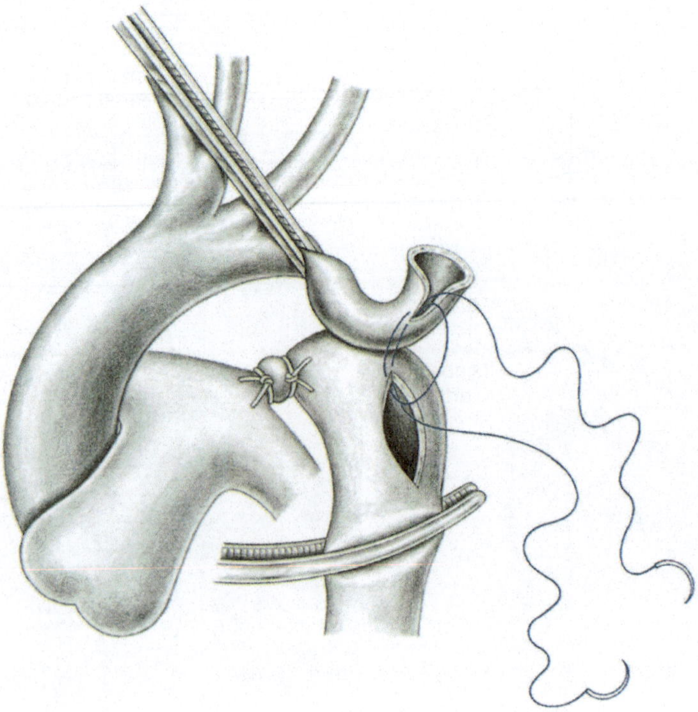

Fig. II-4-3. Blalock–Park procedure: 2. The left subclavian artery is cut back more than 1 cm to obtain a large anastomosis. It is important to avoid ductal tissue during the aortotomy in the descending aorta

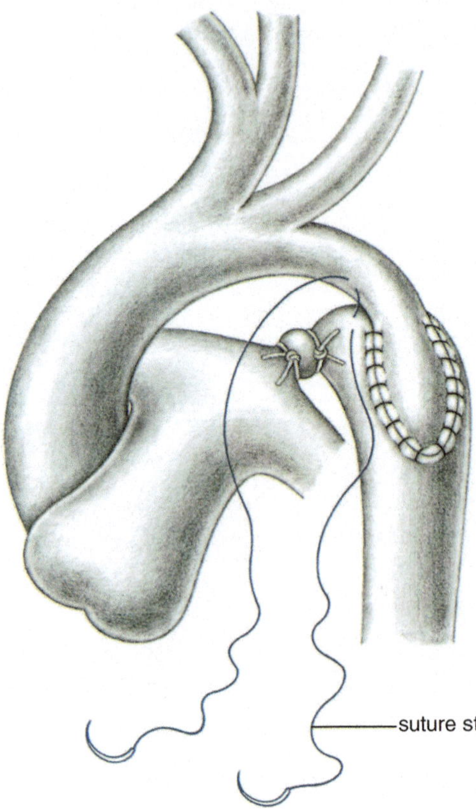

Fig. II-4-4. Blalock–Park procedure: 3. To decrease the tension on the suture line, the adventitia of the ductus and the base of the left subclavian artery are approximated

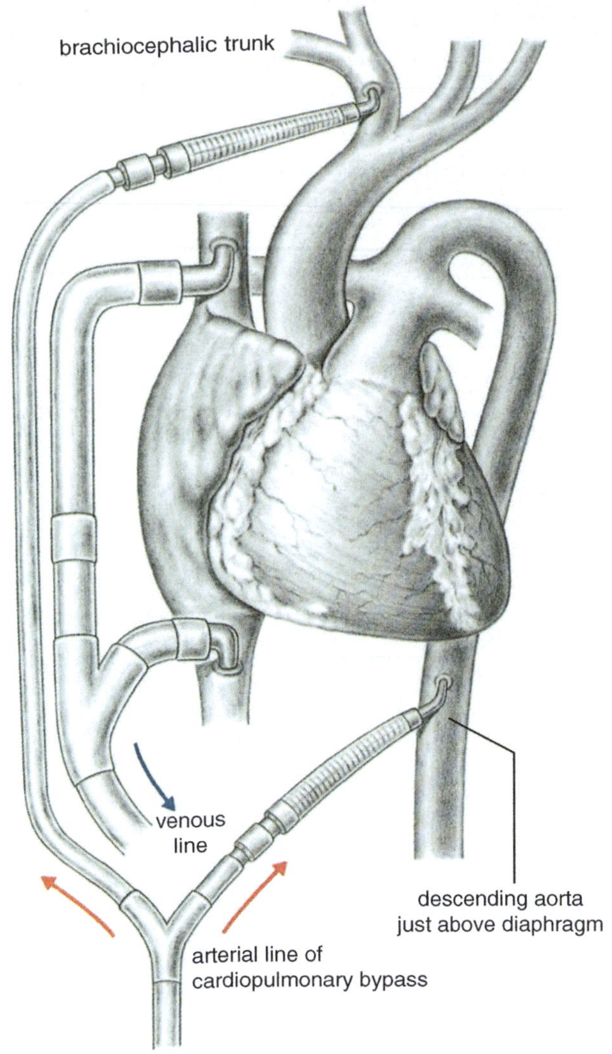

Fig. II-4-5. Aortic arch reconstruction without circulatory arrest: 1. Cardiopulmonary bypass

Because blood flow in the left cerebral hemisphere depends on the blood flow in the right hemisphere through the circle of Willis, to ascertain the perfusion on the left hemisphere, a blood pressure monitor on the left superficial temporal artery is necessary. We therefore monitor lower extremity and left superficial temporal arterial blood pressures. Typically, the difference in mean blood pressure is less than 5 mmHg. The flow rate of bypass is between 180 and 200 ml/kg/min. The rectal temperature is lowered to 32°C [5].

Preparation of Cardiopulmonary Bypass

After median sternotomy, half the thymus is resected to optimize visualization of the operative field. The ascending aorta, aortic arch, arch branches, branch pulmonary arteries, and ductus are dissected. For aortic cannulation, a fine purse-string suture is placed on the brachiocephalic artery, and a right-angle metal tip cannula (2.1 mm; JMS) is inserted distally. The venous cannulae are inserted into the superior and inferior vena cavae, and cardiopulmonary bypass is started. Both branch pulmonary arteries are temporarily occluded with tourniquets. The heart is kept beating until perfusion through the descending aorta is begun. To keep the heart beating, the level of calcium should be kept normal and the perfusate kept at normothermia.

Cannulation into the Descending Aorta

The heart is retracted superiorly to expose the pericardium, which is incised between the inferior vena cava and left phrenic nerve. Division of the inferior pulmonary ligament improves the visualization of the mediastinum. After the esophagus is pushed to the right, the descending aorta is identified, but not encircled, to avoid damage to the intercostal artery and the esophagus. After the superficial adventitia is removed, a purse-string suture is placed in the descending aorta (Fig. II-4-6). Cannulation is straightforward, the same way as is performed for the ascending aorta or brachiocephalic artery. After arch repair, only the cannula to the descending aorta will be retained, so the tip of the cannula should be placed toward the proximal side [5,6]. To improve visualization of the operative fields, the first assistant pushes the diaphragm inferiorly with a retractor while also retracting the heart cephalad. After establishment of perfusion to the lower half of the body, arch reconstruction is started.

Arch Reconstruction

If the proximal arch is not hypoplastic, and the arch and the descending aorta are directly anastomosed, the anastomosis can be performed with the heart beating. After ligation of the duct, a clamp is placed across the arch between the brachiocephalic artery and left carotid artery. The left carotid and subclavian arteries are clamped simultaneously with the same vascular clamp (Fig. II-4-7). The descending aorta is clamped, and the duct is divided. All ductal tissue is resected from the descending aorta. Further dissection of the descending aorta is performed, and the arch is opened longitudinally. An absorbable fine monofilament suture is used for anastomosis (Fig. II-4-8). Because the proximal clamp may compromise a coronary artery or kink the aortic cannula and compromise coronary perfusion during arch reconstruction with the heart beating, careful attention must be paid to the heart rate, color of the heart, and changes in the electrocardiogram. After arch repair, the aortic cannula in the brachiocephalic artery is removed and only the cannula in the descending aorta is employed during intracardiac repair. If normal coronary perfusion is impossible with this approach, a clamp is placed on the brachiocephalic artery proximal to the cannulation site, and the arch is repaired during cardioplegic cardiac arrest (Fig. II-4-9).

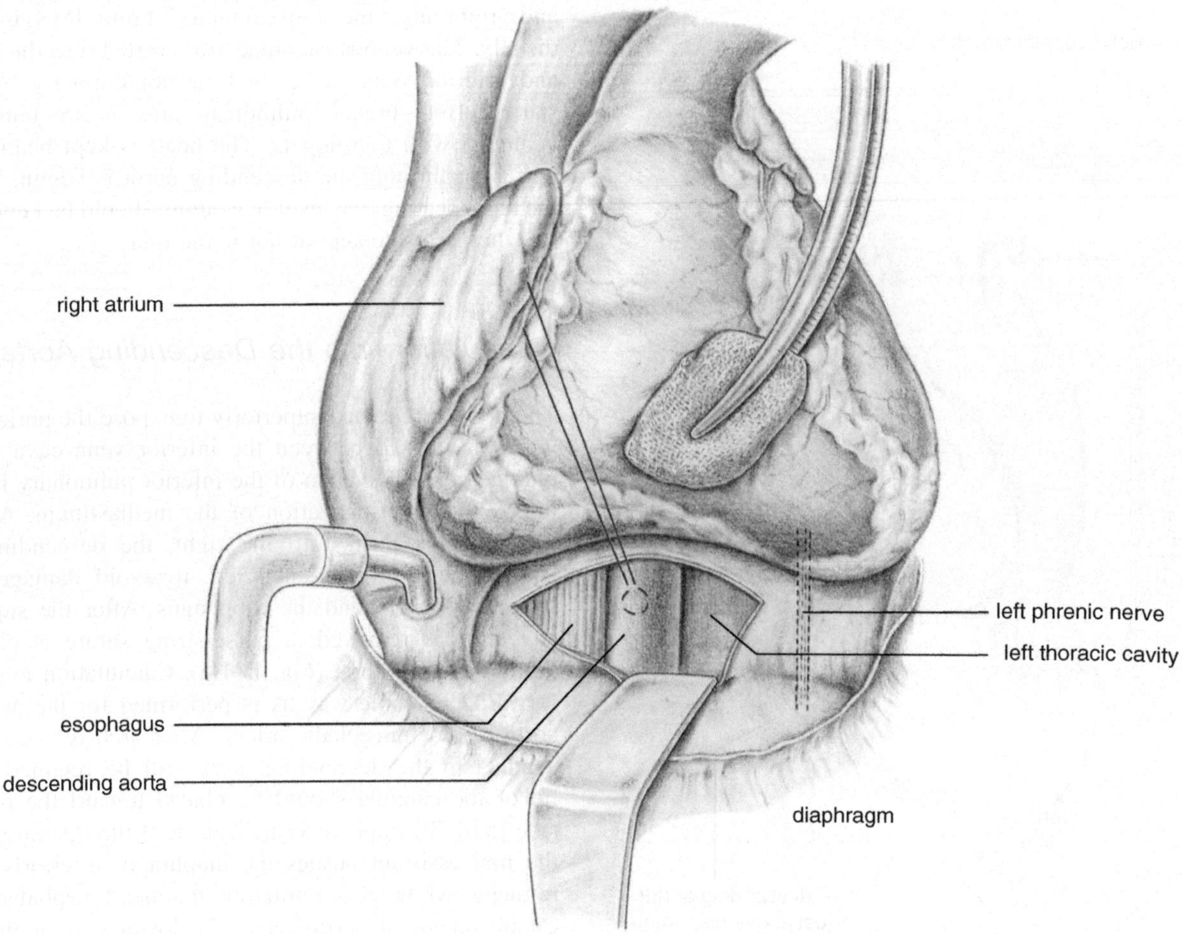

Fig. II-4-6. Aortic arch reconstruction without circulatory arrest: 2. Descending aortic cannulation

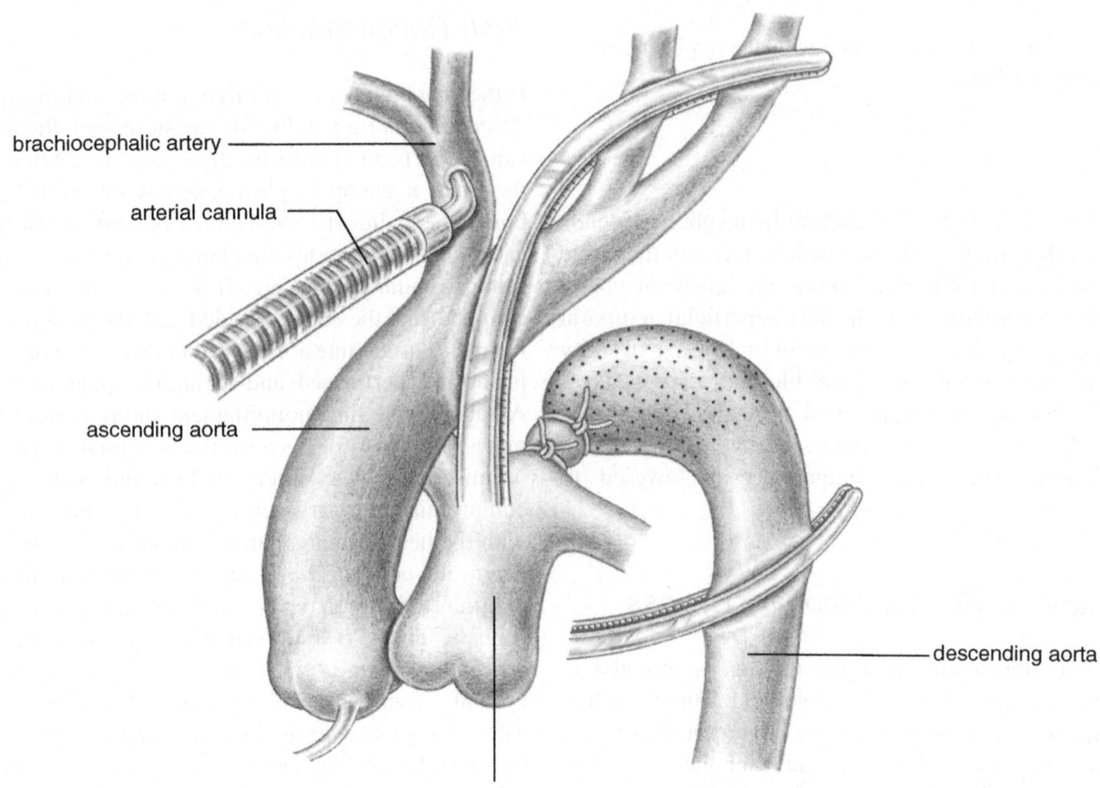

Fig. II-4-7. Aortic arch reconstruction without circulatory arrest: 3. Vascular clamp placement on the aortic arch. The potential to compromise coronary and cerebral perfusion during proximal clamp placement must be considered

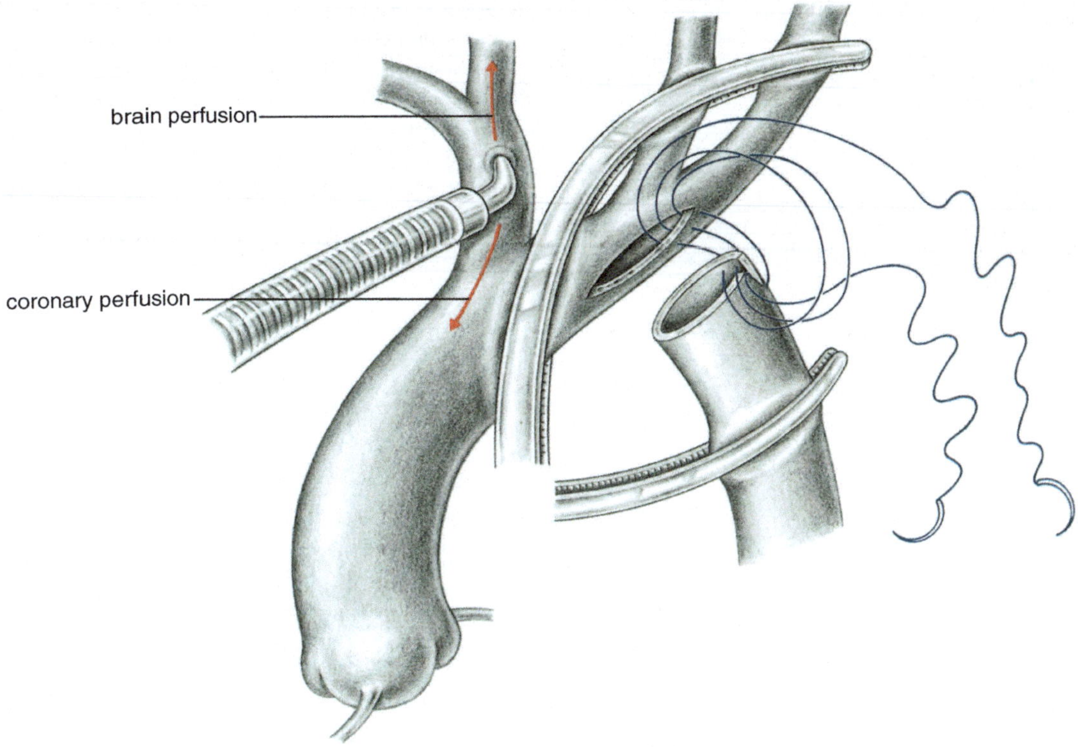

Fig. II-4-8. Aortic arch reconstruction without circulatory arrest: 4. Anastomosis. During anastomosis, cerebral perfusion and cardiac perfusion are maintained. A longitudinal incision is placed on the left side of the descending aorta

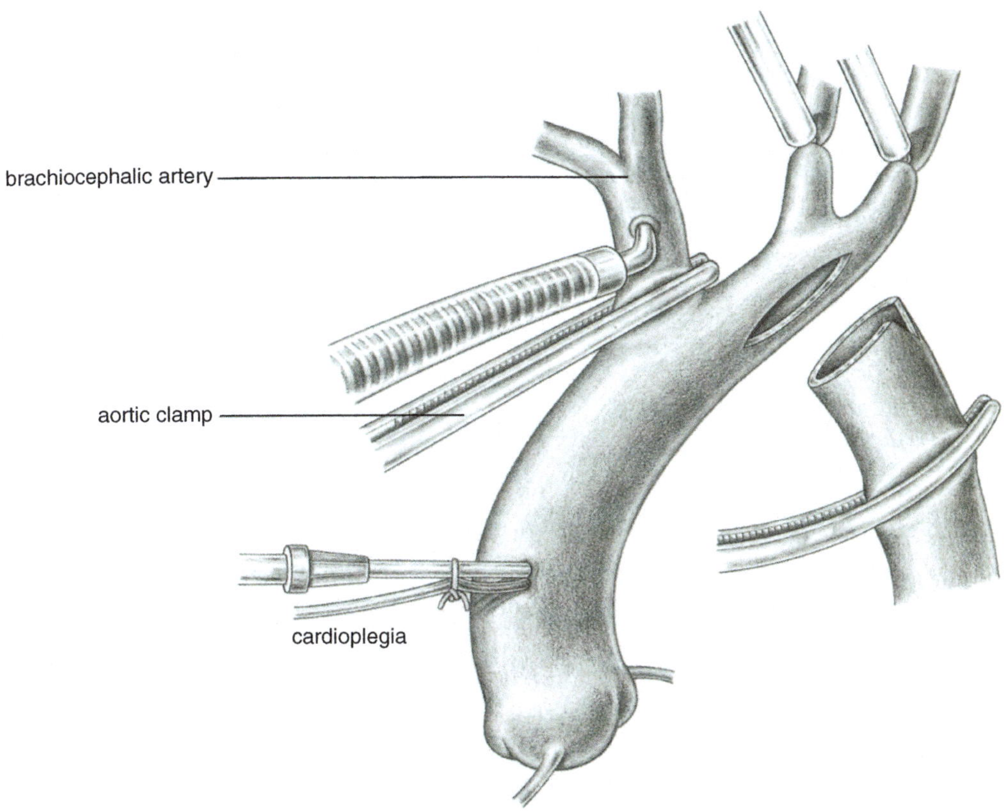

Fig. II-4-9. Aortic arch repair with perfusion through the brachiocephalic artery and descending aorta, but employing cardioplegic arrest

References

1. Celoria GC, Patton RB (1959) Congenital absence of the aortic arch. Am Heart J 58:407–413
2. Karl TR, Sano S, Brawn W, et al (1992) Repair of hypoplastic or interrupted aortic arch via sternotomy. J Thorac Cardiovasc Surg 104:688–695
3. Asou T, Kado H, Imoto Y, et al (1996) Selective cerebral perfusion technique during aortic arch repair in neonates. Ann Thorac Surg 61:1546–1548
4. Yasui H, Kado H, Yonenaga K, et al (1993) Revised technique of cardiopulmonary bypass in one-stage repair of interrupted aortic arch complex. Ann Thorac Surg 55:1166–1171
5. Imoto Y, Kado H, Shiokawa Y, et al (1999) Norwood procedure without circulatory arrest. Ann Thorac Surg 68:559–561
6. Imoto Y (2000) Cannulation of the distal descending thoracic aorta: Reply to the Editor. Ann Thorac Surg 70:2187

II-5. Vascular Ring

Surgical Indication

If the presence of a vascular ring is suspected, the diagnosis should be confirmed and surgery considered. This malformation increases chronic aspiration and tracheomalacia or tracheal stenosis.

To understand the development of vascular ring, a functional aortic arch model proposed by Edwards [1] is useful, as is the classification of vascular ring proposed by Stewart et al. [2].

Vascular rings requiring surgical intervention were analyzed by Hartyanszky and Bertolini [3]. The incidence of double aortic arch was 63%; right aortic arch with left ligamentum, 19%; and aberrant right subclavian artery, 11%.

Operative Procedure

Double Aortic Arch (Fig. II-5-1)

The trachea and esophagus are encircled and compressed by bilateral aortic arches. Hartyanszky and colleagues reported that in 55% of patients both aortic arches are patent, and in the rest, one arch is atretic. In 10% of cases, both arches are the same size; in 70% the right side is larger, and in 20% the left is larger.

The operation is performed with the patient in right lateral decubitus position. The chest is entered via the third or fourth intercostal space. The lung is covered with a sponge and retracted anteriorly. The descending aorta and ductal ligamentum are visualized. The parietal pleura overlying the descending aorta is opened longitudinally, and traction sutures are placed on both edges of the pleural incision. Care is taken not to injure the phrenic and vagus nerves. Dissection is started 1 cm distal from the site of duct attachment to the descending aorta and is advanced proximally. The ductal ligament is dissected and doubly ligated with 2-0 silk sutures. The ligamentum is divided, and the descending aorta is further mobilized. Further dissection facilitates visualization of both aortic arches. It is preferable to leave the larger aortic arch and divide the smaller arch.

After mobilizing the left arch, dissection is advanced to the base of the left subclavian artery. Clamps are placed on the smaller arch distally and proximally. The middle of the smaller arch is divided and both ends are closed using 5-0 Prolene sutures. The right aortic arch is further dissected behind the esophagus to reduce the compression of the esophagus by the right arch. To decrease the compression, the left arch is also occasionally fixed to the sternum.

Right Aortic Arch and Left Ligamentum

There are two types of right aortic arch and left ligamentum. In the first, there is mirror-image branching of the arch, the descending aorta has an aortic diverticulum, and the ligamentum reaches from this diverticulum to the left pulmonary artery (Fig. II-5-2). In the other, the left subclavian artery arises from the descending aorta, and the ligamentum starts from an aortic diverticulum or from the base of the left subclavian artery (Fig. II-5-3).

After the patient is placed in the right lateral decubitus position, the chest is entered through the third or fourth intercostal space. It is typically easy to reach the descending aorta even with the right aortic arch. The descending aorta and ligamentum are dissected. The ligamentum is doubly ligated and divided. Usually this division relieves esophageal and tracheal compression. The esophagus is dissected from the descending aorta to create more space. The aberrant left subclavian artery may still compress the esophagus, and so this artery is divided proximally and re-anastomosed to the left carotid artery, creating mirror-imaging arch branching.

Left Aortic Arch with Aberrant Right Subclavian Artery (Fig. II-5-4)

Via a left thoracotomy, the origin of the right aberrant subclavian artery is divided at the origin. In adults, for whom subclavian steal syndrome or upper extremity ischemia is a concern, the aberrant subclavian artery is divided at its origin and then anastomosed to the ascending aorta via a right thoracotomy.

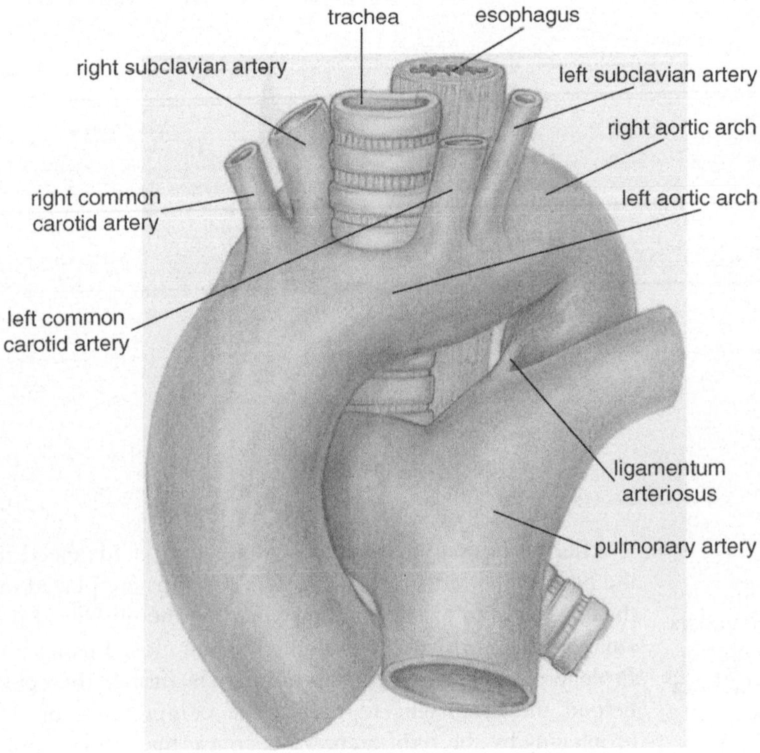

Fig. II-5-1. Double aortic arch

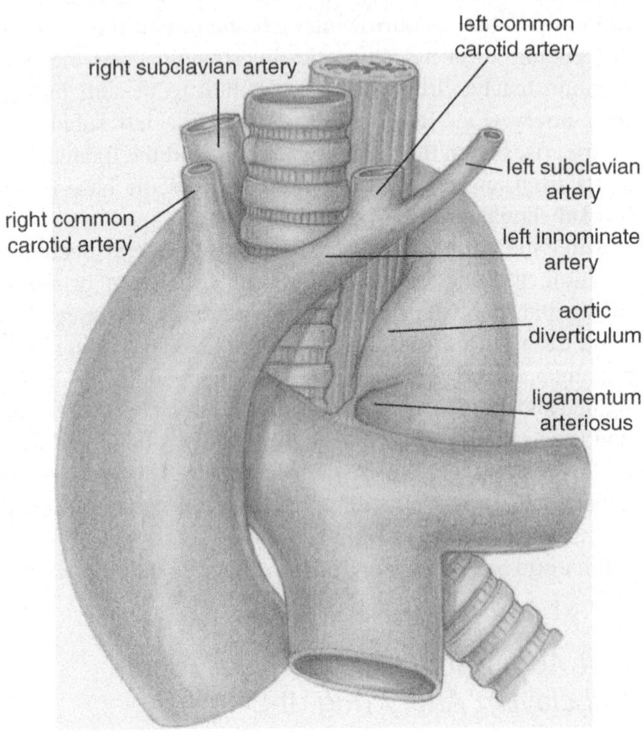

Fig. II-5-2. Right aortic arch with mirror-image branching and left-side ligamentum arteriosus

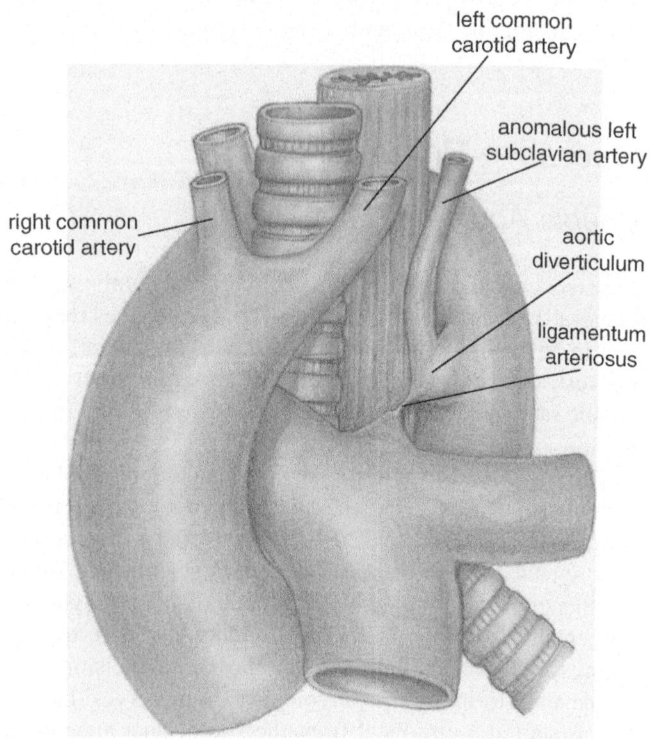

Fig. II-5-3. Right aortic arch and left-side ligamentum with aberrant left subclavian artery

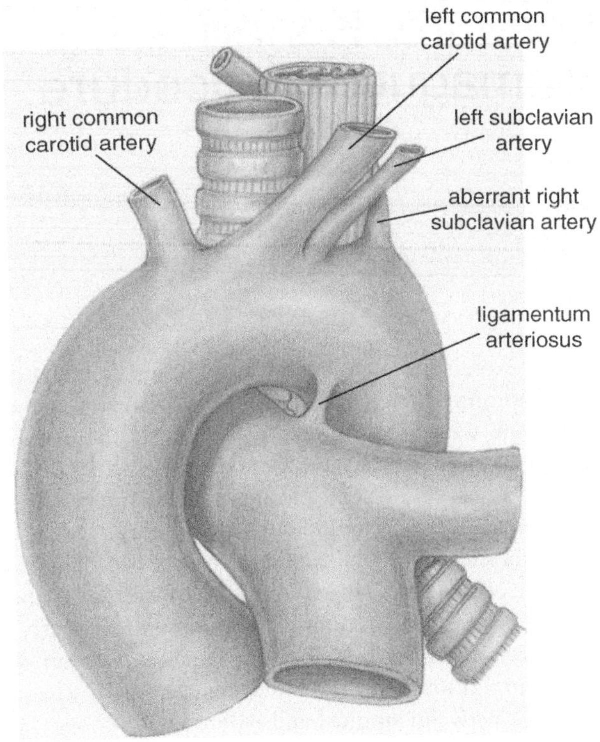

Fig. II-5-4. Aberrant right subclavian artery

References

1. Edward JE (1953) Malformation of the aortic arch system manifested as vascular ring. Lab Invest 2:56–75
2. Stewart JR, Kincaid OW, Edwards JE (1964) An atlas of vascular ring and related malformations of the aortic arch system. Thomas, Springfield, pp 3–129
3. Hartyanszky IL, Lozsadi K, Marcsek P, et al (1989) Congenital vascular rings: surgical management of 111 cases. Eur J Cardiothorac Surg 3:250–254

II-6. Aortic Stenosis: Ross Procedure, Konno Procedure, Nicks Procedure, Yamaguchi Procedure, and Ross–Konno Procedure

Aortic stenosis in a child may be observed in isolation or in combination with other complex congenital heart disease, and consequently the pathophysiology of this disease is diverse. The method of surgical intervention should be decided bearing in mind the anticipated growth of the patient. Occasionally, a staged approach should be considered.

Surgical Indication

Critical Neonatal Aortic Stenosis

In the presence of severe aortic stenosis in the neonate or young infant, the patient may often require an emergent surgery because of the development of acute cardiogenic shock caused by severe congestive heart failure. Left ventricular dilatation, thinning of the left ventricular wall, decrease in left ventricular ejection fraction, and reduced flow through the aortic valve are observed. In severe cases, hemodynamics may be improved with prostaglandin E_1 (PGE_1) infusion to open the ductus arteriosus. Historically, inflow occlusion was used for open surgical valvotomy. In the modern era, open valvotomy has been performed using cardiopulmonary bypass. However, the surgical results remain suboptimal. Even in very experienced centers, early mortality has been 15% to 20%, and late survival rate was only 66% to 74% [1,2]. In the past 10 years, transcatheter balloon valvotomy has become an alternative to the surgical open valvotomy, with recent reports demonstrating early mortality of 12% and late survival of 88% [3,4]. Thus, these results are somewhat superior to the surgical results. Even so, the rates of complication after this approach are still relatively high. In particular, acute aortic regurgitation is a lethal condition, and emergent Ross operation may be necessary. Open valvotomy does permit direct visualization of the valve, and so valvotomy can be tailored to the unique anatomy of each valve. Transcatheter valvotomy has the advantages that it is less invasive, requiring neither cardiopulmonary bypass nor cardioplegic arrest, and is relatively simple to perform from the aspects of staff and equipment required. It is likely that each technique is superior for certain patients, whereas for others, both techniques may work equally well.

Pediatric Aortic Stenosis

Indications for surgery in noncritical aortic valve stenosis include electrocardiographic evidence of ischemia during moderate exercise, systemic systolic pressure gradient more than 50–60 mmHg under resting condition, or the presence of symptoms caused by aortic valve stenosis [5]. Recently, balloon valvuloplasty has been used in the early phase to reduce the stress on the ventricle and is usually very effective in the absence of the calcification at the aortic valve. The timing of aortic valve replacement can thus be delayed, and a larger-sized mechanical valve may be inserted. It should be emphasized, however, that the balloon valvuloplasty is a blind valvotomy procedure that may create or worsen aortic valve regurgitation, causing acute ventricular dysfunction. The choice between surgical and balloon valvotomy should be made based on a through assessment of valve morphology and function in each case. Surgical valvotomy may be preferred in selective cases, such as for an older infant with a degenerated valve, in a case with more than moderate aortic valve regurgitation, in the presence of a small annulus, in the patient who has had previous balloon valvuloplasty, in the patient with severe pulmonary hypertension, or in those with decreased left ventricular function.

For aortic valve replacement in small children, adult-sized mechanical valves may not be feasible. If a smaller-sized valve is used, late reoperation is inevitable. The smallest currently available mechanical valves are those from ATS (16 mm), Carbomedics (16 mm), and St. Jude Medical (17 mm) (Table II-6-1). Because in small patients even the smallest sized valve may not fit in the native aortic annulus, enlargement of the annulus is frequently required.

With the relatively recent introduction of the Ross procedure [6] for small children with aortic stenosis, treatment strategy has changed [7]. The Ross procedure, which uses the autologous pulmonary valve for aortic valve replacement, can avoid several of the previously mentioned problems with aortic valve replacement with mechanical valves in small children. The indications for the Ross procedure are still controversial, but include the presence of a contraindication to anticoagulation, size too small to allow mechanical valve usage, and active infective endocarditis. In a patient who may wish to become pregnant in the future or who does not have access to mechanical valves, the Ross procedure is a good choice. If the patient has an abnormal pulmonary valve or severe pulmonary hypertension, this operation should not be chosen. The presence of previous surgery, however, does not preclude this operation. Considerations weighing against the Ross procedure include its technically demanding nature, its unknown long-term prognosis, especially in the neonate, and the requirement for pulmonary valve replacement after pulmonary autograft removal.

Table II-6-1. Comparison of available small-sized bileaflet mechanical valves

Type of artificial valve	Size	Diameter of annulus (mm)	Diameter of sewing cuff (mm)	Diameter of orifice (mm)	Effective orifice area (cm^2)
ATS AP series	16	16.2	21.5	14.8	1.55
Carbomedics standard	16	16.2	20.6	14.7	1.59
SJM HP	17	17.2	21.6	14.7	1.63
Bicarbon slimline	17	17.2	22.5	15.2	1.76
ATS AP series	18	18.2	23.6	16.8	2.02
Carbomedics standard	18	18.8	21.6	14.7	1.59
SJM HP	19	19.2	23.6	16.7	2.10
Bicarbon slimline	19	19.2	24.5	17.2	2.27

SJM HP, St. Jude Medical HP

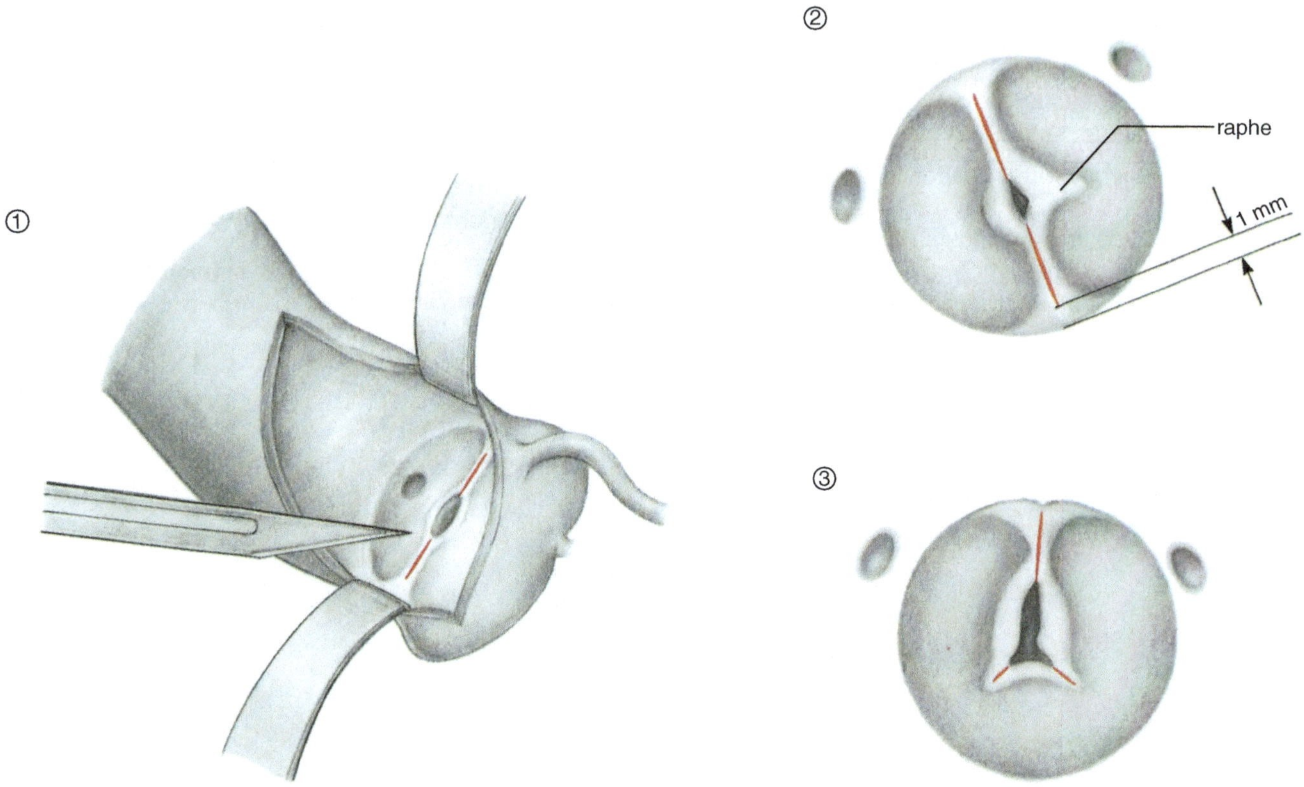

Fig. II-6-1. Open commissurotomy

Because the homograft is not available in Japan, reconstruction of the right ventricular outflow tract requires nonallograft material such as a hand-made or commercially available valved conduit. There is a justified criticism that the Ross procedure creates two-valve disease for the patient with one-valve disease. Therefore, longer-term follow-up is mandatory to justify applying this procedure.

Open Valvotomy (Fig. II-6-1)

Median sternotomy is utilized, and cardiopulmonary bypass is initiated using cannulation through the ascending aorta and right atrium. A vent catheter is inserted into the left atrium. In the neonate, the ductus is ligated soon after bypass initiation because most neonates have a patent ductus arteriosus. After aortic cross-clamping, cardioplegic solution is administered and cardiac arrest is obtained. An aortotomy is performed and extended obliquely toward the noncoronary cusp. The condition of the aortic valve is carefully inspected and the fused commissure is identified. In a majority of cases, a bicuspid aortic valve is observed and a raphe is present in the middle of one of the cusps. Both commissures are opened with a No. 11 scalpel. This incision is stopped 1 mm from the aortic wall to avoid postoperative aortic valve regurgitation. To avoid aortic valve regurgitation, the raphe is not opened. In rare cases, the valve may be unicuspid, and the raphe must be partially opened to obtain an adequate valve orifice.

Ross Procedure

Autograft Harvest

After the distal ascending aorta and superior and inferior vena cava are cannulated, cardiopulmonary bypass is initiated. The ductus is divided to facilitate subsequent pulmonary artery reconstruction. With the heart beating, the main pulmonary artery is transected just proximal to the bifurcation. The condition of the pulmonary valve is inspected to exclude any abnormality. A right-angle clamp is passed retrogradely through the pulmonary valve, and its tip is placed through the anterior wall of the right ventricular outflow tract 5 mm proximal to the pulmonary valve annulus. At this location in the infundibulum, a small ventriculotomy is placed and extended leftward and rightward. The dissection of the posterior conal muscle is started several millimeters beneath the pulmonary valve annulus. The superficial layer of the septum is shaved (Fig. II-6-2-1). Care is taken not to damage the first septal perforating branch of the left anterior descending coronary artery, which is running at the transition area between the right ventricular free wall and the ventricular septum. Such an injury can be avoided by excising the autograft with a shallow cuff. The advantages of harvesting the autograft before aortic cross-clamp are shortening of aortic cross-clamping time, easy discernment of the layer between the right ventricle free wall and the ventricular septum, and clear identification of any bleeding from the harvest site. The harvested autograft is placed into the pericardial well behind the heart to prevent it from drying out. Then, the aorta is cross-clamped with administration of cardioplegia. An aortotomy is created and the aortic valve leaflets are removed from the aortic wall.

Coronary Buttons Removal

The ascending aorta is transected 3–4 mm above the sinotubular junction. After identification of both coronary orifices, the sinus of Valsalva is cut, and the coronary buttons are created (Fig. II-6-2-2). The aortic wall is left about 3–4 mm from the aortic annulus. The aortic wall remnant can be used to wrap the suture line after autograft anastomosis, facilitating hemostasis. After coronary button creation, the dissection of the coronary arteries should be minimized to avoid kinking the coronary arteries.

Autograft Anastomosis

The anterior commissure of the pulmonary autograft is placed as the neo-aortic commissure between right and left

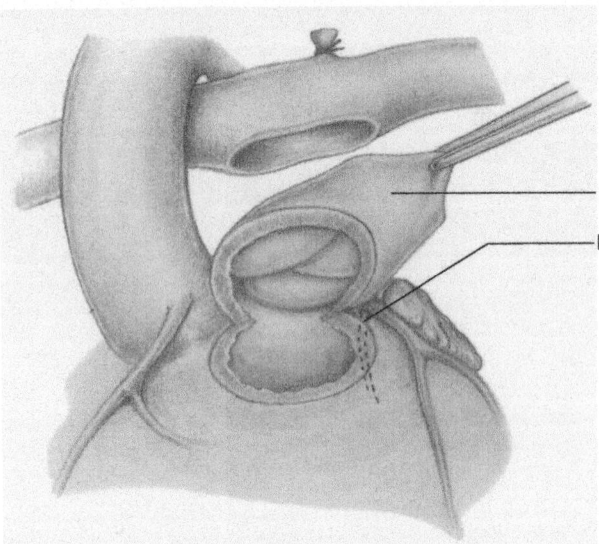

Fig. II-6-2-1. Ross procedure: harvest of autograft

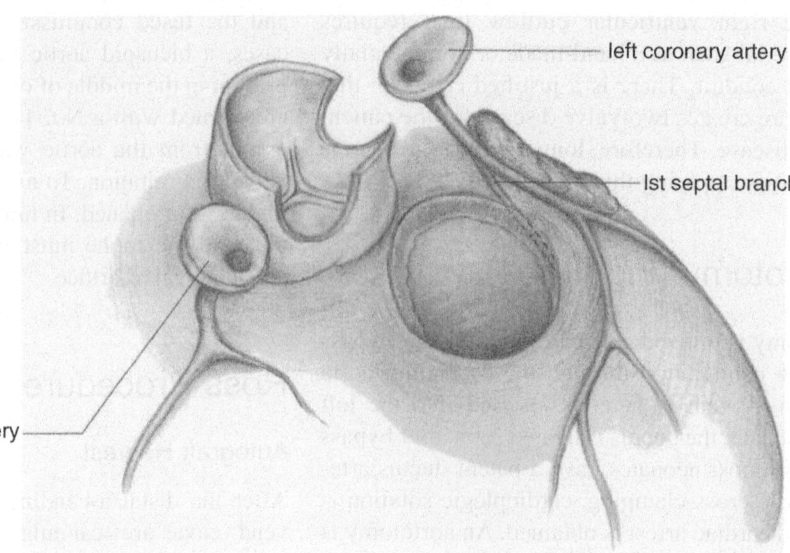

Fig. II-6-2-2. Ross procedure: coronary button creation

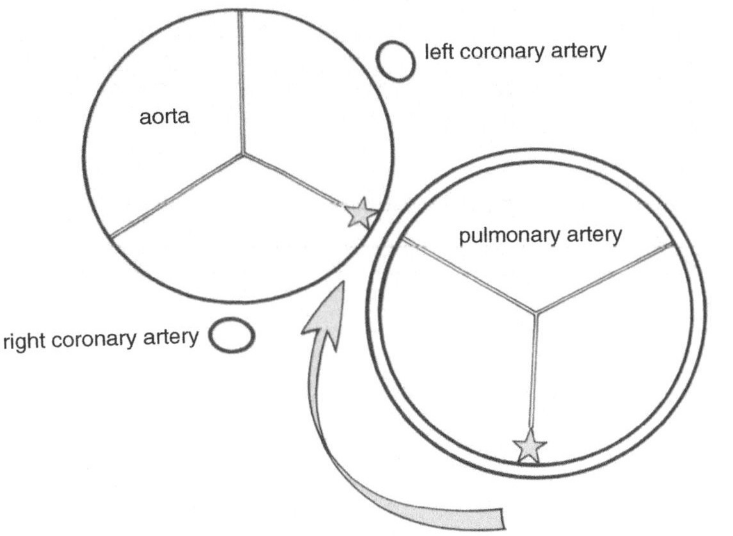

Fig. II-6-2-3. Ross procedure: positioning of the autograft. *LCA*, left coronary artery; *RCA*, right coronary artery; *AO*, aorta; *PA*, pulmonary artery

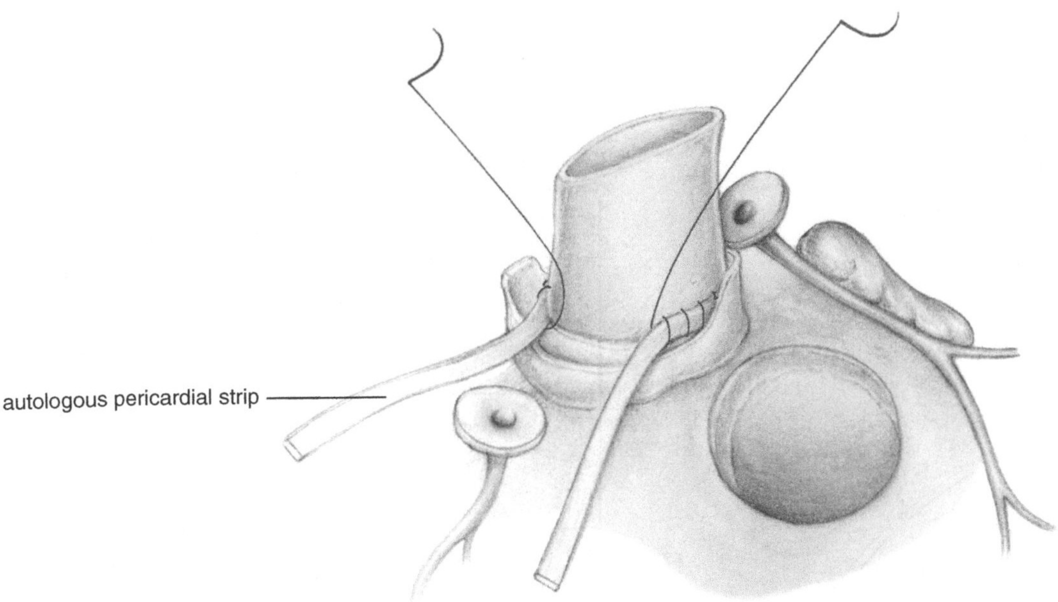

Fig. II-6-2-4. Ross procedure: inflow suture reinforced with pericardial strip

coronary sinus (Fig. II-6-2-3). Two-thirds of the anastomosis of the autograft to the aortic annulus is completed with a fine monofilament running suture. The remaining one-third of the annulus is completed with interrupted sutures. An autologous pericardial strip is placed in the anastomosis as a buttress (Fig. II-6-2-4). To minimize bleeding and prevent annular dilation, the residual native aortic wall is sutured to the pulmonary autograft free wall (Fig. II-6-2-5).

Adjustment of the Autograft Annulus to the Aortic Annulus

If the aortic annulus is smaller than the pulmonary autograft by 10%, simple annular adjustment is utilized. Annular mismatch of more than 20% is managed with a limited anterior enlargement of the aortic annulus (Konno) or posterior annulus enlargement (Nicks). When the difference is more than 20%, the Ross–Konno operation should be chosen. If the aortic annulus is larger than the autograft, late annular dilation is more likely, and to prevent this, the autograft should be implanted with a plication of the native aortic root to downsize the annulus.

Coronary Button Implantation and Ascending Aortic Reconstruction

The left coronary button is implanted into the posterior sinus. The right coronary button is implanted into the anterior sinus. The holes in the autograft are made above the sinotubular junction. The button is anastomosed to the autograft with a fine monofilament running suture (Fig. II-6-2-6). The autograft and ascending aortic anastomosis are similarly completed with fine monofilament running suture.

Right Ventricular Outflow Tract Reconstruction

If a homograft is not available for the patient more than 1 year of age, a 0.1-mm-thick expanded polytetrafluoroethylene (ePTFE) tricuspid valved conduit (Fig. II-6-2-7) is

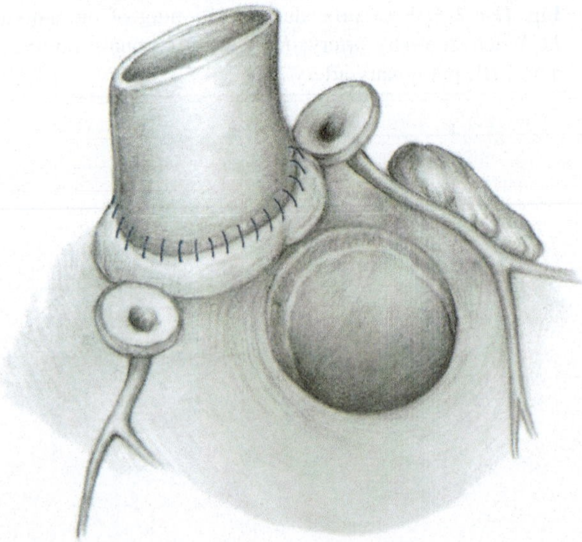

Fig. II-6-2-5. Ross procedure: remnant aortic wall sutured to reinforce inflow suture line

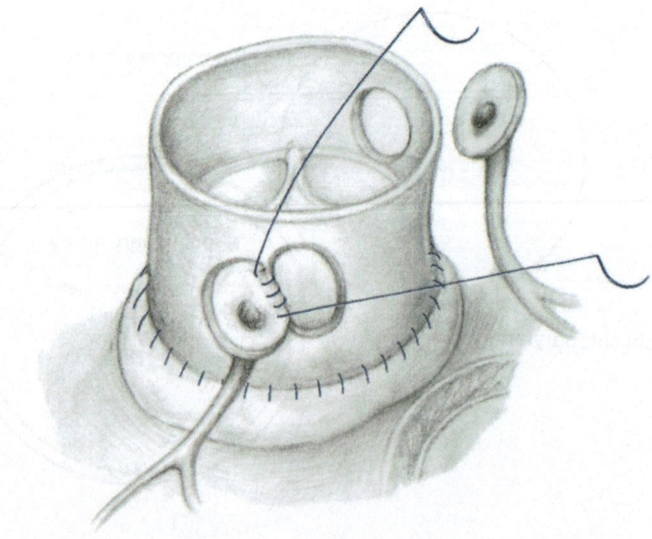

Fig. II-6-2-6. Ross procedure: coronary button implantation

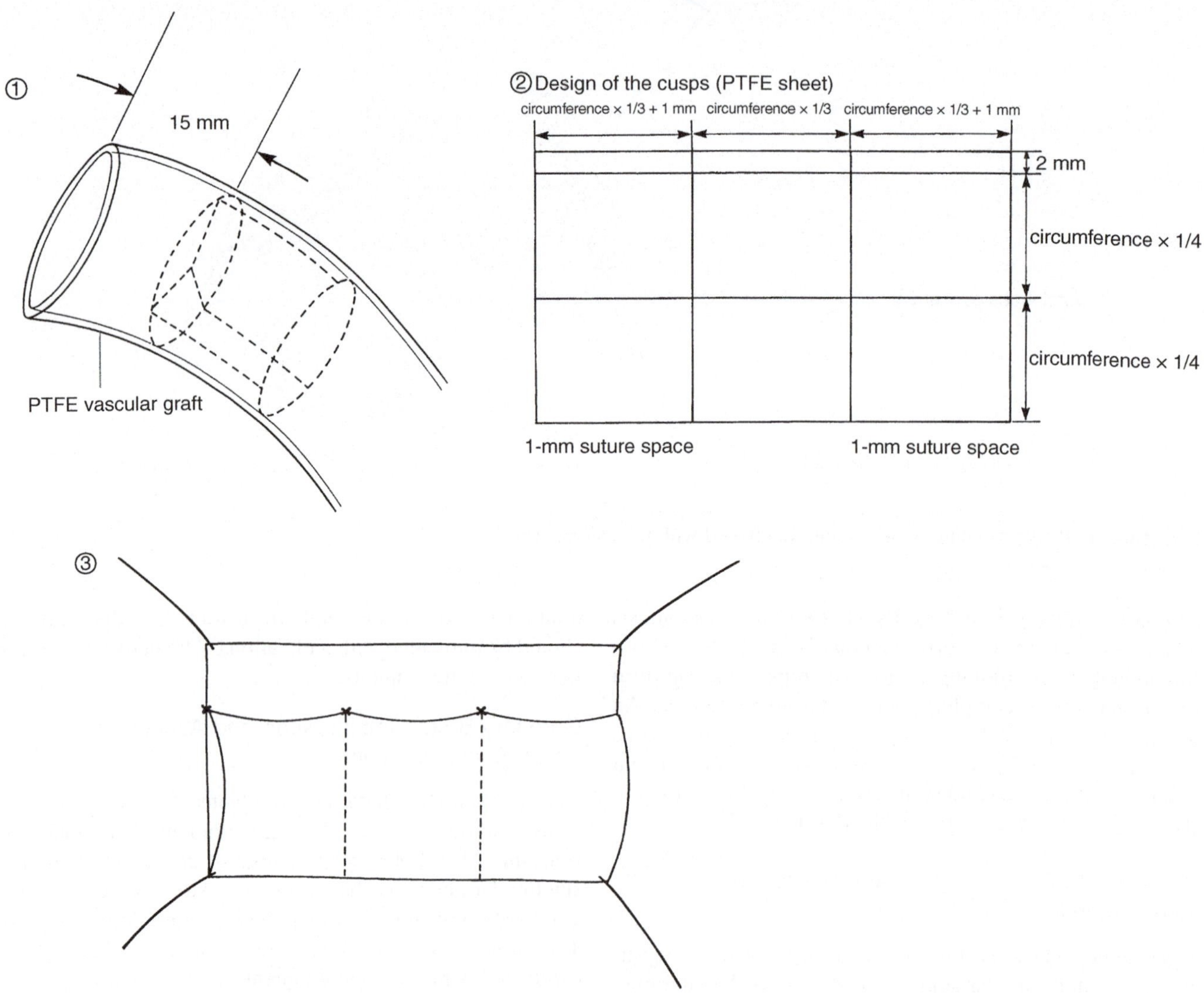

Fig. II-6-2-7. Ross procedure: creation of tricuspid valved conduit. Technique of polytetrafluoroethylene (*PTFE*) valve construction: to place the three valve cusps inside a conduit, a PTFE tube is everted. Three cusps are created using a 0.1-mm-thick PTFE sheet, folded with a depth of one-quarter of circumference of the conduit. The *dotted lines* indicate suture lines used to attach the sheet to the wall of the tube. Care is taken not to place stitches full thickness to avoid bleeding. The valve is placed 15 mm from the distal end of the conduit. After sewing the cusps, the tube is everted again, placing the cusps inside the conduit [8]. ① Position of the cusps in the conduit; ② design of the cusps; ③ suturing of the cusps

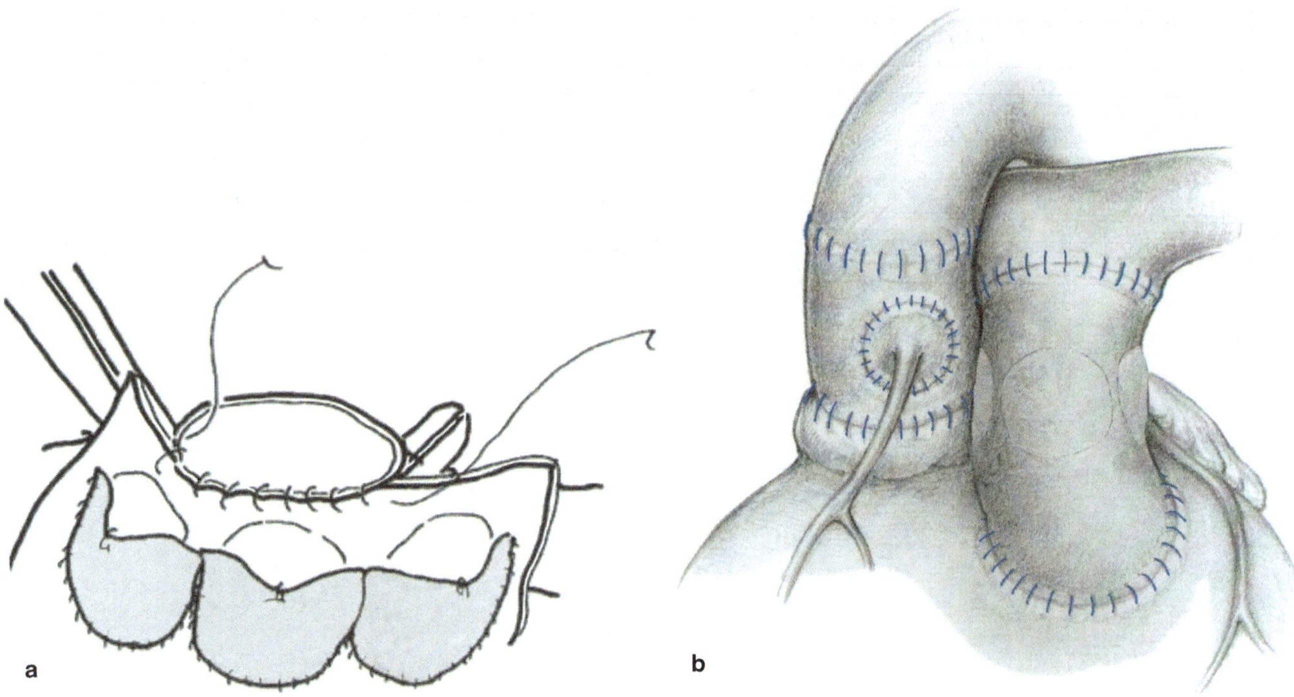

Fig. II-6-2-8. Ross procedure: right ventricular outflow tract (RVOT) reconstruction using a fan-shaped expanded polytetrafluoroethylene (ePTFE) valved conduit with bulging sinuses. We have used a fan-shaped ePTFE valved conduit with bulging sinuses as a right ventricular outflow conduit in the Ross procedure since 2004. This conduit was designed by Yamagishi et al. of Kyoto Prefectural University of Medicine in 2001. Three bulging sinuses are formed on a sheet of ePTFE using a specially designed mold. Fan-shaped ePTFE sheets (0.1 mm thick) are anastomosed to the edge of the bulging sinuses as valve leaflets. These valved conduits with bulging sinuses show excellent early to midterm results and seem to be promising alternatives to homografts in right ventricular outflow tract reconstruction [9]. **a** Anastomosis of the conduit; **b** complete reconstruction of great arteries

constructed (Fig. II-6-2-8). In neonates and small infants, the right ventricular outflow tract is reconstructed by direct anastomosis or autologous pericardial roll interposition, and a monocusp patch is used anteriorly.

Aortic Valve Replacement with Annular Enlargement

The locations of annular enlarging incisions are shown in Fig. II-6-3. In the Nicks approach [10], annular enlargement is toward the noncoronary sinus close to the commissure between the left and noncoronary sinuses. In the Konno approach [11], the anterior annular enlargement is toward the right coronary sinus close to the commissure between right and left coronary sinuses. The Manouguian approach [12] consists of opening the commissure between the noncoronary and left coronary sinuses. With increasing application of the Ross–Konno procedure for severe subaortic stenosis, the indication for the Konno operation has decreased. However, in the patients with an abnormal pulmonary valve and severe left ventricular outflow tract obstruction, this operation is a very useful surgical approach. The Yamaguchi approach [13] combines the Nicks and Konno approaches (partial Konno incision). The Manouguian approach is frequently used if mitral valve replacement is also necessary.

Nicks Procedure

Via a median sternotomy, cardiopulmonary bypass is initiated with aortic and bicaval cannulation. A vent catheter is placed in the left atrium. After aortic cross-clamping and cardioplegic arrest, an aortotomy is placed from the anterior surface of the ascending aorta into the middle of the noncoronary sinus. After removal of the aortic valve leaflets, the incision is extended to the aortic annulus slightly toward the left coronary cusp. This incision is advanced beyond the aortic annulus and reaches the anterior wall of the left atrium (Fig. II-6-4①). If this incision is extended beyond the fibrous aortic–mitral valvar continuity, the orifice is created on the anterior wall of the left atrium. We usually stop the incision at the fibrous aortic–mitral continuity and, although the incision is not placed into the anterior leaflet of the mitral valve, we are able to upsize the aortic annulus by one or two sizes. A teardrop-shaped Hemashield patch is used to patch to the aortotomy from its deepest point with a running suture. When the suture line reaches the level of the sinotubular junction, the size of the annulus is checked to ensure the enlarged annulus is large enough, using a sizer. If the annulus is not large enough, an anterior Konno annular enlargement is added, as with a Yamaguchi procedure. At the level of the annulus of the patch, several 3-0 pledgetted mattress sutures are placed from the outside of the patch (Fig. II-6-4②).

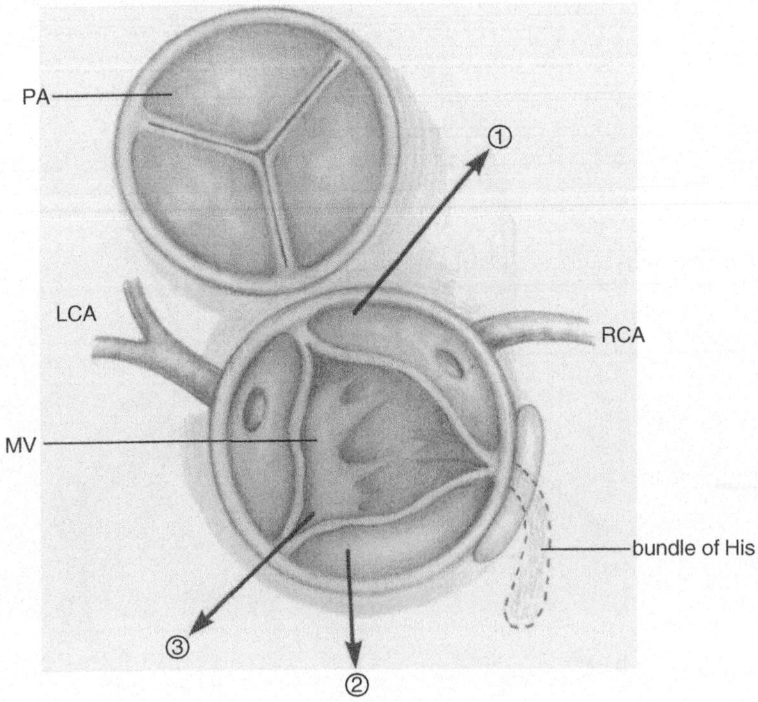

Fig. II-6-3. Incisions for annular enlargement: ①, Konno procedure; ②, Nicks procedure; ③, Manouguian procedure; ① + ②, Yamaguchi procedure. *PA*, pulmonary artery; *LCA*, left coronary artery; *RCA*, right coronary artery; *MV*, mitral valve

Everting mattress pledgetted sutures are placed along the rest of the annulus, and the valve is implanted (Fig. II-6-4③). The remaining patch is used to close the aortotomy (Fig. II-6-4④).

Yamaguchi Procedure

As mentioned earlier, a Nicks approach is utilized, and when the desired size valve does not fit in the enlarged annulus, this approach is chosen. An additional incision is made toward the commissure between the right and left coronary cusps (Fig. II-6-5①). When this incision reaches to the right ventricular free wall and ventricular septum, the incision is stopped. Care is taken not to enter the right ventricular cavity. A teardrop-shaped patch is anastomosed to the posterior incision previously described. A similarly shaped patch is also used for the anterior incision. Aortic valve replacement is performed in the usual fashion (Fig. II-6-5②). With this approach, a valve two or three size larger than the original valve can be inserted.

Konno Procedure

The Konno procedure is useful for the patient with subvalvular and valvar stenosis. Before the initiation of cardiopulmonary bypass, the tissue around the origin of the right coronary artery and the base of the main pulmonary artery is dissected. The cardiopulmonary bypass is initiated with ascending aortic and bicaval cannulation. After aortic cross-clamping and cardioplegic arrest, the anterior surface of the ascending aorta is opened longitudinally. This incision is extended toward the base of the main pulmonary artery. The orifices of the right and left coronary arteries are identified from the inside of the ascending aorta. The incision is extended to the commissure between the right and left coronary cusps. Next, a right ventriculotomy is placed 10 mm beneath the lowest end of the pulmonary valve sinus (Fig. II-6-6-1).

Care is necessary to maintain this distance between the pulmonary valve and right ventriculotomy, because it is easy to make this distance too short. The right ventriculotomy is transversely extended toward the base of the aortic valve until it reaches the lower end of the aortotomy. The aortotomy is now extended inferiorly to reach the upper end of the ventricular septum. The incision in the ventricular septum is extended to a line down the middle of the posterior pulmonary valve annulus and is parallel to the pulmonary valve annulus (Fig. II-6-6-2). The length of the ventriculotomy is similar to the enlargement of the circumference of the aortic valve annulus. [The length of the ventriculotomy (mm) = $\pi \times$ utilizing aortic valve diameter—native aortic valve annulus]. If membranous left ventricular outflow tract obstruction is also present, resection of the tissue causing the obstruction is performed with care from the mitral apparatus.

The ventriculotomy and aortotomy are closed with a teardrop-shaped Hemashield patch or Dacron patch reinforced with a xenopericardium. Pledgetted 4-0 monofilament mattress sutures are utilized. To avoid turbulence in the left ventricular outflow tract, the needle is passed through the following order: right ventricle endocardium → left ventricle endocardium → left ventricle side patch → right ventricle side patch. At the aortic annulus the right ventricular

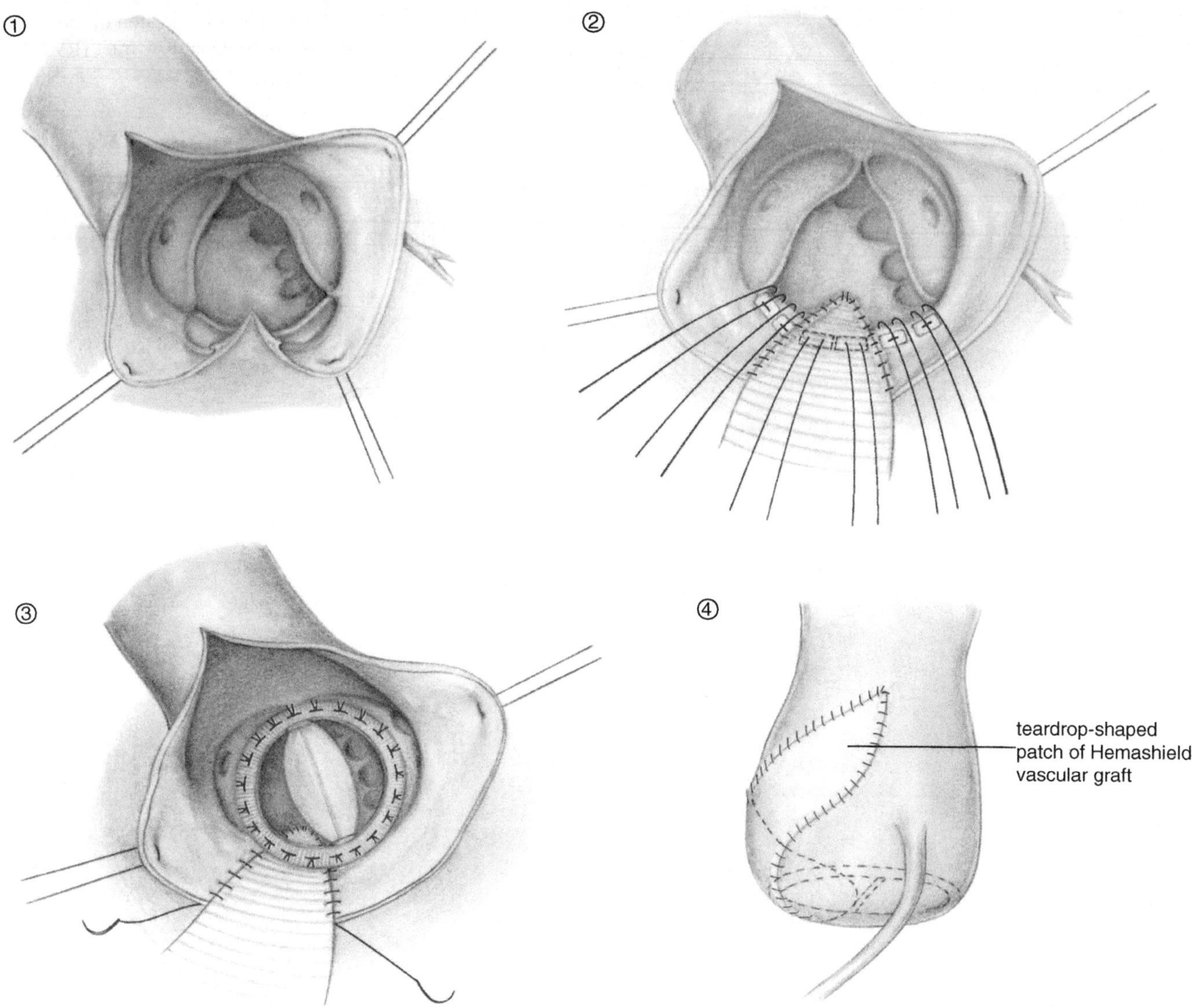

Fig. II-6-4. Nicks procedure

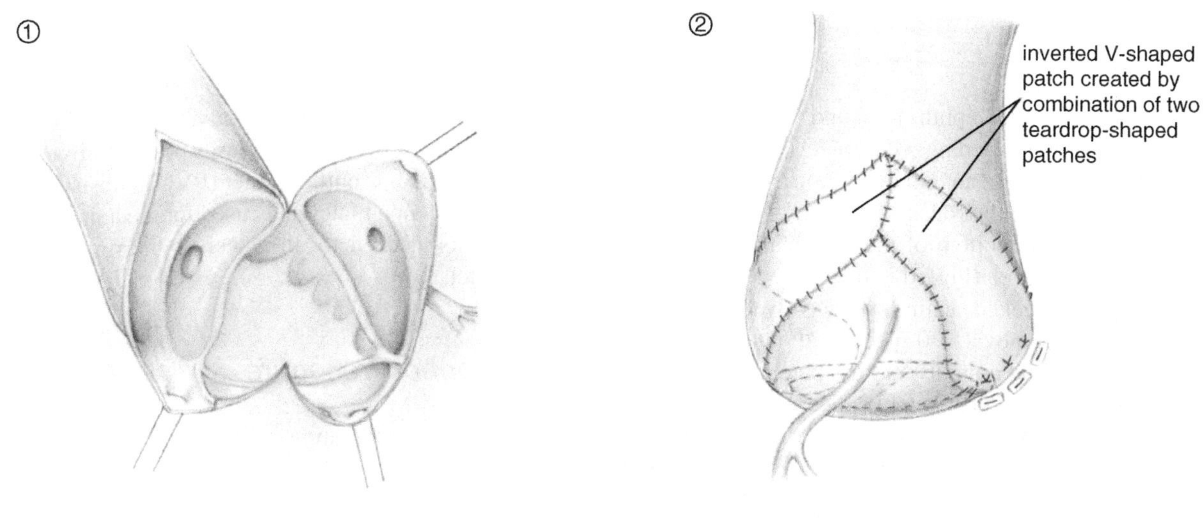

Fig. II-6-5. Yamaguchi procedure

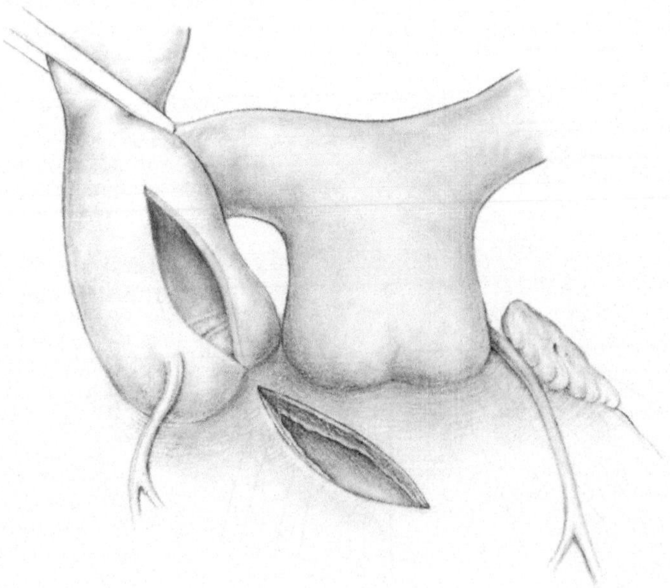

Fig. II-6-6-1. Konno procedure: incision in the ascending aorta and right ventricular outflow tract (RVOT)

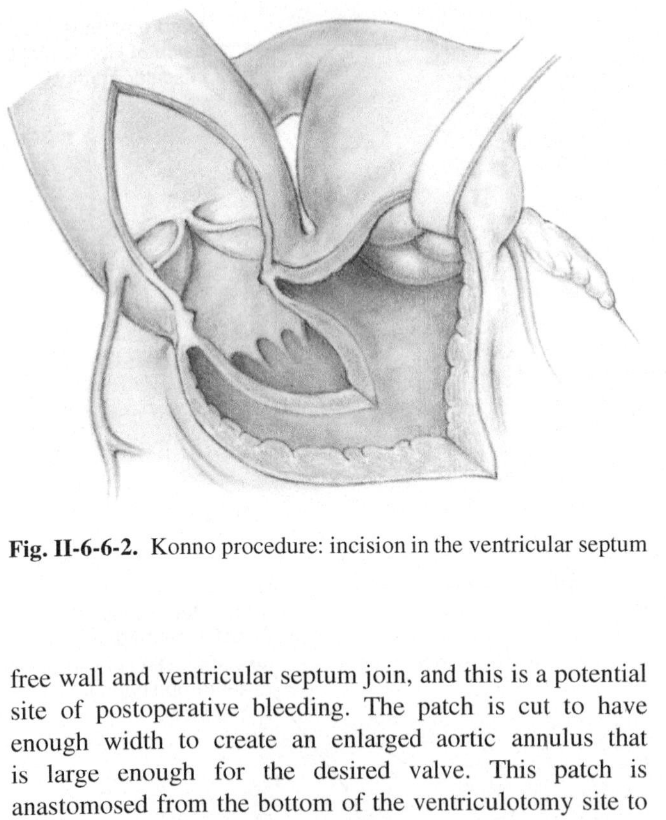

Fig. II-6-6-2. Konno procedure: incision in the ventricular septum

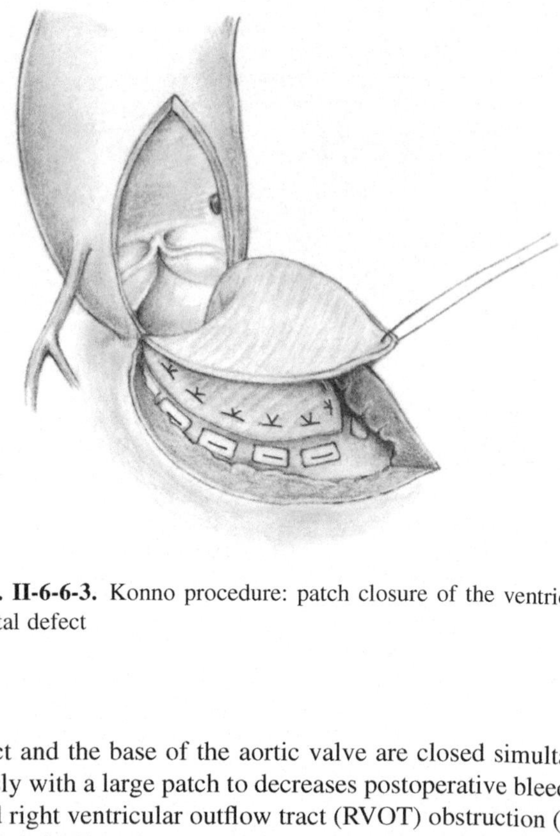

Fig. II-6-6-3. Konno procedure: patch closure of the ventricular septal defect

free wall and ventricular septum join, and this is a potential site of postoperative bleeding. The patch is cut to have enough width to create an enlarged aortic annulus that is large enough for the desired valve. This patch is anastomosed from the bottom of the ventriculotomy site to the aortic annulus level (Fig. II-6-6-3). At this stage the aortic annulus is checked again with a valve sizer. After aortic valve leaflet removal, 4-0 pledgetted mattress sutures are placed in the aortic annulus and the patch. Aortic valve replacement is performed using a bileaflet mechanical valve in the usual fashion (Fig. II-6-6-4). The aortotomy is closed with the remaining sutures (Fig. II-6-6-5). After release of the aortic cross-clamp, the right ventricular outflow tract is closed with the heart beating. The right ventricular outflow tract and the base of the aortic valve are closed simultaneously with a large patch to decreases postoperative bleeding and right ventricular outflow tract (RVOT) obstruction (Fig. II-6-6-6). The same material as used for the annular enlargement patch is utilized for the patch in the right ventricular outflow tract.

Ross–Konno Procedure

The Ross–Konno operation is applicable in the neonate or infant with a small aortic valve annulus [14]. The right ventricular outflow tract is utilized for the incision in the ventricular septum as in the Konno operation.

Pulmonary Autograft Harvest

Cardiopulmonary bypass is established using ascending aortic and bicaval cannulation. After division of the ductus, the pulmonary confluence is mobilized to facilitate subsequent pulmonary artery reconstruction. With the heart beating, the main pulmonary artery is transected at its bifurcation and the pulmonary valve is inspected. In infants, the autograft is then harvested under cardiac arrest, whereas in the older child it is harvested with the heart beating. Because in this surgery the right ventricular outflow tract free wall is utilized to augment the left ventricular outflow tract, a relatively longer "skirt" of right ventricular outflow tract free wall is harvested than in a standard Ross operation. A right-angle clamp is placed through the pulmonary valve retrogradely into the right ventricle and used to mark the site of the ventriculotomy (Fig. II-6-7-1). From this marked point, the ventriculotomy is started and advanced superiorly to create an anterior flap. As in neonates the distance between the left anterior descending coronary artery and the autograft is small, harvest is performed carefully from the inside of the right ventricle after identification of both the left anterior descending coronary artery and the pulmonary valve annulus. The posterior wall incision is started 2 mm beneath the pulmonary valve cusp site, and the middle layer of the right ventricle is carefully enucleated (Fig. II-6-7-2). Care is taken not to damage the first septal branch of the left anterior descending coronary artery, which covers leftward and posterior to the pulmonary annulus. After harvest, the autograft is placed in the pericardium behind the heart.

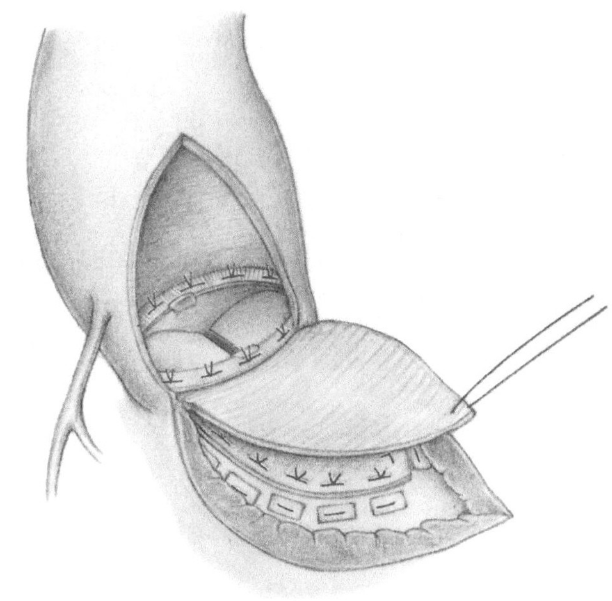

Fig. II-6-6-4. Konno procedure: aortic valve replacement with a mechanical valve

Coronary Button Preparation and Annular Enlargement (Konno Incision)

The ascending aorta is transected 2–3 mm above the sinotubular junction. The orifices of both coronary arteries are identified, and coronary buttons are created from the sinuses of Valsalva (Fig. II-6-7-3). The aortic wall is left 3–4 mm long for subsequent reinforcement of the inflow suture line. After removal of aortic valve leaflets, the incision is placed into the ventricular septum through the anterior commissure of the aortic valve to enlarge the left ventricular outflow tract. This incision is in effect a left ventriculotomy in the superior portion of the ventricular septum (Fig. II-6-7-4).

Autograft Anastomosis

The autograft is anastomosed in the following configurations: (1) the right ventricular free wall is placed to patch

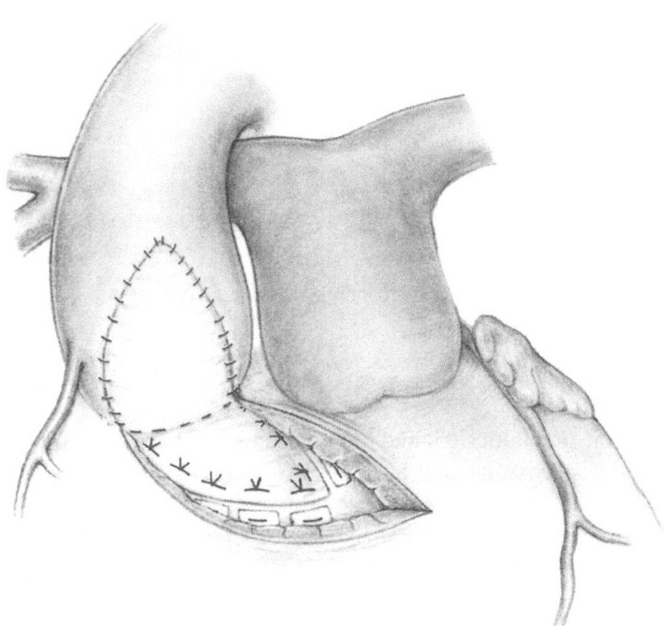

Fig. II-6-6-5. Konno procedure: patch closure of the ascending aorta

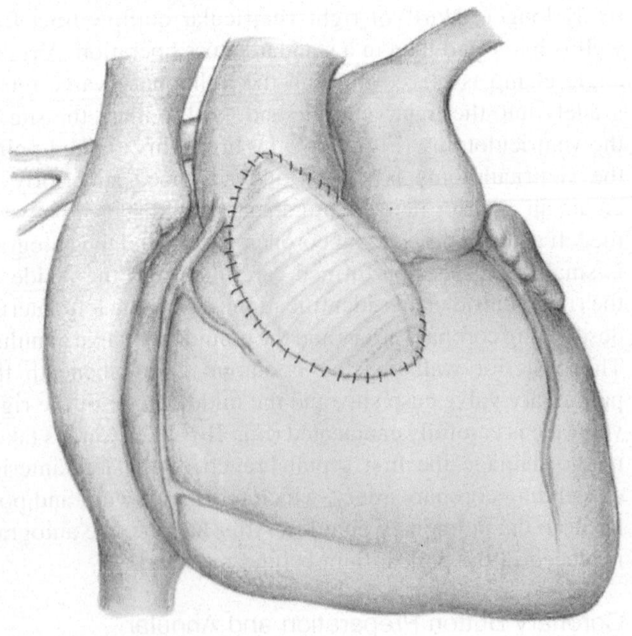

Fig. II-6-6-6. Konno procedure: RVOT patch closure

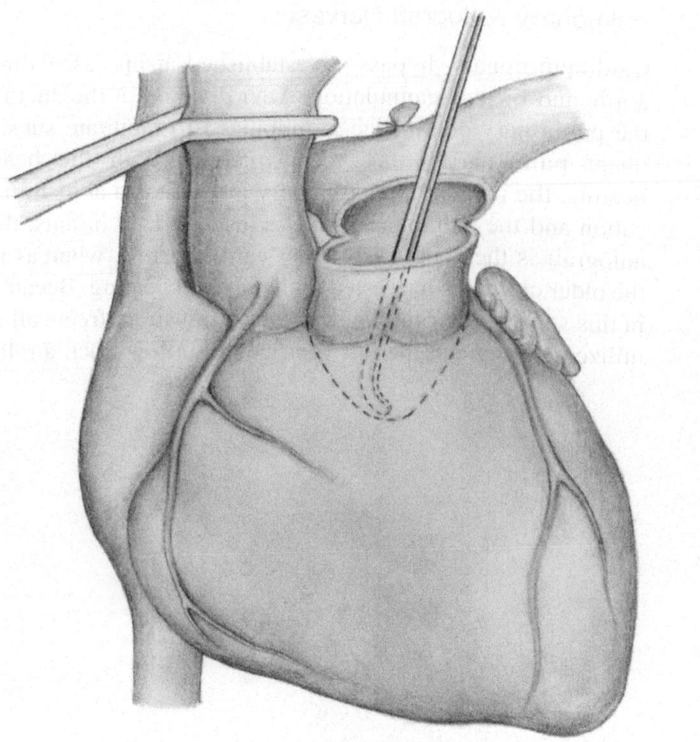

Fig. II-6-7-1. Ross–Konno procedure: marking of right ventriculotomy site

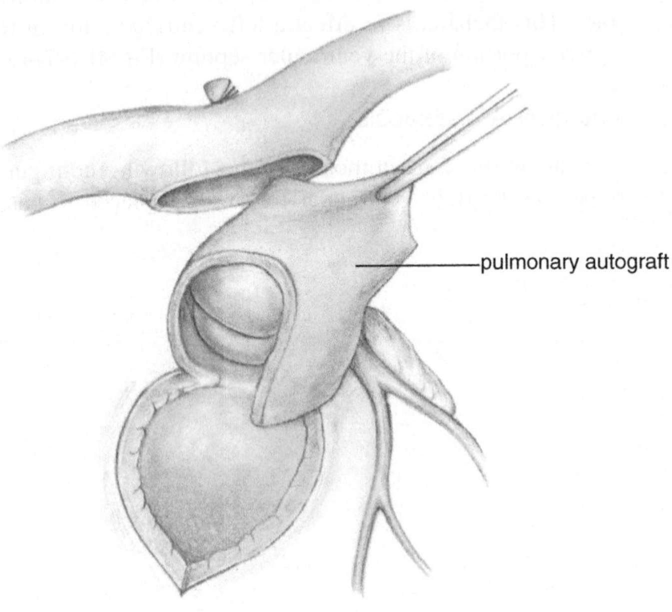

Fig. II-6-7-2. Ross–Konno procedure: excision of autograft

the ventricular septum; or (2) the left coronary button is placed in the posterior sinus. As the right coronary button is reimplanted in a relatively high position, this should not necessarily be placed in the sinus of Valsalva. The Konno ventriculotomy site is closed with 4-0 or 5-0 monofilament running suture reinforced with an autologous pericardial strip. The anastomosis is started from the nadir of the incision, and both right and left ventricular endocardial surfaces are approximated (Fig. II-6-7-5). Posteriorly, the autograft is placed to the aortic annulus using 5-0 monofilament running suture with an autologous pericardial strip (Fig. II-6-7-6). To prevent bleeding or late autograft annular dilation, the inflow suture line is wrapped with the preserved remnant of the native aortic wall (Fig. II-6-7-7).

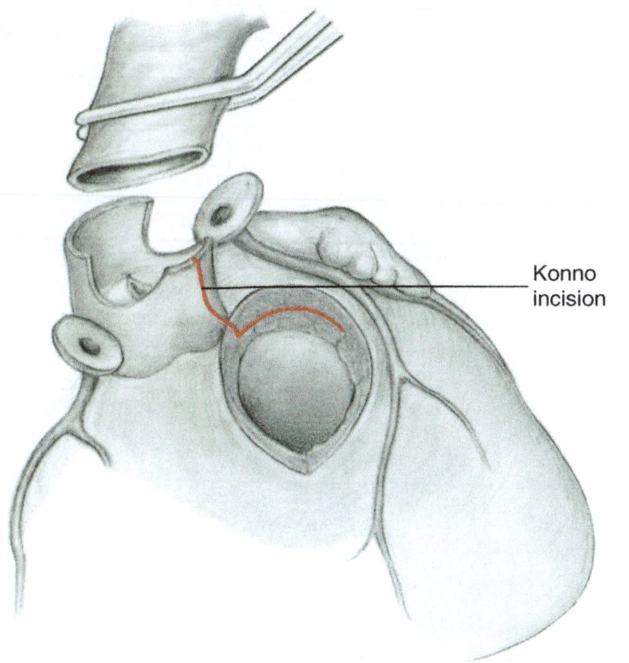

Fig. II-6-7-3. Ross–Konno procedure: creation of coronary button

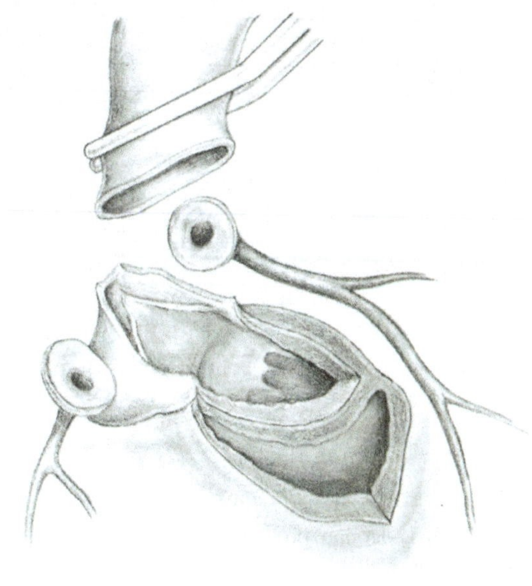

Fig. II-6-7-4. Ross–Konno procedure: Konno incision

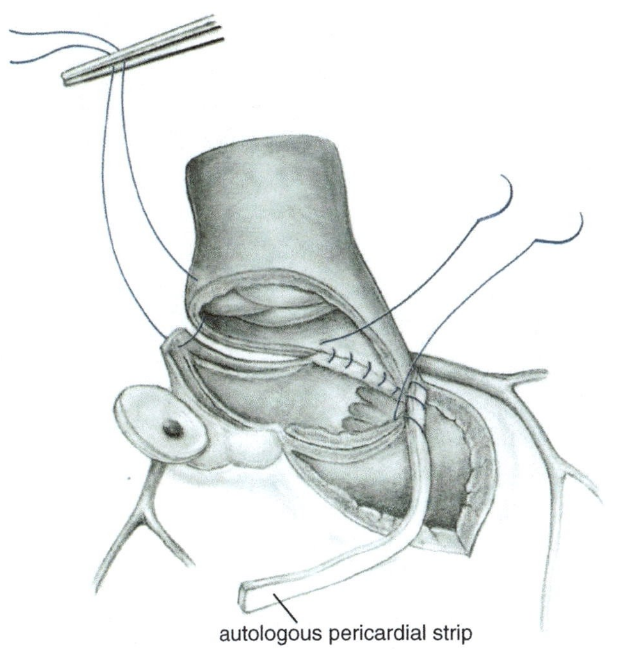

Fig. II-6-7-5. Ross–Konno procedure: autograft implantation at the Konno incision

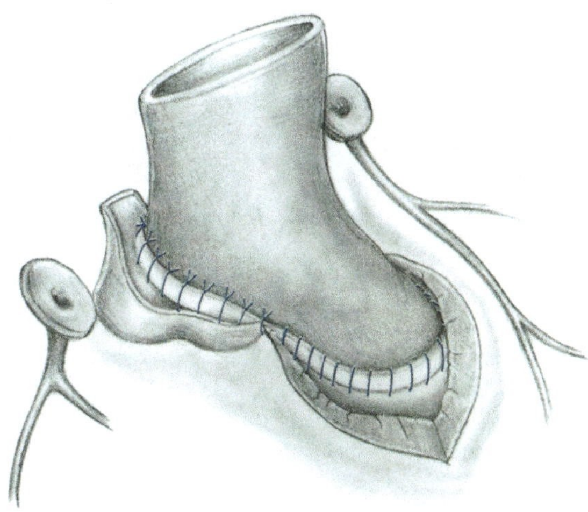

Fig. II-6-7-6. Ross–Konno procedure: autograft implantation

Coronary Button Implantation and Ascending Aortic Reconstruction

The reimplantation site for the coronary button is usually placed above the sinotubular junction in the neo-aorta. The coronary buttons are anastomosed using 6-0 running suture (Fig. II-6-7-8). The ascending aorta is reconstructed by anastomosis of the native ascending aorta to the pulmonary autograft with 6-0 running suture.

Right Ventricular Outflow Tract Reconstruction

After removal of the aortic cross-clamp, an autologous pericardial extension is placed along the posterior half of the right ventriculotomy to bridge to the pulmonary artery. The anterior wall is created with a second patch fashioned of ePTFE with a 0.1-mm-thick ePTFE monocusp leaflet (Fig. II-6-7-9). The outflow tract is constructed to create a cross-sectional area of 2.5–3.0 cm^2/m^2 BSA (body surface area).

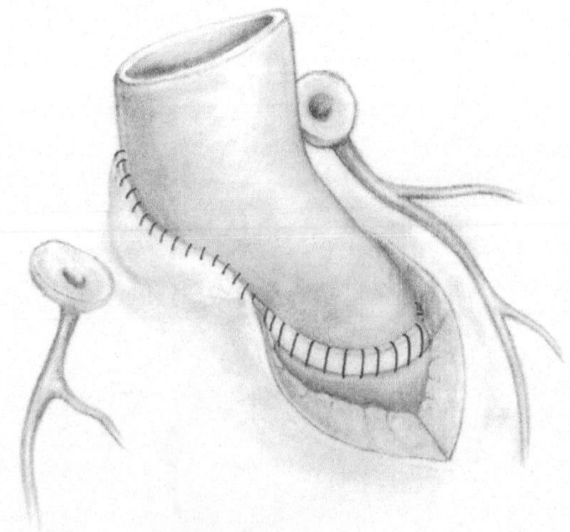

Fig. II-6-7-7. Ross–Konno procedure: wrapping of suture line with residual aortic wall

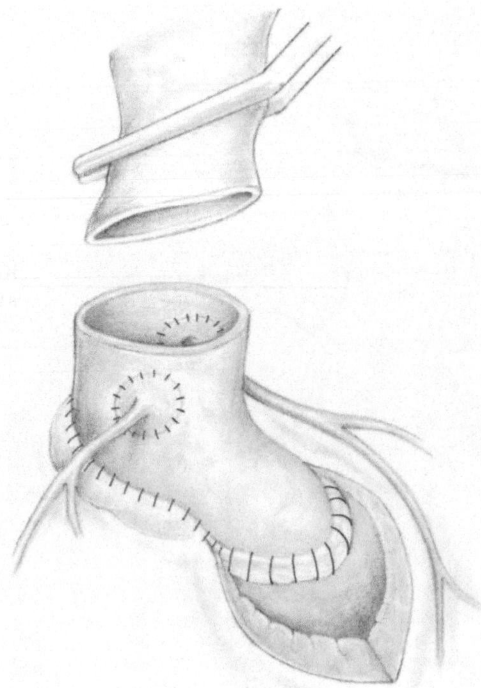

Fig. II-6-7-8. Ross–Konno procedure: coronary button implantation

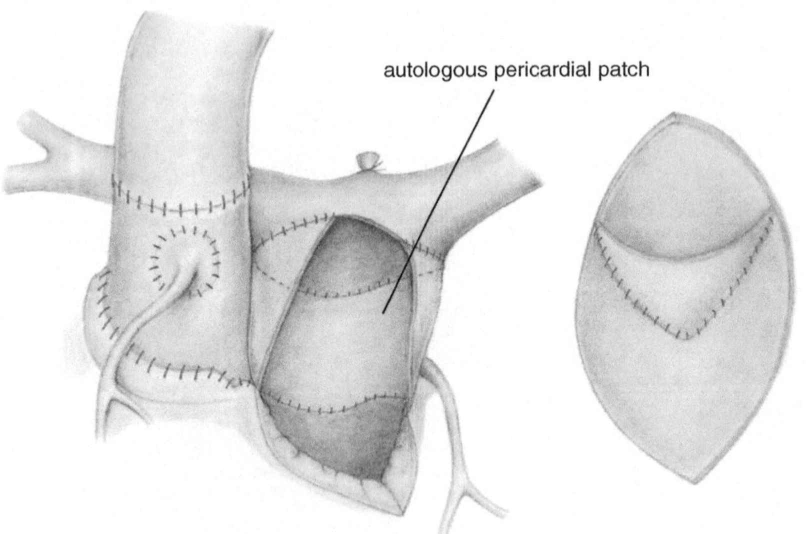

Fig. II-6-7-9. Ross–Konno procedure: RVOT reconstruction

References

1. Cobanoglu A, Thyagarajan GK, Dobbs J (1997) Konno-aortoventriculoplasty with mechanical prosthesis in dealing with small aortic root: a good surgical option. Eur J Cardiothorac Surg 12:766–770
2. Gildein HP, Kleinert S, Weintraab RG, et al (1996) Surgical commissurotomy of the aortic valve: outcome of open valvotomy in neonates with critical aortic stenosis. Am Heart J 131:754–759
3. Lababidi Z, Weinhaus L (1986) Successful balloon valvuloplasty for neonatal critical aortic stenosis. Am Heart J 112:913–916
4. Egito ES, Moore P, O'Sullivan J, et al (1997) Transvascular balloon dilation for neonatal critical aortic stenosis: early and midterm results. J Am Coll Cardiol 29:442–447
5. Kirklin JK, Barrat-Boyes BG (1986) Aortic valve disease. In: Cardiac surgery. Wiley, New York, p 414
6. Ross DN (1967) Replacement of aortic and mitral valves with a pulmonary autograft. Lancet 2:956–958

7. Elkins RC, Knott-Craig CJ, Randolph JD, et al (1994) Medium-term follow-up of pulmonary autograft replacement of aortic valves in children. Eur J Cardiothorac Surg 8:379–383
8. Ando M, Takahashi Y (2009) Ten-year experience with handmade trileaflet polytetrafluoroethylene valved conduit used for pulmonary reconstruction. J Thorac Cardiovasc Surg 137:124–131
9. Miyazaki T, Yamagishi M, Nakashima A, et al (2007) Expanded polytetrafluoroethylene valved conduit and patch with bulging sinuses in right ventricular outflow tract reconstruction. J Thorac Cardiovasc Surg 134:327–332
10. Nicks R, Cartmill T, Bernstein L (1970) Hypoplasia of the aortic root. The problem of aortic valve replacement. Thorax 25:339–346
11. Konno S, Imai Y, Iida Y, et al (1975) A new method for prosthetic valve replacement in congenital aortic stenosis associated with hypoplasia of the aortic valve ring. J Thorac Cardiovasc Surg 70:909–917
12. Manouguian S, Seybold-Epting W (1979) Patch enlargement of the aortic valve ring by extending the aortic incision into the anterior mitral leaflet. New operative technique. J Thorac Cardiovasc Surg 78:402–412
13. Yamaguchi M, Ohashi H, Imai M, et al (1991) Bilateral enlargement of the aortic valve ring for valve replacement in children. New operative technique. J Thorac Cardiovasc Surg 102:202–206
14. Reddy MV, Hiranya A, Rajasinghe, et al (1996) Aortoventriculoplasty with autograft: the Ross-Konno procedure. J Thorac Cardiovasc Surg 111:158–167

II-7. Aortic Regurgitation—Trusler Procedure

In children, the most frequently encountered form of aortic regurgitation is that which is related to a ventricular septal defect (VSD). As the outlet portion of the ventricular septum supports the aortic annulus, doubly committed VSD creates inadequate aortic valve support, with a weakened aortic annulus. The jet through the VSD beneath the aortic valve promotes the prolapse of the aortic valve cusps, especially the right coronary cusp. The combination of inadequate annular support and cusp prolapse causes aortic valve regurgitation [1]. In patients with perimembranous VSDs, occasionally there may be aortic valve regurgitation resulting from cusp prolapse. In these cases, the noncoronary cusp is usually the cusp that prolapses. In patients with a perimembranous VSD and aortic regurgitation, very rarely the aortic valve itself may be congenitally malformed, as is seen with isolated bicuspid aortic valve disease.

Surgical Indication

Because most doubly committed VSDs do not close spontaneously, surgical closure is almost always recommended. Simultaneous intervention on a regurgitant aortic valve is recommended for the patient with moderate or more regurgitation. In the patient with mild or lesser aortic regurgitation, surgical intervention should be undertaken less commonly, bearing in mind the potential for iatrogenic injury because the valve leaflet tissue is thin and fragile. In fact, most patients do not demonstrate progression of aortic regurgitation after VSD closure without intervention on the aortic valve, probably because VSD closure itself reinforces the aortic annulus. It is better for the patients to undergo surgery in early life, and typically, the surgery is performed in the early school-age years.

Trusler Procedure [2]

This technique is the repair most commonly used for aortic cusp prolapse. Via a median sternotomy, standard cardiopulmonary bypass is instituted. To improve visualization, the aortic cannula is placed in the ascending aorta at the base of the innominate artery. A vent catheter is placed in the left atrium through the left atrial appendage or the right upper pulmonary vein. The cardioplegia needle is placed in the root of the ascending aorta in the usual fashion. If the antegrade cardioplegic delivery does not produce cardiac arrest as a result of aortic regurgitation, the aortotomy is performed, and cardioplegic solution is injected directly into the coronary orifices.

Usually the aortotomy is begun distally on the left side of the aorta and extended obliquely into the noncoronary sinus. Alternatively, a transverse aortotomy incision is used. Two retractors for the VSD closure are placed on the edge of the aortic wall, with care not to damage the aortic cusp. The aortic valve is inspected. A fine monofilament suture is placed through the nodule of Aranti of all three cusps (Frater stich [3]), and the all cusps are retracted. This step improves the identification of the prolapsing part of the aortic cusp (Fig. II-7-1). In patients with doubly committed VSD, the right coronary cusp is usually prolapsing. The normal noncoronary cusp is then used as the standard for comparison of the pathological cusp. The redundant and elongated right coronary aortic cusp is suspended to the aortic wall using a pledgetted mattress suture (Fig. II-7-2). The commissure is opened, and a commissure plasty stitch is placed using a pledgetted mattress suture (Figs. II-7-3, II-7-4). If the commissure between the right and left coronary sinus is also redundant, suspension is performed at this commissure. The saline test is performed to evaluate the function of the repaired aortic valve, although occasionally this test is not reliable. After removal of the aortic cross-clamp, definitive assessment of the repair is performed by transesophageal echocardiography.

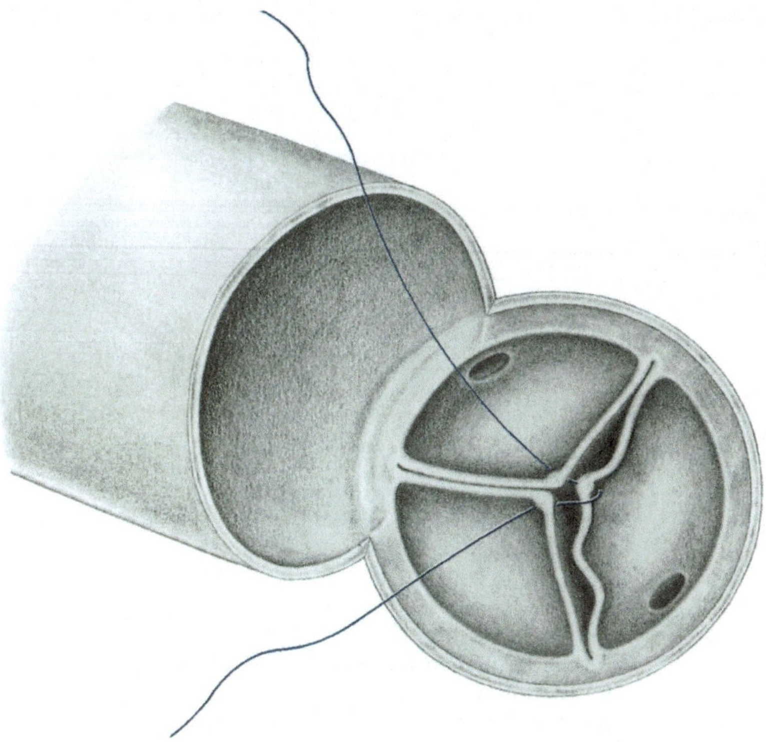

Fig. II-7-1. Trusler procedure: Frater stitch

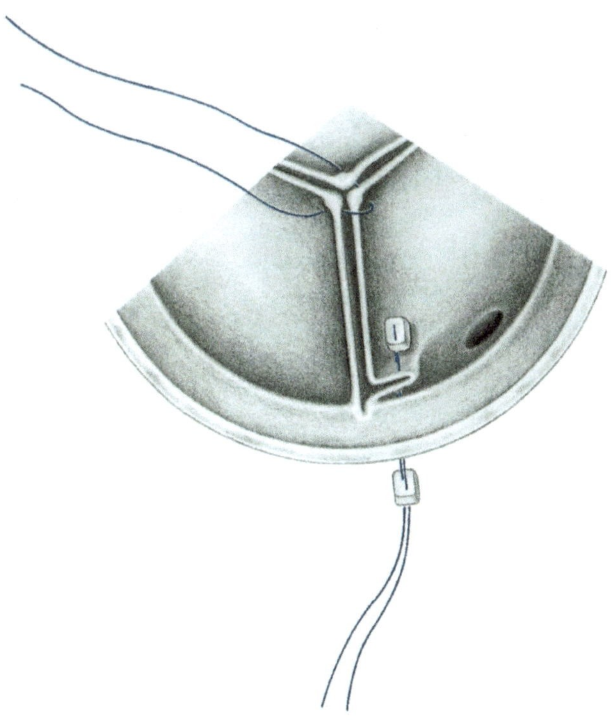

Fig. II-7-2. Trusler procedure: suspension of cusp. To suspend the prolapsing right coronary cusp, the unaffected noncoronary cusp is used for comparison. A pledgetted mattress suture is used to suspend the right coronary cusp

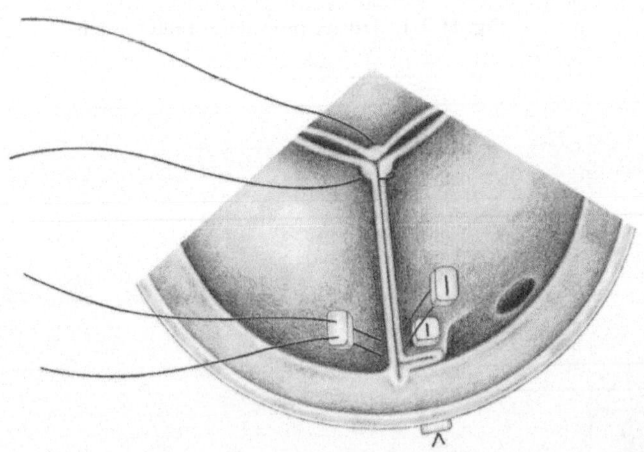

Fig. II-7-3. Trusler procedure: closure of the commissure. The commissure is closed using a pledgetted mattress suture

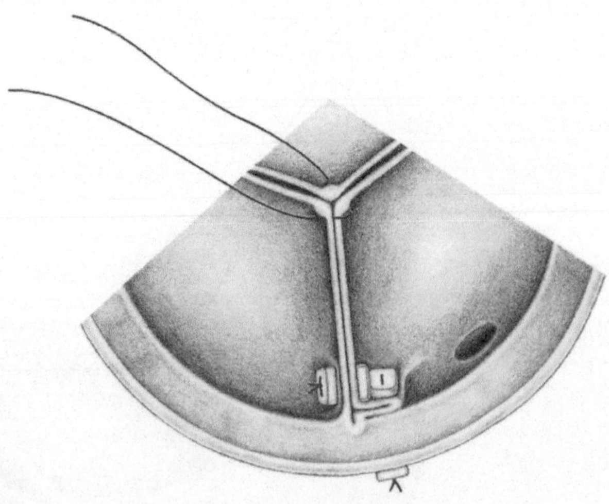

Fig. II-7-4. Trusler procedure: completed repair

References

1. Tatsuno K, Konno S, Ando M (1973) Pathogenetic mechanisms of prolapsing aortic valve and aortic regurgitation associated with ventricular septal defect. Circulation 48:1028–1037
2. Trusler GA, Moes CA, Kidd BS (1973) Repair of ventricular septal defect with aortic insufficiency. J Thorac Cardiovasc Surg 66:394–403
3. Kirklin JW, Barratt-Boyes BG (1993) Ventricular septal defect. In: Kirklin JW, Barratt-Boyes BG (eds) Cardiac surgery, 2nd edn. Churchill Livingstone, New York, p 807

II-8. Supravalvular Aortic Stenosis: Doty Procedure (Two-Sinus Reconstruction), Brom Procedure and Myers Procedure (Three-Sinus Reconstruction)

Supravalvular aortic stenosis, the least common form of congenital left ventricular outflow tract obstruction, is classified into discrete and diffuse types [1]. In the discrete type, there are hourglass and membranous types. The hourglass type is caused by fibrous hyperplasia at the sinotubular junction. In Japan, the membranous type is very rare. In patients with the diffuse type, the whole ascending aorta is hypoplastic, and there is ostial stenosis in the aortic branches. Patients who have supravalvular aortic stenosis, elfin face, mental retardation, hypercalcemia, and chromosome abnormality are diagnosed as Williams syndrome [2]. The aortic wall itself is often thick, and a bicuspid aortic valve is occasionally identified. Intimal thickening, aortic leaflet fusion to the narrowed sinotubular ridge, and coronary ostial stenosis or occlusion are occasionally observed [1,3,4]. As a consequence of hypertension in the coronary artery, these vessels are often dilated and tortuous. The most common associated anomaly is peripheral pulmonary artery stenosis. Occasionally coarctation of the aorta or ventricular septal defect is also seen, although much less commonly.

Surgical Indication

Surgical indications for supravalvular aortic stenosis include a pressure gradient of more than 50 mmHg, coronary artery stenosis or occlusion, and provokable ischemia during exercise stress testing.

Operative Procedure

Doty Procedure [5]

The heart is accessed via median sternotomy, and the root of the ascending aorta is dissected. Cardiopulmonary bypass is initiated with bicaval cannulation and the aortic cannula placed at the base of the brachiocephalic artery. A clamp is placed on the ascending aorta quite distal to the stenosis area. The initial incision is placed in the noncoronary sinus, and the next incision is placed into the right coronary sinus (Fig. II-8-1). The incision on the right coronary sinus is placed between the right and left coronary arteries, with care taken to keep enough distance from the right coronary orifice. Any fibrous ridge at the sinotubular junction is carefully excised. Dacron or xenopericardium is used as the patch material.

An inverted Y-shape patch is created in two parts. First, the noncoronary sinus is augmented using an elliptically shaped patch (Fig. II-8-2). If the right coronary sinus patch is too large, the right coronary artery may develop kinking. A retraction stitch is placed at the tip of the created flap at the base of the ascending aorta. The running suture is started at the nadir of the noncoronary sinus incision, using a fine monofilament running suture. The right coronary sinus is enlarged with a second patch (Fig. II-8-3). This technique is reproducible and results in excellent relief of the obstruction.

Brom Procedure: Three-Sinus Reconstruction

The base of the ascending aorta is dissected, and the aortic cannula is inserted at the base of the brachiocephalic artery. After cardioplegic cardiac arrest, the ascending aorta is transected a few millimeters above the sinotubular junction (Fig. II-8-4). Longitudinal incisions are placed in each of the three sinuses. An initial incision is placed in the noncoronary sinus. This incision facilitates visualization of the right and left coronary orifices and the aortic valve. The depth of the incisions is half of the depth of the sinus. In the Brom procedure [6], the sinuses are repaired using three patches. The reconstructed proximal ascending aorta and distal ascending aorta are then anastomosed using end-to-end technique. As a patch, fresh or glutaraldehyde-treated autologous pericardium is used. If the patches are too large, this may cause aortic valve insufficiency because of dilatation of the sinotubular junction.

In the Myers procedure [7], the incisions in the sinuses of Valsalva are the same as in the Brom procedure (see Fig. II-8-4). Next, counter-incisions are made in the distal ascending aorta, allowing enlargement without prosthetic material. Three traction stitches are placed at the tips of the three flaps above the aortic valve commissures (Figs. II-8-5). The anastomosis is started with monofilament suture from the base of the left coronary sinus and is advanced counterclockwise (Fig. II-8-6). The assistant holds the stitch with the left hand and holds the clamp on the aorta with the right hand to improve visualization of the operating field. After this suture line is brought anterior, the other suture end is brought around clockwise, and sutures are tied (Fig. II-8-7).

Steinberg [8] reported a modification of the Dotty procedure with an additional patch to the left coronary sinus. A longitudinal incision is placed in the left coronary sinus. An

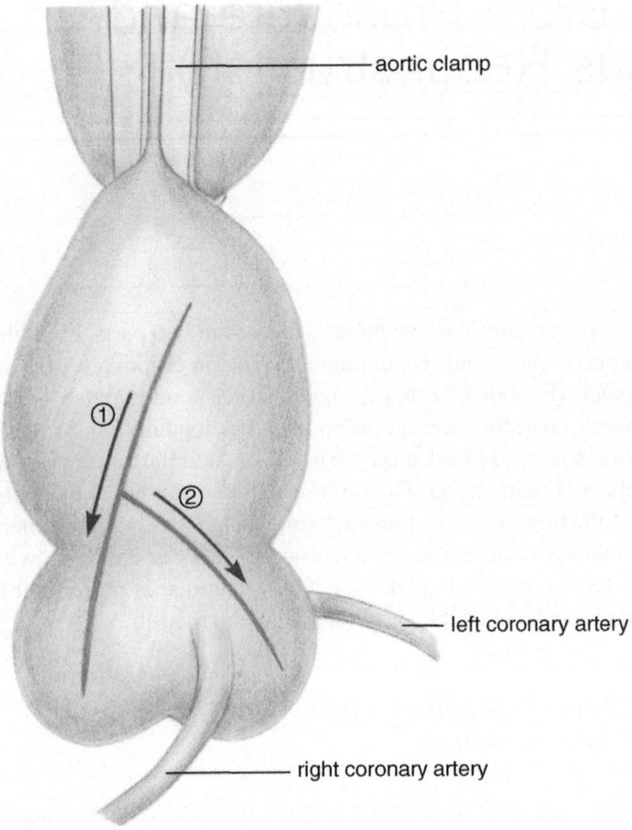

Fig. II-8-1. Doty procedure: incision lines. ① The first incision is placed into the noncoronary sinus. ② The second incision is placed into the right coronary sinus

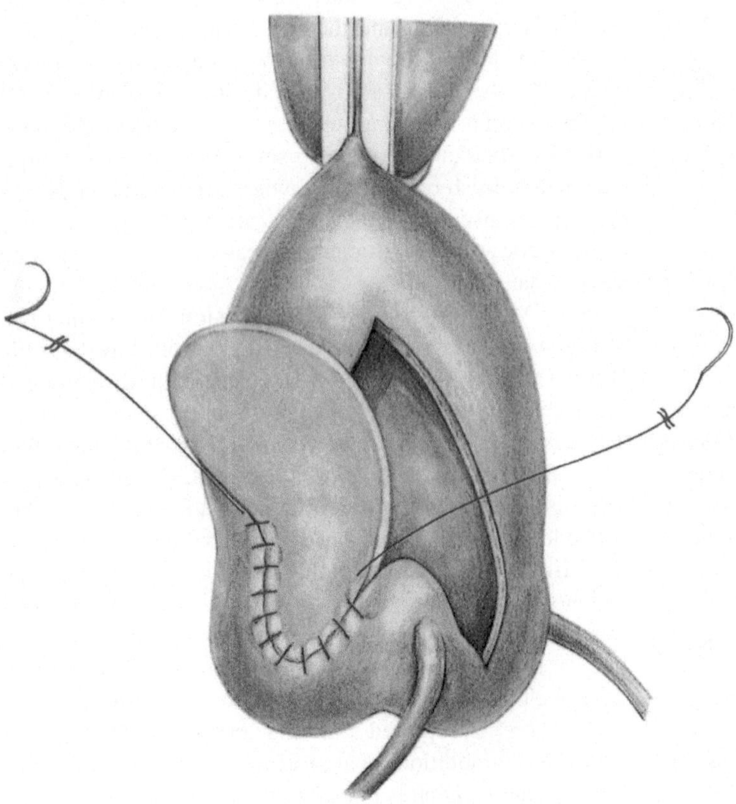

Fig. II-8-2. Doty procedure: patch placement. Suturing of an elliptically shaped patch is started at the base of the noncoronary sinus and carried distally

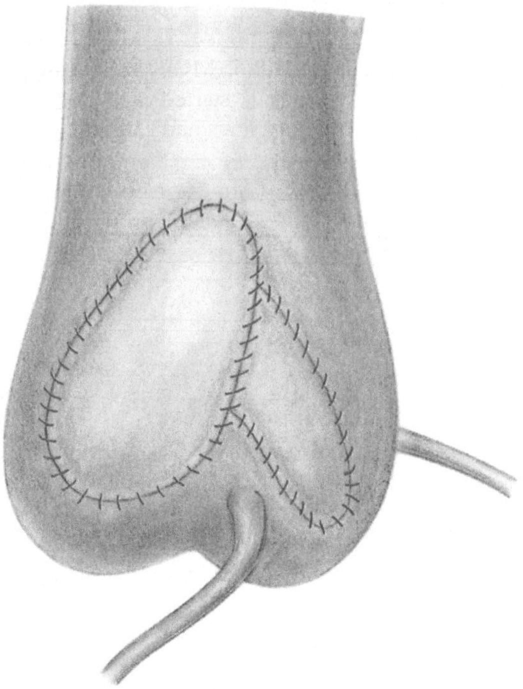

Fig. II-8-3. Doty procedure. Two patches are placed to the noncoronary and right coronary sinuses

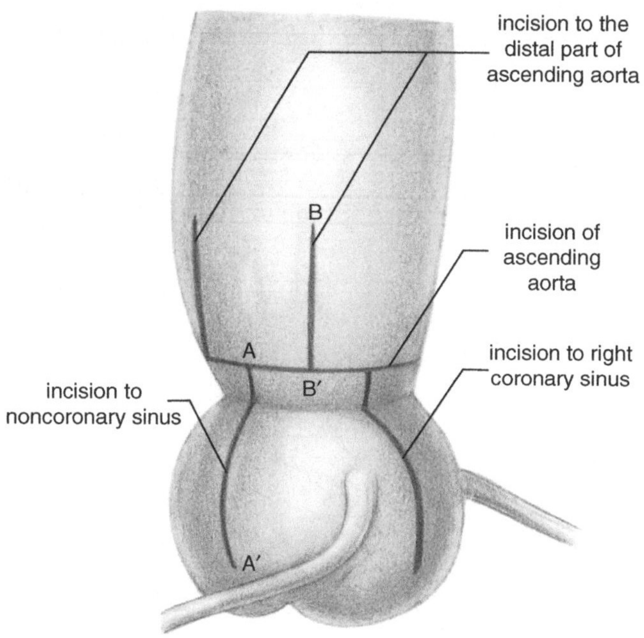

Fig. II-8-4. Myers procedure: incision line. Point *A* and point *A'* are sutured to each other. Points *B* and *B'* are sutured

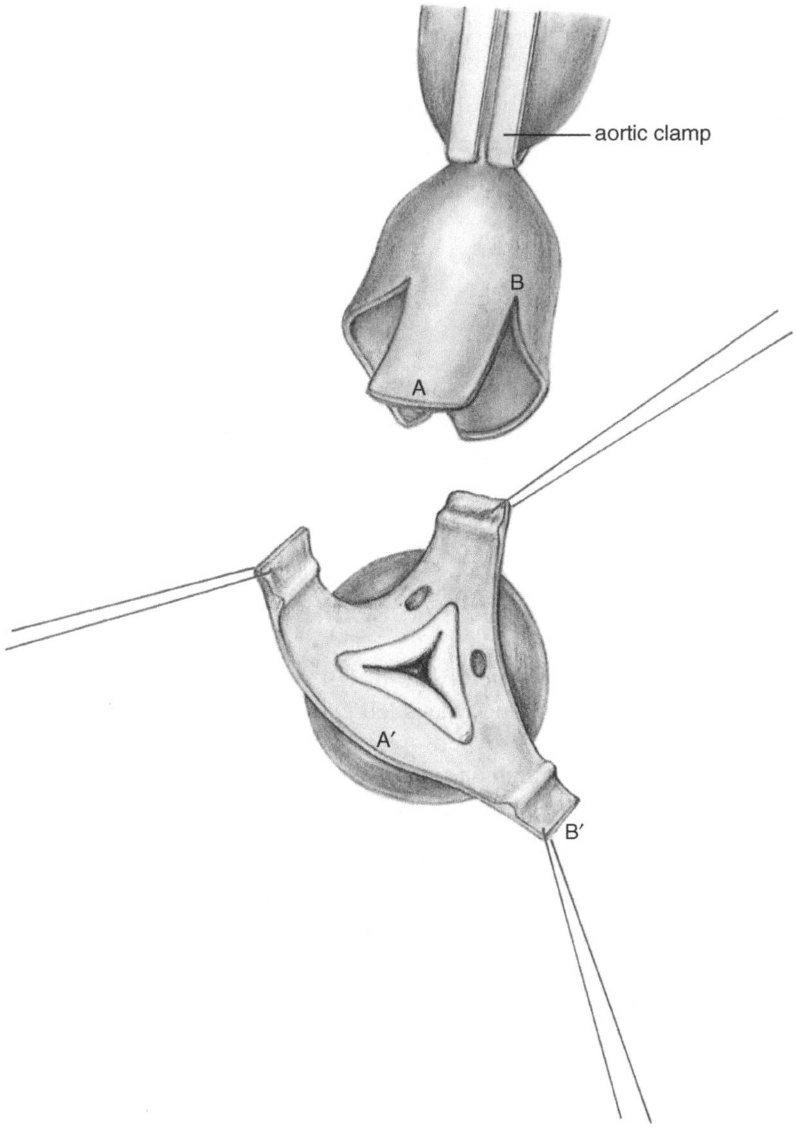

Fig. II-8-5. Myers procedure: after division and longitudinal incision placement. Point *A* and point *A'* are sutured to each other. Points *B* and *B'* are sutured

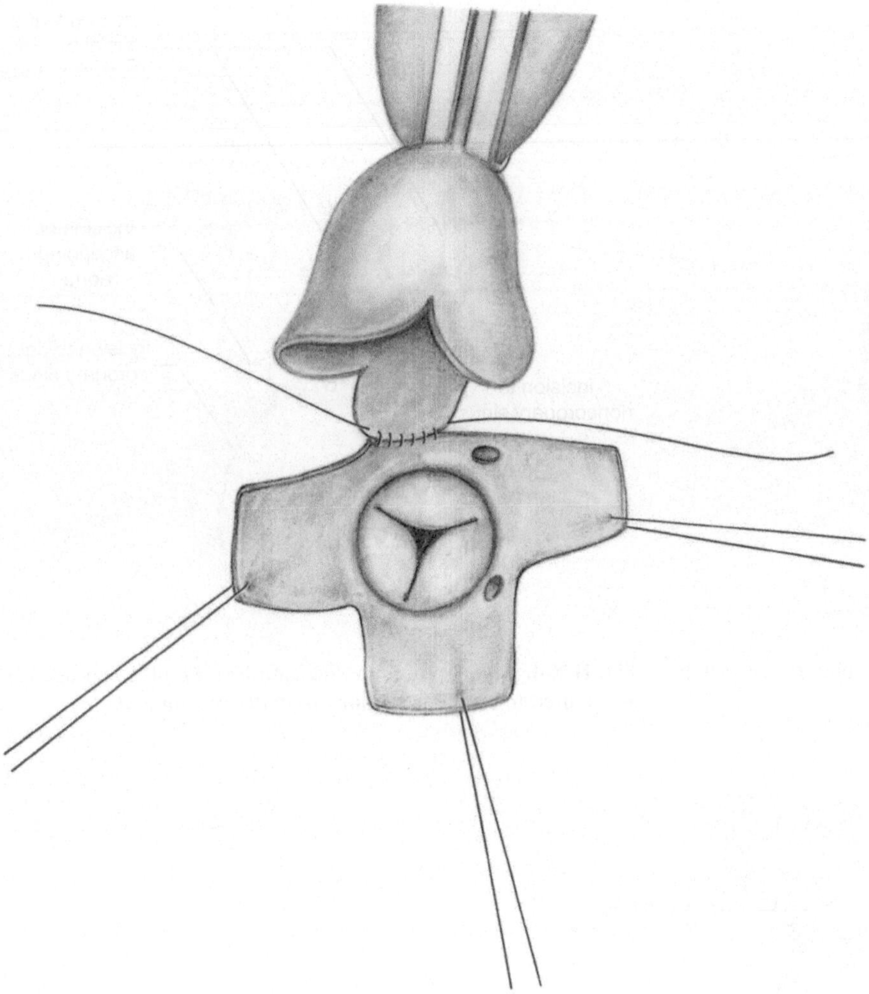

Fig. II-8-6. Myers procedure: suturing. Suturing is started at the base of the left coronary sinus and carried on with running suture

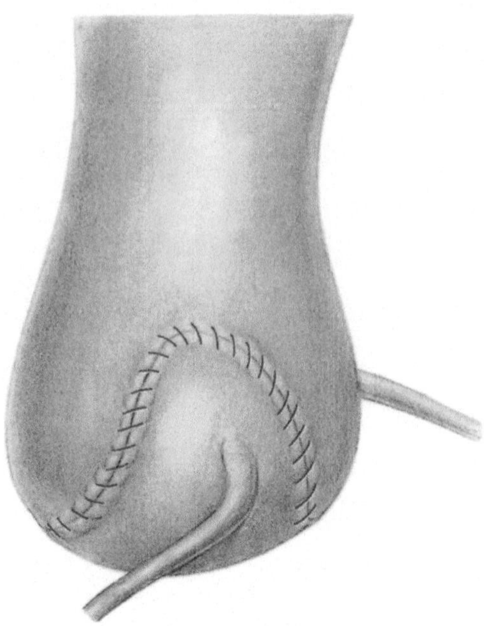

Fig. II-8-7. Myers procedure: after completion of procedure

expanded polytetrafluoroethylene (PTFE) oval-shaped patch is placed in this incision, which creates a three-sinus enlargement technique. The technique differs from the Brom or Myers procedure because there is no transection of the ascending aorta.

Surgery for Associated Anomalies

There are three types of left coronary occlusions [9]. The most common type is left coronary orifice occlusion caused by extreme hypertrophy of the aortic wall thickness. The second common type is caused by fusion of the deformed left cusp to the fibrous ridge of the supravalvular area. The least common type is diffuse stenosis provoked by hypertensive effect on the coronary artery.

Surgical interventions are planned depending on the types of occlusions. In case of orifice stenosis or occlusion, the incision in the left coronary sinus is extended across the coronary orifice onto the left main coronary artery. An autologous pericardial patch plasty is performed on the left main coronary artery and left coronary sinus simultaneously. In patients with diffuse stenosis, coronary artery bypass grafting is performed.

References

1. Rastelli GC, McGoon DC, Ongley PA, et al (1966) Surgical treatment of supravalvular aortic stenosis. Report of 16 cases and review of literature. J Thorac Cardiovasc Surg 51:873–882
2. Williams C, Barratt-Boyes BG, Lowe JB (1961) Supravalvular aortic stenosis. Circulation 24:1311–1318
3. Denie JJ, Verheugt AP (1958) Supravalvular aortic stenosis. Circulation 18:902–908
4. Peterson TA, Todd DB, Edwards JE (1965) Supravalvular aortic stenosis. J Thorac Cardiovasc Surg 50:734–741
5. Doty DB, Polansky DB, Jenson CB (1977) Supravalvular aortic stenosis. Repair by extended aortoplasty. J Thorac Cardiovasc Surg 74:362–371
6. Brom AG (1988) Obstruction of the left ventricular outflow tract: Khonsari S (ed) Cardiac surgery: safeguards and pitfalls in operative technique. Aspen, Rockville, MD, pp 276–280
7. Myers JL, Waldhausen JA, Cyran SE, et al (1993) Results of surgical repair of congenital supravalvular aortic stenosis. J Thorac Cardiovasc Surg 105:281–288
8. Steinberg JB, Delius RE, Behrendt DM, et al (1998) Supra valvular aortic stenosis: a modification of extended aortoplasty. Ann Thorac Surg 65:277–279
9. Thistlethwaite PA, Madani MM, Kriett JM, et al (2000) Surgical management of congenital obstruction of the left main coronary artery with supravalvular aortic stenosis. J Thorac Cardiovasc Surg 120:1040–1046

II-9. Subaortic Stenosis: Subaortic Resection, Modified Konno Procedure, Yasui Procedure, Modified Yasui Procedure

Subaortic stenosis is divided into membranous and fibromuscular stenosis types. More than 50% of patients with this condition have isolated subaortic stenosis. The remainder have membranous or fibromuscular stenosis with concomitant congenital heart disease, such as malalignment of ventricular septum with coarctation of the aorta or interrupted aortic arch, left ventricular outflow tract obstruction after the atrioventricular septal defect repair, narrowing of interventricular septum after double-outlet right ventricle repair, and fibrous granulation accumulation on a ventricular septal defect closure patch [1,2]. A Yasui procedure [3] represents the combination of the Damus–Kaye–Stansel [4] and Rastelli procedures. This procedure has been utilized for single-stage complete repair for coarctation of the aorta or interrupted aortic arch, subaortic stenosis, and ventricular septal defect. The Konno [5] or Ross–Konno procedure [6] was discussed in Chapter II-6.

Surgical Indication

A pressure gradient of more than 50 mmHg between the left ventricle and the ascending aorta is the surgical indication for subaortic stenosis repair. New developing or increasing aortic regurgitation also is the indication. Discrete-type or short-segment fibromuscular-type stenosis may be relieved by membranous or muscle resection. However, in long-segment or tunnel-type stenosis, the techniques of resecting and opening the ventricular septum, such as Konno, Ross–Konno, or modified Konno [7], will be required [8]. In the neonate or young infant, with additional complex congenital heart disease, the preoperative study often does not evaluate the pressure gradient accurately. In the patient with aortic arch anomaly and patent ductus arteriosus, echocardiography may significantly underestimate the gradient. Therefore, the anatomic evaluation is important, and a subaortic area diameter smaller than 60% of the normal value or less than 2.5 mm diameter in a neonate weighing 3 kg is believed to be an indication for surgery for subaortic stenosis.

Subaortic Resection

The operations are performed through a median sternotomy. Cardiopulmonary bypass is initiated using ascending aortic and right atrial cannulation with left atrial venting. After the aortic cross-clamp is applied, aortotomy is performed obliquely from the anterior aspect of the aorta to the noncoronary sinus of Valsalva. The subaortic area is visualized, and the nature of the subaortic stenosis is evaluated.

In the discrete type, a white, disk-shaped shelf is observed. The fibrous shelf is shaved carefully using a No. 11 blade knife from the junction of the ventricular septum and aortic annulus to the fibrous continuity area of the anterior leaflet of the mitral valve and aortic valve cusp (Fig. II-9-1 ①). The conduction system is located in the membranous septum, and deep resection in this area is avoided. After removal of the fibrous tissue, it is beneficial to excise the hypertrophic ventricular septum in a wedge shape and to dilate the subaortic area with a finger or dilator.

In the fibromuscular type, asymmetrical hypertrophy is observed in the left ventricular outflow tract. A traction stitch is placed in the ventricular septum beneath the commissure between the left and right coronary cusps. This stay stitch is pulled up, and the exposed hypertrophied muscle is excised in a wedge shape (Fig. II-9-1 ②).

Modified Konno Procedure

In the case of severe and extended left ventricular outflow tract obstruction, muscle or fibrous tissue resection may not be enough to relieve the obstruction. The patient having subvalvular stenosis, a normal aortic valve without annular stenosis, may undergo a modified Konno procedure, preserving the aortic valve (Fig. II-9-2). Cardiopulmonary bypass is initiated with ascending aortic and bicaval cannulation and left atrial venting. After aortic cross-clamping and cardioplegic arrest, a transverse incision is made on the ascending aorta and the subaortic area is inspected. When diffuse or tunnel-type stenosis is identified, the right ventricular outflow tract is opened transversely. A right-angle clamp is passed retrograde through the aortic valve into the left ventricle. The ventricular septum beneath the left and right coronary cusp is probed. From the left ventricular side, the tip of the right-angle clamp is placed inferiorly along the ventricular septum 10 mm beneath the pulmonary valve annulus, and a small incision is made. The ventricular septal incision is extended parallel to the pulmonary annulus, and the left ventricular outflow tract is inspected. The fibromuscular tissue is excised with care taken not to damage the mitral chordae and papillary muscles. Hypertrophic ventricular septal muscle of the left ventricle is resected. After muscle

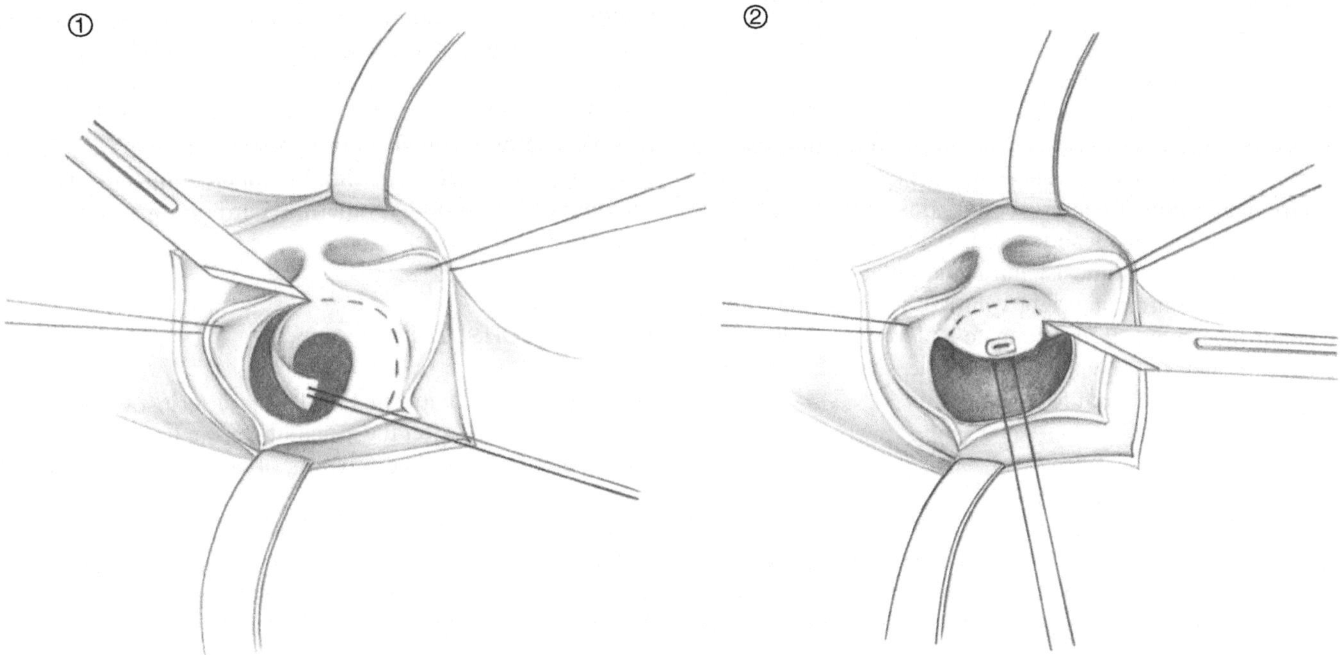

Fig. II-9-1. Subaortic resection. ① Membranous type. ② Fibromuscular type

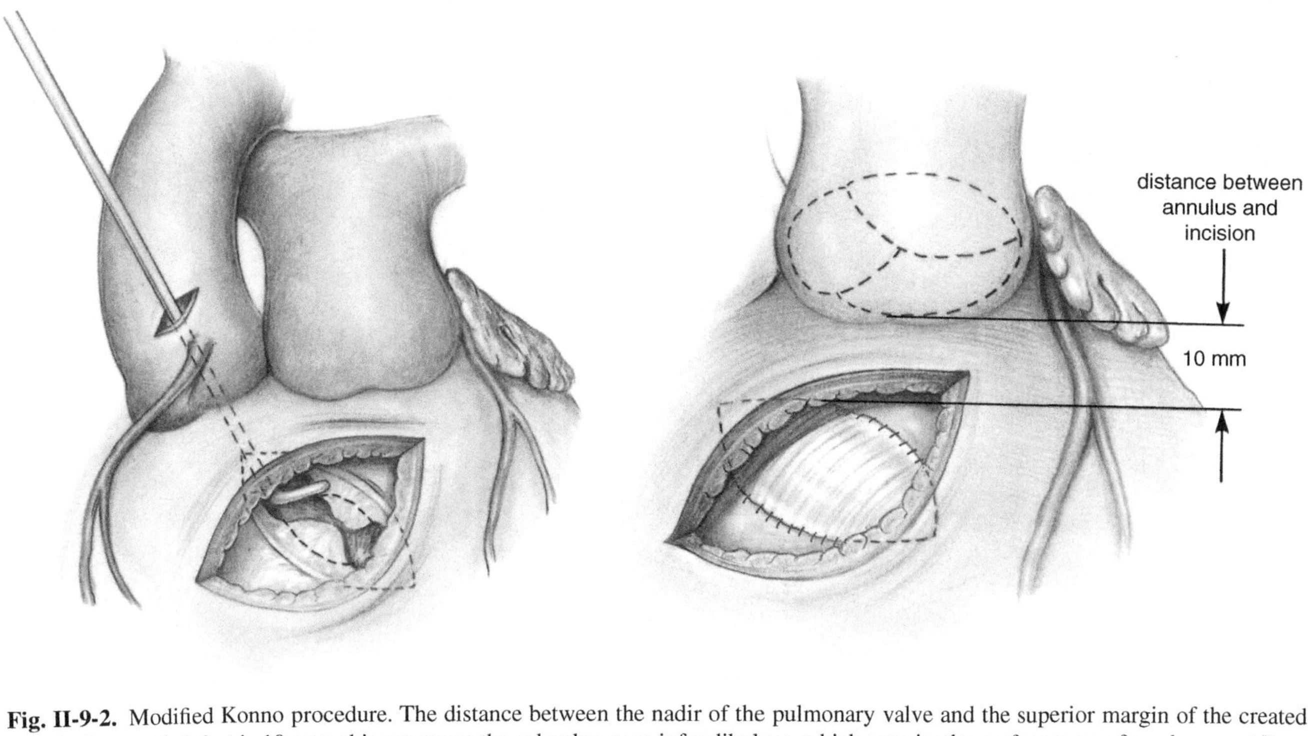

Fig. II-9-2. Modified Konno procedure. The distance between the nadir of the pulmonary valve and the superior margin of the created ventricular septal defect is 10 mm; this preserves the subpulmonary infundibulum, which permits the performance of a subsequent Ross procedure

resection, the resultant ventricular septal defect is closed using a polytetrafluoroethylene (PTFE) patch (Fig. II-9-2).

Yasui Procedure

This procedure is a single-stage repair for the neonate having aortic arch hypoplasia, ventricular septal defect, and left ventricular outflow tract obstruction. Basically the operation is the combination of aortic arch reconstruction, Damus–Kaye–Stansel anastomosis, intraventricular rerouting (LV-VSD-PA rerouting), and right ventricle-to-pulmonary artery conduit placement. In the neonate and young infant with a left ventricular outflow tract diameter less than 2.5 mm, this procedure is considered to be an option.

Cardiopulmonary Bypass

The arterial perfusion is through the brachiocephalic artery and descending aorta, and circulatory arrest is not utilized. A median sternotomy and subtotal thymectomy are performed. A 3-mm PTFE tube graft is anastomosed to the brachiocephalic artery, and an 8 Fr. arterial cannula is inserted into the graft for perfusion of the brain and the upper body. An L-shaped arterial cannula (JMS, 2.1 mm) is placed into the descending aorta above the diaphragm, providing flow to the lower body (as shown in Figs. II-4-5 and II-4-6). The two cannulae are connected to the arterial line of the bypass circuit through a Y-shaped connector. Bicaval cannulation and mild hypothermic cardiopulmonary bypass is used (Fig. II-9-3 ①).

Arch Reconstruction

Following the division of the ductus arteriosus, all ductal tissue is removed. After the ascending aorta is cross-clamped and cardioplegic cardiac arrest is obtained, the descending aorta and distal ascending aorta are anastomosed in a side-to-end fashion using 7-0 polydioxane suture (PDS) (Fig. II-9-3 ②). When the ascending aorta is of adequate size, a side-biting clamp is placed on the distal ascending aorta, and the anastomosis is performed with the heart beating.

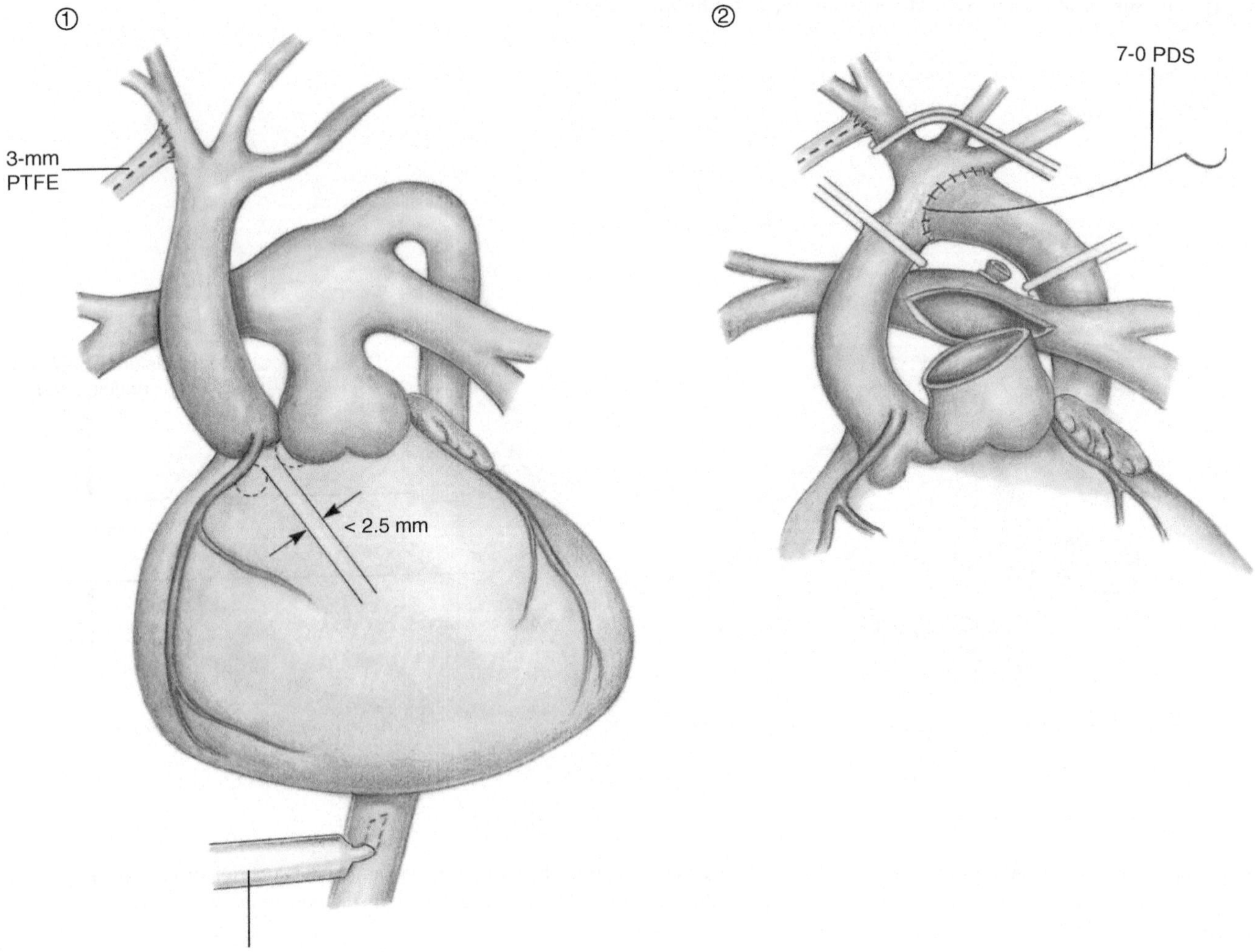

Fig. II-9-3. Yasui procedure. ① Cardiopulmonary bypass for the Yasui procedure. ② Aortic arch reconstruction by direct anastomosis. ③ Creation of intraventricular tunnel. ④ Damus–Kaye–Stansel anastomosis. ⑤ Right ventricular outflow tract reconstruction with valved conduit

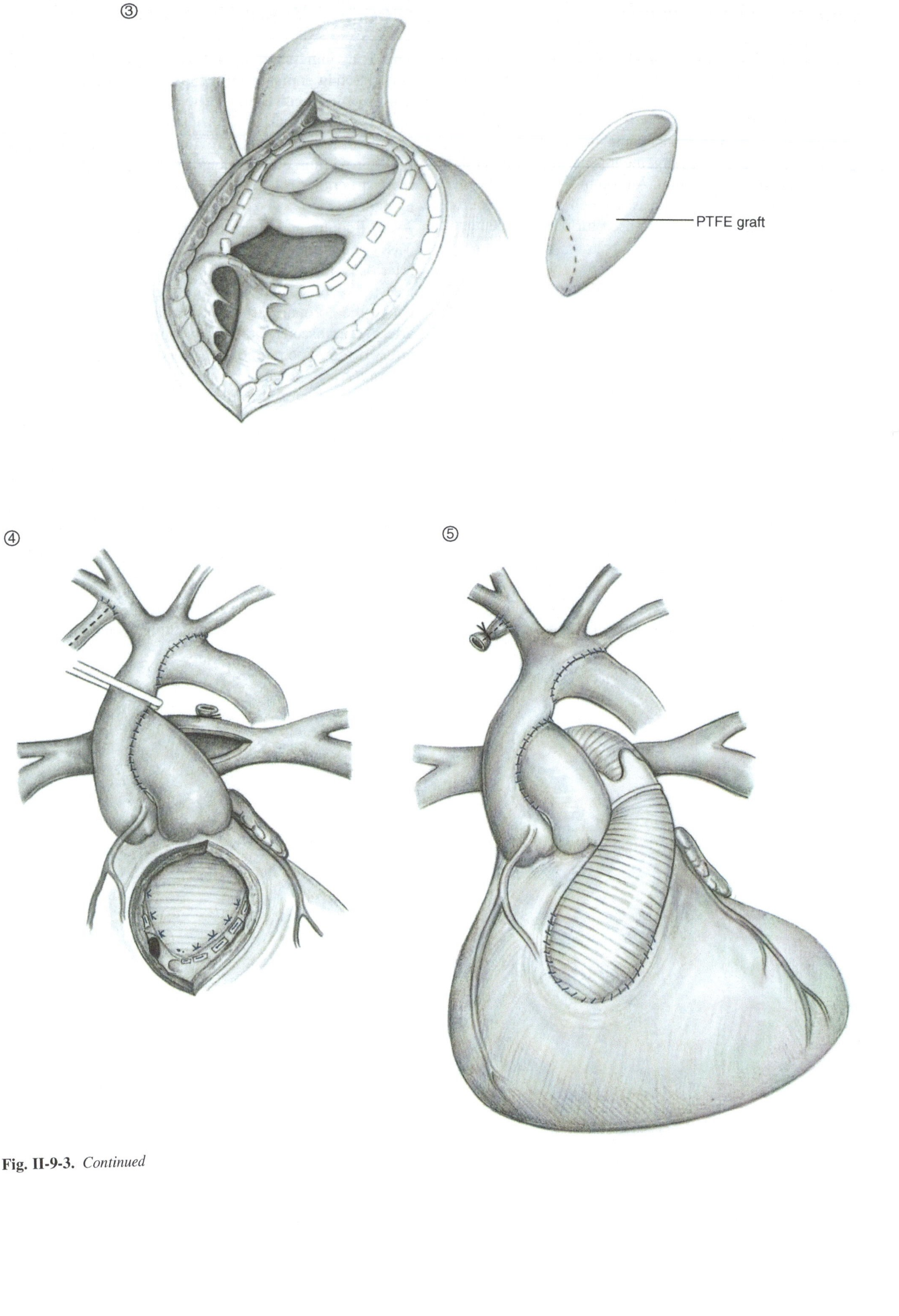

Fig. II-9-3. *Continued*

Intraventricular Rerouting

A longitudinal incision is made in the right ventricular outflow tract, and an intraventricular rerouting pathway is created from the left ventricle to the main pulmonary artery through the ventricular septal defect (Fig. II-9-3 ③). Usually, enlargement of the ventricular septal defect is not necessary. If this is necessary, the enlargement is performed toward the anterior and superior septum. An 8-mm PTFE tube is cut in a spindle shape and is used as a patch for the rerouting. Pledgetted mattress sutures are used for patch placement.

Damus–Kaye–Stansel Anastomosis

The main pulmonary artery is transected at the base of the branch pulmonary arteries. In most cases, the right side of the main pulmonary artery stump is shorter than the left side (Fig. II-9-3 ②). Therefore, an end-to-side direct anastomosis is possible between the main pulmonary artery and ascending aorta. A 7-0 PDS running suture is used (Fig. II-9-3 ④).

Right Ventricular Outflow Tract Reconstruction

After the aortic cross-clamp is released, a porcine valved conduit or a hand-made monocusp PTFE graft tube is anastomosed between the right ventricle and pulmonary artery with the heart beating (Fig. II-9-3 ⑤).

Modified Yasui Procedure

This is a single-stage operation for the patient with severe aortic arch hypoplasia, left ventricular outflow tract obstruction (aortic stenosis or aortic atresia), ventricular septal defect, and normal left ventricular volume. This procedure is a modification of the previously described Yasui operation, providing enlargement of the ascending aorta and reconstruction of the right ventricular outflow tract without a conduit.

Cardiopulmonary bypass technique is the same as for the Yasui operation (Fig. II-9-4 ①). After ligation of the ductus arteriosus, the ascending aorta is cross-clamped and cardiac arrest is obtained. The ascending aorta is transected 10 mm above the coronary artery origin, and the main pulmonary artery is transected at the level of the branch pulmonary artery origin. The pulmonary artery confluence is brought to anterior to the ascending aorta. The proximal ascending aorta is anastomosed to the main pulmonary artery using a side-to-side anastomosis. The left posterior main pulmonary artery is then anastomosed to the ventral surface of the descending aorta in a side-to-side fashion. The length of this anastomosis is one-third of the circumference of the descending aorta. A longitudinal incision is made in the small curvature of the aortic arch, and the arch and neo-proximal aorta are anastomosed. Reconstruction of the aortic arch and neo-aorta are accomplished with autologous tissue (Fig. II-9-4 ②). A longitudinal incision is made in the right ventricular outflow tract. Via this ventriculotomy, patch placement is accomplished for the rerouting from the left ventricle

①

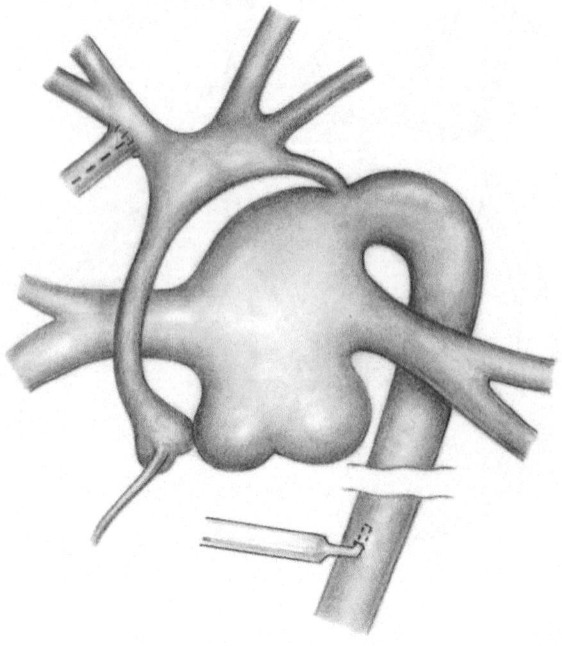

②

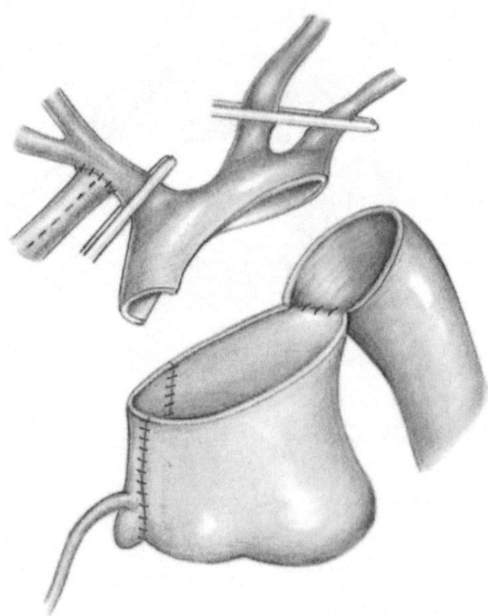

Fig. II-9-4. Modified Yasui procedure. ① Cardiopulmonary bypass for the modified Yasui procedure. ② Aortic arch reconstruction by direct anastomosis.

③

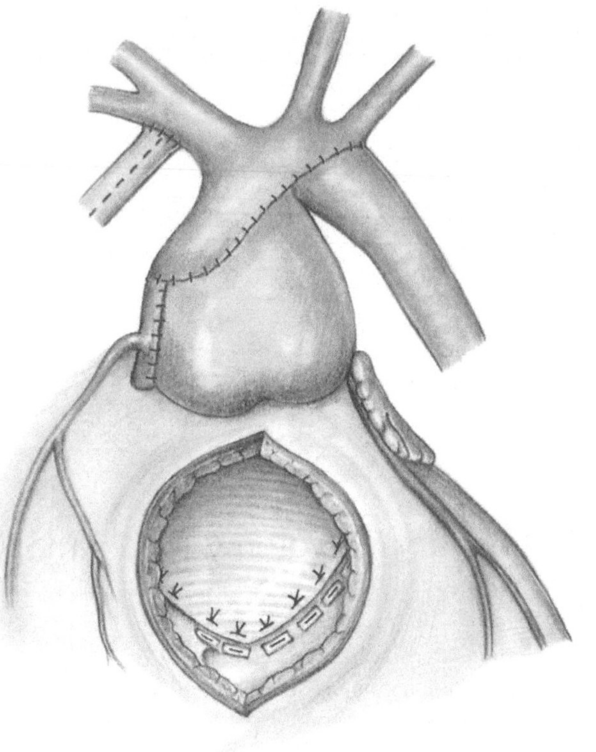

④

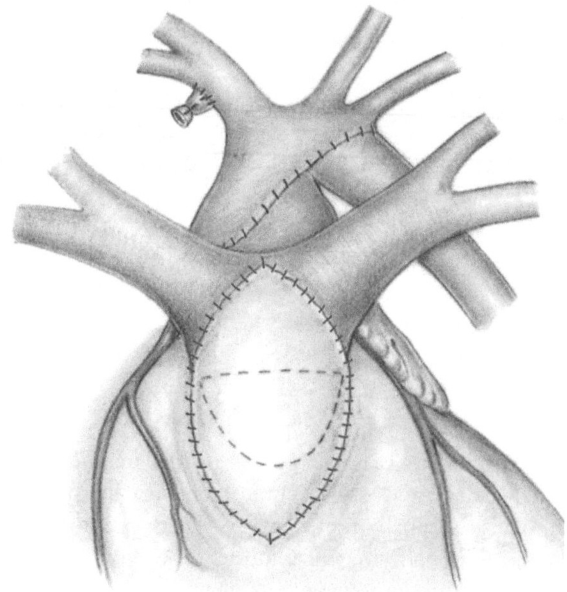

Fig. II-9-4. ③ Creation of intraventricular tunnel. ④ Right ventricular outflow tract reconstruction using Lecompte maneuver

to the main pulmonary artery through the ventricular septal defect (Fig. II-9-4 ③). Following removal of the aortic cross-clamp, the neo-pulmonary artery is reconstructed anterior to the neo-aorta using a Lecompte maneuver. A 0.1-mm-thick PTFE monocusp patch is placed in the right ventricular outflow tract (Fig. II-9-4 ④), as described in Chapter II-23.

References

1. Zielinsky P, Rossi M, Haertel JC, et al (1987) Subaortic fibrous ridge and ventricular septal defect: role of septal malalignment. Circulation 75:1124–1129
2. Shiokawa Y, Becker AE (1997) The left ventricular outflow tract in atrioventricular septal defect revisited: surgical considerations regarding preservation of aortic valve integrity in the perspective of anatomic observations. J Thorac Cardiovasc Surg 114:586–593
3. Yasui H, Kado H, Nakano E, et al (1987) Primary repair of interrupted aortic arch and severe aortic stenosis in neonates. J Thorac Cardiovasc Surg 93:539–545
4. Stansel HC Jr (1975) A new operation for d-loop transposition of the great vessels. Ann Thorac Surg 19:565–567
5. Konno S, Imai Y, Iida Y, et al (1975) A new method for prosthetic valve replacement in congenital aortic stenosis associated with hypoplasia of the aortic valve ring. J Thorac Cardiovasc Surg 70:909–917
6. Reddy VM, Rajasinghe HA, Teitel DF, et al (1996) Aortoventriculoplasty with the pulmonary autograft: the "Ross-Konno" procedure. J Thorac Cardiovasc Surg 111:158–165; discussion 165–167
7. Vouhe PR, Neveux JY (1991) Surgical management of diffuse subaortic stenosis: an integrated approach. Ann Thorac Surg 52:654–661; discussion 661–662
8. Serraf A, Zoghby J, Lacour-Gayet F, et al (1999) Surgical treatment of subaortic stenosis: a seventeen-year experience. J Thorac Cardiovasc Surg 117:669–678

II-10. Pulmonary Stenosis

Pulmonary stenosis is a broad term that includes valvular, supravalvular, and subvalvular stenosis. In strict terms, pulmonary stenosis represents isolated pulmonary valve stenosis. The pathological features of valvular stenosis are thickened pulmonary valve leaflets with or without commissural fusion. Isolated subvalvular stenosis by hypertrophied infundibular muscle is rare, and other intracardiac anomalies are usually observed simultaneously. Supravalvular stenosis, or peripheral pulmonary artery stenosis, is also frequently associated with other cardiac malformations. Peripheral pulmonary artery stenosis may develop anywhere along the pulmonary artery distal from the main pulmonary artery. In patients with cyanotic heart disease, branch pulmonary artery stenosis is often observed at the insertion of the ductus arteriosus [1,2].

Balloon valvuloplasty has become the procedure of choice for pulmonary valve stenosis, with excellent early results [3–5]. The gradient relief and the degree of pulmonary valve insufficiency after treatment are similar or better than with surgical intervention. Presently, surgical interventions are limited to patients who have failed balloon valvotomy or who have additional infundibular stenosis, or atrial septal defects not amenable to catheter intervention [6]. From a hemodynamic point of view, a gradient of 50 mmHg or more is usually considered to be an indication for surgery.

When an adequate effect is not obtained with balloon valvotomy at interventional catheterization, patients usually require a transannular patch. Because cardiac tamponade caused by cardiac perforation has been reported for neonatal balloon pulmonary valvotomy, backup by the surgical team is essential [7].

Surgery for peripheral pulmonary artery stenosis is quite challenging. Patch plasty or cut-back techniques have been attempted with suboptimal results. Currently balloon angioplasty and stent placement are the treatments of choice for peripheral pulmonary artery stenosis [8–10].

Because the need for surgery in pulmonary valve stenosis is rare now, in this chapter commissurotomy for valvular pulmonary stenosis and repair of pulmonary artery stenosis related to the ductus arteriosus are discussed.

Pulmonary Valvotomy for Pulmonary Stenosis

A median sternotomy is performed to expose the heart. Cardiopulmonary bypass is instituted with ascending aortic and bicaval cannulation. The main pulmonary artery is longitudinally opened. This incision is extended proximally with care not to damage the pulmonary valve leaflets (Fig. II-10-1), and 6-0 monofilament stay sutures are placed in each edge of the pulmonary arteriotomy sites to improve visualization. The fused commissures are incised from the orifice toward the pulmonary arterial wall with a fine scalpel. When an adequate orifice is not obtained, the commissure is detached from the pulmonary arterial wall (Fig. II-10-2). If any abnormal muscle bundles are present in the right ventricular outflow tract, these muscle bundles are removed through the pulmonary valve. When supravalvular stenosis is present, a patch of autologous pericardium is placed to augment the pulmonary trunk.

Relief of Pulmonary Artery Stenosis Related to Ductus Arteriosus

The heart is exposed through a median sternotomy. The pulmonary artery around the stenotic area is mobilized as much as possible. To enlarge the stenosis, an autologous pericardial patch is prepared in advance. Stay sutures are placed in this pericardial patch, and this patch is kept between wet sponges. If the patient has not had prior surgery, typically enough pericardium is available. In reoperations, a patch of expanded polytetrafluoroethylene, cut from a tubular graft, is used. Conventional cardiopulmonary bypass is started with ascending aortic and bicaval cannulation. After full flow bypass, a longitudinal incision is placed in the pulmonary artery. This incision is extended well beyond ductal tissue area. A 6-0 or 5-0 monofilament running suture is used for patch placement. In cases of severe stenosis, the stenotic segment of the pulmonary artery is resected and an end-to-end anastomosis using a 6-0 or 5-0 running suture (Fig. II-10-3) is performed.

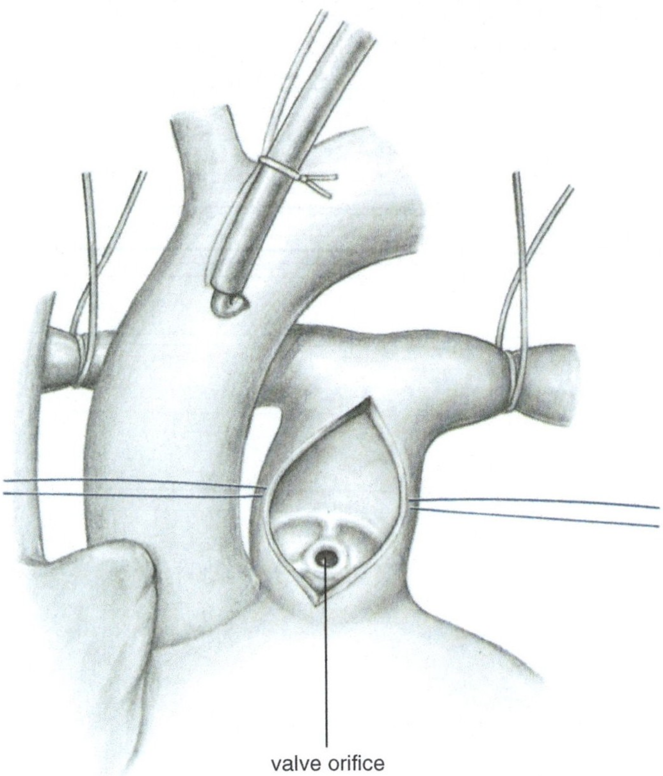

Fig. II-10-1. Commissurotomy for valvular pulmonary stenosis: 1. A longitudinal incision is made on the pulmonary trunk, and traction stitches are placed in each edge

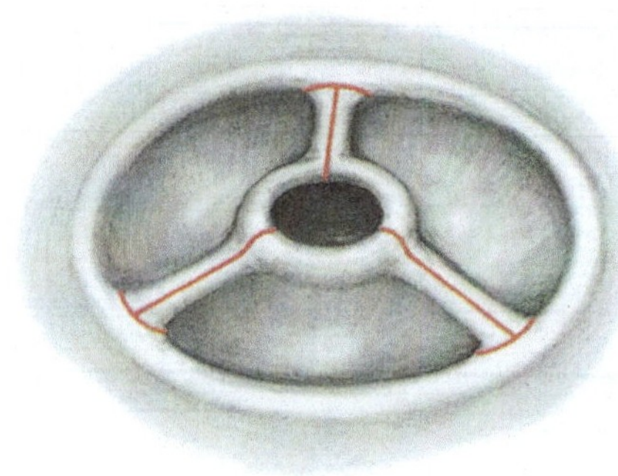

Fig. II-10-2. Commissurotomy for valvular pulmonary stenosis: 2. Fused commissures are incised with a knife toward the pulmonary arterial wall

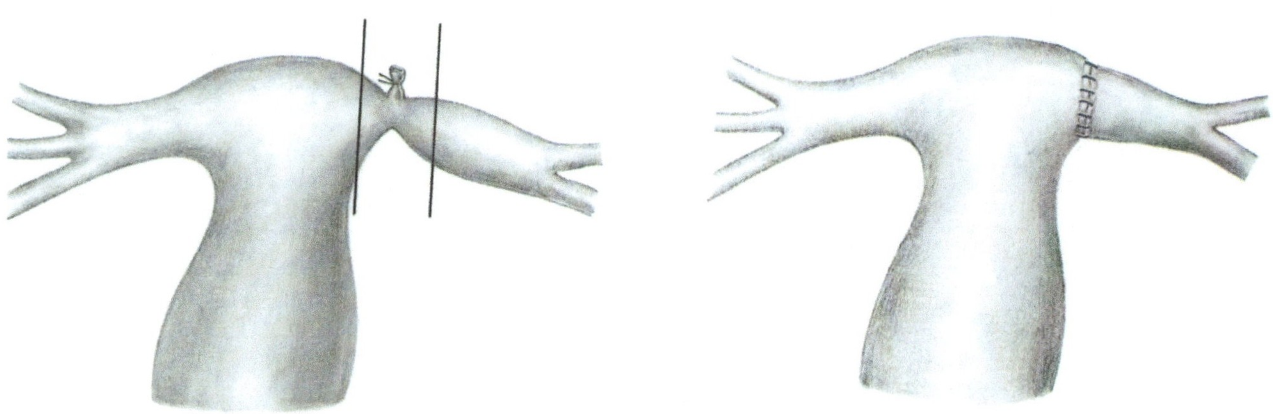

Fig. II-10-3. Relief of branch pulmonary artery stenosis related to the ductus arteriosus. All ductal tissue is removed, and an end-to-end anastomosis is performed with monofilament running suture

References

1. Nugent EW, Freedom RM, Nora JJ, et al (1977) Clinical course in pulmonary stenosis. Circulation 56:sI38–47
2. Hayes CJ, Gersony WM, Driscoll DJ, et al (1993) Second natural history study of congenital heart defects. Results of treatment of patients with pulmonary valvar stenosis. Circulation 87:sI28–37
3. McCrindle BW (1994) Independent predictors of long-term results after balloon pulmonary valvuloplasty. Circulation 89:1751–1759
4. Masura J, Burch M, Deanfield JE, et al (1993) Five year follow-up after balloon pulmonary valvuloplasty. J Am Coll Cardiol 21:132–136
5. Rao PS, Galal O, Patnana M, et al (1998) Results of three to 10 year follow-up of balloon dilatation of the pulmonary valve. Heart 80:591–595
6. Vancini M, Roberts KD, Silove ED, et al (1980) Surgical treatment of congenital pulmonary stenosis due to dysplastic leaflets and small valve annulus. J Thorac Cardiovasc Surg 79:464–468

7. Lock JE, Niemi T, Einzig S, et al (1981) Transvenous angioplasty of experimental branch pulmonary artery stenosis in newborn lambs. Circulation 64:886–893
8. O'Laughlin MP, Slack MC, Grifka RG, et al (1993) Implantation and intermediate-term follow-up of stents in congenital heart disease. Circulation 88:605–614
9. Hosking MC, Thomaidis C, Hamilton R, et al (1992) Clinical impact of balloon angioplasty for branch pulmonary arterial stenosis. Am J Cardiol 69:1467–1470
10. Kan JS, Marvin WJJ, Bass JL, et al (1990) Balloon angioplasty—branch pulmonary artery stenosis: results from the valvuloplasty and angioplasty of congenital anomalies registry. Am J Cardiol 65:798–801

II-11. Pulmonary Atresia with Intact Ventricular Septum

In the patient with pulmonary atresia with intact ventricular septum, the heart has two ventricles, no communication between the right ventricle and pulmonary artery, and no ventricular septal defect. An atrial septal defect or patent foramen oval is present. Tricuspid valve hypoplasia and coronary sinusoids are often seen. Approximately 70%–80% of patients have membranous atresia and the rest have muscular atresia. Most patients with this disease have significant hypoplasia of the right ventricle, although about half of patients have a tripartite right ventricle with inlet, trabecular, and outlet portions [1].

If a right ventricular outflow tract is present, the initial palliative procedure is pulmonary valvotomy and systemic-to-pulmonary artery shunt placement. In the absence of a right ventricular outflow tract, only a systemic-to-pulmonary artery shunt placement is performed. If the development of the right ventricle is not sufficient, a right ventricular overhaul is performed as a second-stage surgery [2,3]. For the final stage of surgery, biventricular repair is performed if the patient has an adequate right ventricle and tricuspid valve (more than 70% of normal size). When the right ventricle and tricuspid valve sizes are not large enough (less than 30% of normal size), Fontan-type surgery is performed. If the sizes of the right ventricle and tricuspid valve are between 30% and 70%, surgical options include biventricular repair, Fontan repair, or one-and-one-half ventricle repair. The last option combines a bidirectional superior cavopulmonary anastomosis with a biventricular repair [4].

Whether pulmonary valvotomy is performed at the time of initial operation is determined by the presence of coronary sinusoid as well as the morphology of the right ventricle. If the right ventricle has communications to the coronary arteries and the coronary arteries have stenosis or interruption, myocardial perfusion is dependent on the right ventricle–coronary artery connection (right ventricle-dependent coronary circulation) [5]. In these patients, because decompression of the right ventricle may result in coronary insufficiency, decompression of the right ventricle is contraindicated. If the presence of right ventricle-dependent coronary circulation is suspected, only a systemic-to-pulmonary artery shunt is performed in the neonate, and further investigation of coronary anatomy is performed later in preparation for subsequent surgery.

Closed Pulmonary Valvotomy: Brock Procedure

When the nature of the pulmonary valve atresia is membranous, a closed pulmonary valvotomy may be appropriate. The heart is exposed through a median sternotomy. A 4-0 horizontal mattress suture buttressed with a pledget is placed in the right ventricular outflow tract. Another pledget is placed opposite the site of the initial sutures, and this suture is attached to a tourniquet. A small stab wound is placed in the middle of this mattress suture with a no. 11 knife. A Brock knife is advanced from this stab across the pulmonary valve (Fig. II-11-1). Hegar dilators are placed into the main pulmonary artery through the pulmonary valve, proceeding from smaller to larger dilators. Ideally, a dilator that is the size of the main pulmonary artery is employed. A systemic-to-pulmonary artery shunt from either the brachiocephalic artery to the right pulmonary artery or from the ascending aorta to the main pulmonary artery is placed (Fig. II-11-2).

Transpulmonary Valvotomy without Cardiopulmonary Bypass [6]

A Blalock–Taussig shunt and pulmonary valvotomy are performed simultaneously. The chest is accessed via a left thoracotomy through the fourth intercostal space. The pericardium is opened longitudinally anterior to the phrenic nerve. The edges of the pericardium are retracted superficially to improve visualization. A vascular clamp is placed on the main pulmonary artery as distally as possible, but proximal to the branching point. The main pulmonary artery is longitudinally opened (Fig. II-11-3). Because there is pulmonary atresia, a bloodless operating field is obtained. A small stab wound is created in the center of the atretic pulmonary valve with a fine scalpel. A 6 Fr. Foley catheter is placed to the right ventricular outflow tract retrograde through the hole in the pulmonary valve. The balloon is inflated, and blood flow from the right ventricle to the main pulmonary artery is controlled. The pulmonary valve is incised at the fused commissures, and care is taken not to damage the balloon. The main pulmonary artery is closed

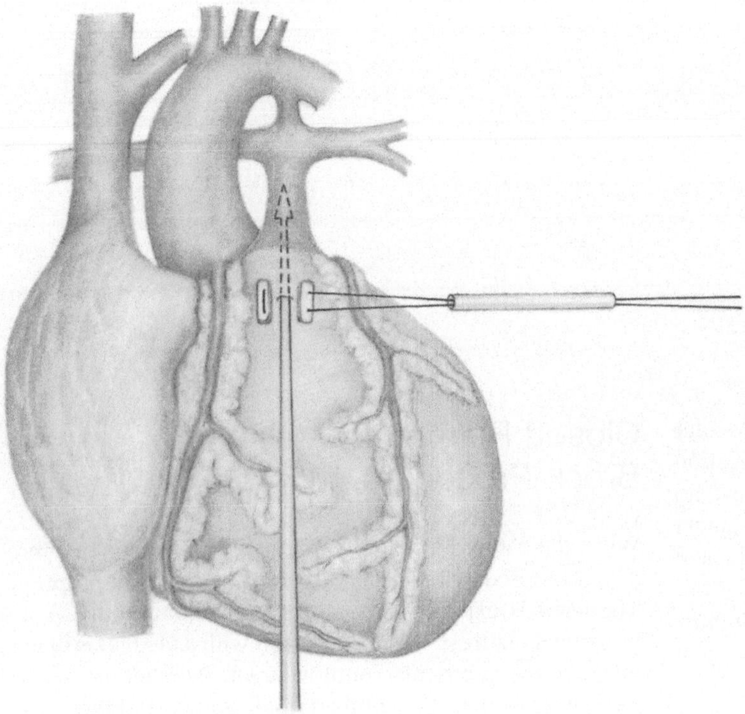

Fig. II-11-1. Closed pulmonary valvotomy: 1

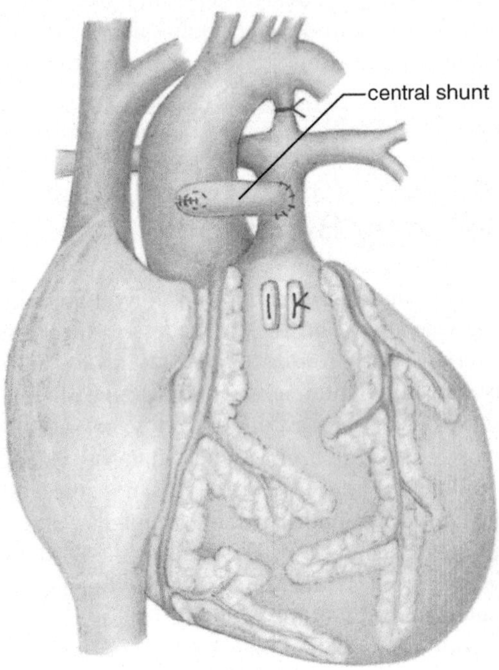

Fig. II-11-2. Closed pulmonary valvotomy: 2

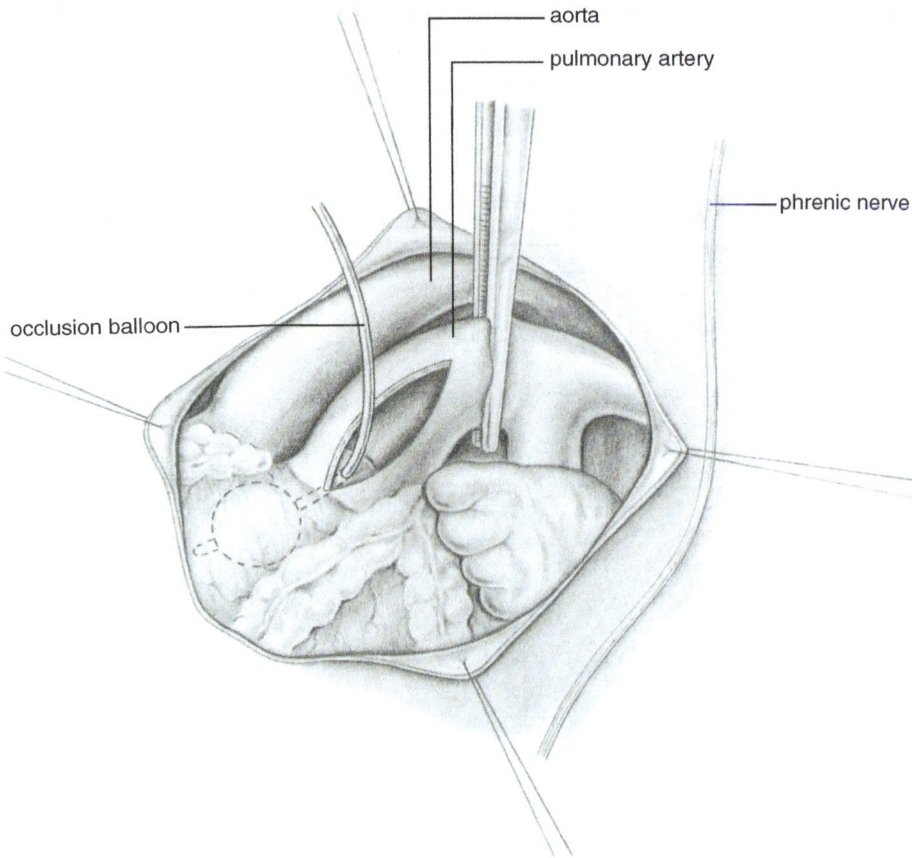

Fig. II-11-3. Transpulmonary valvotomy: 1

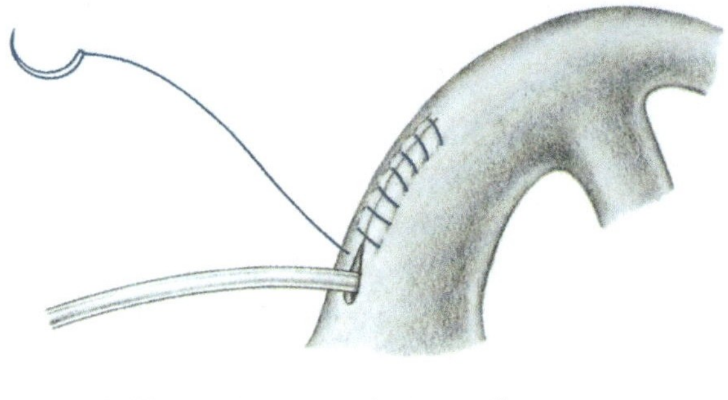

Fig. II-11-4. Transpulmonary valvotomy: 2

with 6-0 monofilament running suture (Fig. II-11-4). The ductus arteriosus is ligated at the end.

Palliative Right Ventricular Outflow Tract Reconstruction

Via a median sternotomy, cardiopulmonary bypass is initiated with ascending aortic and bicaval cannulation. The ductus arteriosus is ligated after bypass initiation. The aortic cross-clamp is placed with cardioplegic arrest and topical cooling. The main pulmonary artery is longitudinally opened. Traction stitches are placed in the edges of the main pulmonary artery to facilitate visualization (Fig. II-11-5). An incision is extended proximally across the pulmonary

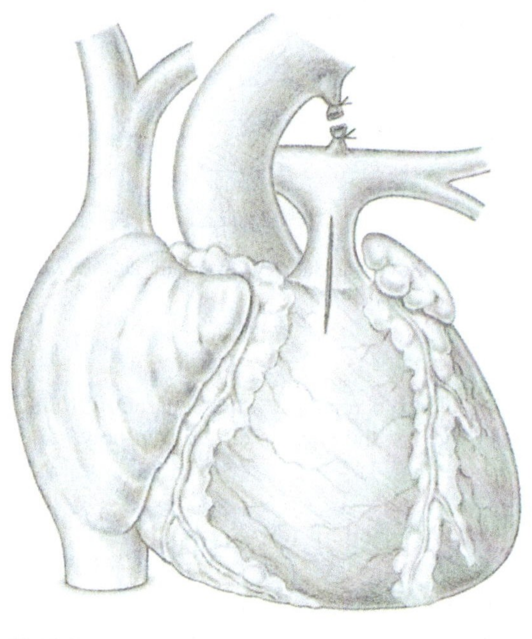

Fig. II-11-5. Palliative right ventricular outflow tract reconstruction: 1

annulus. If the valve tissues are mobile, they are preserved. If the valve tissues are immobile, they are removed. The right ventriculotomy is limited as much as possible. A polytetrafluoroethylene transannular patch is placed using a monofilament running suture (Fig. II-11-6). After de-airing through the cardioplegic site on the ascending aorta, the

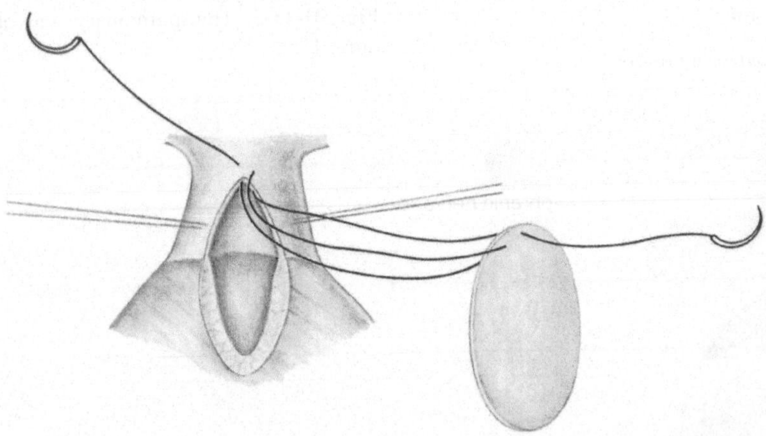

Fig. II-11-6. Palliative right ventricular outflow tract reconstruction: 2

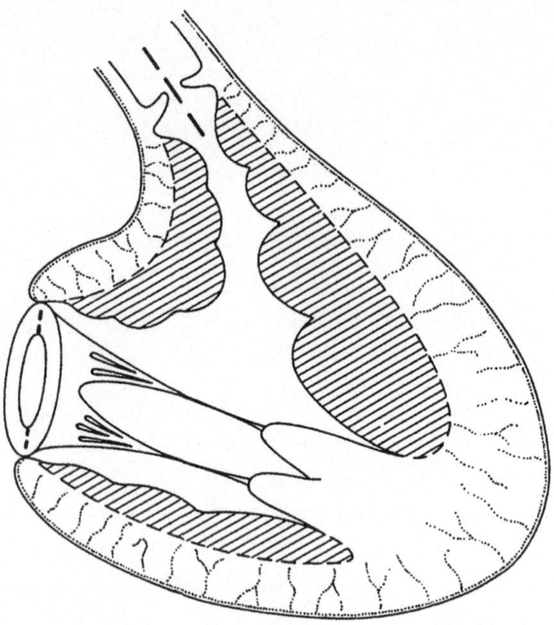

Fig. II-11-7. Right ventricular (RV) overhaul. *Dashed line area* of the right ventricle is resected

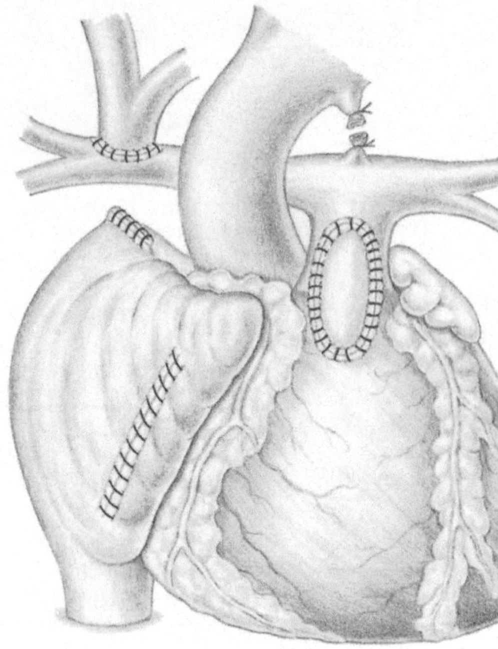

Fig. II-11-8. One-and-one-half ventricle repair

aortic cross-clamp is released. After separation from cardiopulmonary bypass, the chest is closed routinely.

Right Ventricular Overhaul

Except for the papillary muscles supporting the tricuspid valve, any abnormal hypertrophic muscles can be removed from the apical trabecular portion through the tricuspid valve. Care is taken not to create a ventricular septal defect or a defect in the right ventricular (RV) free wall. At the infundibulum, additional muscle resection is performed retrograde through the pulmonary artery. Commissurotomy is performed at the pulmonary valve. If the pulmonary valve is hypoplastic, a transannular patch is placed as in the patient with tetralogy of Fallot. Occasionally, commissurotomy is also necessary on the tricuspid valve (Fig. II-11-7).

One-and-One-Half Ventricular Repair

For patients with normal or slightly small right ventricular volume and tricuspid valve annulus, biventricular repair of right ventricular outflow tract reconstruction and atrial septal defect closure is performed. For the borderline patients with marginal sizes of ventricular volume and tricuspid valve annulus, biventricular repair is performed initially. If central venous pressure exceeds 18 mmHg after separation from cardiopulmonary bypass, a one-and-one-half ventricular repair is performed subsequently by constructing a bidirectional cavopulmonary anastomosis (Fig. II-11-8). An alternative is to partially open the atrial septal defect, which has the disadvantage of resultant desaturation caused by right-to-left shunting through the atrial septal defect. The benefit of a one-and-one-half ventricle repair is the elimination of desaturation after surgery.

References

1. Bull C, de Leval MR, Mercanti C, et al (1982) Pulmonary atresia and intact ventricular septum: a revised classification. Circulation 66:266–272
2. Pawade A, Mee RBB, Karl T (1995) Right ventricular "overhaul": an intermediate step in biventricular repair of pulmonary atresia with intact ventricular septum. Cardiol Young 5:161–165
3. Sano S, Ishino K, Kawada M, et al (2000) Staged biventricular repair of pulmonary atresia or stenosis with intact ventricular septum. Ann Thorac Surg 70:1501–1506
4. Muster AJ, Zales VR, Ilbawi MN, et al (1993) Biventricular repair of hypoplastic right ventricle assisted by pulsatile bi-directional cavopulmonary anastomosis. J Thorac Cardiovasc Surg 105:112–119
5. Giglia TM, Mandell VS, Connor AR, et al (1992) Diagnosis and management of right ventricle-dependent coronary circulation in pulmonary atresia with intact ventricular septum. Circulation 86:1516–1528
6. de Leval M (1994) Pulmonary stenosis and pulmonary atresia with intact ventricular septum. In: Surgery for congenital heart defects, 2nd edn. Saunders, Philadelphia, pp 389–404

II-12. Atrial Septal Defect

There are three types of atrial septal defect (ASD): sinus venosus defects, secundum defects, and primum defects. In this chapter, secundum atrial septal defect is discussed.

The indication for surgery is generally considered to be a pulmonary-to-systemic blood flow ratio of more than 2:1. If the patient is symptomatic, a pulmonary/systemic blood flow ratio of 1.5:1 or more is used as the criterion. The optimal timing of surgery is thought to be just before school age, because of the likelihood of avoiding transfusion, as well as certain psychological benefits. In the infant period, 1%–2% of patients develop heart failure, and early surgery is necessary. In a teenager or adult, pulmonary vascular resistance of more than 14 Wood Units·m^2 is considered to be a contraindication to repair [1,2]. In some cases, the reactivity of the pulmonary vasculature to inhaled oxygen or nitric oxide may need to be evaluated. Rarely, in borderline cases, a lung biopsy may be necessary [3].

Because abnormal pulmonary venous return is occasionally seen in association with a secundum atrial septal defect, pulmonary venous return should be carefully evaluated preoperatively.

Sinus node or atrioventricular (AV) node dysfunction is also occasionally seen, and thus in some patients an electrophysiological study may be needed before surgery.

ASD Closure via Median Sternotomy

A median sternotomy has been the standard approach, although recently a limited midline sternotomy or short skin incision has been utilized more frequently for access to the heart, as described in Chapter 36. The pericardium is opened longitudinally to the right of midline to allow for the possible usage of the pericardium as a patch. After opening the pericardium, cardiac anatomy is inspected externally, especially for the presence of an abnormal pulmonary venous return to the superior vena cava or the right atrium. This inspection should be performed even in patients whose cardiac catheterization study or echocardiography showed no abnormality. Cardiopulmonary bypass is instituted with ascending aortic and bicaval cannulation. In the presence of a left superior vena cava, an additional venous cannula may be inserted into the left superior vena cava directly through the coronary sinus, or a cardiotomy sucker may be inserted. Alternatively, the left superior vena cava may be temporarily occluded during the intracardiac repair.

After aortic cross-clamp, with cardioplegic arrest, the right atrium is opened obliquely along the AV groove from the right atrial appendage to the inferior vena cava (Fig. II-12-1). Retraction stitches are placed in the edges of the atriotomy to improve visualization. The triangle of Koch, which is defined by the base of the septal leaflet of the tricuspid valve, the tendon of Todaro, and the coronary sinus, is identified (Fig. II-12-2). The position and size of the defect are inspected, and the type of defect (sinus venosus, secundum, and primum) is discerned. All the pulmonary veins are identified, and the left atrium is inspected. In patients with atrial fibrillation, the presence of thrombus in the left atrial appendage is checked. A relatively small septal defect may be closed primarily, whereas a large defect should be closed with a patch (Fig. II-12-3). In adult patients, a patch is virtually always used to avoid excess tension on the atrium, which may predispose to arrhythmias.

For direct suture closure, 5-0 or 4-0 monofilament suture is used. Usually the suture closure is started from the inferior corner. At the posterior septal margin, deep bites are utilized. However on the superior margin, deep bites should be avoided to avoid damage to the sinus of Valsalva of the aortic valve. For a defect with a deficient inferior margin, a suture should be placed firmly in the left atrial wall (Fig. II-12-4).

Before finishing defect closure, air in the left atrium is evacuated. The patient is placed with the left side down, and the lung is gently inflated by the anesthesiologist. A hemostat clamp is placed into the left atrium across the superior end of the suture line, and de-airing is accomplished.

Aortic venting is instituted via the cardioplegic cannula. After the right atrium is filled with blood, the suture line is tied. Blood is aspirated from the right atrium to obtain a bloodless field. The lung is inflated by the anesthesiologist again, and the presence of the residual shunt is assessed. If a residual shunt is identified, additional stitches are placed. Before removal of the aortic clamp, the left atrium and ventricle are compressed manually for additional de-airing. After aortic declamping, the right atriotomy is closed using 5-0 monofilament running suture. Before finishing this closure, tourniquets are released and the right atrium is filled with blood to expel air from the right atrium.

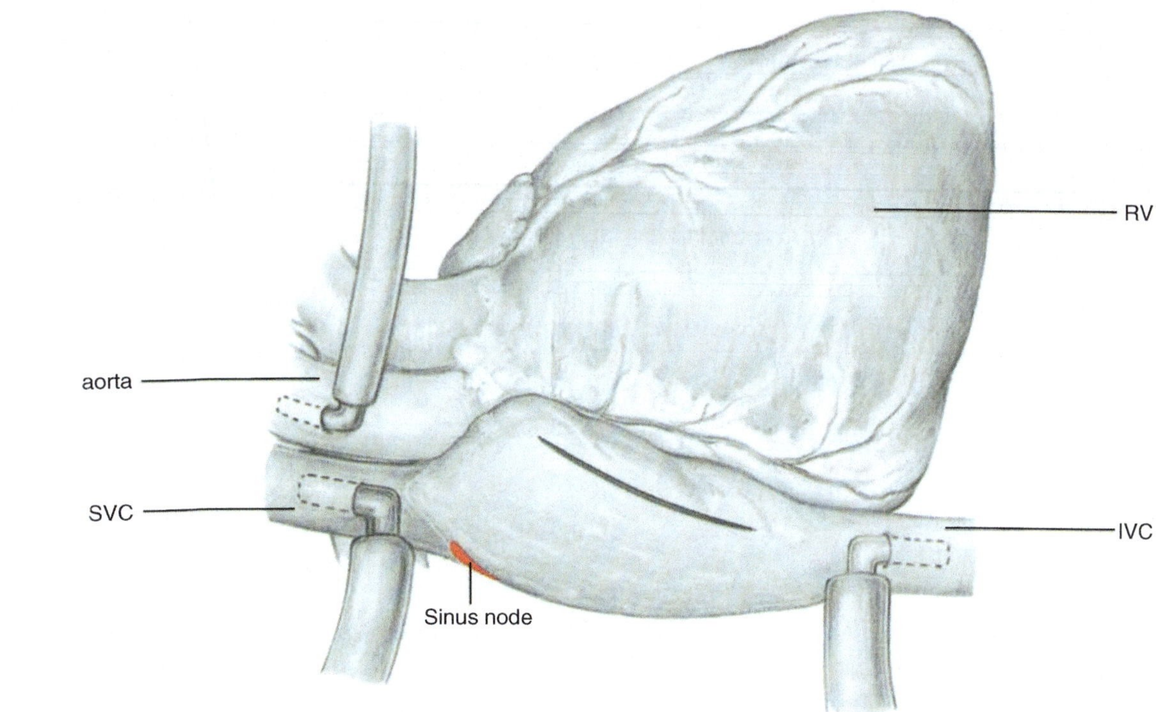

Fig. II-12-1. Institution of cardiopulmonary bypass. Ascending aortic and bicaval cannulation is used. The superior vena cava (SVC) cannula can be inserted from the right atrial appendage into the *SVC*. The right atriotomy is placed 1–2 cm from the atrioventricular (AV) groove from the base of the right atrial appendage to the inferior vena cava (*IVC*). *RV*, right ventricle

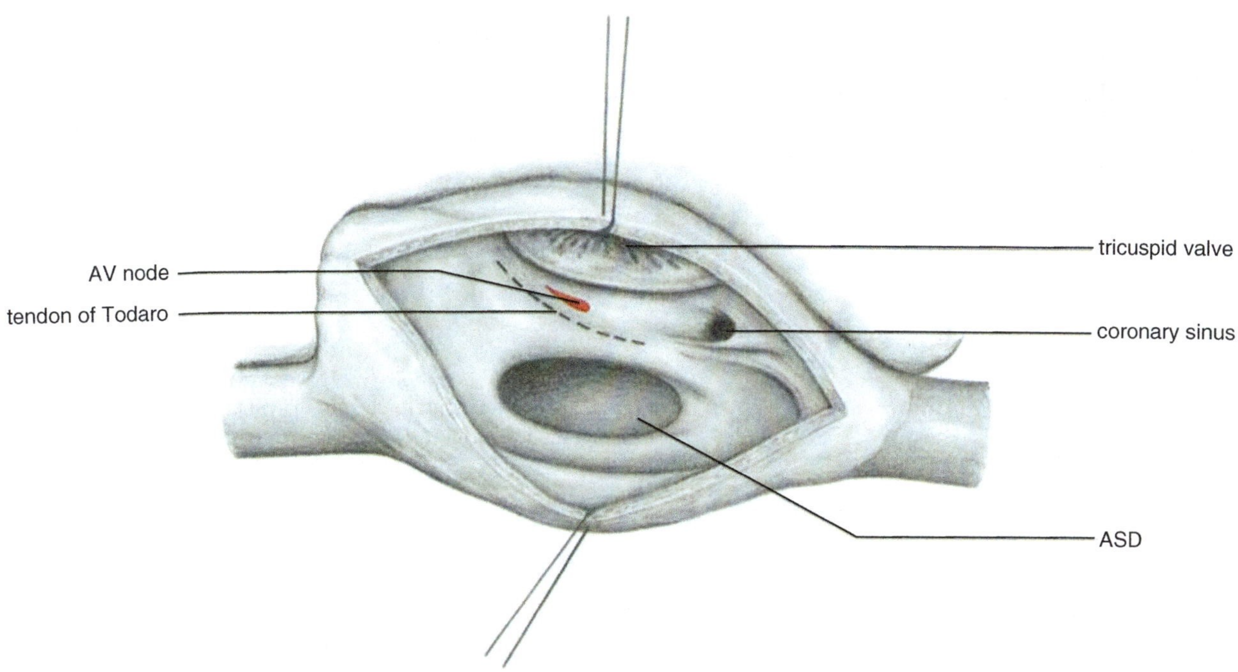

Fig. II-12-2. Anatomy of atrial septal defect (*ASD*). The triangle of Koch is composed of the base of the septal leaflet of the tricuspid valve, coronary sinus, and tendon of Todaro. The *AV* node is located at the apex of this triangle

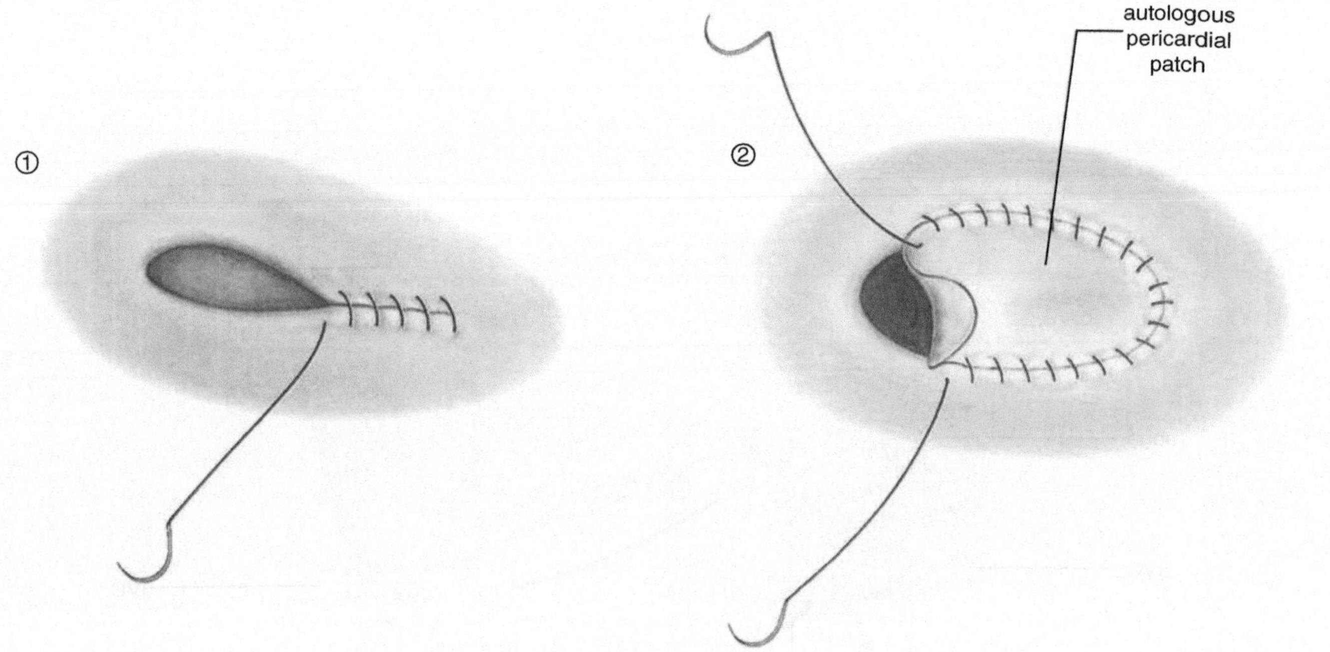

Fig. II-12-3. Technique of ASD closure. An oval hole may be closed by direct suture ①. A large defect should be closed using a patch ②

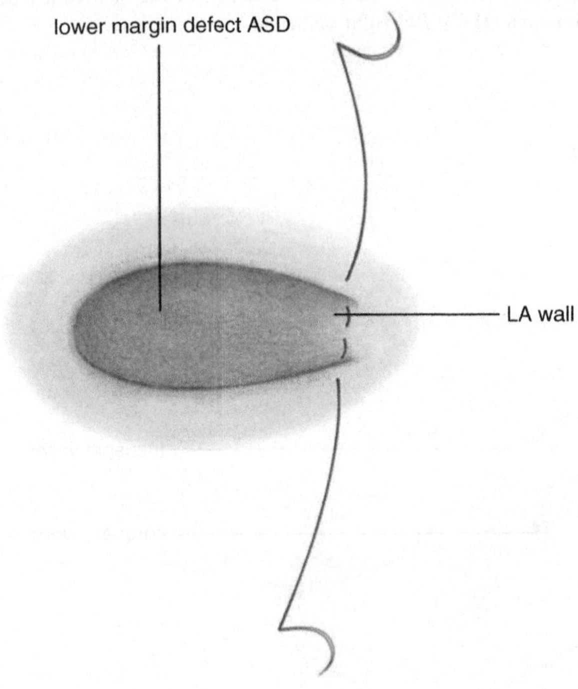

Fig. II-12-4. Direct suture closure of ASD. When the inferior margin is missing, the left atrial (*LA*) wall is used to close the defect at the inferior margin

Choice of Patch Material

An autologous pericardium is used as a first choice, and to avoid thromboembolism, the smooth surface should be placed to the left atrial side [4]. The patch is prepared according to the size and shape of the defect. Fibrous tissue on the pericardium is removed bluntly with a sponge or sharply with scissors. Retraction stitches are placed in the patch at four points. The patch is anastomosed with a running suture (Fig. II-12-5). The redundant part of the patch is removed if necessary.

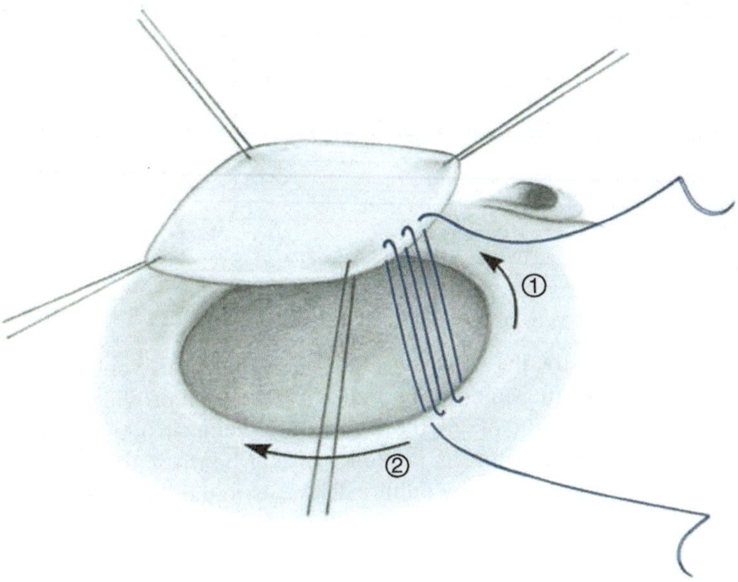

Fig. II-12-5. Patch closure of ASD. Four traction sutures are placed in the patch. Suturing is started at the inferior margin. Running suture is advanced toward the base of the tricuspid valve ①. Then, the other arm is carried along the other margin ②

ASD Closure via Right Thoracotomy

In some cases, for cosmetic reasons a right thoracotomy may be elected for repair of an atrial septal defect [5].

The skin incision is started 1 cm below the inferior margin of the scapula and extended toward the midpoint between nipple and costal arch. Care is taken not to extend the incision beyond the anterior axillary line. The chest is entered through the fourth intercostal space, and the intercostal space is opened longer than the skin incision. The pericardium is opened longitudinally 1–2 cm anterior and parallel to the phrenic nerve. Retraction stitches are placed in the edges of this pericardial opening to facilitate visualization of the great vessels. Retraction stitches are placed slightly deeper than the edges of the opening to the pericardium. Tapes are passed around the ascending aorta and the superior vena cava. A tape around the inferior vena cava is placed after institution of the cardiopulmonary bypass to avoid damage to the inferior vena cava during passage of the tape. Two purse-string sutures are always placed in the ascending aorta as insurance. A flexible straight cannula is used as an aortic cannula.

The major difference from the standard median sternotomy approach is increased difficulty in de-airing from the left side of the heart with the thoracotomy approach. Care must be taken not to aspirate too much blood from the left side of the heart through the atrial septal defect during surgery. If filling of the left side of the heart is not sufficient, the lung is inflated by the anesthesiologist during tying of the repair suture. The operative field is flooded with carbon dioxide during surgery to avoid air embolism. The technique to close the defect is the same as that of median sternotomy. To prevent cardiac tamponade, the pericardium is closed loosely. A single chest tube is placed in the right pleural space with no tubes in the mediastinum.

References

1. Steele PM, Fuster V, Cohen M, et al (1987) Isolated atrial septal defect with pulmonary vascular obstructive disease: long-term follow-up and prediction of outcome after surgical correction. Circulation 76:1037–1042
2. Hashimoto A, Momma K, Hayakawa H, et al (1991) Natural histories of atrial septal defect with pulmonary hypertension, and ventricular septal defect with pulmonary hypertension. Jpn Circ J 55:791–793
3. Yamaki S, Horiuchi T, Miura M, et al (1986) Pulmonary vascular disease in secundum atrial septal defect with pulmonary hypertension. Chest 89:694–698
4. Haas GS, Laks H, Perloff JK (1991) The selection, use, and long-term effects of prosthetic materials. In: Perloff JK, Child JS (eds) Congenital heart disease in adults. Saunders, Philadelphia, pp 213–223
5. Lancaster LL, Mavroudis C, Rees AH, et al (1990) Surgical approach to atrial septal defect in the female. Right thoracotomy versus sternotomy. Am Surg 56:218–221

II-13. Partial Anomalous Pulmonary Venous Return

Hemodynamically, partial anomalous pulmonary venous return (PAPVR) (Fig. II-13-1) is identified as an atrial level or caval level left-to-right shunt. Typically, there is also a true atrial septal defect (ASD) [1]. The amount of shunt depends on the size and number of anomalous pulmonary veins and the size of the ASD. Patients may have no symptoms or may be limited by congestive heart failure secondary to a large left-to-right shunt. Virtually all patients require surgery because of the large left-to-right shunt, even in the absence of symptoms, and the ASD is repaired simultaneously.

Generally, this type of defect is repaired at an older age, compared to the circumstances with total anomalous pulmonary venous drainage. In general, for the partial form, the risk is lower, and the prognosis is considered better. The surgical procedure is based on the type of pulmonary venous return. In this chapter, the more common types of right pulmonary vein returning to the superior vena cava, right pulmonary vein returning to the right atrium, and left pulmonary vein returning to the innominate vein are discussed.

Returning to Superior Vena Cava Type, Ordinary Procedure and Williams Procedure

A majority of patients with this type of PAPVR also have a sinus venosus ASD. In most patients, the abnormal pulmonary veins drain to the proximal superior vena cava (SVC). These defects are repaired by rerouting pulmonary vein flow toward the sinus venosus ASD using an intraatrial tunnel. The SVC is also enlarged to avoid stenosis.

The heart is exposed via median sternotomy. The SVC is mobilized up to its junction of the innominate vein. A tape is placed around the azygous vein. The SVC is typically noted to be enlarged from the junction of abnormal veins. Cardiopulmonary bypass is instituted with ascending aortic and bicaval cannulation. A right-angled cannula is inserted into the high SVC directly. Cardiac arrest is obtained with cardioplegic solution. The right atrium (RA) is opened obliquely from the base of the right atrial appendage. Through this opening, the abnormal pulmonary veins are inspected. The presence of other abnormal veins is sought.

Usually, the ASD is a superior type of sinus venosus ASD missing the superior margin. This approach provides limited visualization of all the pulmonary veins inside the SVC. Even if exposure is possible, it may be difficult to place a patch to reroute the pulmonary veins to the left atrium (LA) without compromising SVC flow. In this situation a second incision is placed longitudinally, in front of the abnormal pulmonary vein and behind and parallel to the sulcus terminalis (Fig. II-13-2). Through this second incision, the pulmonary veins are visualized. Some authors suggest that the caudal part of this incision should be brought anteriorly to cross the crista terminalis [2]. We believe that this kind of extension of incision damages the posterior portion of the sinus node and the preferential pathway between the sinus node and AV node [3]. Although the clinical significance of preservation of the preferential pathway is not clear, on general principles it is preferable to minimize damage to the conduction system.

Through this second incision, the tunnel, which brings blood from the anomalous pulmonary vein to the ASD, is created. An autologous pericardial patch is used because of its flexibility. The anastomosis is started from the top corner of the pulmonary vein orifice. To obtain an adequate tunnel diameter, the posterior surface of the SVC is utilized for the patch placement (Fig. II-13-3). The orifice of the azygous vein will be superior to the pulmonary vein orifice, but if separation of the orifice of the azygous vein is difficult, the azygous vein may be ligated. The posterior suture line is stopped at the superior margin of the ASD. Next, the anterior suture line is carried down along the incision in the SVC. When this suture line comes down to the end of the second incision, the needle is passed into the atrium, and the rest of the suture line is completed through the first atriotomy incision (Fig. II-13-4). If the patient has a more central type ASD, the superior margin of the ASD can be removed to shorten the length of the pulmonary venous baffle. If the patient has a small sinus venosus ASD, the ASD should be enlarged inferiorly toward the fossa ovalis to prevent stenosis of the pulmonary vein route.

Next, to obtain an adequate SVC dimension, the second incision is enlarged with a generous oval-shaped autologous pericardial or polytetrafluoroethylene (PTFE) patch (Fig. II-13-5). The second incision should be started higher than the pulmonary vein tunnel and ended 2–3 cm lower from the SVC–RA junction. Finally, the oblique right atriotomy is closed.

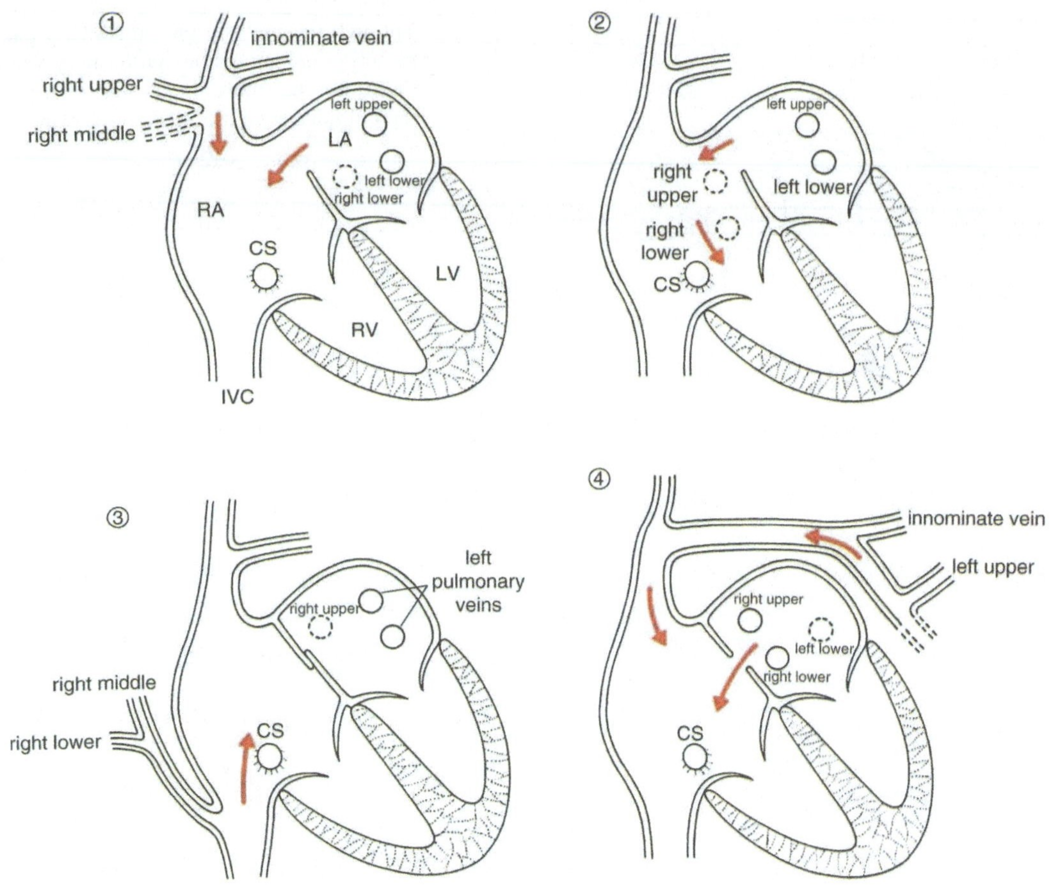

Fig. II-13-1. Partial anomalous pulmonary venous return. ① Right pulmonary veins returning to the superior vena cava (SVC); ② right pulmonary veins returning to the right atrium (*RA*); ③ right pulmonary veins returning to the inferior vena cava (*IVC*) (Scimitar syndrome etc.); ④ left pulmonary veins returning to the innominate vein. *CS*, coronary sinus; *LA*, left atrium; *LV*, left ventricle; *RV*, right ventricle

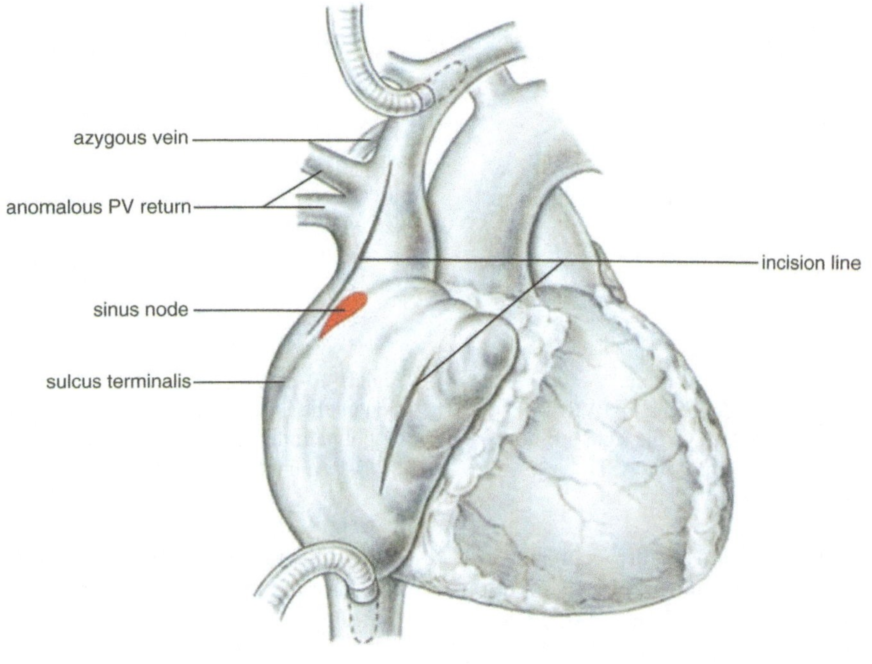

Fig. II-13-2. Right atriotomy for right pulmonary veins returning to the superior vena cava (SVC). The SVC cannula is placed at the SVC–innominate vein junction. Through the standard right atriotomy, the atrial septal defect (ASD) and orifices of the anomalous pulmonary veins are inspected. A second incision is placed toward the SVC–RA junction parallel and posterior to the sulcus terminalis. *PV*, pulmonary vein

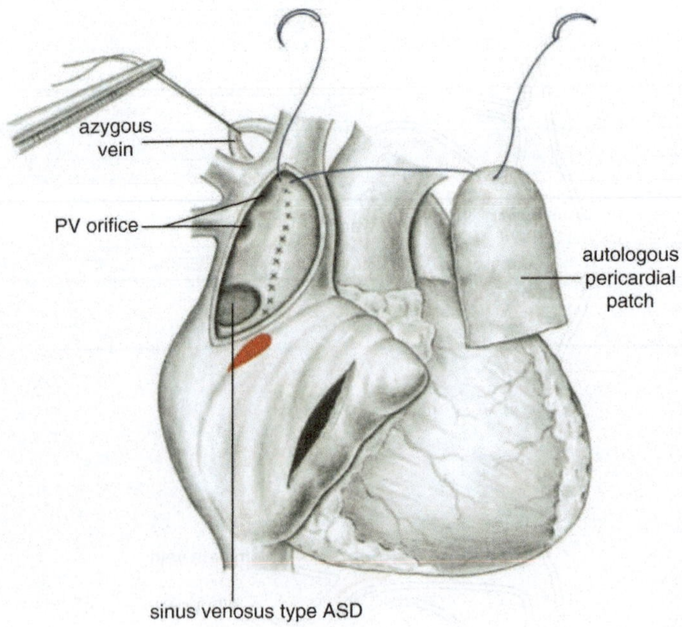

Fig. II-13-3. Patch placement for SVC-type partial anomalous pulmonary venous return (PAPVR): 1. Through the incision on the SVC, a patch is placed for rerouting the anomalous pulmonary venous flow toward the ASD. The suture line is started at the superior end of the pulmonary vein orifice and advanced inferiorly

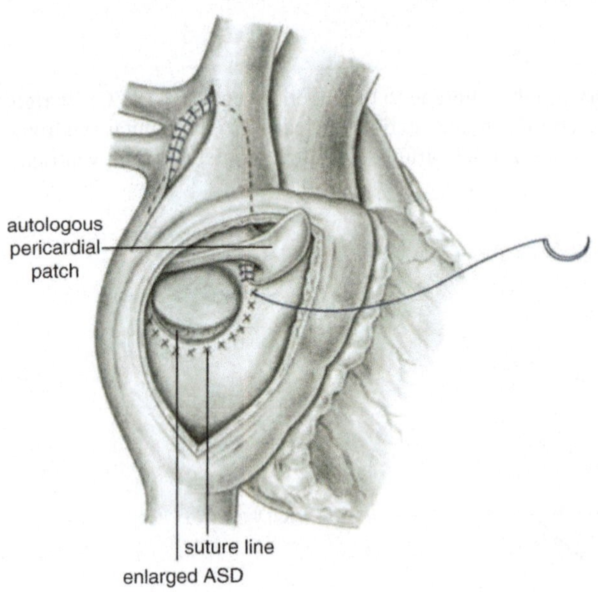

Fig. II-13-4. Patch placement for SVC-type PAPVR: 2. The ASD is enlarged at the superior margin through the right atriotomy. The patch is sutured to the inferior margin of the ASD

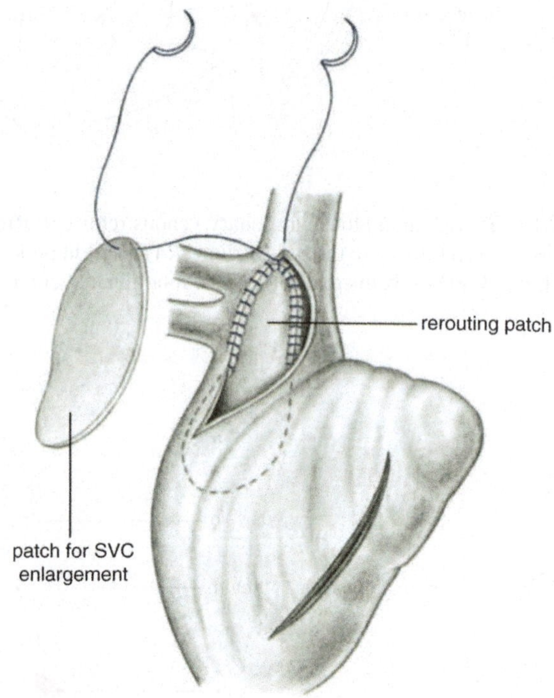

Fig. II-13-5. SVC enlargement for SVC-type PAPVR. The incision on the SVC is closed using an elliptical autologous pericardial or polytetrafluoroethylene (PTFE) patch to avoid stenosis at the SVC–RA junction

If the abnormal pulmonary veins return cephalad to the edge of the right pulmonary artery, the previously mentioned partition of the SVC is difficult to perform. In small patients especially, the risk of postoperative pulmonary vein stenosis or SVC syndrome is quite high. For these cases, a better alternative is to perform the Williams procedure [4], which utilizes the proximal SVC as the pulmonary venous pathway and uses the right atrial appendage as the systemic venous route.

To perform the Williams procedure, extensive mobilization of the SVC and proximal innominate vein is necessary. The azygous vein is doubly ligated and divided. The SVC is pulled down and its mobility is ascertained. It is advantageous to put the venous cannula far cephalad to the anomalous vein, and so the purse-string suture is placed at the junction of the innominate vein and SVC. If necessary, the cannula can be inserted into the innominate vein itself. After initiation of cardiopulmonary bypass, a clamp (instead of the usual tourniquet) is applied to the SVC.

After aortic cross-clamp and cardioplegic arrest, a J-shaped incision is placed in the RA (Fig. II-13-6). The incision is begun at the base of the right atrial appendage. The RA is inspected from this incision, including the position of the ASD. The incision is extended rightward and stopped at the crista terminalis. If necessary, the ASD is enlarged. For a central ASD, the ASD is enlarged superiorly, and in small sinus venosus ASD, the ASD is enlarged inferiorly. The wall of the atriotomy is anastomosed to the anterior margin of the ASD. This suture line is started at the top of the incision and carried caudally, ending at the crista terminalis (Fig. II-13-7). Next, a vent is inserted via the left atrial appendage. Then, the SVC is divided above the anomalous pulmonary vein. The division is started a few millimeters above the anomalous pulmonary vein entrance to avoid pulmonary vein stenosis and placed obliquely to leave a sufficient length of the SVC. The proximal SVC is oversewn, and this completes pulmonary venous rerouting. The anterior edge of the J-shaped incision is used to cover the posterior flap, which completes closure of the RA (Fig. II-13-8). This suture line is started cephalad and carried caudally. To avoid damage to the sinus node, the suture line is kept away from the line of the SVC–RA junction to the sulcus terminalis line. As the suture line is advanced, the

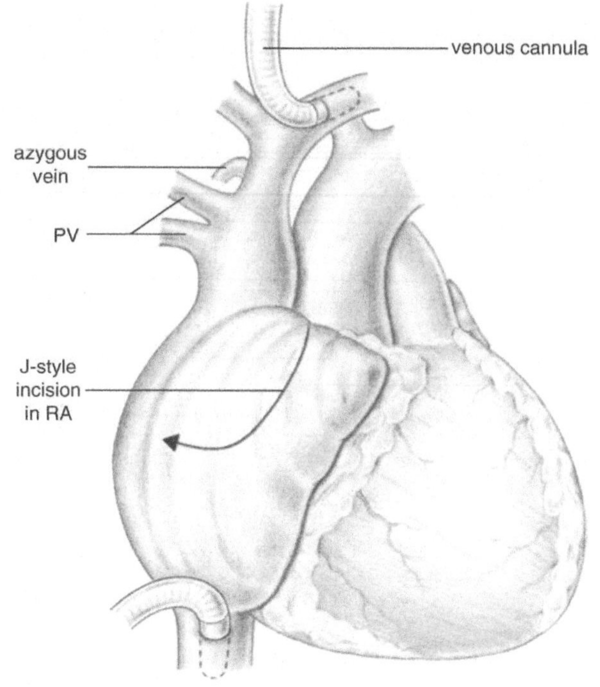

Fig. II-13-6. Williams procedure: an incision to the right atrium. An incision is started at the base of the right atrial appendage and advanced inferiorly. Then the inside of the right atrium is inspected, especially the location and size of the ASD. The incision is brought up to the crista terminalis toward the inferior margin of the ASD to create a J-shaped opening

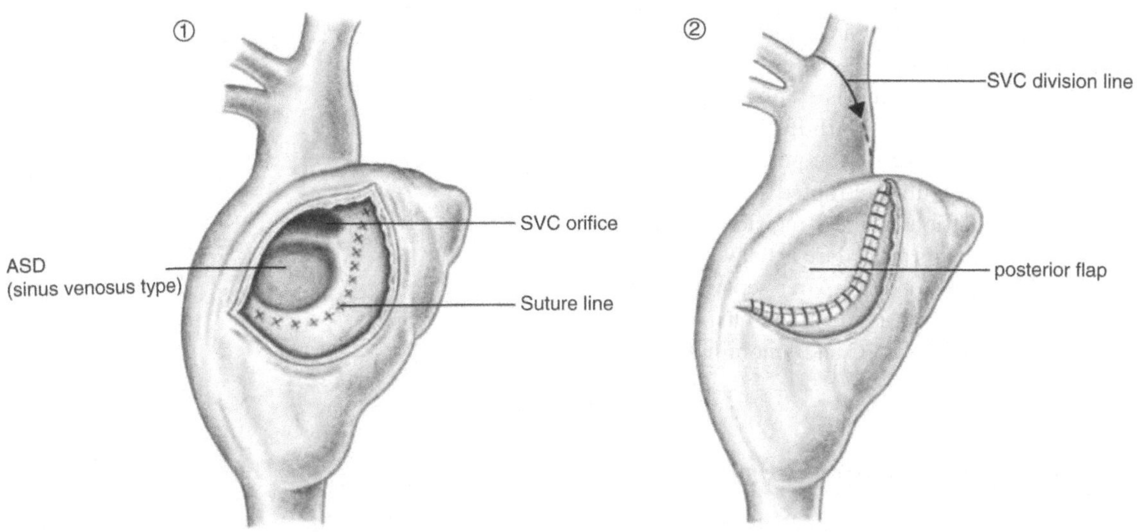

Fig. II-13-7. Williams procedure: posterior flap suture and division of the SVC. Suturing of the posterior flap is started at the superior end to cover the orifice of the SVC and advanced along the anterior and inferior margins of the ASD. This step is finished at the crista terminalis. The division of the SVC is started 2–3 mm above the pulmonary vein entrance site and advanced obliquely toward the left side of proximal SVC

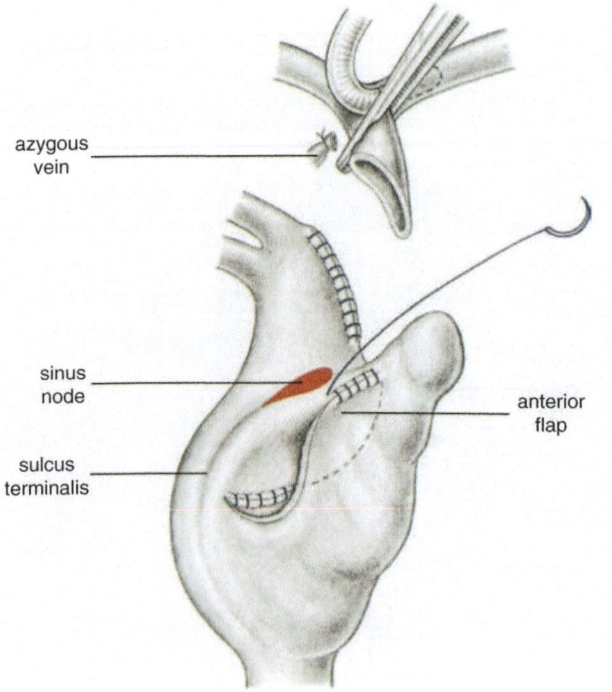

Fig. II-13-8. Williams procedure: anterior flap suture. Suturing is started at the superior end and carried inferiorly, keeping some distance from the sulcus terminalis to protect the sinus node

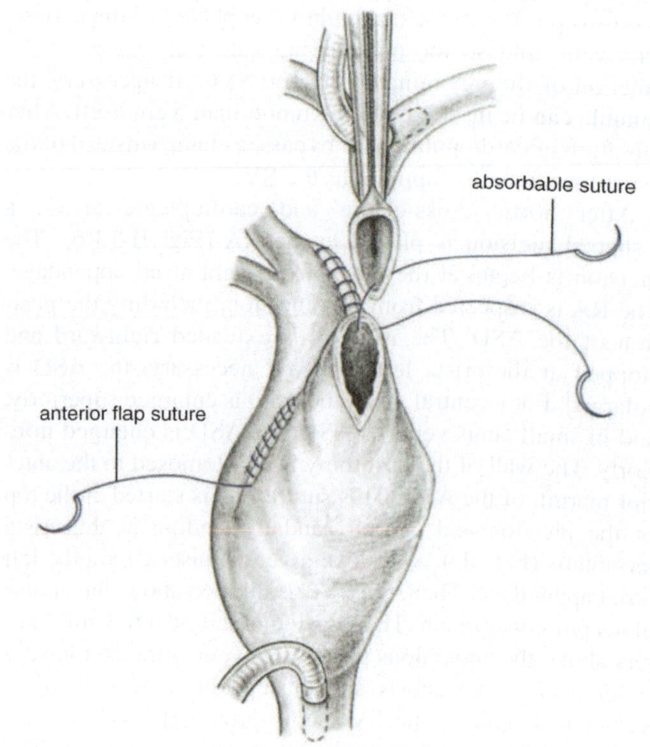

Fig. II-13-9. Williams procedure: anastomosis between the SVC and the right atrial appendage. An incision is placed in the right atrial appendage, larger than the SVC orifice. The pectinate muscles are excised from the right atrial wall. The anastomosis between the SVC and this right atrial opening is performed with a running suture in the posterior wall and interrupted sutures in the anterior wall

right atrial appendage is brought rightward from its original position. This repositioning of the atrial appendage brings the appendage just inferior to the SVC. Before completion of the final third of this suture line, the SVC is anastomosed to the right atrial appendage. To accomplish the SVC–RA appendage anastomosis, an opening is created in the right atrial appendage, larger than the size of the SVC. Through this opening, the pectinate muscles are removed. Then, it is helpful to pass a Hegar that is at least the same size as the SVC to confirm that the anastomosis is of adequate size. Then, anastomosis is started (Fig. II-13-9) using a fine absorbable monofilament suture for the posterior wall. The anterior wall is completed with interrupted sutures. Finally, the closure of the last portion of the J-incision is finished (Fig. II-13-10). The key to this procedure is to avoid stenosis of the appendage–SVC anastomosis. After separation from the bypass, if excessive tension is identified at this anastomosis, further dissection of the SVC and innominate vein is instituted.

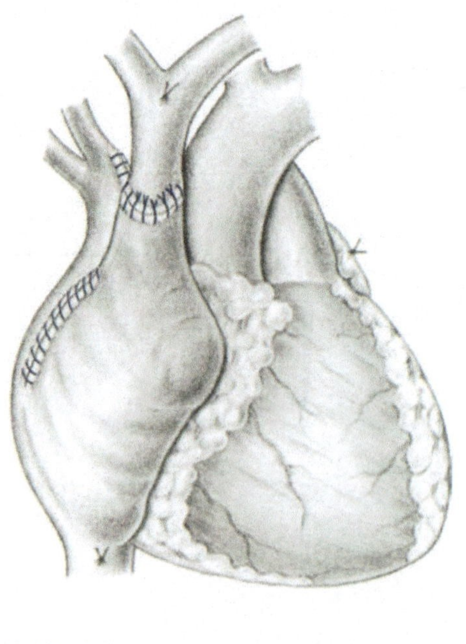

Fig. II-13-10. Williams procedure: after completion of repair. When excessive tension is present at the anastomosis between the SVC and right atrial appendage, the SVC–innominate junction is dissected to decrease the tension to the anastomosis

Returning to Right Atrium Type

In this most common type of partial anomalous pulmonary venous return, the right pulmonary veins drain to the sinus part of the right atrium. Preoperatively these patients are diagnosed as having a large shunt ASD, and partial anomalous pulmonary venous drainage is often overlooked. Surgery is relatively straightforward, and additional dissection is not necessary. Standard cardiopulmonary bypass is utilized. A venous cannula for the SVC through the right atrial appendage is acceptable. Approach via right thoracotomy or limited sternotomy are equally efficacious. After aortic cross-clamp, the RA is opened obliquely from the base of the right atrial appendage (Fig. II-13-11). Through the RA, abnormal pulmonary venous return is inspected, and through the ASD, normal left-sided pulmonary venous return in the LA is identified. If the ASD is central and small, the fossa ovalis tissue and the posterior limbus are removed, enlarging the ASD (Fig. II-13-12). In the case of sinus venosus ASD, usually the ASD is located next to the abnormal pulmonary veins. Atrial septal tissue is often missing between the ASD and orifices of the abnormal pulmonary vein. An autologous pericardial patch is used for intraatrial baffle, and ASD and abnormal pulmonary vein orifices are covered. The atriotomy is directly closed in the end.

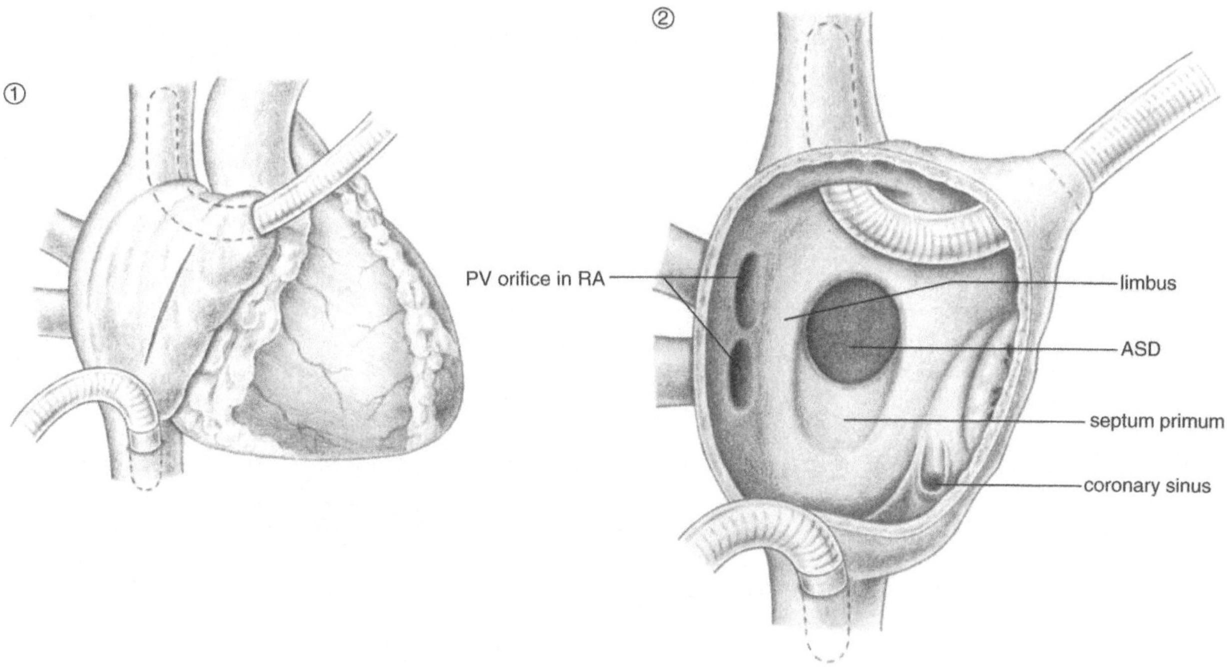

Fig. II-13-11. Right pulmonary veins returning to the right atrium (**1**). After a standard right atriotomy, the intracardiac anatomy is inspected (**2**)

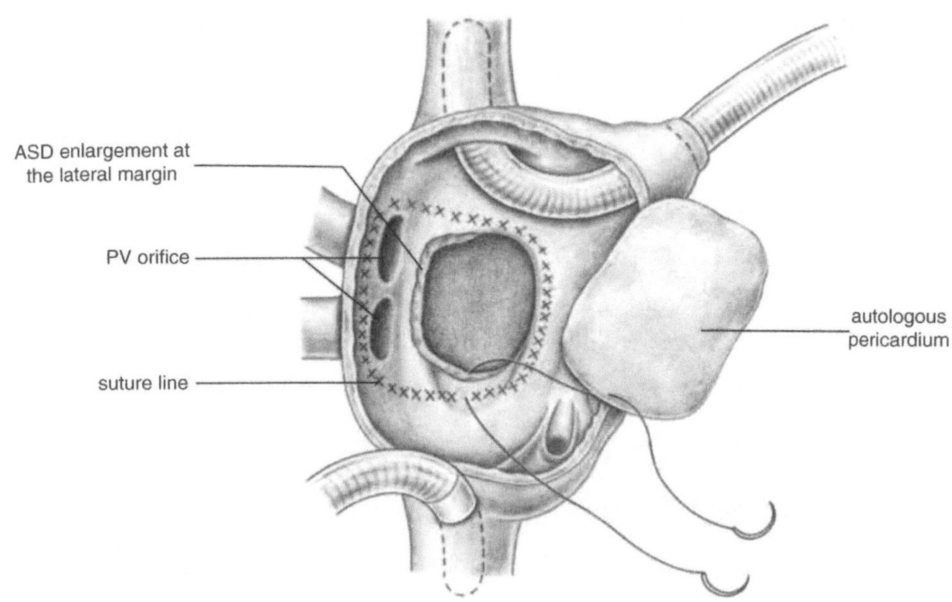

Fig. II-13-12. Patch placement for the anomalous right pulmonary venous (PV) return. The ASD is enlarged

An alternative technique employs the right atrial free wall to create an intraatrial tunnel. The atriotomy is placed slightly closer to the AV groove, and from each end of this incision, transverse incisions are placed superiorly and inferiorly toward the crista terminalis. A rectangular-shape flap is thus created (Fig. II-13-13 ①). This flap is used as a patch to baffle the anomalous pulmonary veins to the LA. If there is a septum primum, the septum primum is utilized as a flap from the anterior margin (Fig. II-13-13 ②). Finally, the right atrial wall is anastomosed to the anterior surface of the flap, and the RA is closed (Fig. II-13-14).

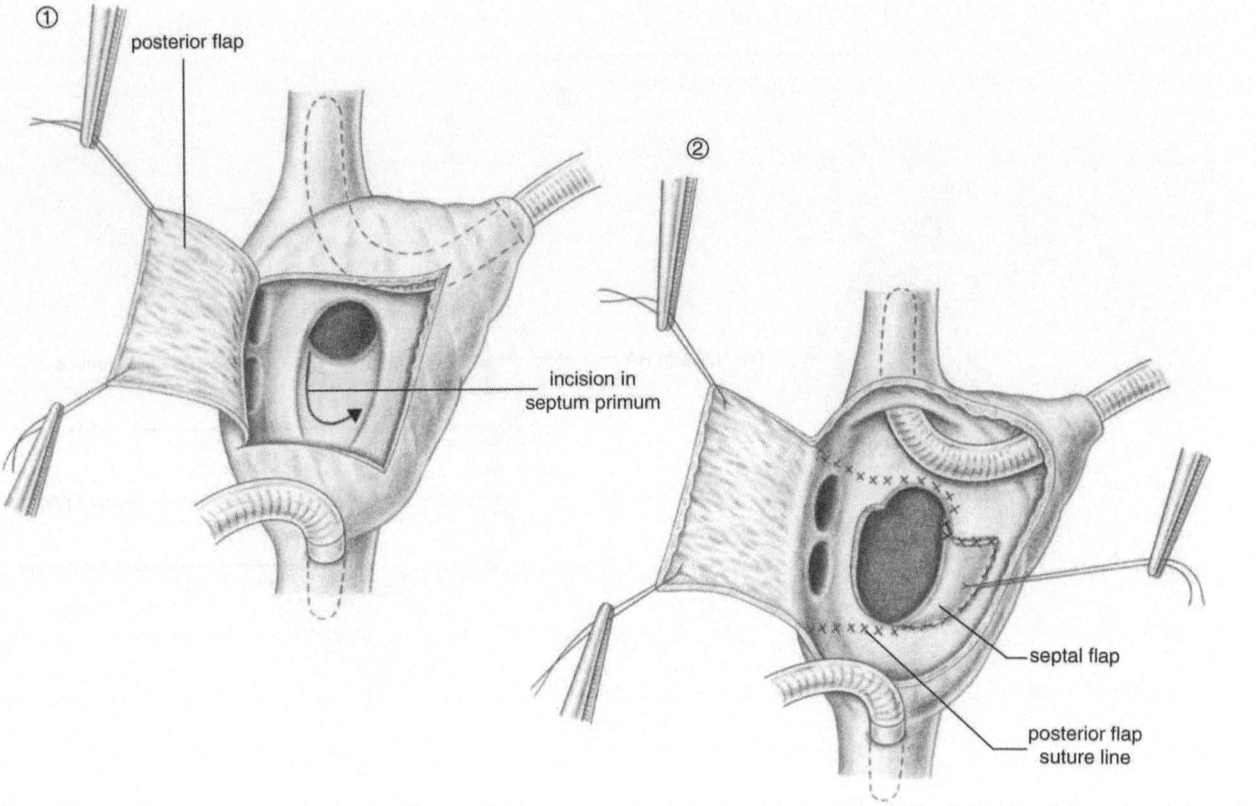

Fig. II-13-13. Repair using right atrial wall: 1. The septum primum is mobilized ① to enlarge the ASD and facilitate baffle construction ②

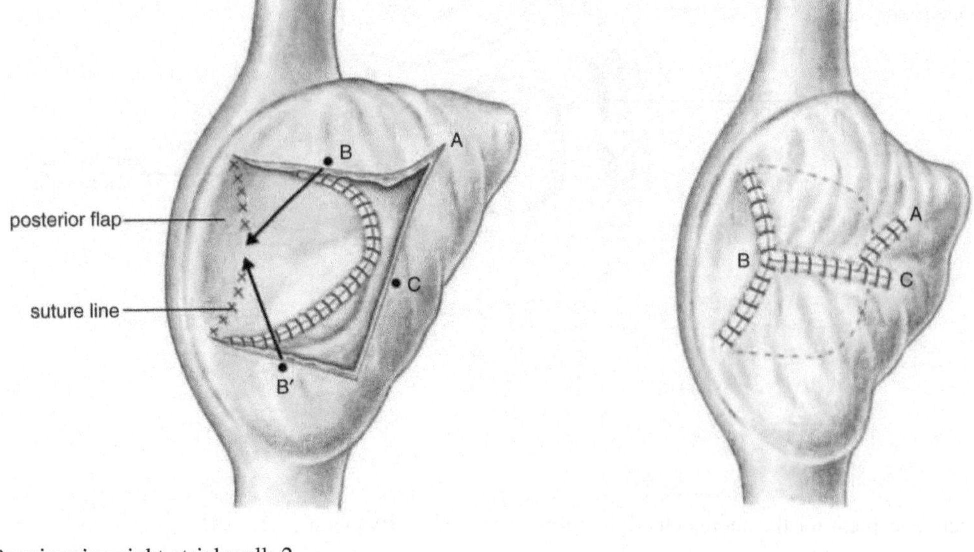

Fig. II-13-14. Repair using right atrial wall: 2

Left Pulmonary Vein Returning to Innominate Vein Type

This is a rare anomaly that is usually associated with other cardiac defects. Surgical repair consists of anastomosis between the anomalous vein and the left atrial appendage. The likelihood of anastomotic stenosis is relatively high. Therefore, if the patient is young or the amount of shunt is very small, the abnormality may be left uncorrected [5].

Surgery is performed via median sternotomy. Before initiation of cardiopulmonary bypass, the area of left pulmonary vein returning to the innominate vein is dissected. The abnormal vein ascends in front of the left PA. After the left lobe of the thymus is bluntly dissected, the junction of the abnormal pulmonary vein to the innominate vein is visualized. A silk string is put around this abnormal vein for later ligation (Fig. II-13-15). From this point the abnormal vein is bluntly dissected distally, with care taken to avoid the damage to the phrenic nerve. Dissection from outside the pericardium facilitates the visualization of whole abnormal pulmonary vein. Occasionally the edge of pericardium may be cut down toward the left hilum, which improves exposure of the operative field. Cardiopulmonary bypass is instituted in the usual fashion. After cardioplegic arrest, the abnormal pulmonary vein is anastomosed to the left atrial appendage. The technique of cannulation is determined depending on other cardiac defects.

The abnormal pulmonary vein is ligated as close as possible to the innominate vein and divided. The pulmonary vein end is brought toward the left atrial appendage. A defect is created in the pericardium behind the phrenic nerve to bring the pulmonary vein into the pericardium, and this defect should be large enough to avoid stenosis of the pulmonary vein. Care is taken to avoid kinking of the pulmonary vein. The length of the pulmonary vein is adjusted to fit the LA. Two traction sutures are placed to the edges of the pulmonary vein cephalad and caudal to preserve orientation. The end of the pulmonary vein is longitudinally incised to create a large opening. If blood return is excessive, a bulldog clamp is placed on the abnormal pulmonary vein to allow a bloodless field. Next, a hole is created in the left atrial appendage. The surgeon changes position to the left side of the patient at this stage. The assistant elevates the apex of the heart toward the right side of the table to improve visualization of the base of the left atrial appendage.

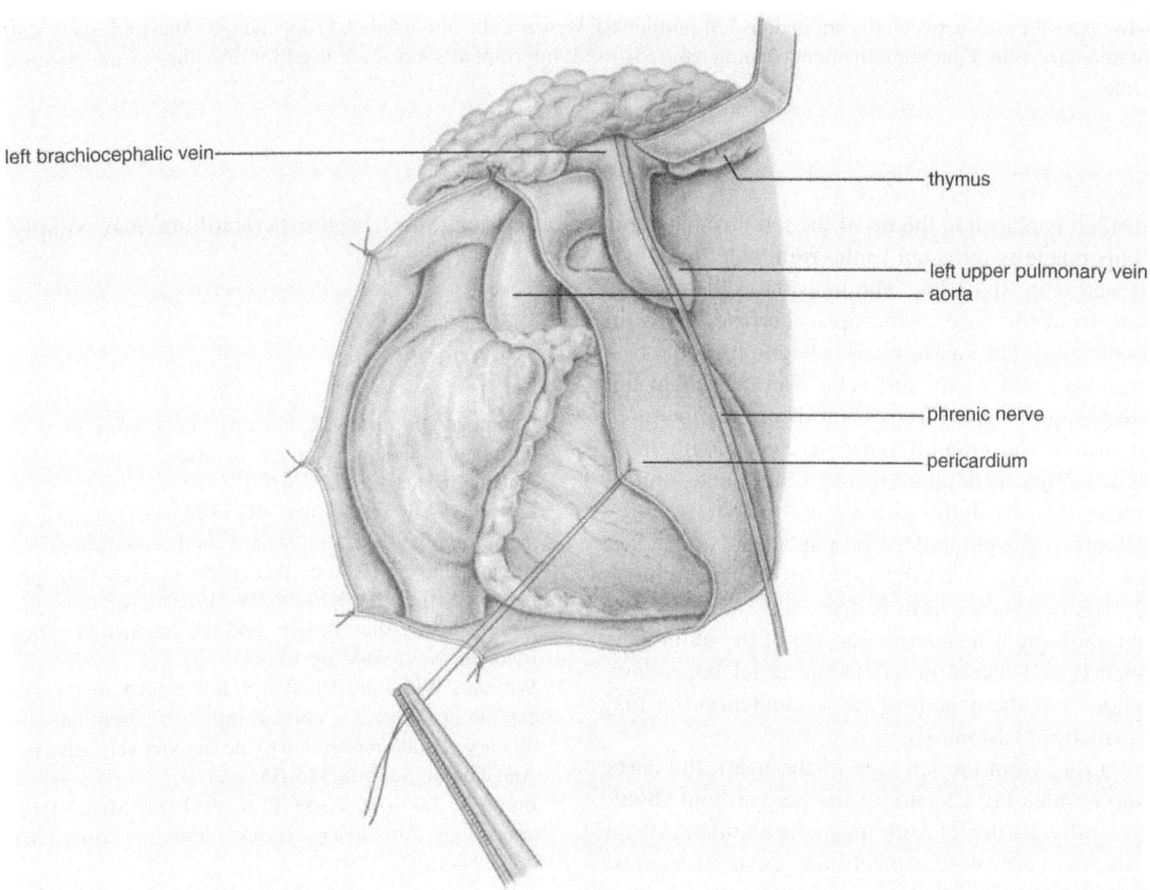

Fig. II-13-15. Left pulmonary vein draining to the innominate vein. After dissection of the left lobe of the thymus, the communication between the left pulmonary vein and the innominate vein is visualized. Care is taken to avoid damage to the phrenic nerve

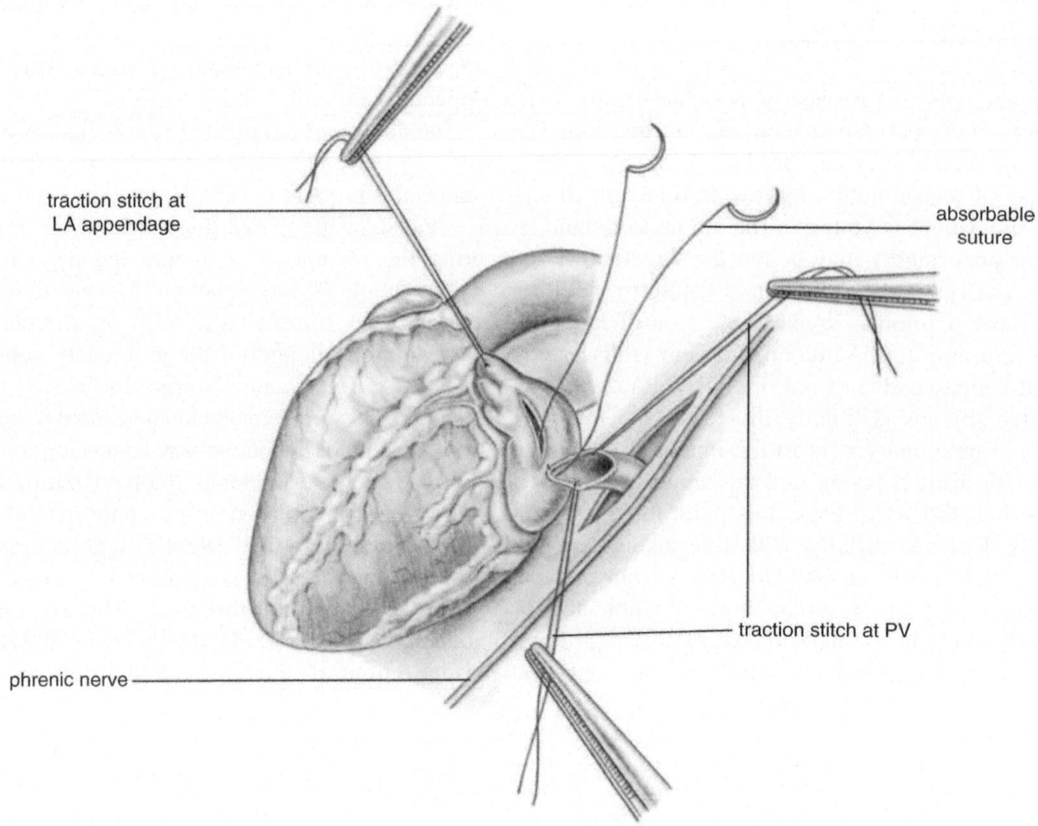

Fig. II-13-16. Anastomosis between the anomalous left pulmonary vein and the left atrial (*LA*) appendage. Anastomosis is started at the toe of the pulmonary vein. Fine monofilament running suture is used. Interrupted sutures are used for one-third of the circumference of the suture line

A traction stitch is placed in the tip of the left atrial appendage. The appendage is retracted to the right side, fixed and visualized well (Fig. II-13-16). The incision at the appendage is made from the base to the tip to correspond to the opening in the vein. The anastomosis is begun from the base of the appendage and toe of the vein. An absorbable fine monofilament suture is used for two-thirds of the circumference. The rest of the circumference is closed with interrupted sutures. This technique creates a large anastomosis and minimizes the possibility of kinking the vein.

Alternatively, if the pulmonary vein and atrial appendage are already adjacent to each other, side-to-side anastomosis is utilized. The pulmonary vein is dissected and is brought into the pericardium. The anterior surface of the pulmonary vein is opened and anastomosed to the atrial appendage. This technique has the benefit of easy orientation but may result in a smaller anastomosis.

After de-airing from the left side of the heart, the aortic cross-clamp is released. Closure of the pericardium should be done carefully, as this closure may cause kinking of the anastomosis. In such cases, a patch may be used to close the pericardium, or the pericardium may simply be left open.

References

1. Gotsman MS, Astley R, Parsons CG (1965) Partial anomalous pulmonary venous drainage in association with atrial septal defect. Br Heart J 27:566–571
2. Kirklin JW, Barratt-Boyes BG (1993) Atrial septal defect and partial anomalous pulmonary venous connection. In: Cardiac surgery, 2nd edn. Churchill Livingstone, New York, pp 609–644
3. Bharati S, Lev M, Kirklin JW (1983) Operations in the right atrium. In: Cardiac surgery and the conduction system. Wiley Medical, New York, pp 14–44
4. Williams WH, Zorn-Chelton S, Raviele AA, et al (1984) Extracardiac atrial pedicle conduit repair of partial anomalous pulmonary venous connection to the superior vena cave in children. Ann Thorac Surg 38:345–355
5. Imoto Y, Kado H, Asou T, et al (1998) Mixed type of total anomalous pulmonary venous connection. Ann Thorac Surg 66:1394–1397

II-14. Total Anomalous Pulmonary Venous Return

Patients with total anomalous pulmonary venous return (TAPVR) typically develop symptoms as neonates and require surgery early in life. Especially in the presence of pulmonary venous obstruction, the patient typically develops severe progressive pulmonary congestion and heart failure, and emergent surgery is necessary shortly after birth. In these situations, echocardiography is the only preoperative study necessary. Precise descriptions of pulmonary vein anatomy may not be obtained before surgery, and intraoperative evaluations for the pulmonary veins are always mandatory. In supracardiac- or infracardiac-type TAPVR patients, the shape of the common pulmonary vein is important because the common pulmonary vein will be anastomosed to the left atrium. Occasionally, the shape of the common pulmonary vein is atypical and anastomosis is difficult [1].

Improvements in infant cardiopulmonary bypass (CPB) and cardioplegia, and advancements in postoperative management, including inhaled nitric oxide, have dramatically decreased early operative mortality. Postoperative pulmonary vein obstruction remains a significant problem after surgery for this disease [2].

Operative Procedure for Darling Type IA, III [3]

For patients with Darling types IA and III TAPVR (Fig. II-14-1), the common pulmonary vein and left atrium are anastomosed. There are two approaches for this surgery: posterior and superior. A posterior approach is applicable to all types. This approach has one benefit of a wide visualization of all pulmonary veins. The superior approach is applicable to type IA. This approach has a merit of easy orientation of the pulmonary vein and left atrium at the time of anastomosis.

Posterior Approach

The heart is exposed via median sternotomy. If patent ductus arteriosus is present, the ductus is dissected from the pulmonary artery. After the recurrent nerve is pushed to the aortic side, a string is placed around the ductus. In the Darling IA type patient, the vertical vein is dissected at its junction with the innominate vein. Usually the vertical vein lies in front of the left pulmonary artery, but rarely this vein is identified behind the left pulmonary artery. After the left lobe of the thymus is dissected bluntly, the vertical vein–innominate vein junction is visualized. A string is placed around the vertical vein for later ligation. It is not necessary to dissect the entire vertical vein. Care is taken to avoid the tension on this string (which would cause pulmonary vein obstruction). It is important to inspect the pulmonary vein before initiation of CPB. In cases of mixed-type TAPVR, elucidation of the pulmonary vein anatomy reduces the CPB time. With elevation of the apex, orientation of the pulmonary veins is confirmed. The right side of the right atrium (RA) is dissected, and the right pulmonary veins are identified. The two pulmonary veins should be visualized and dissected at the point of junction to the common pulmonary vein.

Cardiopulmonary bypass is started with ascending aortic and bicaval cannulation. Placement of the superior vena cava (SVC) cannula from the right atrial appendage works well, although direct cannulation of the SVC may facilitate elevation of the apex of the heart. After bypass is initiated, the ductus arteriosus is ligated. Additional dissection of the common pulmonary vein is accomplished. As already mentioned, the right pulmonary veins are dissected from the right side of the heart up to the common pulmonary vein. The left pulmonary veins and common pulmonary vein are visualized by elevation of the heart. During this procedure, the surgeon moves to the left side of the operating table. The assistant stands at the right side of the table to elevate the apex of the heart. Care is taken to avoid arrhythmias or impeding venous return. If necessary to prevent these conditions, this procedure is interrupted intermittently. Dissection is completed of the four pulmonary veins, as well as the common pulmonary vein. This extensive dissection decreases the tension on the anastomosis due to kinking at the anastomosis. In type IA, the left pulmonary veins and vertical vein are clearly identified and distinguished from each other. This identification is very important to determine the incision line. In type III, the vertical vein is dissected thoroughly inside the pericardium.

At this stage, the ascending aorta is cross-clamped and cardioplegic solution is injected. After atriotomy the vertical vein is ligated, and the common pulmonary vein is opened. In types IA and III, the vertical vein is ligated at its junction with the innominate vein and at the diaphragm, respectively. The assistant elevates the apex of the heart toward the right side with a wet sponge soaked with cold saline. During readministration of cardioplegic solution, the heart is put back into the pericardium. Topical cooling is maintained

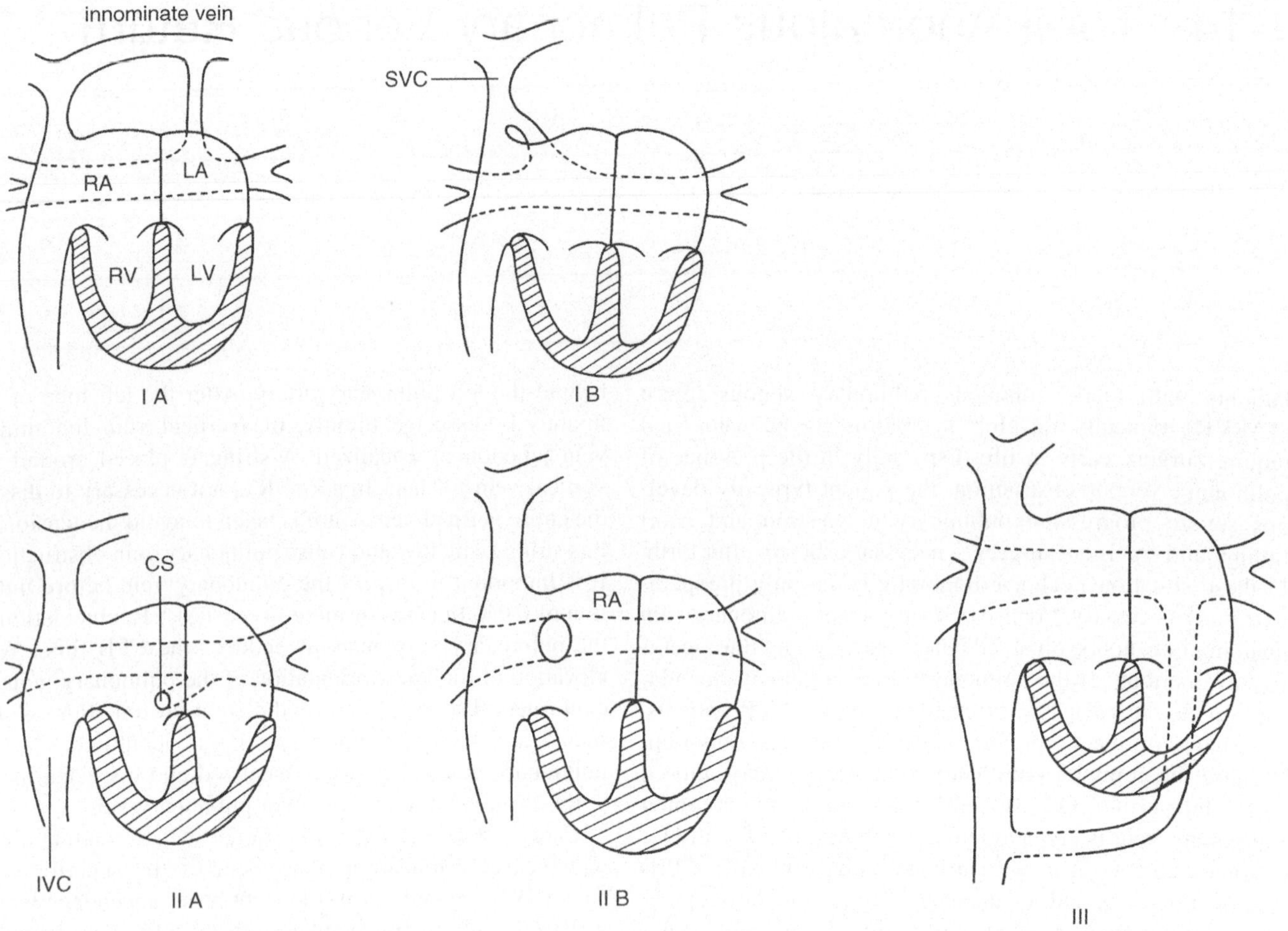

Fig. II-14-1. Darling classification (IA, IB, IIA, IIB, III). *RA*, right atrium; *LA*, left atrium; *RV*, right ventricle; *LV*, left ventricle; *CS*, coronary sinus; *SVC*, superior vena cava; *IVC*, inferior vena cava

during anastomosis with cold saline in the sponge used for retraction.

In neonates, an incision to the common pulmonary vein should not be extended into the individual pulmonary veins, but must be at least 10 mm in length. In type IA, the middle of the common pulmonary vein is transversely opened. Care is taken to avoid making the incision too close to the individual veins. If the incision is not long enough, it is extended into the vertical vein (Fig. II-14-2). In type III, an incision is made from the common pulmonary vein to the vertical vein toward the diaphragm inferiorly (Fig. II-14-3). This incision is started precisely in the middle of the common pulmonary vein. Care is taken to avoid deviation from the middle of the common pulmonary vein. The length of the incision on the common pulmonary vein is decided according to the size of the left atrium (LA). If an additional incision to the common pulmonary vein is necessary, the incision is extended toward the left side (Fig. II-14-3). In patients with a short common pulmonary vein, extending the incision leftward increases the risk of pulmonary vein stenosis. In these patients, the incision is extended straight to the roof of the common pulmonary vein. If the incision does not reach 10 mm with these maneuvers, the vertical vein is divided just above the ligation site, and the divided end is incorporated into the anastomosis.

The incision to the LA is started at the base of the left atrial appendage and is extended rightward to the atrial septum. Before this incision, a traction suture is placed to the left atrial appendage. Retraction of this suture helps visualization of opening and anastomosis. The final position and length of the incision on the LA are decided according to the position of the common pulmonary vein incision. In type IA, the incision is extended to the atrial septum (see Fig. II-14-2). In type III the incision is brought rightward at first and extended inferiorly toward the inferior vena cava (IVC) (see Fig. II-14-3). To avoid damaging the coronary sinus during anastomosis, a 5-mm distance is kept from the AV groove. The tape on the IVC is used as a target for extending the incision. The incision is stopped at the inferior end of the atrial septum.

The anastomosis between the LA and common pulmonary vein is performed with running suture technique using an 7-0 absorbable monofilament suture. Five to seven interrupted sutures are utilized in the suture line. To reconfirm the starting point for the anastomosis, the elevated apex of the heart is returned to the original position, to prevent possible kinking of the anastomosis. In type IA, the right-side end of the left atrial incision meets the right-side end of the incision of the common pulmonary vein. The anastomosis is started from the right side. A suture is placed inside-out

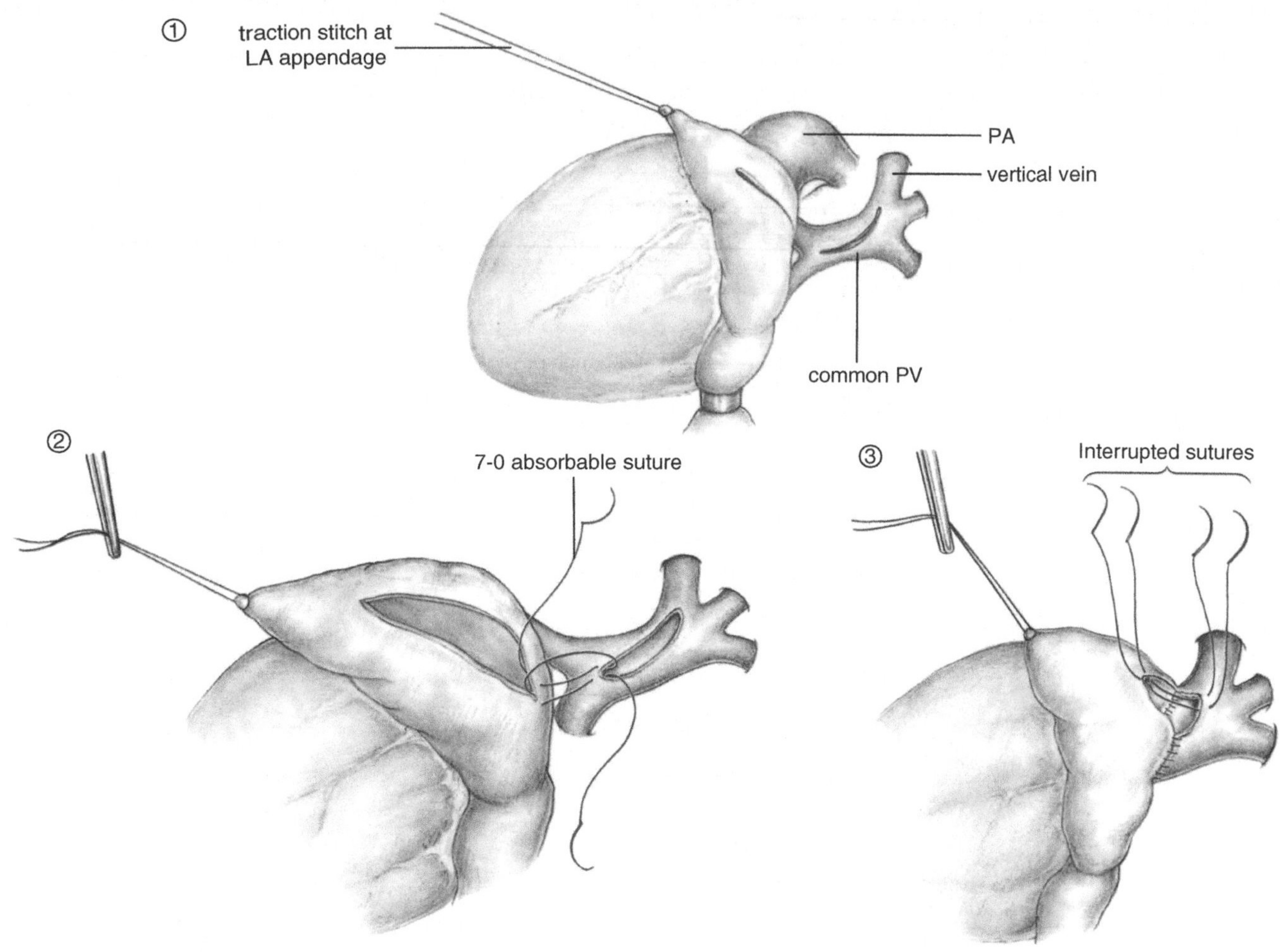

Fig. II-14-2. Posterior approach for Darling IA. ① In neonates, an incision to the common pulmonary vein should not be extended to each pulmonary vein, but must be at least 10 mm in length. If the common pulmonary vein incision is not long enough, it is extended into the vertical vein. The incision in the left atrium (*LA*) is started at the base of the left atrial appendage and is extended rightward to the atrial septum. ② The anastomosis is started from the right side. After four or five stitches are placed, the left atrium is lowered down into place. ③ At the left side of the anastomosis, several interrupted sutures are placed. *PA*, pulmonary artery

from the pulmonary vein. After four or five stitches are placed with two-bite technique, both ends of the sutures are pulled and the LA is pushed down to the common pulmonary vein. Half of the posterior suture line is completed, and then the anterior suture line is started. At the end of the suture line, five or six interrupted sutures are placed (see Fig. II-14-2). In type III, the two incisions are not completely parallel. The endpoint of the pulmonary vein incision meets the right lower end of the left atriotomy site. The anastomosis is started from this point. The anastomosis is performed in a similar fashion to that of type IA, using running suture with several interrupted sutures in the end of anastomosis (see Fig. II-14-3). After anastomosis, a pressure-monitoring catheter is placed into the left atrium through the atrial septum and the atrial septal defect (ASD) is closed. After de-airing through the root of the ascending aorta, the aortic cross-clamp is released. The right atriotomy is closed at the end. At the time of separation from bypass, the pulmonary artery pressure is monitored. Typically, at the time of separation from bypass, the pulmonary artery pressure is 60%–70% of the systemic systolic pressure. In the majority of cases, the pulmonary arterial pressure comes down to normal during chest closure. If pulmonary hypertension persists, inhaled nitric oxide is started after pulmonary vein stenosis is ruled out by echocardiography.

Superior Approach [4]

The common pulmonary vein is dissected between the superior vena cava and ascending aorta (Fig. II-14-4). First, the ascending aorta and superior vena cava are fully mobilized. Then the common pulmonary vein is dissected between these two vessels. Because the dissection of the common pulmonary vein may compromise hemodynamics, further dissection is performed during bypass with ascending aortic and IVC cannulation. The common pulmonary vein is visualized after the right pulmonary artery is retracted superiorly with a vessel loop. The right atrial appendage is retracted with a traction stitch. The dissection of the pulmonary vein is performed thoroughly behind both the SVC and the ascending aorta (Fig. II-14-4). Occasionally this approach may provide

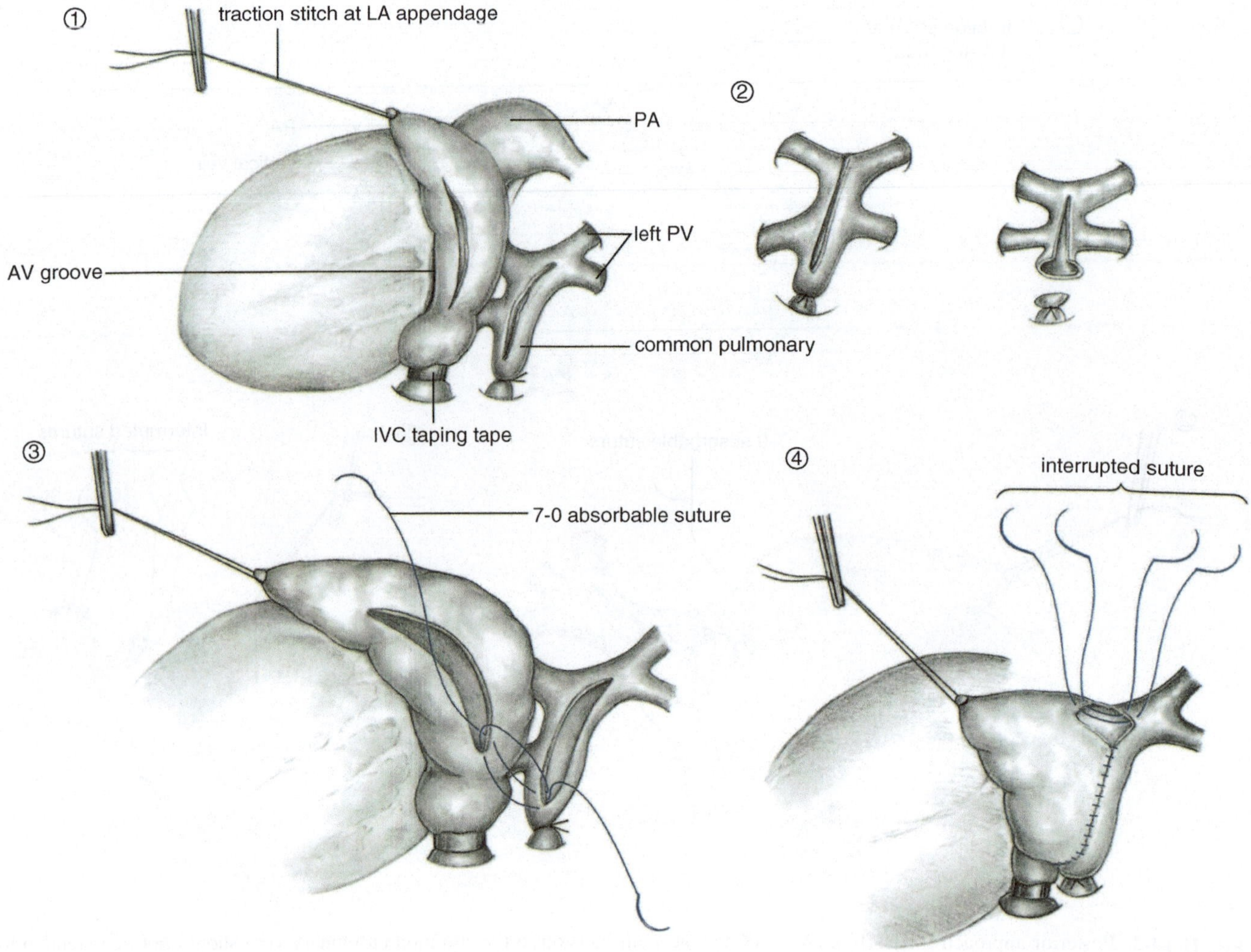

Fig. II-14-3. Posterior approach for Darling III. ① The common pulmonary vein (*PV*) is opened downward toward the diaphragm. The incision at the left atrium (*LA*) is started from the base of the appendage and advanced rightward, then carried downward toward the inferior vena cava (*IVC*), keeping a distance of 5 mm from the atrioventricular (AV) groove. ② When the incision at the common pulmonary vein cannot be extended, the incision can be advanced to the roof of the common pulmonary vein; then, the vertical vein can be divided above the ligation site and the division site can be used for anastomosis. ③ The anastomosis is started at the most inferior point. After four or five stitches are placed, the left atrial wall is lowered down into place. ④ At the left side of the anastomosis, several interrupted sutures are applied

inadequate exposure. At this stage the apex of the heart is elevated as in the posterior approach. The pulmonary vein anatomy is inspected, and dissection of the pulmonary vein is performed. Some surgeons have recommended division of the ascending aorta [5], but we believe that by usage of the posterior approach for visualization and dissection, division of the ascending aorta can usually be avoided.

A cannula is inserted in the SVC. After aortic cross-clamping, the right atrium is opened and decompression of the heart is instituted. The incision in the common pulmonary vein is placed on the anterior surface between the SVC and ascending aorta. With the retraction on the SVC toward the right side, this incision is extended rightward. Similarly, with retraction of the ascending aorta toward the left side, the incision is extended leftward. Each branching point of the pulmonary vein is ascertained from the right side of the right atrium and from the left side of the left atrium by elevating the apex of the heart. With the heart arrested, the LA is decompressed, which may make orientation of the LA difficult. In such cases, a traction stitch is placed on the left atrial appendage to facilitate the left atriotomy. The two incisions are placed adjacent to each other, and the anastomosis is started along the posterior suture line with 7-0 monofilament running suture. At the end of the anastomosis, the SVC or ascending aorta is retracted and visualization is facilitated. Traction sutures placed on the anterior surface of the left atrial and common pulmonary vein incision sites facilitate exposure (Fig. II-14-5). Before completion of the suture line, five or six interrupted sutures are used. The ASD is closed through a right atriotomy.

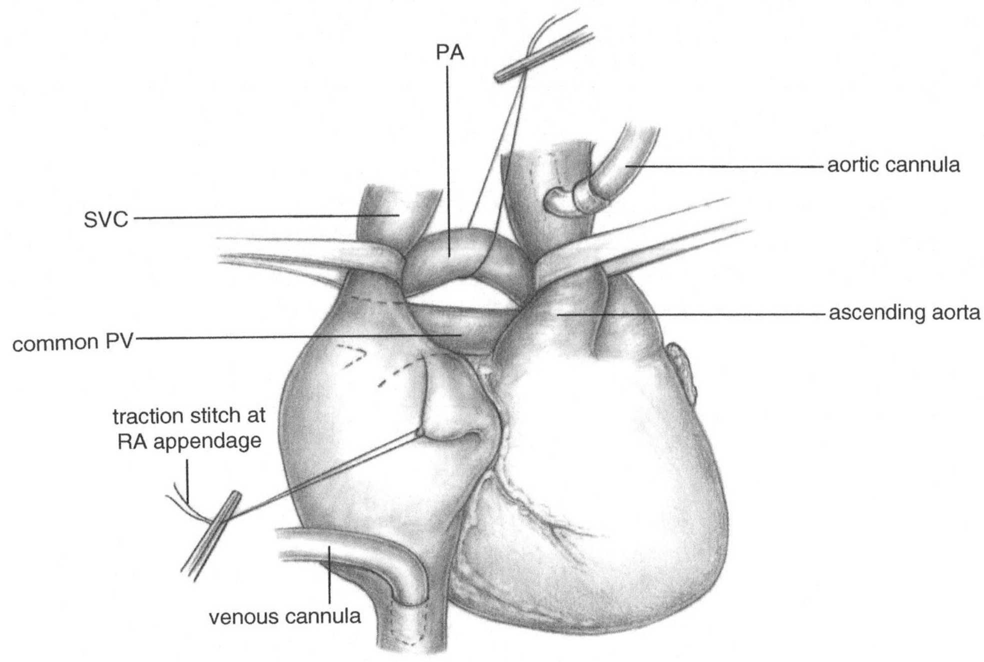

Fig. II-14-4. Superior approach: dissection of the common pulmonary vein (PV). On cardiopulmonary bypass, the common pulmonary vein is dissected between the superior vena cava (*SVC*) and ascending aorta. Retraction tapes are applied to the right pulmonary artery (*PA*), ascending aorta, and the SVC. To optimize the operative field, the right atrial (*RA*) appendage is retracted inferiorly and rightward using a traction stitch. To allow complete dissection of the left side of the common pulmonary vein, the apex of the heart may be elevated as in the posterior approach

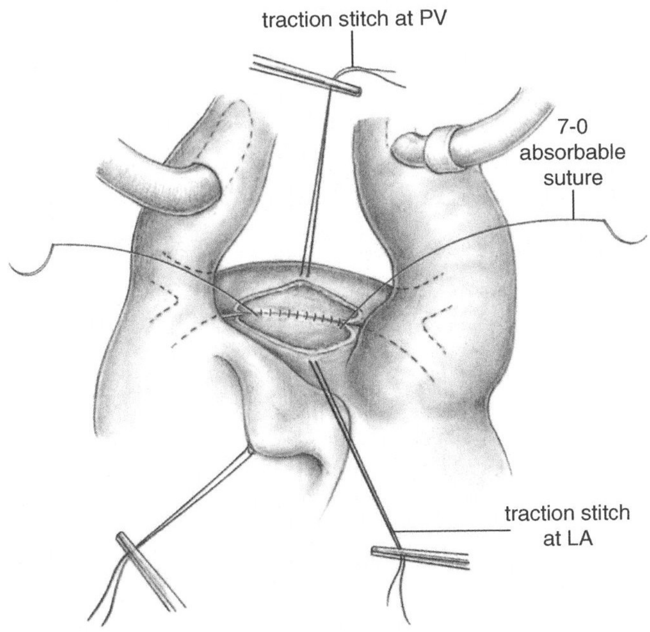

Fig. II-14-5. Superior approach: anastomosis. At the anterior walls of the common pulmonary vein (*PV*) and the left atrium (*LA*), traction stitches are applied to facilitate visualization of the suture line. At the end of the anterior suture line, several interrupted sutures are placed

Operative Procedure for Darling Type IIA

In this type, the common pulmonary vein returns to the coronary sinus. The wall between the coronary sinus and LA is removed, and the ASD and the coronary sinus are closed with an autologous patch. An alternate technique is to use the right atrial wall for patch material. Another technique described by Van Praagh et al. is the creation of the communication between the coronary sinus and LA, followed by direct closure of both the ASD and the coronary sinus [6]. This technique is not applicable in small babies because of an inability to create a large enough communication between the LA and coronary sinus. These techniques have a slight risk of pulmonary vein stenosis at the junction of the common pulmonary vein to the coronary sinus. Occasionally, these patients later require relief of stenosis. The risk of recurrence of pulmonary vein stenosis is fairly high in such cases.

Cardiopulmonary bypass is initiated with bicaval cannulation. After aortic cross-clamp, the RA is opened obliquely. The RA is inspected, and the dilated coronary sinus and the ASD are identified (Fig. II-14-6). From the coronary sinus, the inferior margin of the ASD is excised, and the LA should be visualized through this excision. Before this excision, it is important to identify the atrioventricular (AV) node by the position of the triangle of Koch composed of the tricuspid

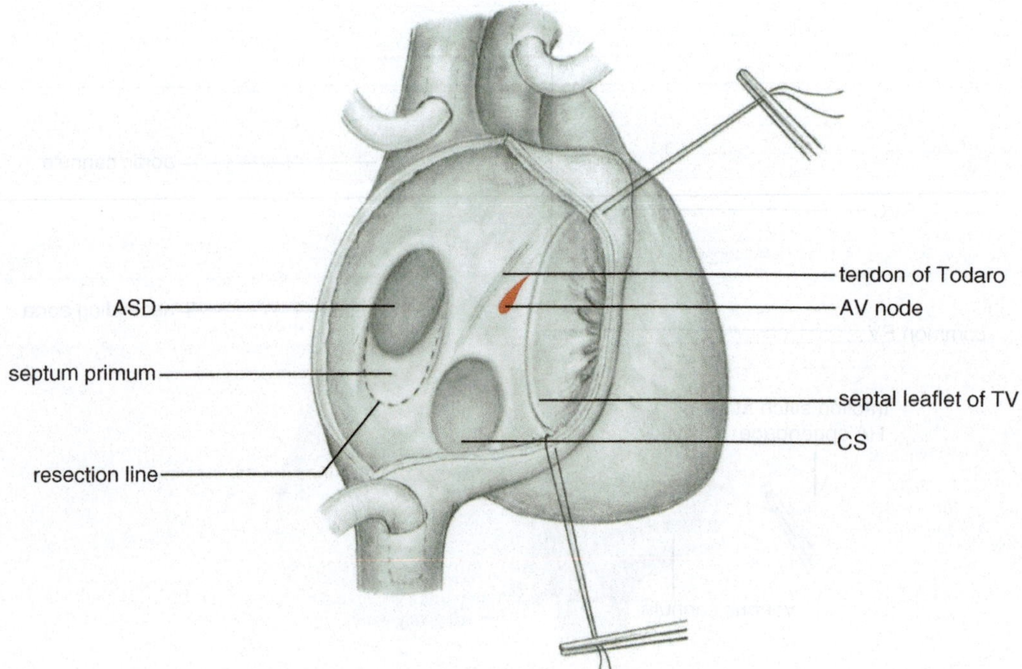

Fig. II-14-6. Right atrial approach for Darling IIA. The atrial septal defect (*ASD*) and the large coronary sinus are identified. The inferior margin of the ASD is excised. The separating wall between the coronary sinus and the left atrium is visualized well. Before excision of the coronary sinus wall, anatomic landmarks of the triangle of Koch [composed of the tricuspid valve (*TV*) annulus, coronary sinus (*CS*) orifice, and tendon of Todaro] are identified, and the position of the atrioventricular (*AV*) node is ascertained

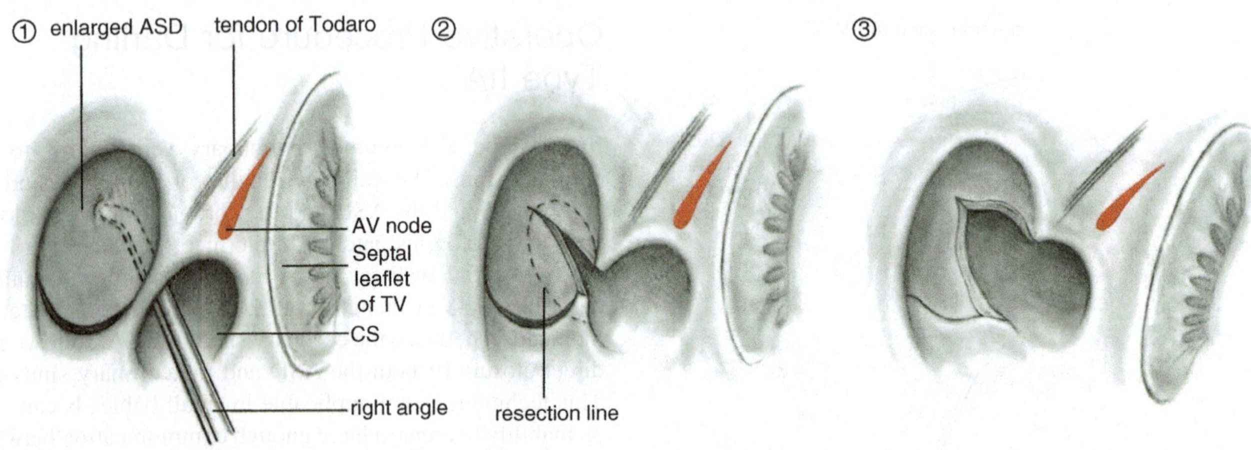

Fig. II-14-7. Coronary sinus excision for Darling IIA-1. ① A right-angle clamp is placed into the coronary sinus to confirm the location of the coronary sinus wall, and the incision to the coronary sinus is advanced carefully. The incision should not be brought too close to the pulmonary vein orifices. ② At the orifice of the coronary sinus (*CS*), to avoid the damage to the *AV node*, excision is not advanced superiorly. In the wall between the left atrium and coronary sinus, care is taken to avoid perforation of the left atrial wall. ③ A large communication between the coronary sinus and the left atrium is created

annulus, orifice of the coronary sinus, and tendon of Todaro. After excision of the atrial septum, the position of these structures easily becomes unclear. The first incision is placed to the wall between the coronary sinus and the LA (Fig. II-14-7 ①). This incision is close to the triangle of Koch, so care is necessary to avoid damage to the AV node. A right-angled clamp is placed from the coronary sinus and the direction of the coronary sinus is ascertained. Then, the incision is gradually advanced, but it should not be advanced too close to the pulmonary vein orifice. The importance is that this procedure is an excision of the common wall tissue between the left atrium (LA) and coronary sinus and is not a mere cut-back. Excision is not advanced anteriorly to prevent damage to the AV node. For excision to the posterior wall toward the LA, care is taken to avoid perforating the LA (Fig. II-14-7 ②). If a perforation is suspected, the endocardium is approximated with fine absorbable sutures. A large communication is created between the ASD and the coronary sinus (Fig. II-14-7 ③). This communication hole is covered with a patch. For the anterior suture, a line 1–2 mm inside the coronary sinus is used to avoid damage to the AV node. Care is taken to avoid occlusion of the major coronary vein orifices (Fig. II-14-8), but otherwise the suture line proceeds along the margins of the defect. Last, the right atriotomy is closed. The ideal patch material allows bulging toward the right side and has growth potential. For these reasons, a right atrial wall flap can be applied to close the defect [7]. When the right atrial wall is used as a flap, the right atriotomy incision is made close to the AV groove. From this incision toward the crista terminalis, two transverse incisions are placed superior and inferior, which create an oblong flap (Fig. II-14-9). The width of this flap is deter-

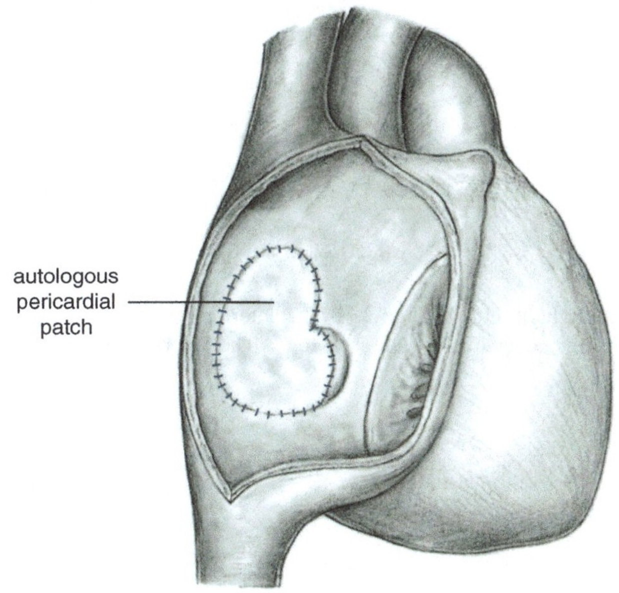

Fig. II-14-8. Coronary sinus excision for Darling IIA-2. The original ASD and coronary sinus are closed with a single patch of autologous pericardium. To protect the AV node, at the anterior edge of the coronary sinus orifice, the suture line is placed 1–2 mm inside the coronary sinus. At the other margins, the edges of the ASD are used

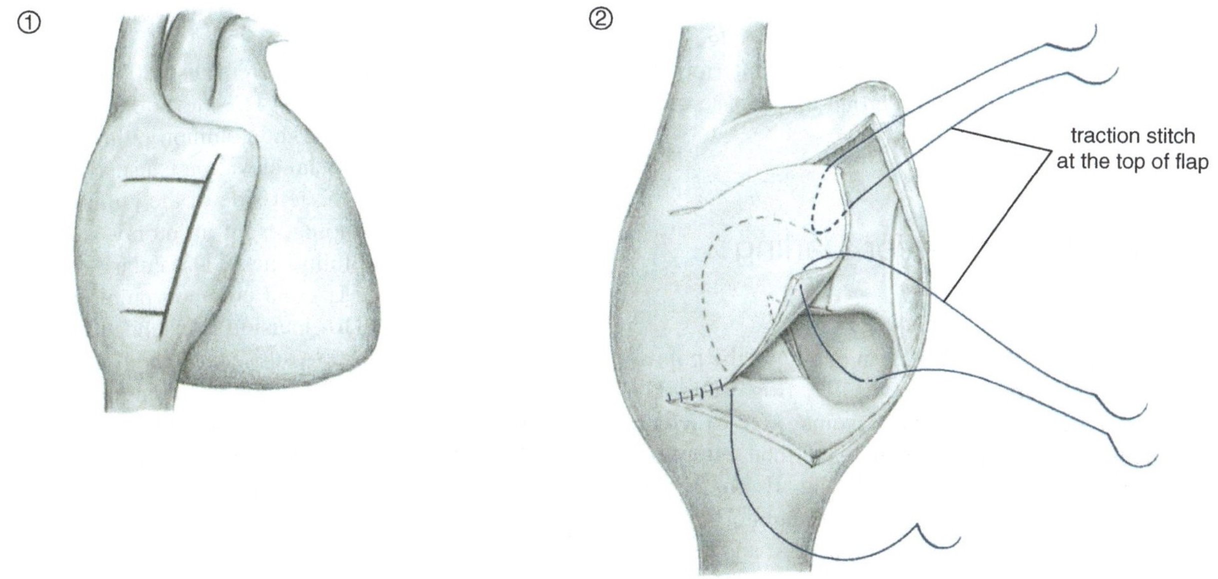

Fig. II-14-9. Darling IIA: repair with right atrial flap: 1. A right atriotomy is placed close to and parallel to the AV groove. To create a flap with the right atrial wall, two additional incisions are made, superiorly and inferiorly, toward the crista terminalis (①, ②)

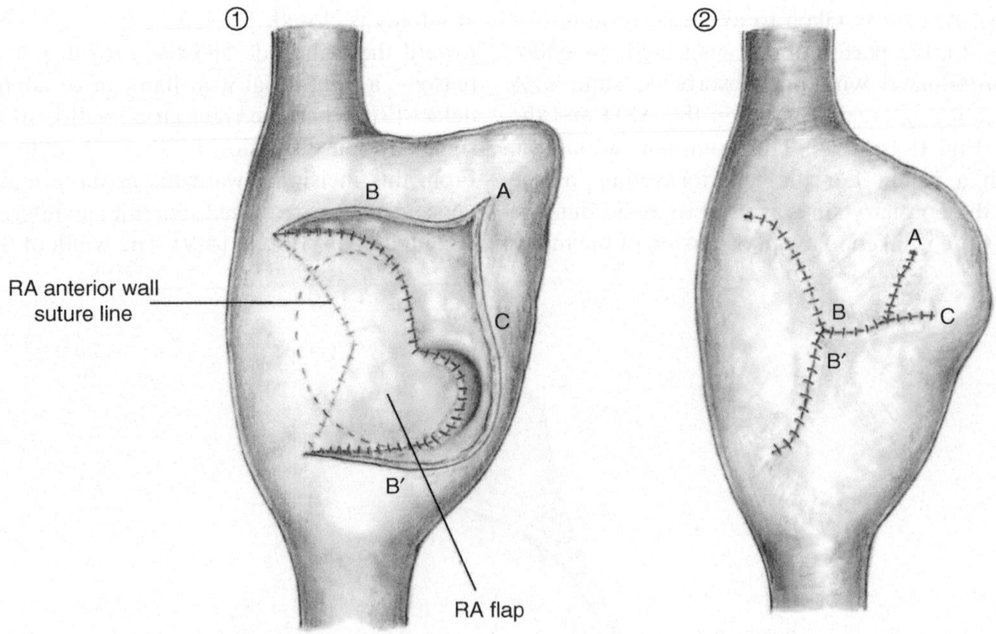

Fig. II-14-10. Darling IIA: repair with right atrial (*RA*) flap: 2. ① The anterior edge of the flap is sutured to the coronary sinus 1–2 mm inside the orifice. At the other margins the edges of the ASD is used. ② The anterior edge of the right atriotomy is sutured on the flap to close the RA

mined by the length between the superior and inferior ends of the previously created large hole (composed of the ASD and the coronary sinus). Traction sutures are placed at the edge of the flap, and the hinge point of the flap is determined. The suture lines are started from the hinge points and advanced anteriorly. Fine absorbable monofilament running sutures are used. The suture line at the anterior edge is the same as in patch closure technique. Finally, the anterior edge of the right atriotomy covers the flap up to the base of the flap (Fig. II-14-10).

Operative Procedure for Darling Type IIB

There are two types of Darling IIB. In one type, the pulmonary veins return individually to the RA (Fig. II-14-11). In the other type, the pulmonary veins join to create a common pulmonary vein, which itself then returns to the RA, usually superior to the ASD (Fig. II-14-12). The first type is similar to partial anomalous pulmonary vein with right pulmonary vein returning to the RA, and its treatment is also similar: the ASD is enlarged if necessary, and rerouting is performed using a patch or a flap (see Fig. II-14-11).

In the common pulmonary vein type, a cut-back or excision-and-patch technique is known to have a high incidence of postoperative pulmonary vein obstruction. For this type, anastomosis of the common pulmonary vein to the left atrium is considered the technique of choice because the anastomosis results in the largest opening with the least turbulent blood flow.

During bypass, pulmonary vein dissection is performed as in the posterior approach. The elevation of the heart is slightly restricted, because the common pulmonary vein is connected to the RA. Partial elevation is usually enough, as the main dissection is the left side of the pulmonary veins. After aortic cross-clamping, right atriotomy is performed. Through the right atriotomy, the ASD is enlarged superiorly. The wall between the LA and common pulmonary vein is opened and excised. This incision is extended leftward and reaches outside the heart. At this stage, the heart is elevated and incisions are extended in the common pulmonary vein to its branching point and correspondingly on the left atrium. With these extensions, a very large anastomosis is obtained (Fig. II-14-13). The anastomosis is started from the inside, approximating the intima. After this suture line comes to the outside, the heart is elevated and anastomosis is advanced behind the heart (Fig. II-14-14). The common pulmonary vein orifice and the ASD are closed simultaneously with an autologous pericardial patch (Fig. II-14-15).

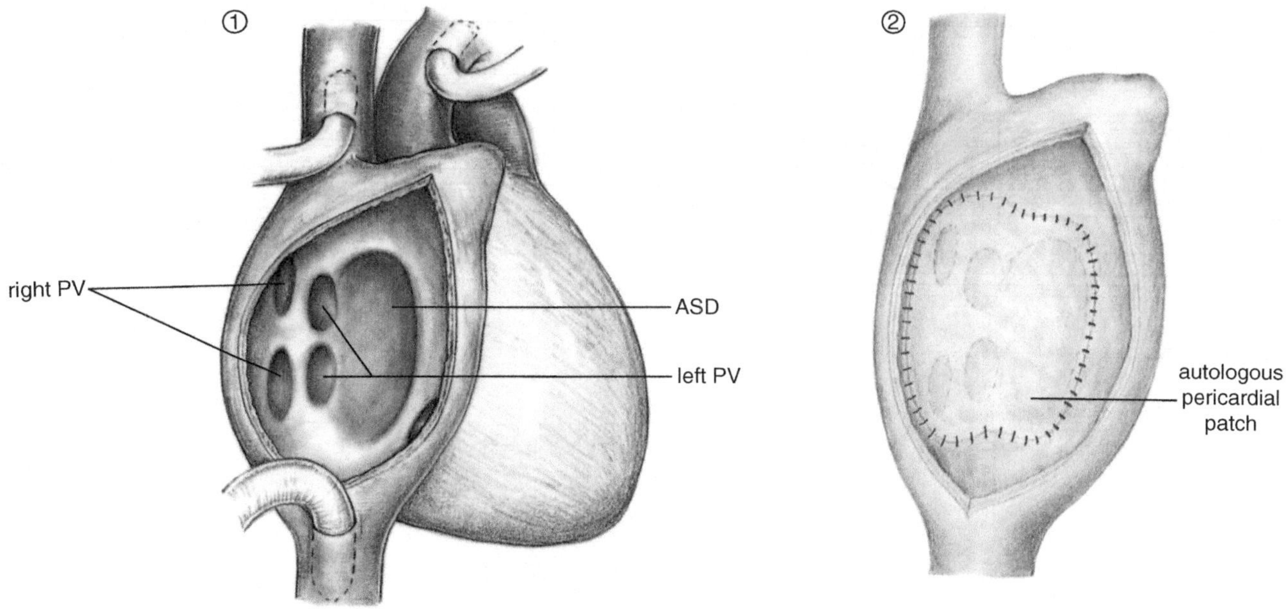

Fig. II-14-11. Darling IIB: pulmonary vein (*PV*) returning to the right atrium. ① All pulmonary veins are returning into the right atrium (*RA*) posterior to the *ASD*. ② The ASD is enlarged if necessary. All pulmonary veins are rerouted toward the left atrium (LA) through the enlarged ASD

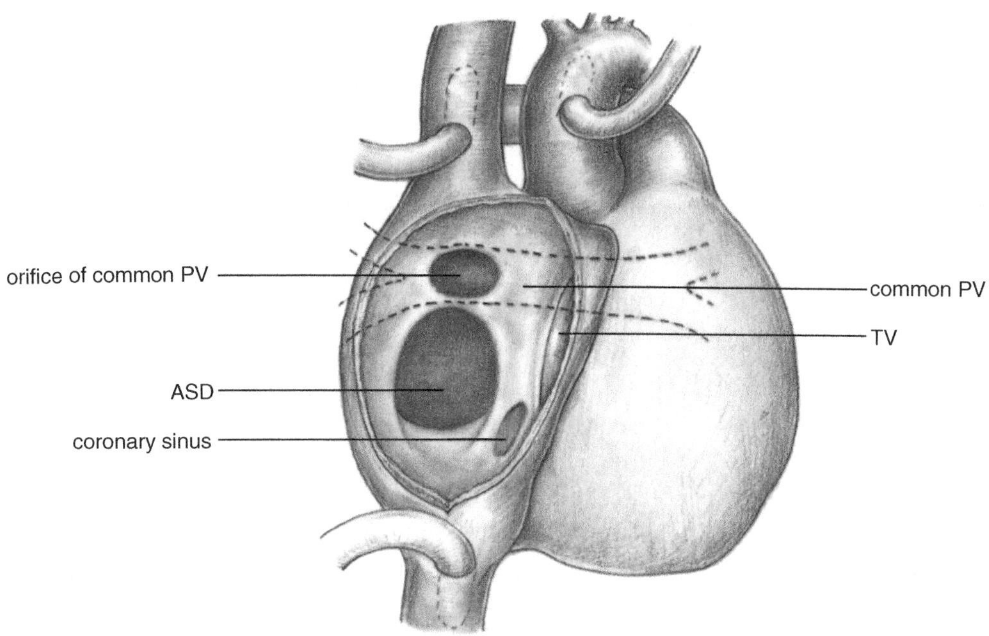

Fig. II-14-12. Darling IIB: anatomy of common *PV* type. Pulmonary veins join and create the common pulmonary vein. This common chamber communicates with the right atrium superior to the ASD. *TV*, tricuspid valve

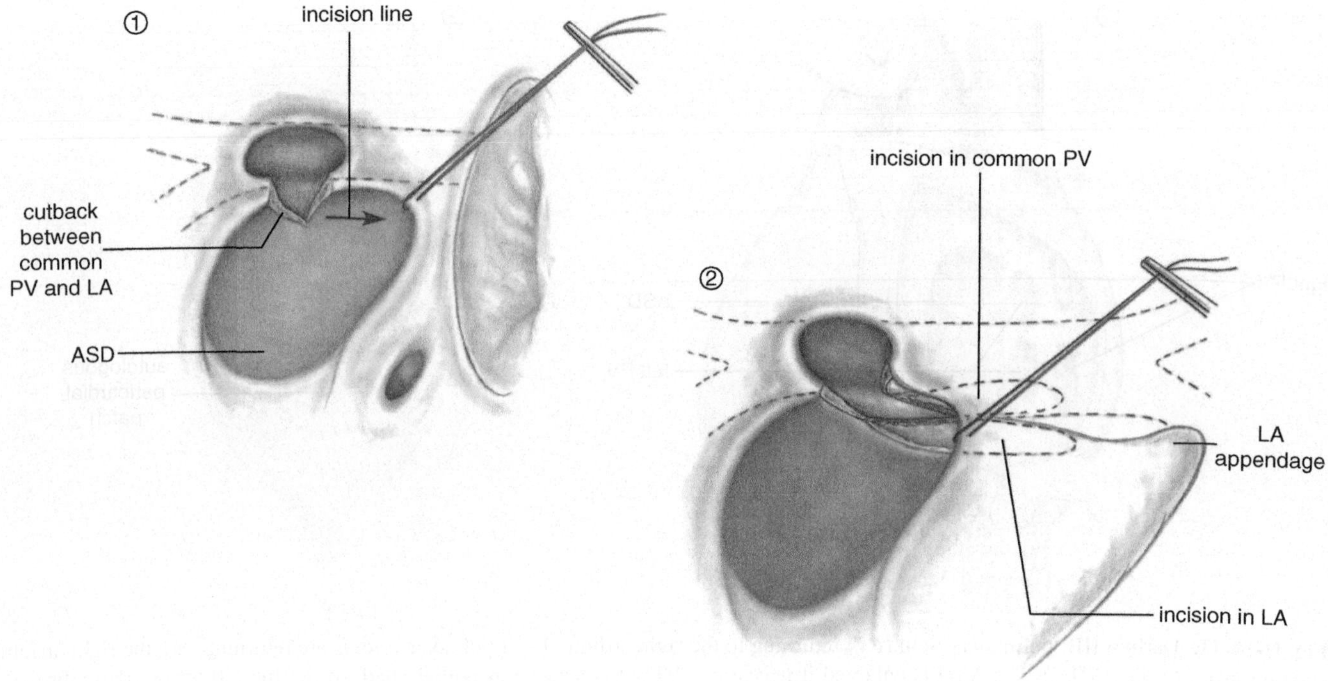

Fig. II-14-13. Darling IIB: repair of common PV type: 1. ① The ASD is enlarged superiorly and the membrane between the common pulmonary vein and the right atrium (RA) is resected. ② This incision is extended to the left side using a posterior approach intermittently. *LA*, left atrium

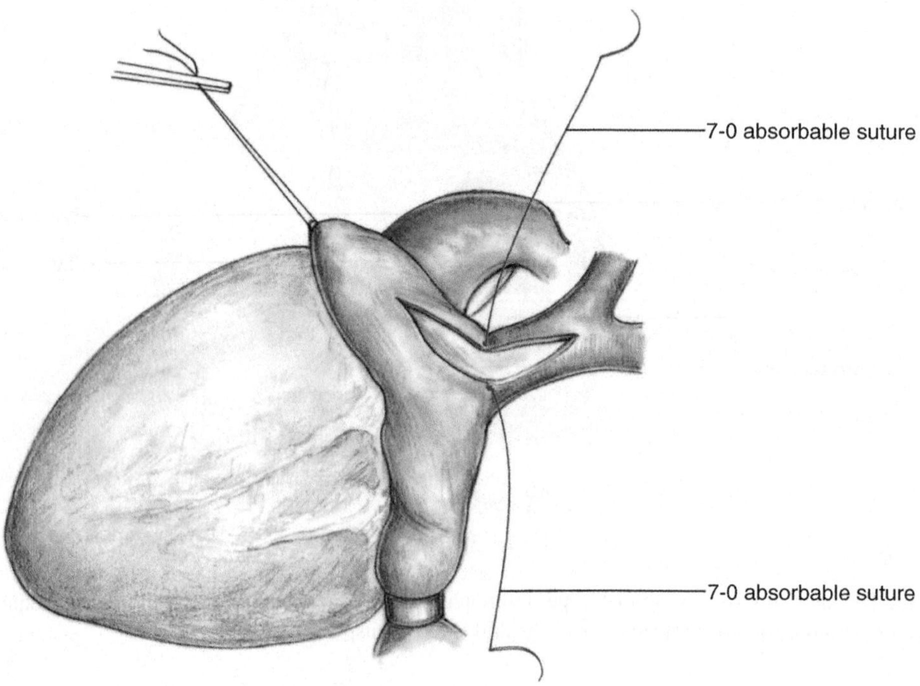

Fig. II-14-14. Darling IIB: repair of common pulmonary vein (*PV*) type: 2. Suturing is started from the inside the RA to approximate the intima of the RA and the common PV. The left side of the common PV and LA are anastomosed from outside the heart as with the posterior approach

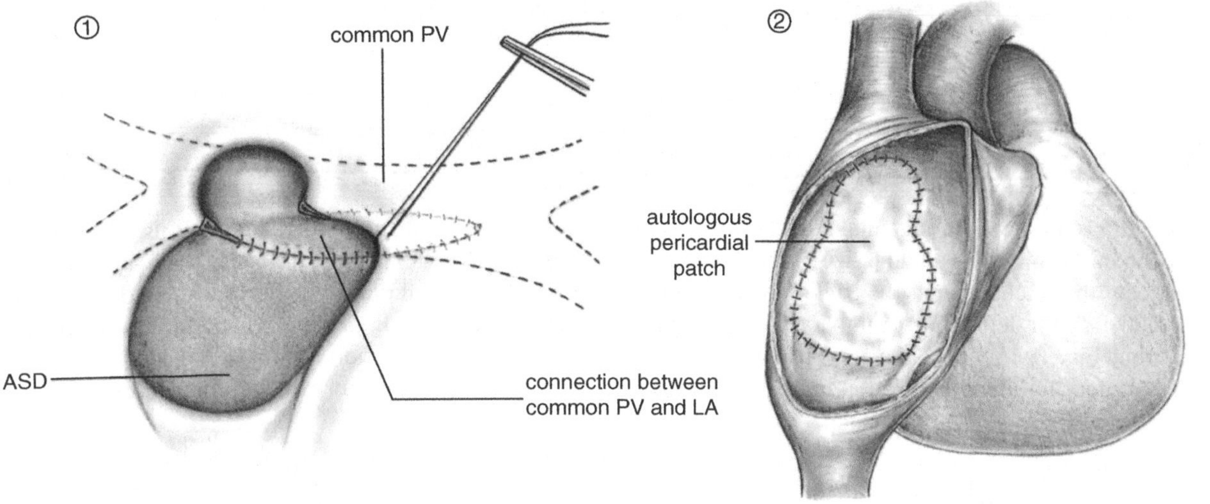

Fig. II-14-15. Darling IIB: repair of common PV type: 3. The enlarged orifice of the common chamber and the *ASD* are closed together with an autologous pericardial patch through the right atriotomy

Operative Procedure for Darling Type IB

There are two types of Darling IB TAPVR. In one type, the individual veins join to form a common pulmonary vein, and this common vein drains to the SVC. In the other type, the pulmonary veins return individually to the SVC. In the presence of a common pulmonary vein, the surgical procedure is similar to that used for type I A. In our experience, because extensive dissection is usually required for this type, we prefer the superior approach. In the patient with individual pulmonary veins returning to the SVC, the Williams technique for partial anomalous pulmonary venous return to the SVC is applicable [8]. In this type of patient, the pulmonary vein–SVC junction site occasionally is stenotic, and additional stenosis relief may be required [9].

References

1. Delisle G, Ando M, Calder AL, et al (1976) Total anomalous pulmonary venous connection: report of 93 autopsied cases with emphasis on diagnostic and surgical considerations. Am Heart J 91:99–122
2. Ando H, Yasui H, Kado H, et al (1990) Surgical repair of total anomalous pulmonary venous connection in neonates and infants: prevention for pulmonary venous obstruction at the site of anastomosis. Nippon Kyobu Geka Gakkai Zasshi 38:618–624
3. Darling RC, Rothney WB, Craig JM, et al (1957) Total pulmonary venous drainage into the right side of the heart: report of 17 autopsied cases not associated with other major cardiovascular anomalies. Lab Invest 6:44–64
4. Trucker BL, Lindesmith GG, Stiles QR, et al (1976) The superior approach for correction of the supracardiac type of total anomalous pulmonary venous return. Ann Thorac Surg 22:374–377
5. Serraf A, Belli E, Roux D, et al (1998) Modified superior approach for repair of supracardiac and mixed total anomalous pulmonary venous drainage. Ann Thorac Surg 65:1391–1393
6. Van Praagh R, Harken AH, Delisle G, et al (1972) Total anomalous pulmonary venous drainage to the coronary sinus. A revised procedure for its correction. J Thorac Cardiovasc Surg 64:132–135
7. Imoto Y, Tominaga R, Morita S, et al (1999) Fate of atrial flap used in repair of total anomalous pulmonary venous connection. Jpn J Thorac Cardiovasc Surg 47:288–290
8. Williams WH, Zorn-Chelton S, Raviele AA, et al (1984) Extracardiac atrial pedicle conduit repair of partial anomalous pulmonary venous connection to the superior vena cave in children. Ann Thorac Surg 38:345–355
9. Tsuruhara Y, Kado H, Nakano H, et al (1990) A case report of total anomalous pulmonary venous drainage corrected with Vargas' method. Nippon Kyobu Geka Gakkai Zasshi 38:523–527

II-15. Cor Triatriatum

Cor triatriatum is a very rare congenital heart disease. Symptoms depend on the presence and the size of the communication between three chambers: the right atrium and the superior and inferior left atrial chambers (Lucas–Schmidt classification; Fig. II-15-1) [1]. Severe pulmonary congestion or respiratory failure may develop in the early neonatal period, as is seen in total anomalous pulmonary venous return (TAPVR) with pulmonary vein obstruction. Therefore, differential diagnosis becomes important. Diagnosis is made by echocardiography or catheterization, by identifying a septum inside the left atrium (LA). The surgical procedure is removal of an abnormal septum and closure of an atrial

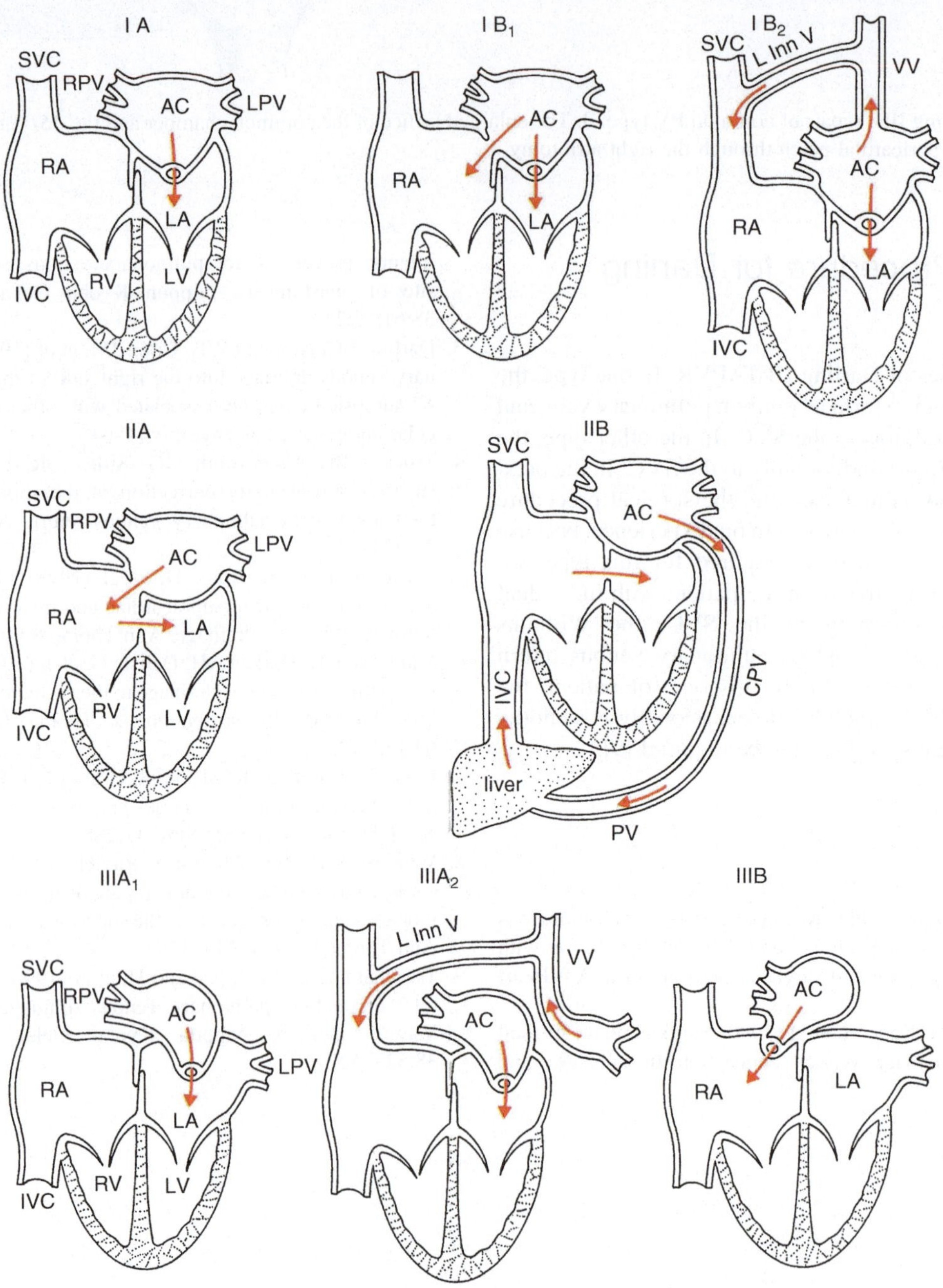

Fig. II-15-1. Classification of cor triatriatum by Lucas and Schmidt. *AC*, accessory chamber; *InnV*, innominate vein; *VV*, vertical vein; *CPV*, common pulmonary vein

septal defect. In neonates, the identification of the LA and an accessory chamber is not easy.

At the time of pericardial opening, a pericardial patch is prepared. Even in the patient with a small atrial septal defect (ASD), patch placement is often required because of the enlargement of the ASD or atrial septal tissue resection. Standard bypass technique is used. To improve visualization, direct cannulation to the superior vena cava (SVC) is utilized. A large purse-string suture is placed to the left atrial appendage for vent placement, and this purse-string is also used for the placement of a Hegar dilator to identify the true chamber. Under mild hypothermia, an aortic cross-clamp is placed with administration of cardioplegic solution. An oblique incision is placed in the right atrium, and the right atrium is inspected. Usually the ASD is identified at the fossa ovalis. If this ASD is not identified, a longitudinal incision is made in the fossa ovalis. It is important to note that the abnormal wall is perpendicular to the atrial septum. When the ASD is opening to the accessory chamber, abnormal wall is at the anterior from the ASD. ASD is enlarged anterior toward the mitral valve. If the ASD is opening to the true chamber of the LA, the abnormal wall stays posterior to the ASD, and the incision is placed posteriorly from the ASD (Fig. II-15-2).

To identify the true chamber, the mitral valve and the left atrial appendage are used as landmarks. Preoperative evaluation of the size of the communication from the accessory chamber is usually not reliable. Placement of a small Hegar dilator through the left atrial appendage is helpful to identify the true chamber of the LA. If the dilator is seen from the ASD, the ASD is opened to the true chamber (Fig. II-15-3). If the dilator is identified over the wall, the ASD is opened to the accessory chamber (Fig. II-15-3). The incision is extended at the base of the abnormal wall to the atrial septum. Then, the ASD is opened to both chambers over the abnormal wall (Fig. II-15-4). The abnormal wall tissue is removed from the LA with care to avoid perforation. To remove the abnormal wall tissue completely from the atrial septum, the fossa ovalis tissue is excised (Fig. II-15-5). The enlarged ASD is closed with an autologous pericardial patch with a running suture. A vent is inserted from the left atrial appendage, the aortic cross-clamp is released with de-airing, and the right atriotomy is closed.

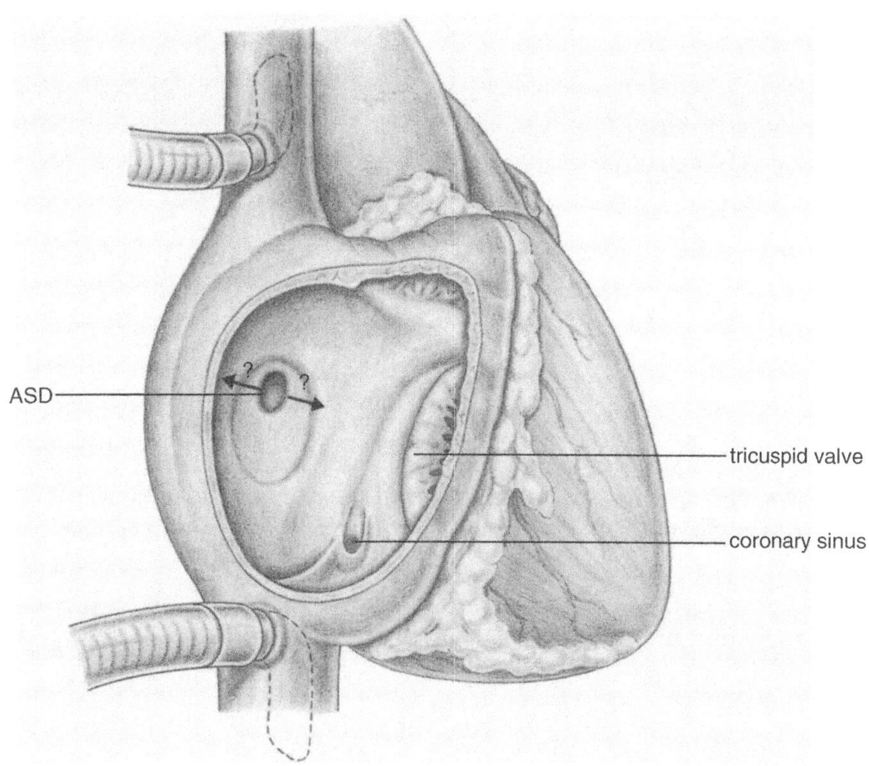

Fig. II-15-2. Approach to the left atrium through the right atrium. The enlargement of the atrial septal defect (*ASD*) is determined depending on the opening of the accessory chamber

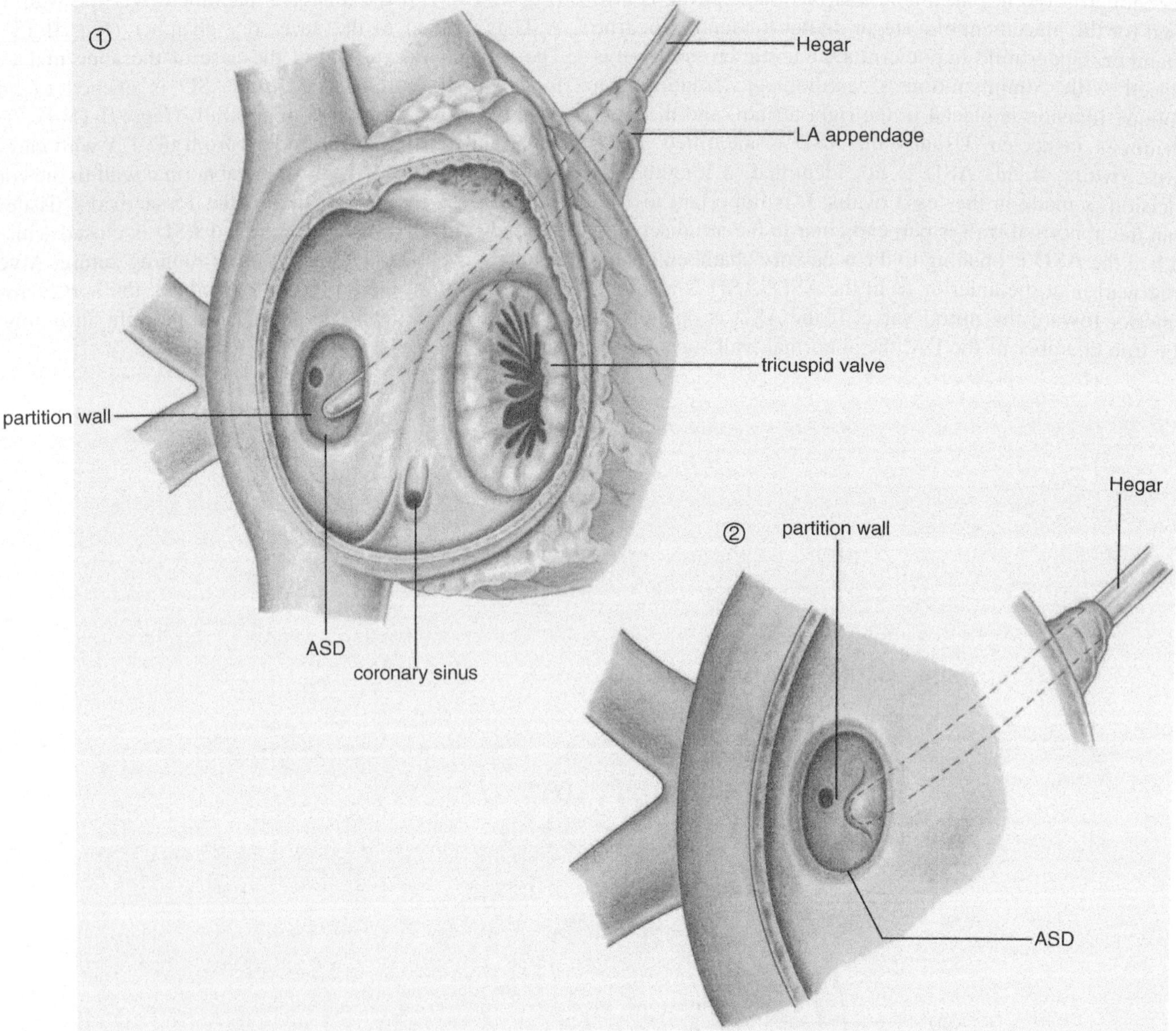

Fig. II-15-3. Identification of the left atrial (LA) chamber. A small Hegar probe is inserted from the left atrial appendage to identify the communication between the accessory chamber and the ASD. When the tip of the Hegar probe is found through the ASD, the ASD is opening to the true chamber. When the tip of the probe is not visualized directly through the ASD and is found beneath the atrial wall, the ASD is opening to the accessory chamber. ① ASD is opening to the true chamber. ② ASD is opening to the accessory chamber

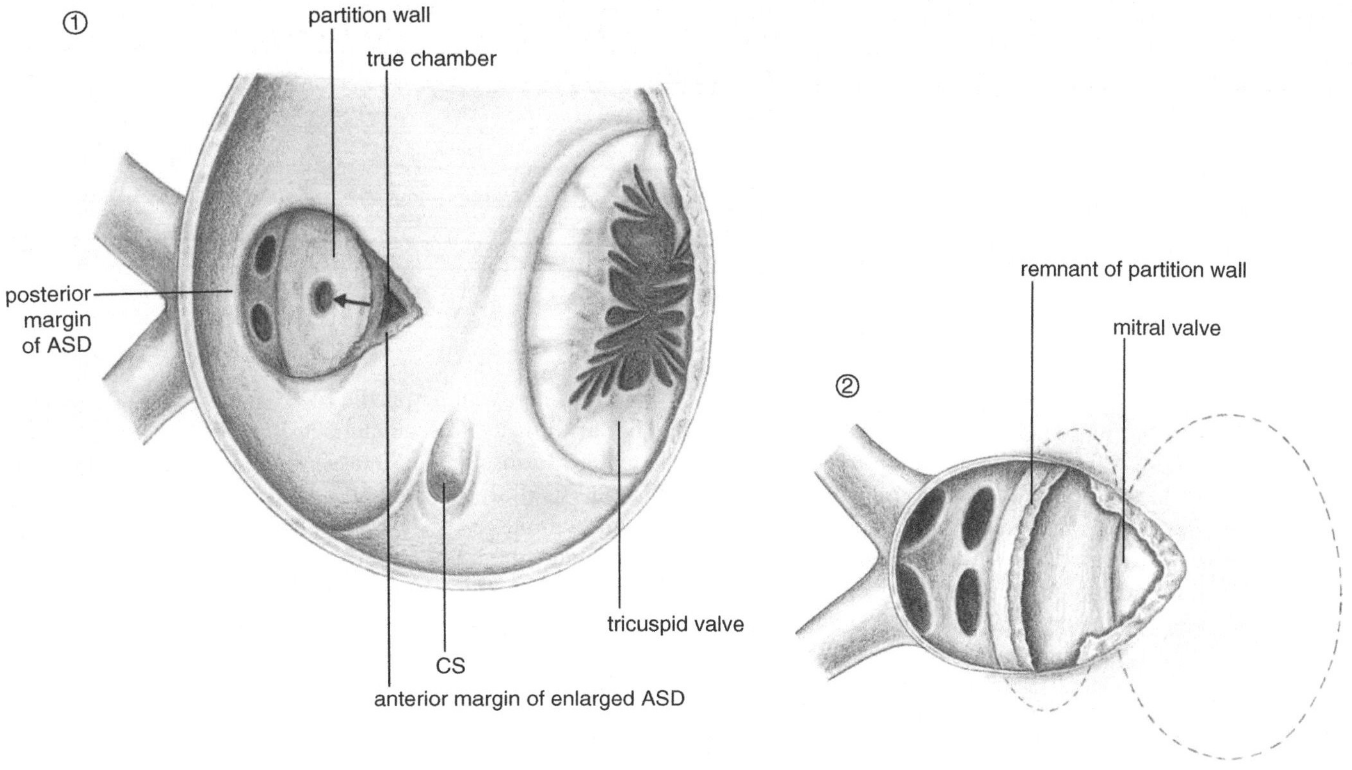

Fig. II-15-4. ASD enlargement. When the ASD is opening to the accessory chamber, the ASD is enlarged anteriorly. ① This incision is advanced to both the true chamber and the accessory chamber. This opening is extended to the communication of the accessory chamber and ASD. ② The membranous structure is resected from the left atrium and accessory chamber. *CS*, coronary sinus

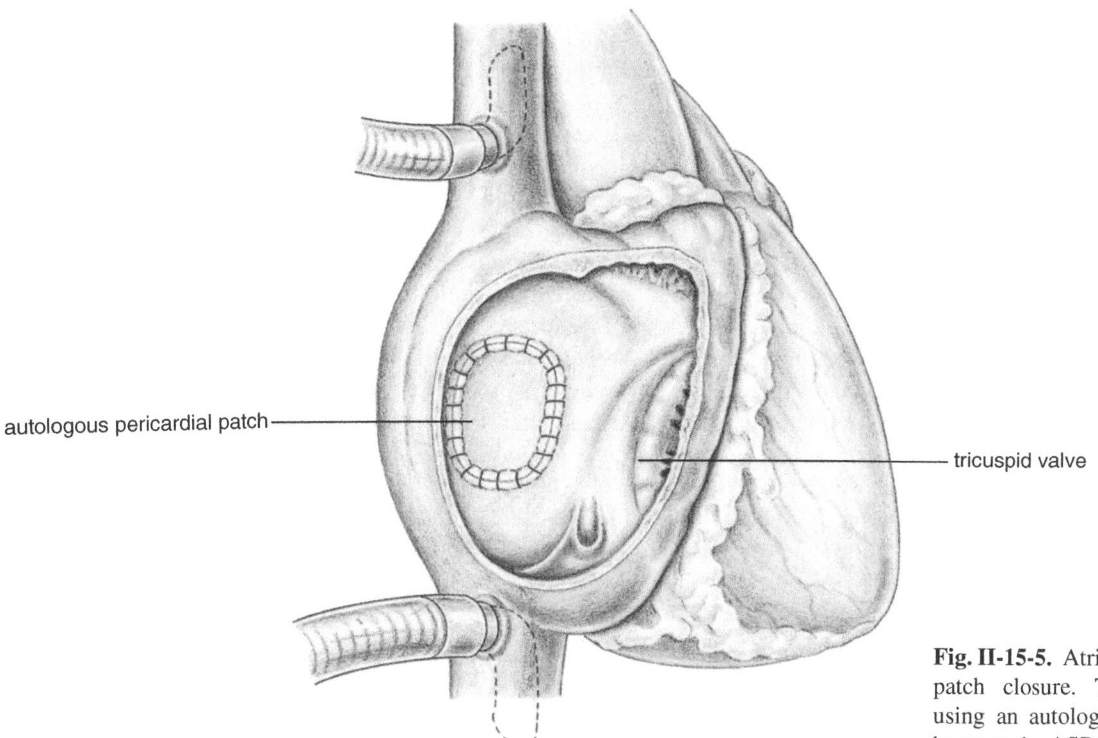

Fig. II-15-5. Atrial septal defect (ASD) patch closure. The ASD is closed using an autologous pericardial patch because the ASD is large

Reference

1. Lucas RV, Schmidt RE (1977) Anomalous venous connections: pulmonary and systemic. In: Moss AJ, Adams FH, Emmanouilidis GC (eds) Heart disease in infants, children and adolescents. Williams & Wilkins, Baltimore, pp 437–470

II-16. Atrioventricular Septal Defect: Partial, Intermediate, and Complete Type

Underdevelopment of the endocardial cushion causes atrioventricular (AV) septal defects, including AV valve deformity and atrial septal defect, with or without ventricular septal defect. The tricuspid valve and mitral valve are located at the same level and create a common AV connection. In normal hearts, the aortic valve is usually situated between the tricuspid and mitral valves, the so-called wedge position. In AV septal defects, the aortic valve is located anterior to the AV valve. The normal mitral valve is composed of two valve leaflets and has two papillary muscles, the anterolateral and posteromedial. In AV septal defects, the left AV valve typically has three leaflets, and two papillary muscles, which are anterior and posterior. The superior aspect of the muscular septum is deficient or "scooped out." In a normal heart, the distance between the apex and the semilunar valve is the same as the distance from the apex to the AV valve. In AV septal defects, the inlet portion of the ventricular septum is missing and the inlet is therefore significantly shorter than the outlet [1,2]. Left ventriculography shows a so-called "gooseneck" sign corresponding to left ventricular outflow tract elongation, which may also be associated with varying degrees of left ventricular outflow tract obstruction.

Generally, AV septal defects are classified as complete, partial, or intermediate types based on the morphology of the atrioventricular valve (Fig. II-16-1). The partial type is often called a primum atrial septal defect (ASD). In this form of AV septal defect, the common superior and inferior leaflets are attached together by a connecting tongue. There is a commissure in the left AV valve between the superior and inferior leaflets, often termed a cleft, and there is no ventricular septal defect (VSD). In the complete type, the connecting tongue is absent and the superior and inferior leaflets are thus not attached to each other. There is a primum ASD and a VSD. Complete AV septal defects are classified into three types according to the shape of the superior bridging leaflet (Rastelli classification). In type A, the superior bridging leaflet is divided above the ventricular septum and its chordae are attached to the ventricular septum. In type B, the division point is shifted slightly rightward. In type C (free-floating type), the division point is shifted extremely to the right, and the chordae are not attached to the ridge of the ventricular septum (Fig. II-16-2). As described by Anderson et al. [1], the third type of AV septal defect, the intermediate type, has a connecting tongue, but lacks connection between the ventricular septum and the AV valve; this creates a small VSD beneath the connecting tongue.

The hemodynamic profile of a partial AV septal defect is similar to that of a secundum ASD. For the partial or intermediate forms, if the shunt is large, surgery is indicated. In addition, if the patient has significant left AV valve regurgitation, congestive heart failure may result in early life, mandating surgery in early infancy. In the complete type of AV septal defect, patients typically develop severe heart failure early because of the presence of both a large ventricular level shunt as well as an atrial level shunt. Especially in the patient with Down's syndrome, pulmonary vascular obstructive disease may develop relatively early [3], and early intervention is required to prevent this [4–6].

Partial AV Septal Defect

Via a median sternotomy, a piece of pericardium is harvested. Cardiopulmonary bypass (CPB) is initiated with ascending aortic and bicaval cannulation. After aortic cross-clamping and cardioplegia administration, the right atrium is opened obliquely. Two traction sutures are placed on each edge of the atriotomy (Fig. II-16-3). To avoid postoperative bleeding, these traction sutures are not full-thickness bites. The cardiotomy sucker is inserted into the left atrium across the atrial septum.

The primum ASD and cleft at the left AV valve are inspected. Crystalloid cardioplegic solution is injected to the left ventricle, and left AV valve regurgitation is evaluated. At this stage, de-airing is performed through the ascending aorta. In a majority of cases regurgitation is identified through the cleft. In the presence of an accessory mitral orifice, regurgitation should be checked from this orifice as well [7].

In AV septal defects, the conduction system is located differently than in the normal heart, in that the AV node and His bundle are displaced inferiorly; this must be taken into account to avoid conduction system injury in the placement of the patch for the ASD (see Fig. II-16-3). U-shaped stitches are placed in the base of the septal leaflet of the right AV valve (Fig. II-16-4). Anterior to the cleft the stitches are placed in the ventricular septum and posterior to the cleft the stitches are placed in the valve leaflet itself, to avoid damage to the conduction system. At the posterior end, a last stitch is placed at the valve annulus 5 mm anterior to the crux of the heart; a 5-mm margin is left from the valve annulus (Fig. II-16-5). After passage of the suture through the valve, these stitches are placed in the autologous peri-

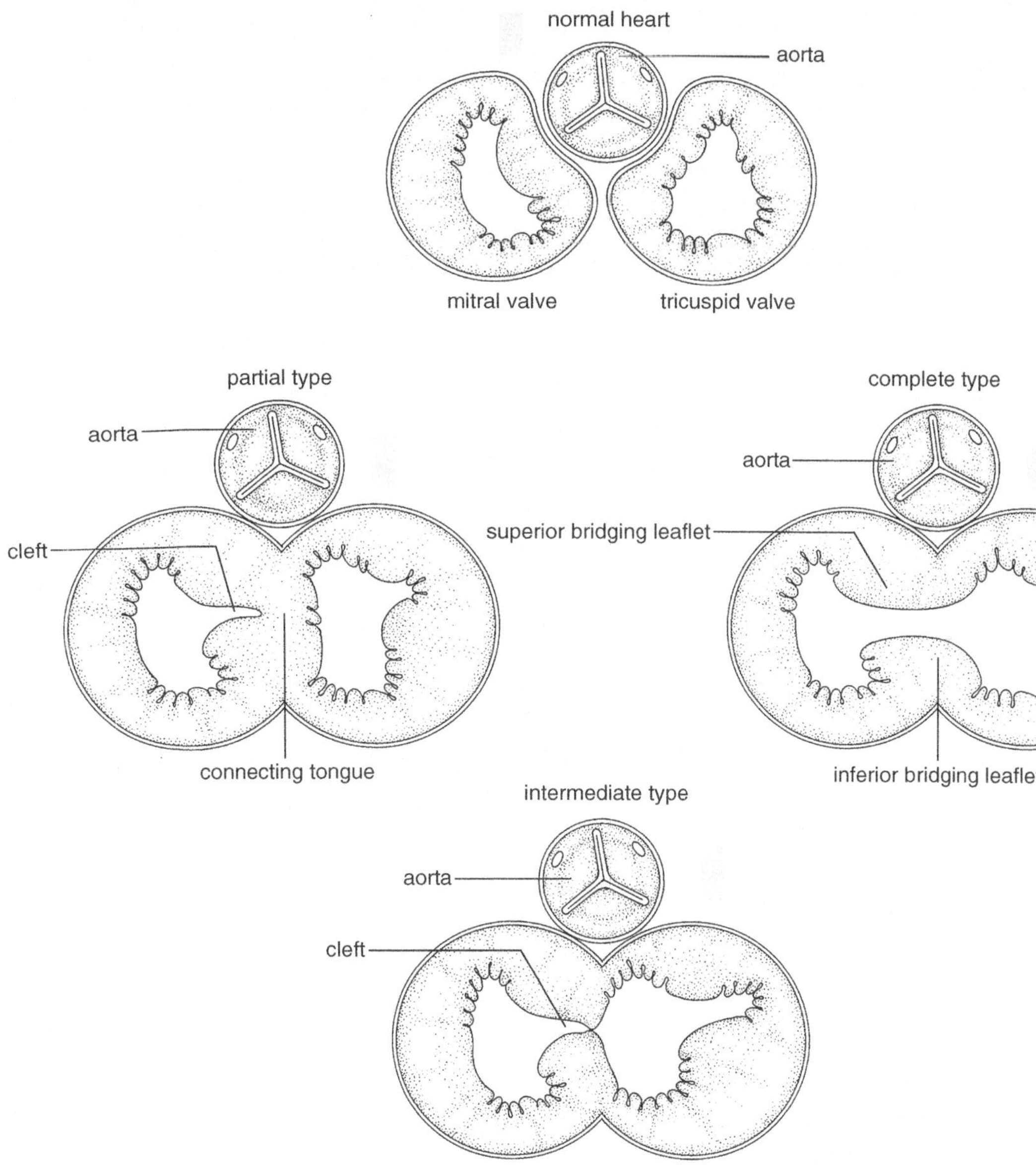

Fig. II-16-1. Classification of atrioventricular septal defects

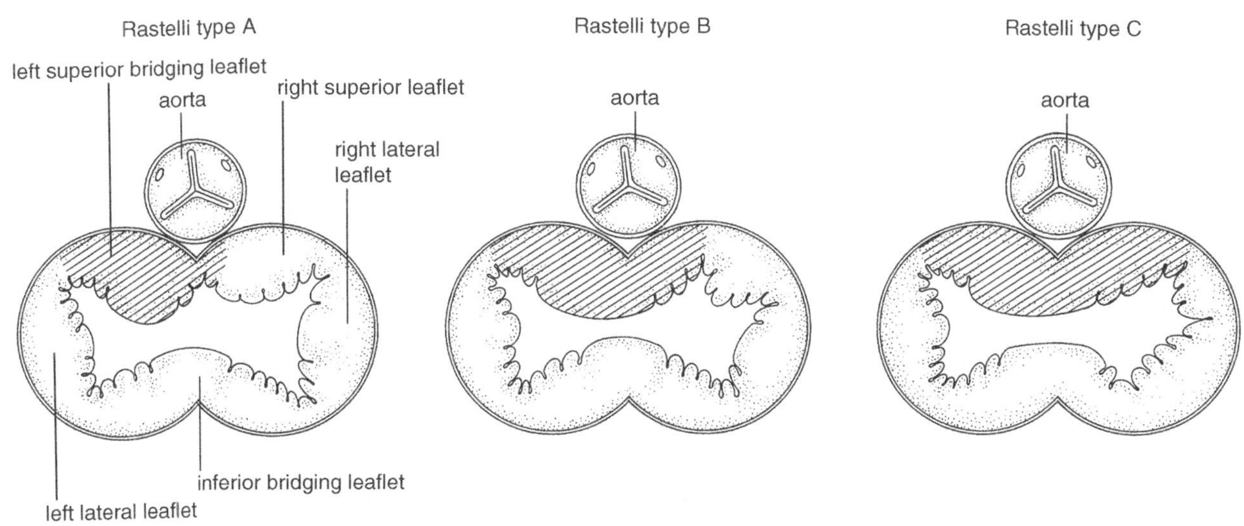

Fig. II-16-2. Rastelli classification of complete atrioventricular septal defect

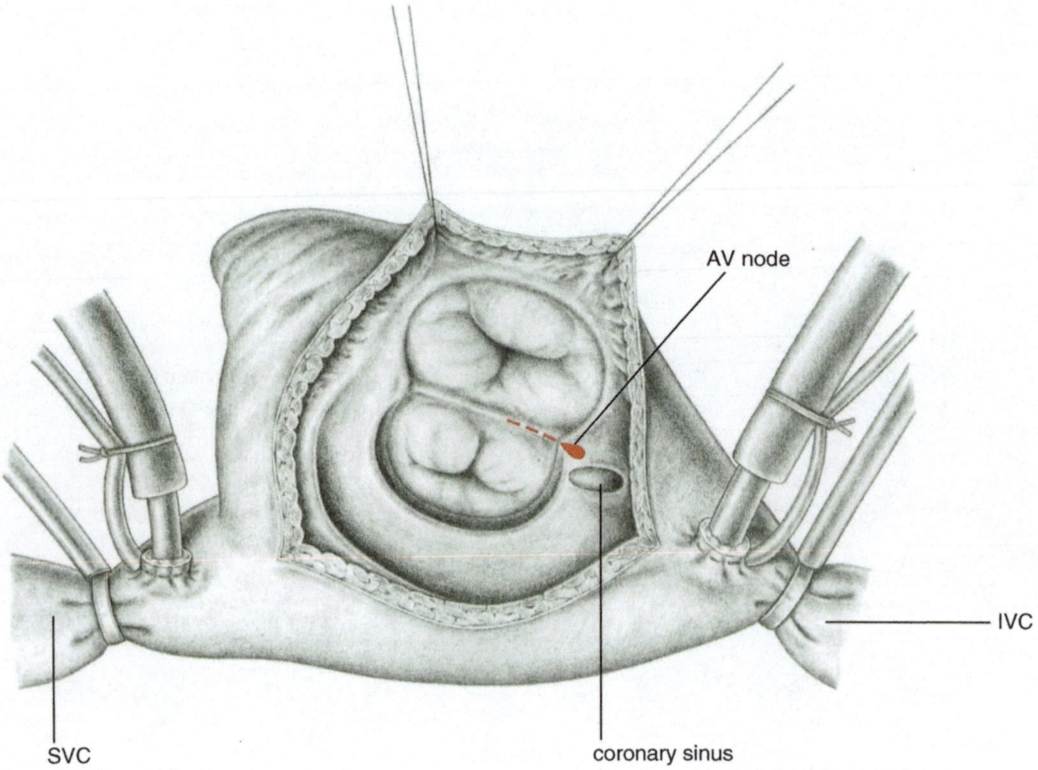

Fig. II-16-3. Partial atrioventricular septal defect: 1. Operative view after right atriotomy. *SVC*, superior vena cava; *IVC*, inferior vena cava

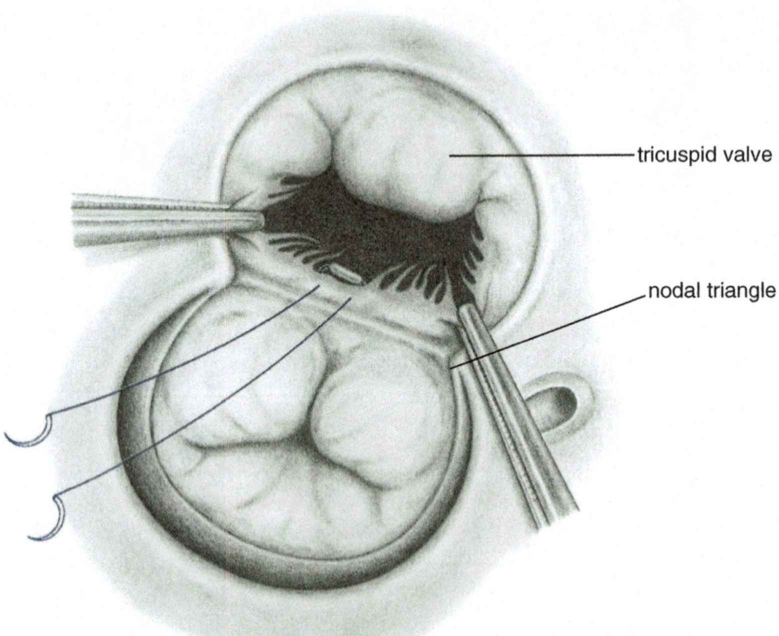

Fig. II-16-4. Partial atrioventricular septal defect: 2. U-shaped stitches are placed in the base of the septal leaflet of the tricuspid valve

cardial patch with the smooth side of the patch placed to the left side to avoid thrombus formation (Fig. II-16-6).

Next, the cleft of the left AV valve is closed. A traction suture of fine monofilament suture is placed at the tips of the anterior leaflets where the true chordae are attached. From the annulus of the valve, a series of mattress sutures with autologous pericardial pledgets are placed to close the cleft. The valve is tested by injecting fluid into the left ventricle (Fig. II-16-7). Hegar dilators are then inserted across the valve to ensure that the valve diameter is at least 90% of normal. In small babies, to avoid left AV valve stenosis, occasionally the cleft may not be closed completely.

Then, the ASD closure is completed. In the presence of the secundum ASD, this is closed simultaneously. A running

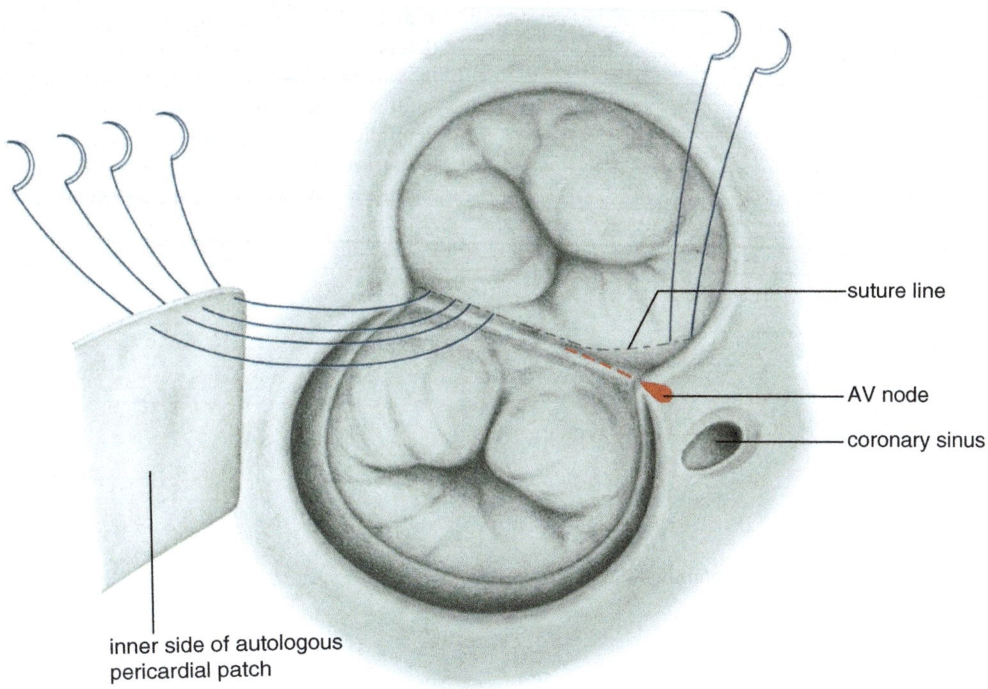

Fig. II-16-5. Partial atrioventricular septal defect: 3. U-shaped stitches are placed in the autologous pericardial patch. Anterior to the cleft, the stitches are placed in the ventricular septum, and posterior to the cleft, the stitches are placed in the valve leaflet itself, to avoid damage to the conduction system. At the posterior end, a last stitch is placed at the valve annulus 5 mm anterior to the crux of the heart. *AV node*, atrioventricular node

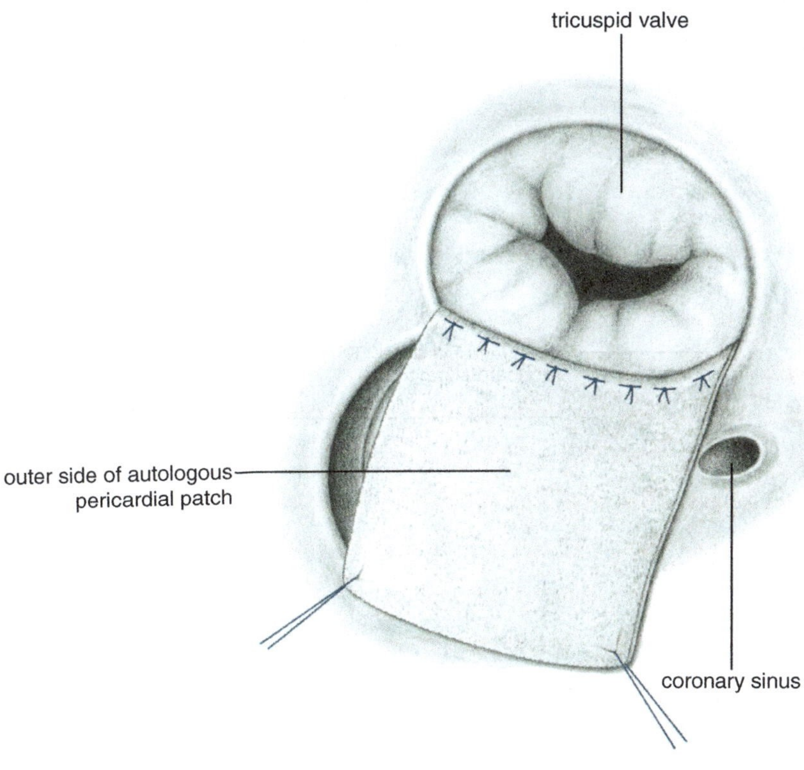

Fig. II-16-6. Partial atrioventricular septal defect: 4. The patch is lowered into place, and all sutures are tied

suture is begun in front of the coronary sinus and the edge of the primum ASD. The coronary sinus is thus left draining to the left atrium (Fig. II-16-8) [8]. To avoid obstruction of the coronary sinus orifice, the posterior wall of the coronary sinus is cut back. In the case of the presence of a persistent left superior vena cava, the suture line is placed inside the orifice of the coronary sinus, rather than anterior to it, still leaving the AV node to the left (Fig. II-16-8). An alternative technique is to bring the suture line along the annulus of the left AV valve and place the coronary sinus to the right. To preserve left AV valve function and minimize the chance of conduction system damage, and because leaving the coronary sinus leftward does not affect systemic saturation, we prefer the former technique in the absence of a persistent left superior vena cava. Before finishing patch placement, the left side of the heart is filled with blood. To avoid air embolism, de-airing is accomplished through the cardioplegic needle by connecting it to the vent line. Before tying the suture line for the ASD patch, a mosquito clamp is used to hold the suture line open. During this period, the lung is

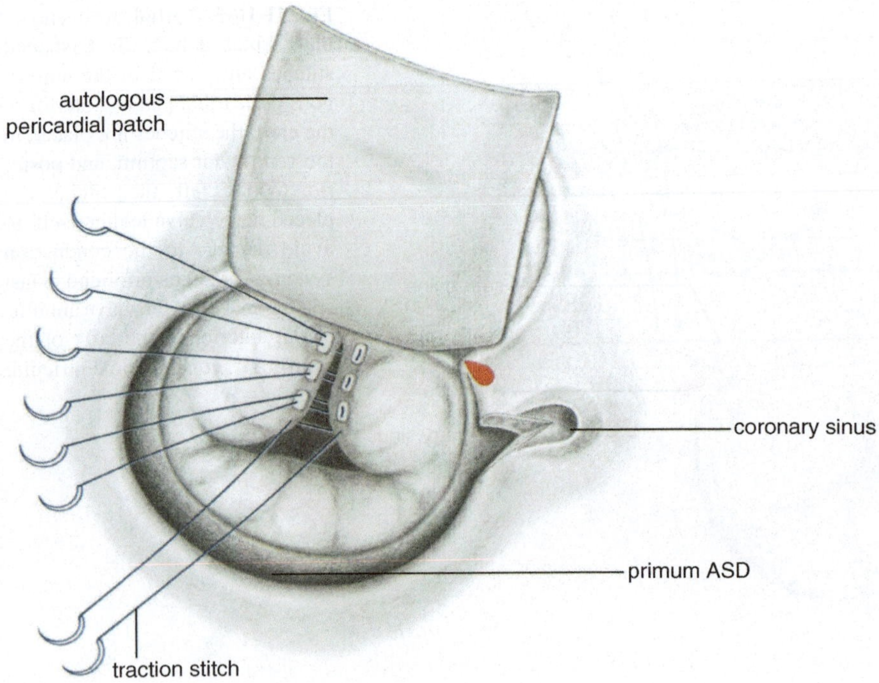

Fig. II-16-7. Partial atrioventricular septal defect: 5. The cleft of the left atrioventricular valve is closed using pledgetted mattress sutures. Cold saline is injected into the left ventricle to evaluate the competence of the left atrioventricular valve. The orifice of the coronary sinus is cut back and enlarged

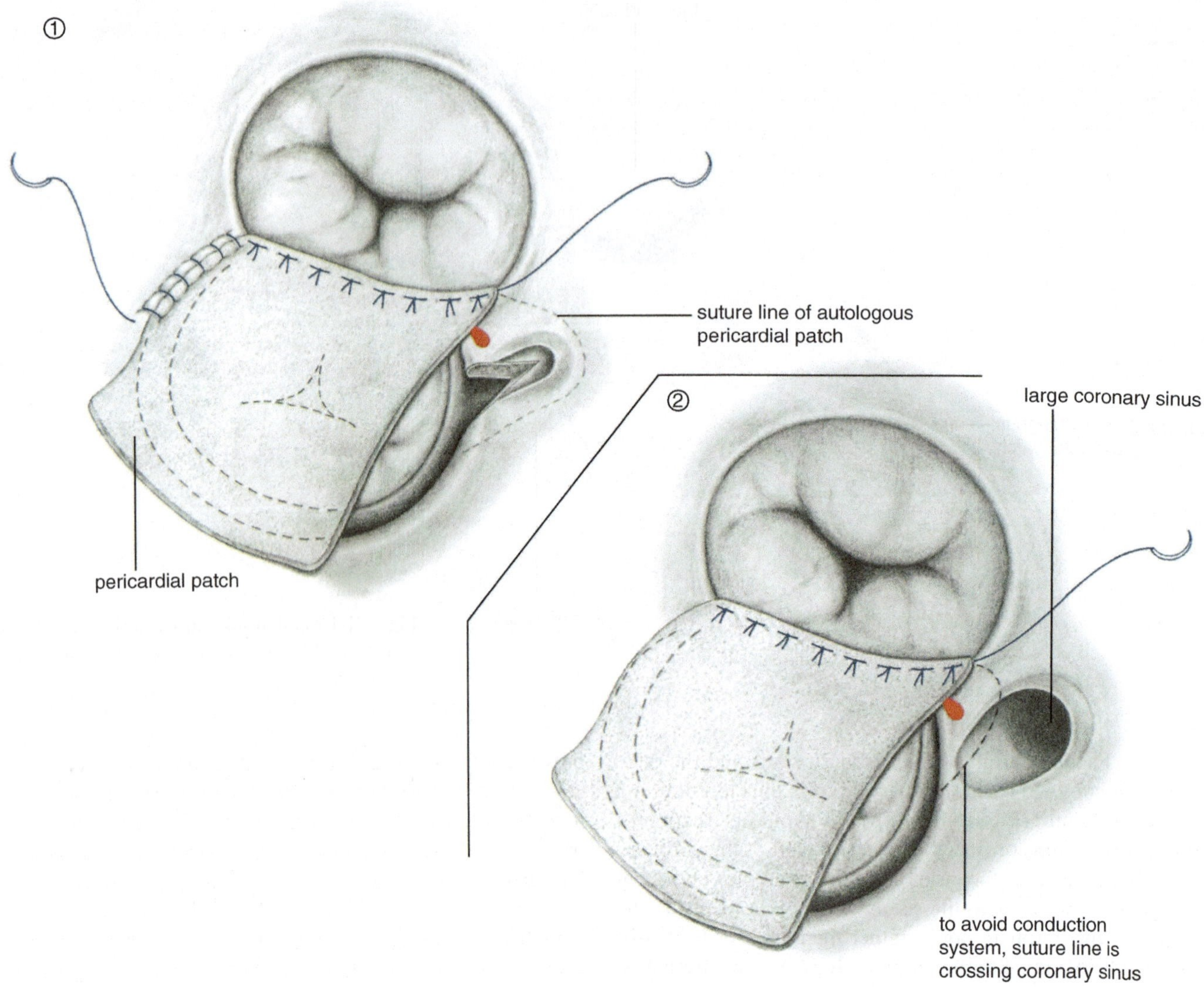

Fig. II-16-8. Partial atrioventricular septal defect: 6. The primum atrial septal defect is closed using an autologous pericardial patch. ① The coronary sinus is left draining into the left atrium. ② The coronary sinus is left draining into the right atrium. The posterior wall of the coronary sinus is used as a suture line in the presence of a persistent left superior vena cava

inflated by the anesthesiologist to help de-airing. If the patient has a patent foramen ovale, or a hole was created in the septum for venting, this site is used to de-air and is then closed directly.

After completion of de-airing, the aortic cross-clamp is removed, and the right atriotomy is closed. A left atrial pressure line is placed, to guide separation from CPB.

Intermediate AV Septal Defect

This type of AV septal defect is similar to the partial type, in that a connecting tongue is attached to both bridging leaflets, creating two AV valves. However, the AV valves are not completely attached to the ventricular septal crest, which creates a VSD. The surgical procedure is essentially the same as for the partial type. A pledgetted mattress suture is placed on the right side of the ventricular crest beneath the VSD. One stitch is placed in the superior bridging leaflet and another is placed in the inferior bridging leaflet. Both are placed in the pericardial patch. The rest of the repair is the same as for the partial type. In unusual cases, if the VSD is large, it is closed using a patch as is done with the complete type. In the intermediate type, frequently there are abnormal chordae beneath the aortic valve, which should be removed, as they may predispose to left ventricular outflow tract obstruction.

Complete AV Septal Defect (Rastelli Type A and C)

The surgical exposure is the same in the intermediate or partial type. To repair these defects, we primarily use a two-patch technique. Because repair surgical maneuvers for VSD closure and tricuspid valve are different in Rastelli type A and C, these are described separately.

Rastelli Type A

The ventricle is inflated with cold cardioplegic solution and the apposition point of the bridging leaflets is identified. A marking stitch of fine monofilament suture (Fig. II-16-9) is placed to mark the apposition point [8].

Pledgetted mattress sutures are used to anchor the patch to the ventricular septum. The first stitch is placed on the middle and the right side 2–3 mm from the ventricular septal crest (Fig. II-16-10 ①). Anterior to this point, the stitches are placed on the septal crest because the area is remote from the conduction system. The most anterior portion is the fibrous connection between the aortic valve and common AV valve. It is important to put a stitch in this fibrous skeleton to avoid a postoperative residual VSD. If the chordae from the crest impede visualization, the chordae can be removed to facilitate VSD patch placement. At the posterior area, to avoid conduction system damage stitches are put 2–3 mm away from the crest of the septum. At the right AV valve annulus, stitches are placed 5 mm from the crux (Figs. II-16-10 ②, II-16-11 ①). This last stitch is important to avoid a residual VSD.

The size of the VSD is measured to determine the size of the patch. The width of the patch is 80% of the width of the VSD, which decreases the tension on the sutures used for cleft closure. By "creating" enough tissue for cleft closure, the undersizing of the VSD patch helps avoid dehiscence and improves left AV valve function after surgery. The shape

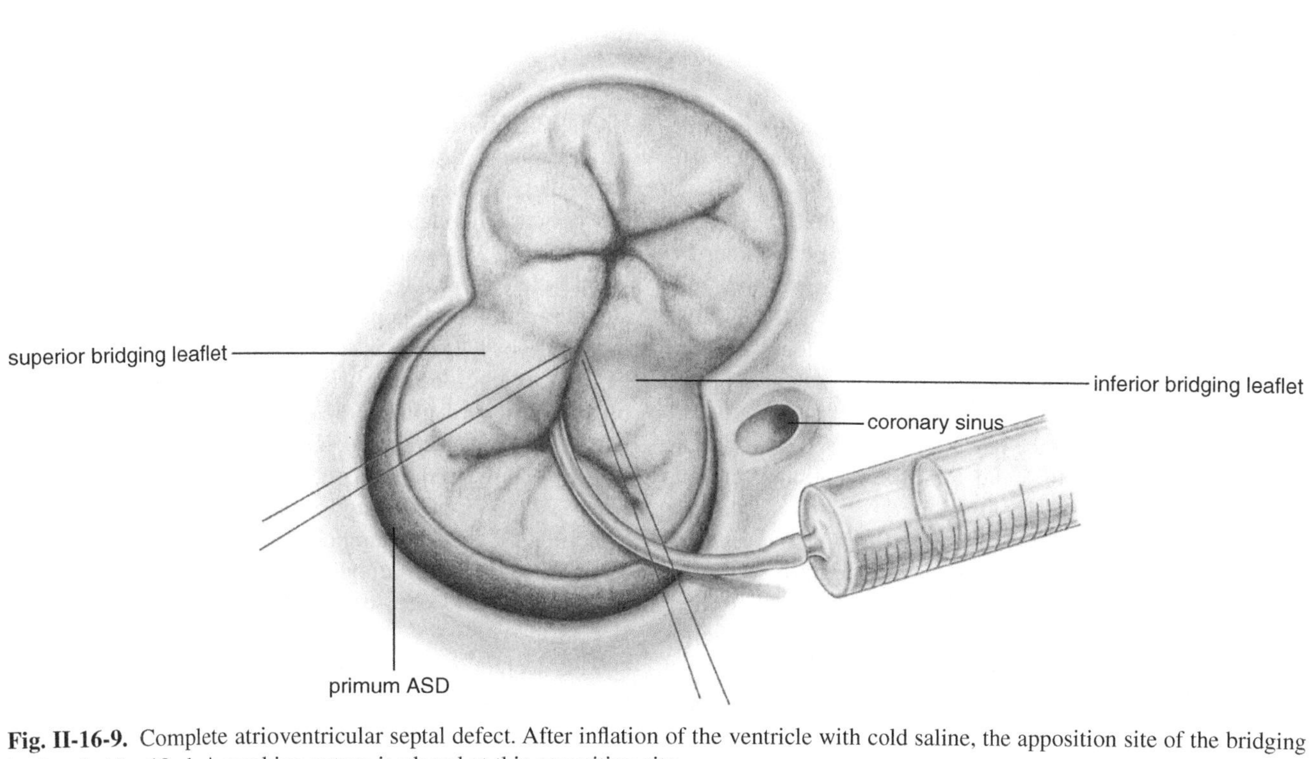

Fig. II-16-9. Complete atrioventricular septal defect. After inflation of the ventricle with cold saline, the apposition site of the bridging leaflets is identified. A marking suture is placed at this apposition site

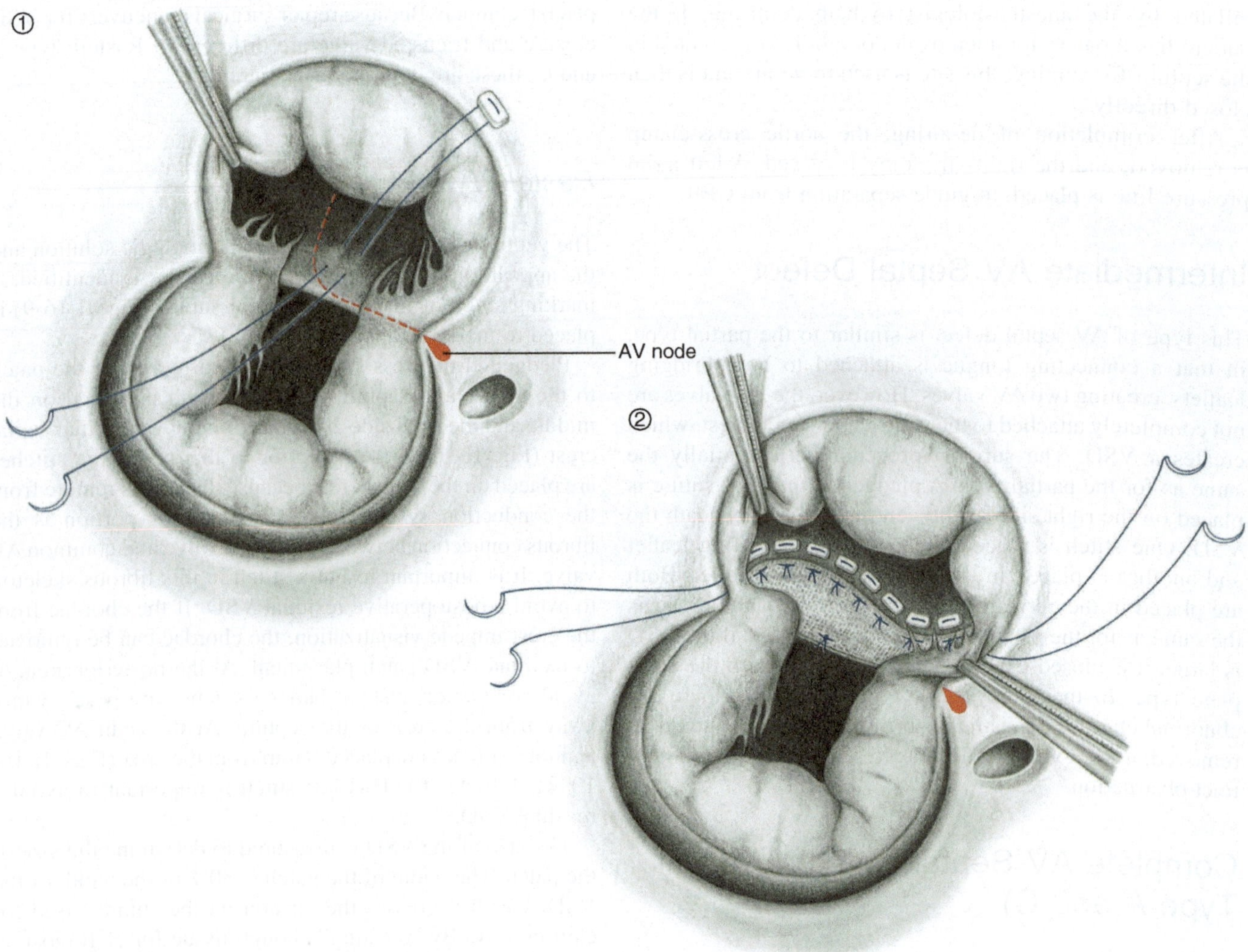

Fig. II-16-10. Complete atrioventricular septal defect (Rastelli type A): 1. ① Pledgetted mattress sutures are placed on the right side of the ventricular septal crest. ② All sutures are put in the patch, and the patch is lowered into place

of the patch is wider beneath the superior bridging leaflet and more narrow under the inferior bridging leaflet. The patch is curved at the bottom and straight at the top. Sutures are put in the inferior margin of the patch, and the patch is lowered into position; then, the sutures are tied. Under the superior bridging leaflet, the patch is placed to the right side of any chordae to avoid compromise of the left AV valve orifice. It is important not to compromise function of chordae of the inferior bridging leaflet, and so the patch is placed between the inferior bridging leaflet and chordae before placement of sutures in the patch. Then the VSD stitches are placed in the patch, to avoid the aforementioned chordal dysfunction (see Fig. II-16-11 ①).

Next, 6-0 monofilament U-shaped sutures are placed through the top end of the VSD patch, then through the AV valve, and finally through an autologous pericardial patch for ASD closure (see Fig. II-16-11 ②). At first, one stitch is placed in the VSD patch just beneath the apposition point of the bridging leaflets as marked by the stay stitch. Care is taken that the U stitches fit the patch and valve so as to create redundancy in the cleft to reduce tension on the cleft closure stitch (Fig. II-16-11). The smooth side of the pericardial patch is placed toward the left atrium. At the superior bridging leaflet, stitches are placed about 5 mm from the edge of the pericardial patch, and this redundant portion is later sutured to the right side of the bridging leaflet.

The cleft of the left AV valve is closed with mattress sutures using autologous pericardial pledgets. As with the partial type, the cleft is closed up to the attachment site of the true chordae (Fig. II-16-12). If regurgitation is still present observed after cleft closure (Fig. II-16-13 ①), an annuloplasty is performed. One or two commissuroplasty sutures (Kay–Reed procedure) or a half-annulus annuloplasty is chosen according to the site of regurgitation. It is important to place the annuloplasty sutures of 3-0 pledgetted mattress sutures deep enough. Care is taken not to damage the conduction system or circumflex coronary artery (Fig. II-16-13 ②).

This technique creates space between the anterior and posterior bridging leaflet at the right side after septation of the ventricle which may cause right AV valve regurgitation. The previously prepared redundant part of autologous peri-

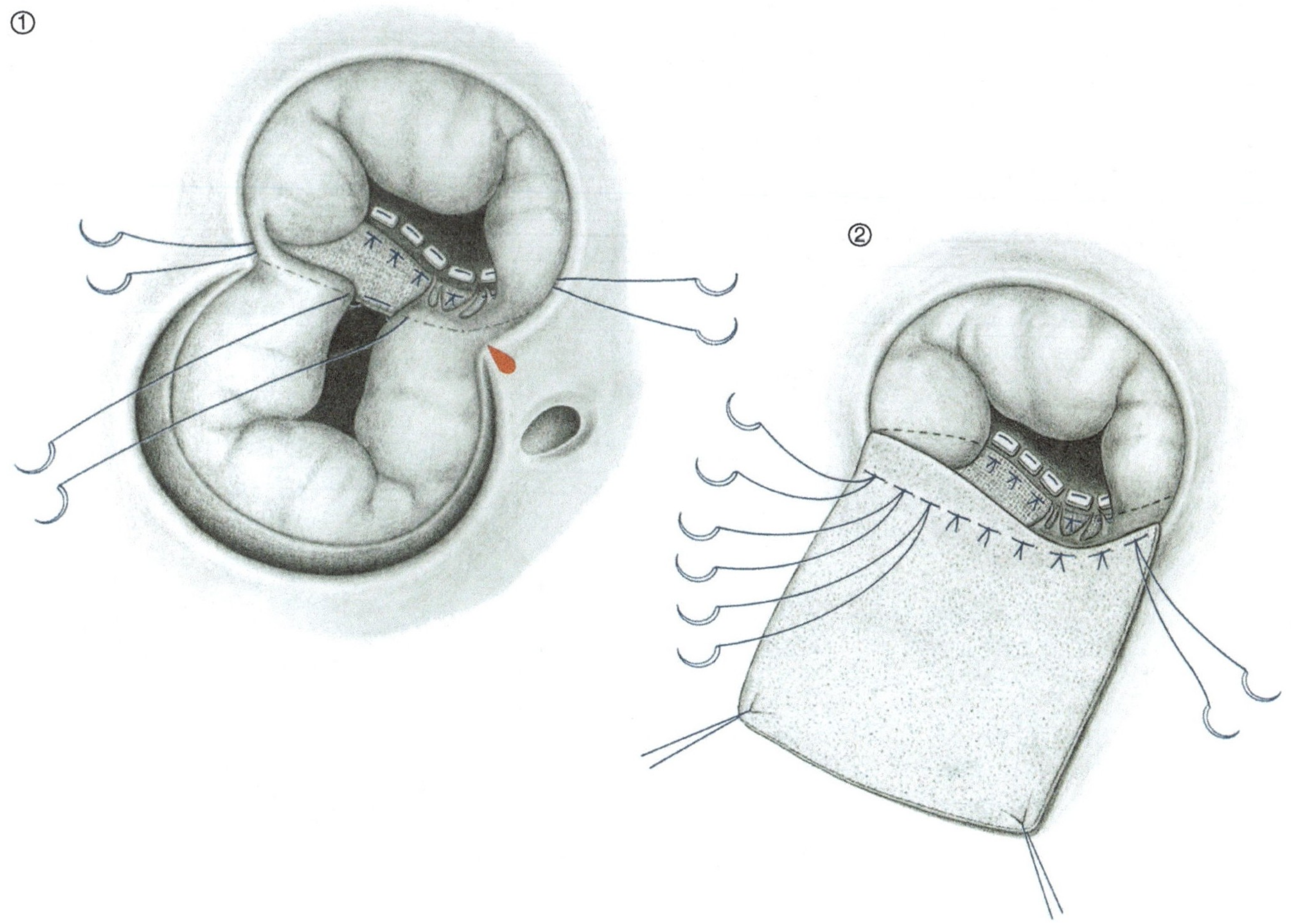

Fig. II-16-11. Complete atrioventricular septal defect (Rastelli type A): 2. ① Mattress sutures are placed in the superior edge of the VSD patch. ② These stitches are then placed through the above bridging leaflets and an autologous pericardial patch

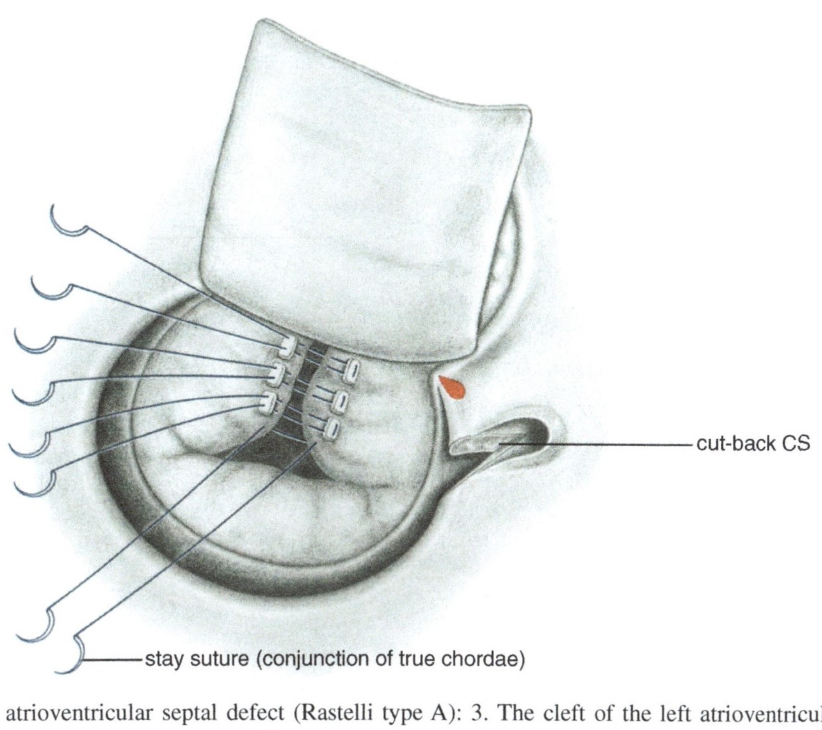

Fig. II-16-12. Complete atrioventricular septal defect (Rastelli type A): 3. The cleft of the left atrioventricular valve is closed using autologous pericardial pledgetted mattress sutures. *CS*, coronary sinus

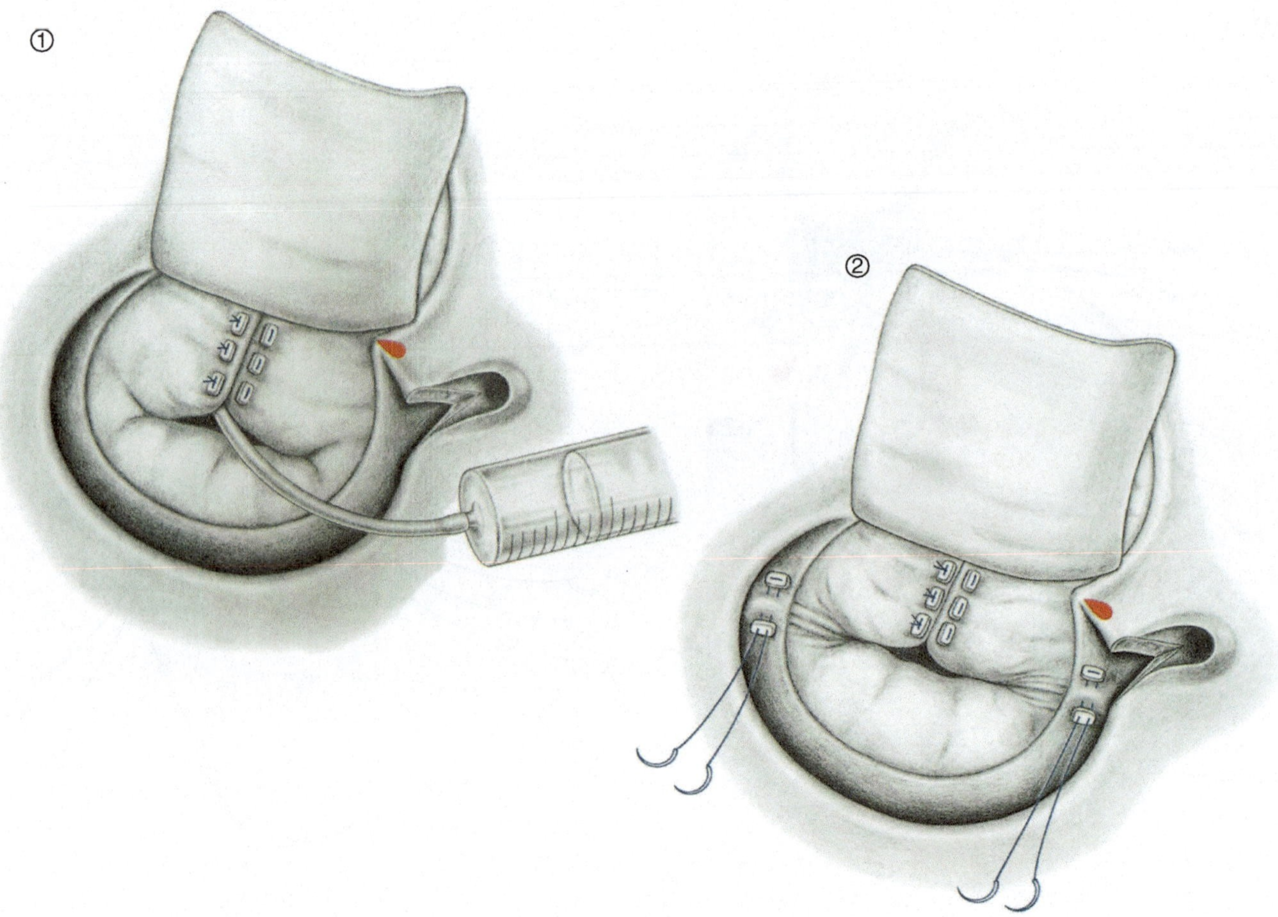

Fig. II-16-13. Complete atrioventricular septal defect (Rastelli type A): 4. ① Regurgitation test by injecting cold saline solution into the left ventricle. ② Annuloplasty stitches

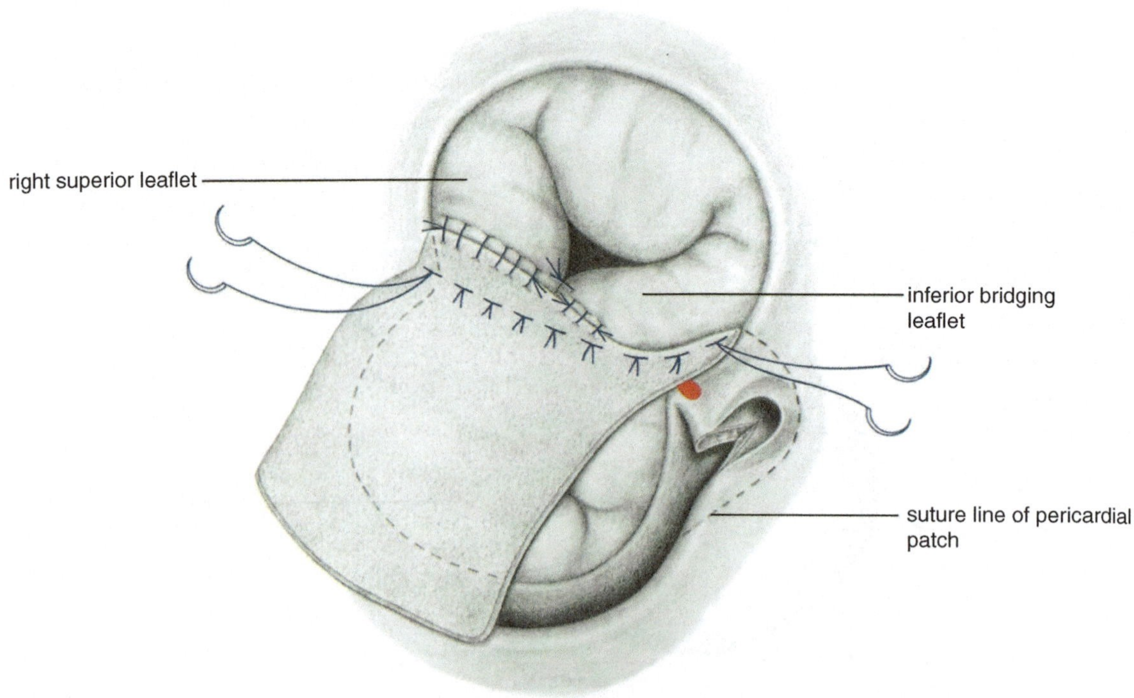

Fig. II-16-14. Complete atrioventricular septal defect (Rastelli type A): 5. The edge of autologous pericardial patch is sutured to the superior or inferior bridging leaflet to augment the deficient commissure site. The orifice of the coronary sinus is cut back, and is left draining to the left atrium by placement of autologous pericardial patch

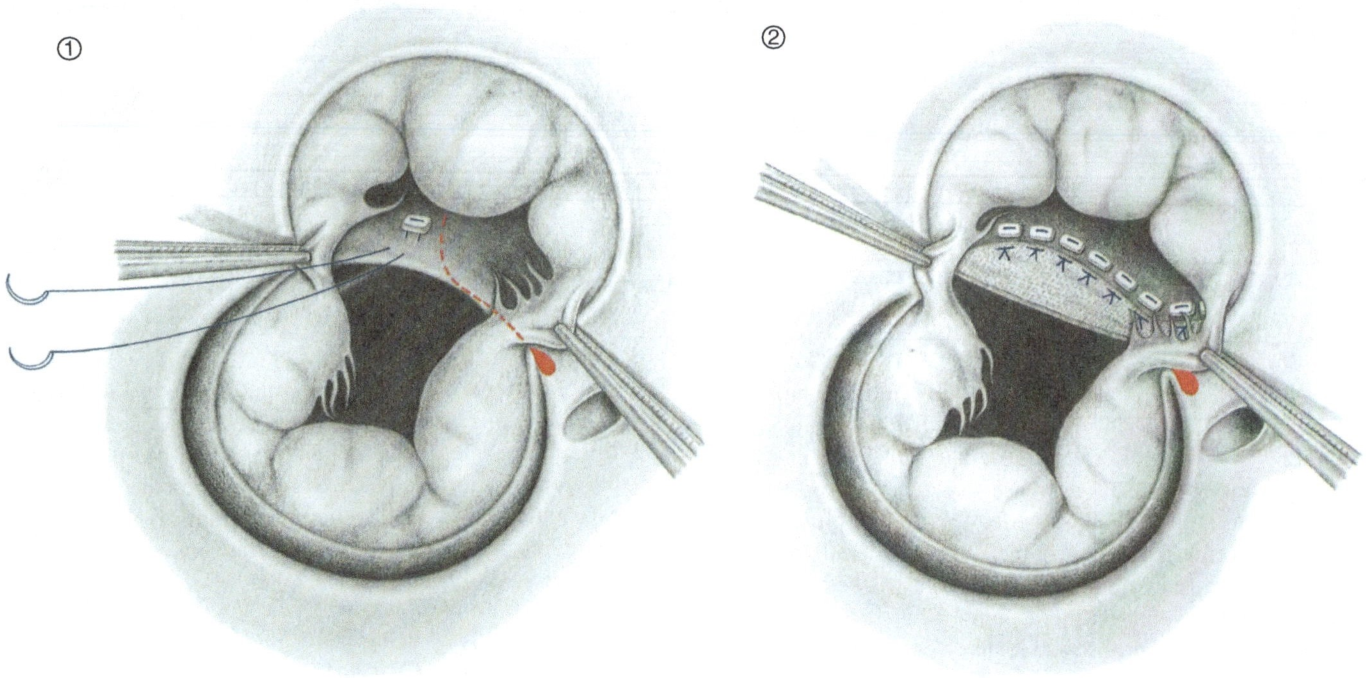

Fig. II-16-15. Complete atrioventricular septal defect (Rastelli type C) ①. Pledgetted mattress sutures are placed in the right side of the ventricular septal crest. ② Because of the absence of chordae beneath the valve, visualization is better than Rastelli type A

cardium and right AV valve are therefore sutured and regurgitation is avoided (Fig. II-16-14). Right AV valve function is checked with injection of solution as with the left AV valve.

The primum ASD is closed as with the partial type, and the coronary sinus is usually left draining to the left atrium.

Rastelli Type C

Stitch placement along the ventricular septum is the same as for type A. Because the superior bridging leaflet is floating, the visualization of the superior margin of the VSD is actually better than in type A (Fig. II-16-15). The shape of the patch is the same as in type A. The patch is positioned beneath the superior bridging leaflet. Under the inferior bridging leaflet, the maneuver in which the patch is placed under the leaflet and sutures are put in the patch later is the same as in type A. The U-shaped stitches are placed as in type A in the superior end of the VSD patch, the bridging leaflet, and the autologous pericardial patch for ASD closure using 6-0 monofilament sutures. The left AV valve is treated as in type A. If right AV valve regurgitation is observed, the right AV valve is treated with apposition of the bridging leaflets to each other using mattress sutures with autologous pericardial pledgets. The primum ASD is closed as in type A.

References

1. Ho SY, Baker EJ, Rigby ML, et al (1995) Atrioventricular septal defect. In: Ho SY, Baker EJ, Rigby ML, Anderson RH (eds) Color atlas of congenital heart disease, 1st edn. Mosby-Wolfe, London, pp 65–76
2. Wilcox RB, Anderson RH (1985) Atrioventricular septal defect. In: Wilcox RB, Anderson RH (eds) Surgical anatomy of the heart, 1st edn. Raven Press, New York, pp 610–616
3. Yamaki S, Yasui H, Kado H, et al (1993) Pulmonary vascular disease and operative indications in complete atrioventricular canal defect in early infancy. J Thorac Cardiovasc Surg 106:398–405
4. Yasui H, Nakamura Y, Kado H, et al (1990) Primary repair for complete atrioventricular canal. Recommendation for early primary repair. J Cardiovasc Surg 31:498–504
5. Masuda M, Kado H, Kajihara N, et al (2001) Early and late results of total correction of congenital cardiac anomalies in infancy. Jpn J Thorac Cardiovasc Surg 49:497–503
6. Masuda M, Kado H, Tanoue Y, et al (2005) Does Down syndrome affect the long-term results of complete atrioventricular septal defect when the defect is repaired during the first year of life? Eur J Cardiothorac Surg 27:405–409
7. Nakano T, Kado H, Shiokawa Y, et al (2002) Surgical results of double-orifice left atrioventricular valve associated with atrioventricular septal defects. Ann Thorac Surg 73:69–75
8. Pacifico AD (1994) Atrio-ventricular septal defect. In: Stark J, de Leval M (eds) Surgery for congenital heart defects, 2nd edn. Saunders, Pennsylvania, pp 373–388

II-17. Ventricular Septal Defect

Surgical Indication

1. A pulmonary-to-systemic blood flow ratio of more than 1.5 is considered an indication for surgical closure. In patients with a restrictive ventricular septal defect (VSD), the majority of defects decrease in size or close spontaneously over the first 2 years of life. Therefore, optimal timing of surgery for restrictive defects is considered to be 2–3 years of age. To avoid transfusion, surgery is best performed when patient weight is more than 10 kg. If progression of pulmonary vascular obstructive disease is a concern, surgery should be performed before the age of 2 years.

2. If the patient develops heart failure as a consequence of the large shunt during early infancy, surgery is indicated because there is little likelihood of spontaneous closure. Growth failure is certain in such cases, and premature death may occur in extreme cases. Surgical mortality for isolated VSD closure is less than 1%–2%. Another benefit of surgery at this age is a much less prominent scar than if surgery is performed at an older age.

3. If aortic valve prolapse is present with a doubly committed VSD or a perimembranous subarterial VSD, surgery is indicated regardless of the degree of shunt flow, to avoid permanent damage to the aortic valve.

4. In the presence of pulmonary hypertension, a pulmonary vascular resistance of less than 8 Wood units·m^2 is considered an indication for surgery. In marginal conditions, assessment with oxygen, tolazoline infusion, inhaled nitric oxide, and open lung biopsy may be helpful in estimating surgical risk.

Preoperative Evaluation

The position of the VSD, the presence of additional VSDs, and the presence of malalignment of the outlet septum should be evaluated carefully before surgery. If there is a patent ductus arteriosus, the operative field will be obscured by blood return during surgery, so the presence of a patent ductus arteriosus should be assessed before initiation of cardiopulmonary bypass (CPB).

Operative Procedure

Figure II-17-1 shows a classification of VSD proposed by Soto et al. [1], with several landmarks to identify the conduction system, including atrioventricular (AV) node and His bundle (Fig. II-17-2).

Cardiopulmonary bypass is instituted in the usual fashion. A left atrial vent cannula is inserted from the right side of the left atrium or left atrial appendage. To avoid postoperative pulmonary vein stenosis, we prefer the left atrial appendage for small babies. The aortic cross-clamp is placed, and cardioplegic solution is delivered in the root of the ascending aorta (Fig. II-17-3).

Exposure of the Operative Field

A special "VSD drape" with a large central opening is used to help organize the operative field. The right atrium is opened obliquely [2]. Partial-thickness traction sutures are placed in the inner wall of the right atrium. These stitches are fixed to the sheet to improve exposure of the VSD. A small retractor is placed to the anterior leaflet of the tricuspid valve to further facilitate exposure. The position of the VSD, triangle of Koch, medial papillary muscle, and anterior papillary muscle and the shape of the VSD are assessed. Then, the expected position of the conduction system is evaluated [3,4] (Figs. II-17-1, II-17-2, II-17-4; see Fig. II-17-6).

Perimembranous Inlet-Type VSD

Shape of VSD

This type of VSD has extension from the membranous area to the inlet area. The posterior margin of the defect is located inferior to the commissure between the anterior and septal leaflets of the tricuspid valve. The angle composed of the tricuspid valve annulus and inferior margin of the VSD is acute or a right angle (see Fig. II-17-4, angle y. The medial papillary muscle is located at the anterior margin of the VSD.

Conduction System

The bundle of His is present at the inferior margin of the VSD at the junction of the tricuspid valve annulus. It then runs down the left side of the ventricular crest. The degree of the left shift of the penetrating bundle depends on the

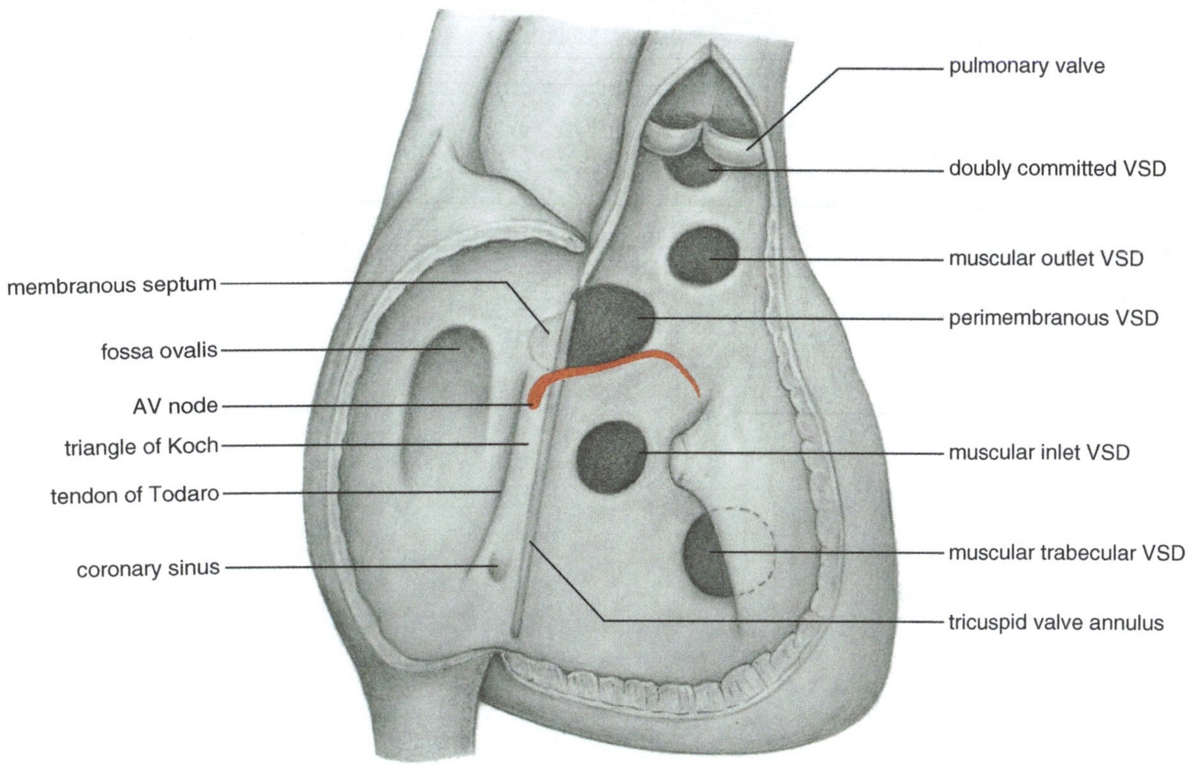

Fig. II-17-1. Classification of ventricular septal defect (*VSD*)

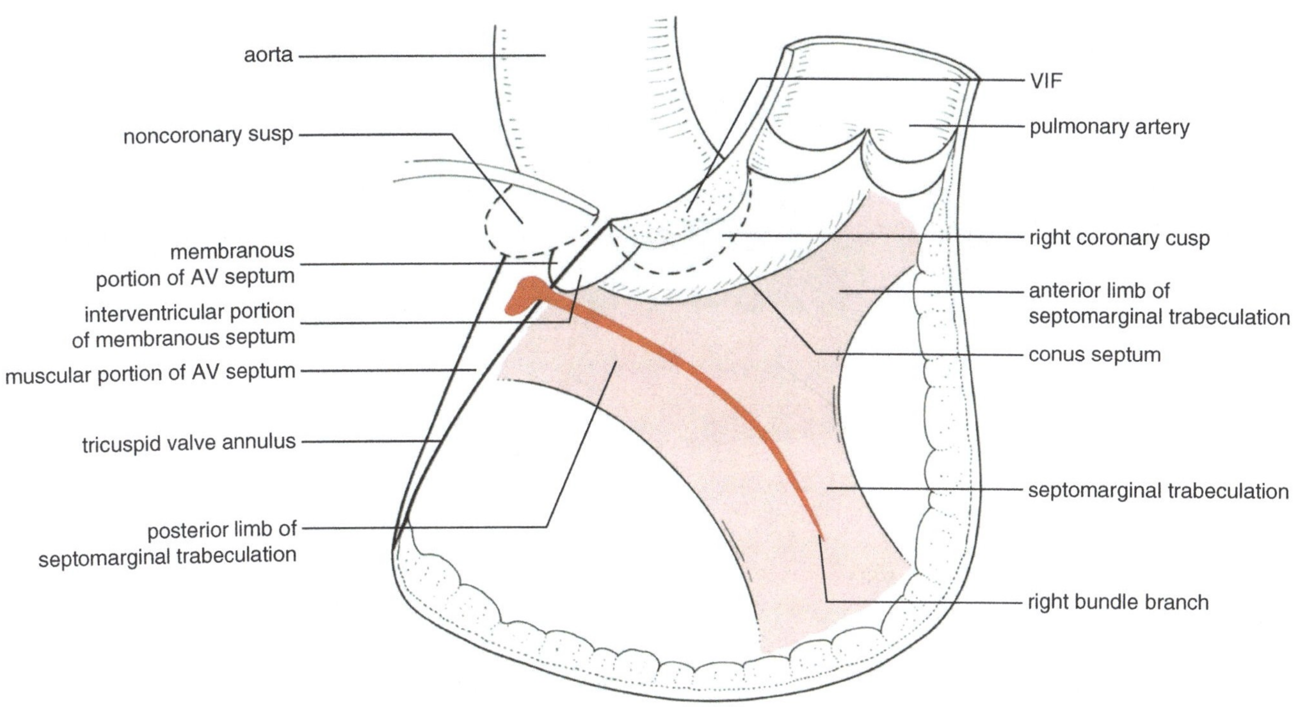

Fig. II-17-2. Anatomy of the right-side ventricular septum. *AV*, atrioventricular

degree of development of the posterior limb of the septomarginal trabeculation (see Fig. II-17-2). In this type of defect, its development is poor, and left-side deviation of the bundle is minimal. The inferoposterior margin is the most dangerous area. In the case of infants, needles are placed 5 mm from the inferior margin superficially in the depth of 0.5–1.0 mm and brought out 2.0 mm from the VSD margin at the right ventricular side.

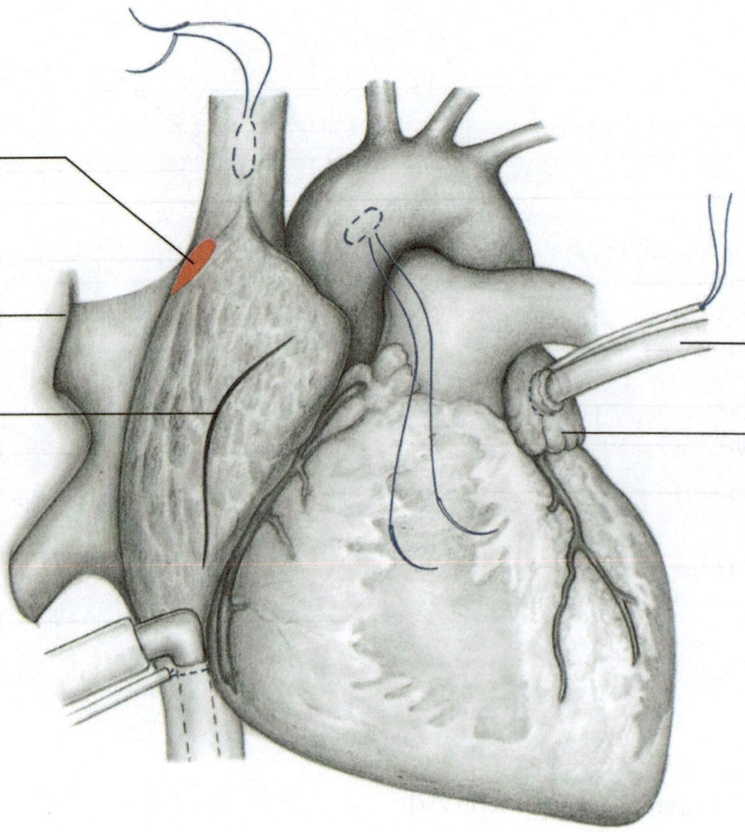

Fig. II-17-3. Operation overview. *LA*, left atrium

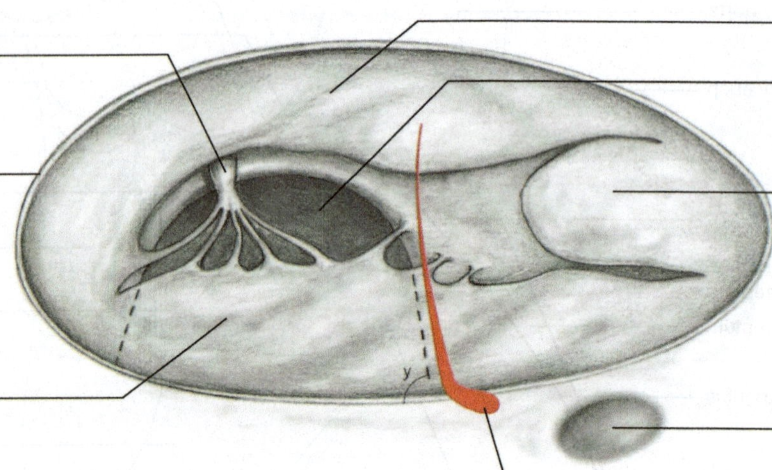

Fig. II-17-4. Inlet-type perimembranous VSD

Operative Procedure

Because the medial papillary muscle is located at the anterior and superior margin of the defect in this type of VSD, the numerous chordae of the tricuspid valve may obscure the VSD (Fig. II-17-5). A silk string is used to gather these chordae to facilitate visualization (Fig. II-17-5). The first pledgetted suture is placed on the base of the septal leaflet 2 mm inferior to the inferoposterior margin of the VSD, from the right atrium to the right ventricle. Care should be taken so as not to bite the tricuspid valve annulus (Fig. II-17-5; stitch A). The next stitch is placed 3 mm from the first stitch, from the right atrium to the right ventricle (Fig. II-17-5; stitch B). Then, these stitches are secured to the drape using a rubber-shod clamp; this improves visualization of the VSD. The next stitch is placed to the base of the tricuspid valve superior to the previous stitch (Fig. II-17-5; stitch C). The following stitch is placed 3 mm from the first stitch (Fig. II-17-5; stitch D). This second pair of stitches is also affixed to the drape.

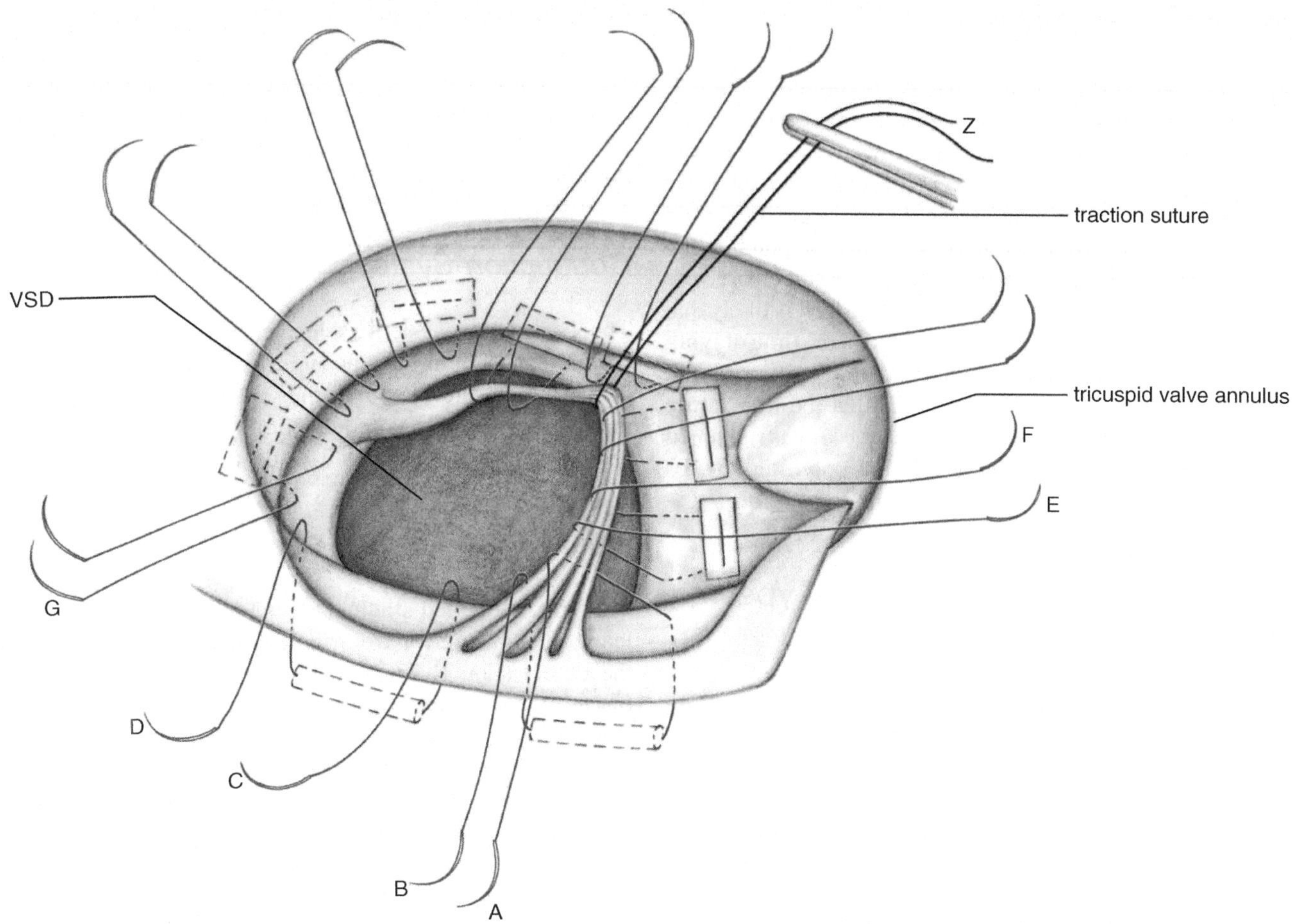

Fig. II-17-5. Interrupted suture closure of inlet-type perimembranous VSD

Attention is turned to the inferior margin. Stitches are placed superficially 5 mm from the inferior margin to 2 mm from the edge in the depth of 0.5–1.0 mm starting 0.5–1.0 mm from the tricuspid valve annulus (Fig. II-17-5; stitch E). In this type of VSD, the inferoposterior margin of the septum is thin, and care is necessary to avoid damage to the conduction system. The bundle is located at the rim of the left ventricular side of the posteroinferior margin of the VSD. The next stitch is started 5 mm from the VSD margin and brought out 3 mm from the first stitch (Fig. II-17-5; stitch F). Along the inferior margin the stitches are placed in a similar fashion. Stitches are placed in the margin of the defect at the anterior margin as there is no risk to the conduction system there.

At the superior margin of the defect in this type of defect, there is usually no outlet extension. If outlet extension is present, identification of the margin is important. At the superior margin, a pledgetted stitch is released 0.5–1 mm from the previously placed tricuspid valve annulus stitch (Fig. II-17-5; stitch G). At the superior margin, care is taken not to damage the aortic valve cusp.

Stitches to close the VSD are affixed to the drape one by one in order. This method simplifies and speeds correct ordering of the sutures as they are subsequently placed through the patch.

Suture Placement to the Patch

Stitches are placed in the patch 1–1.5 mm from the edge of the patch. Therefore, the size of the patch is about 3 mm larger than the size of the VSD. The oversized patch minimizes suture tension and so has less tendency to dehiscence and cause a residual shunt. It is better to keep the distance of suture pairs on the patch slightly shorter than that in the tissue. Adjacent suture pairs do not need to be placed immediately adjacent to each other, and a 1-mm distance is acceptable. If the distance of each pair of sutures at the patch site is wider than in the tissue, the suture may tear out of the tissue during tying because the myocardium is weaker than a patch.

Patch Material

As mentioned, because myocardium is more fragile than the patch material, so long as the patch material has enough strength, a thinner and more flexible material is better. A soft and compliant material is desirable, especially for the VSD with irregular margins. Material that facilitates fibrin deposition also may be advantageous in encouraging spontaneous closure of small residual defects.

How to Tie the Sutures

After all sutures are placed in the patch, the surgeon holds half the sutures and the assistant holds the other half. The tension is kept on the sutures as the patch is lowered into position. Care is taken to avoid compromising the leaflets and chordae of the tricuspid valve. During tying, knot placement should be gentle, guided by the feeling of adjusting the patch to the myocardium. If sutures are tied with excessive force, the myocardium may tear, causing a residual VSD. It is likely that the majority of residual defects are created at the time of tying sutures. Delicate and careful tying is important to avoid tearing the myocardium. A key point is that the first suture throw is used for approximation and then the knot is tightened gradually with subsequent throws. Teflon polyester sutures need at least five or six ties to be secured into position.

Perimembranous Trabecular-Type VSD

A perimembranous trabecular-type VSD, as shown in Fig. II-17-2, is defined relative to the septomarginal trabeculation. The medial papillary muscle is located at the anterior margin of the VSD. The angle made between the tricuspid valve annulus and the inferior margin of the defect is obtuse. The conduction system is located in the triangle of the septum facing the tricuspid valve. The septomarginal trabeculation is underdeveloped, not strong, and this portion of the ventricular septum is thin. The conduction system is embedded just posterior at the margin, and so this portion should not be used for closure. Stitches are placed as in the technique for the perimembranous inlet-type VSD, with sutures placed 5 mm from the inferior margin and superficially.

Perimembranous Outlet-Type VSD

Shape of VSD

The septomarginal trabeculation extends posteriorly, and the angle made between the inferior margin of the VSD and tricuspid valve annulus is a dull angle. The ventricular septum of this portion is thick. A remnant of the membranous septum, called a membranous flap, is often observed (Fig. II-17-6). This type of VSD has an extension toward the outlet septum, and the medial papillary muscle is located at the inferior margin of the VSD.

Conduction System

The conduction system is located on the left side of the ventricular septum at the inferior margin of the VSD, because the posterior rim of the septomarginal trabeculation is well developed. The conduction system does not stay at the margin of the defect and is located slightly posteriorly.

Operative Procedure

The first pledgetted stitch is placed at the base of the septal leaflet 3 mm inferior from the inferior-posterior margin of the defect (Fig. II-17-7; stitch A). The following stitch is placed 3 mm superiorly at the base of the tricuspid valve (Fig. II-17-7; stitch B). If there is a membranous flap, this stitch is placed in the flap. These sutures are affixed to the drape with a rubber-shod clamp, and this fixation facilitates exposure of the operative field (Fig. II-17-7). The next superior stitch is placed 1 mm from the previous stitch spot as for the inlet-type defect (Fig. II-17-7; stitch C). For the inferior margin, a stitch is placed 5 mm from the margin, passed superficially at a depth of 1.0–0.5 mm, and then brought out 1.5–2.0 mm from the margin of the VSD and 0.5 mm from the annulus of the septal leaflet of the tricuspid valve. It is put through the membranous flap if present (Fig. II-17-7; stitch D). The next stitch is started 3 mm from the previous stitch and 5 mm from the VSD margin and brought out 1.5–2.0 mm from the margin (Fig. II-17-7; stitch E).

At the anterior and superior margins of the defect, the technique is similar to closure of the inlet type of defect. However, in this type of defect, the aortic valve tends to be very close to the VSD. To avoid damage to the aortic valve cusp, clear visualization of the superior margin is important. An assistant places a retractor at the commissure between

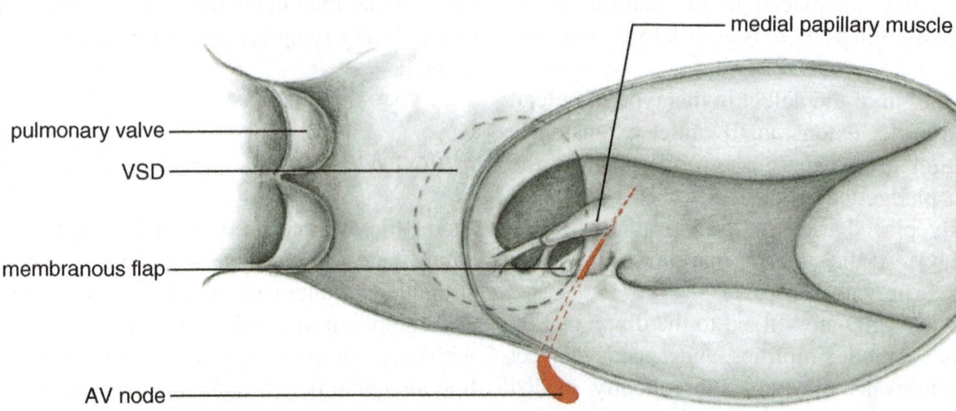

Fig. II-17-6. Outlet-type perimembranous VSD

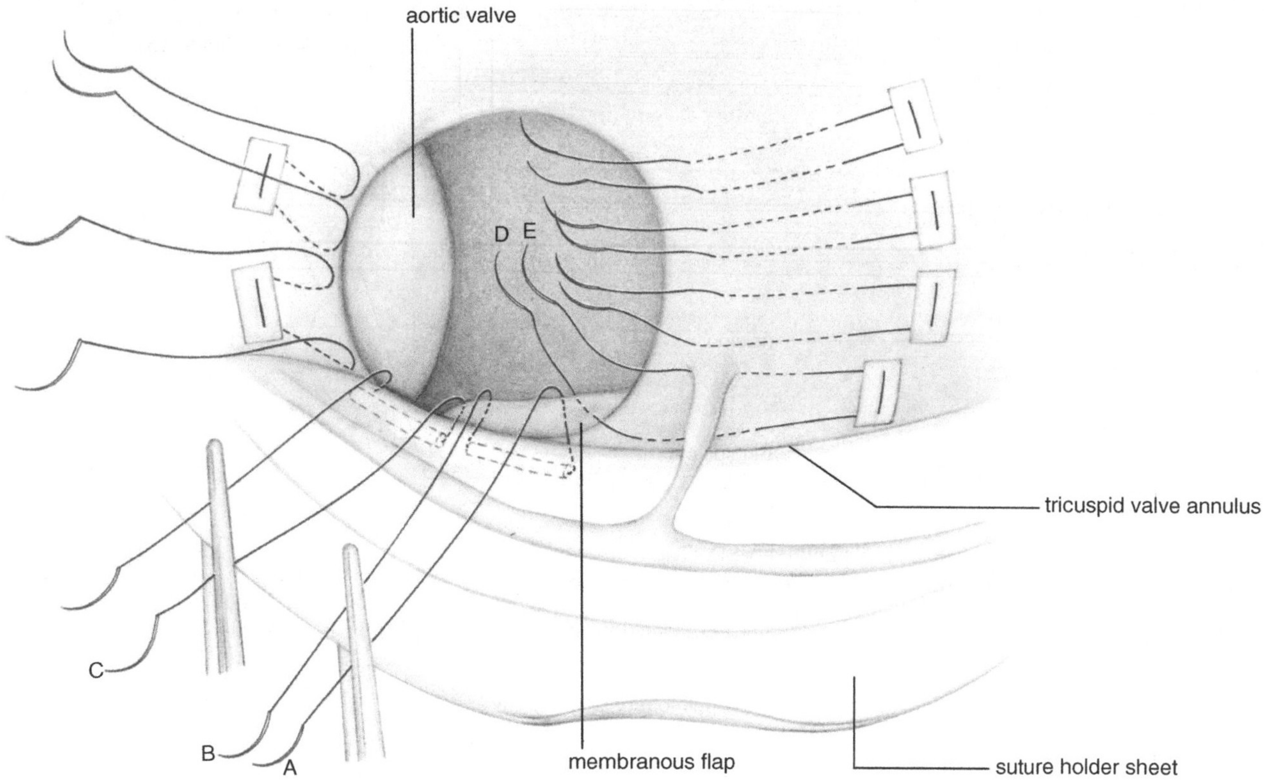

Fig. II-17-7. Interrupted suture closure of outlet-type perimembranous VSD

the anterior and septal leaflets with the right hand and another retractor in the VSD with the left hand with an inferiorly directed tension. Alternatively, the base of the aortic valve or right ventricular outflow tract may be pushed inferiorly and posteriorly from outside the heart to better expose the upper margin of the defect and its relationship to the aortic cusp. A pledgetted suture is placed 0.5–1 mm from the previous tricuspid valve annulus stitch at the superior margin of the VSD. As mentioned before, care is taken to avoid damaging the aortic valve. When discrimination of the aortic valve cusp is difficult, cardioplegic solution is injected, and the annulus of the aortic valve and margin of the VSD are identified clearly.

Avoidance of Right Bundle Branch Block

Right bundle branch block causes ventricular dysfunction, especially in the presence of pulmonary hypertension and right ventricular hypertrophy [5]. There are two types of right bundle branch block, the peripheral and proximal types. The mechanism of right bundle branch block is usually the proximal type, because a ventriculotomy is rarely necessary to close the defect. The location of the right bundle is variable depending on the position of the VSD, and no clear landmark is present. Generally, the right bundle emerges from the His bundle, penetrates the septum, and runs toward the anterior papillary muscle. At 5 mm from the inferior margin of the defect, the bundle is still situated superficially. At the inferior and anteroinferior margins of the VSD, stitches are placed superficially within 5 mm of the margin of the defect [6].

Doubly Committed VSD

Shape of VSD

This VSD is located beneath the pulmonary valve. The aortic valve cusp may prolapse into the defect and decrease the actual shunt through the defect. The prolapsing aortic valve cusp may result in aortic valve regurgitation in the future.

Exposure of VSD

A longitudinal incision is begun in the main pulmonary artery, 10–15 mm above the pulmonary valve annulus. This incision is extended with care not to damage the pulmonary valve (Fig. II-17-8). To avoid damage to the pulmonary valve by this incision and to have the ability to extend the incision to improve visualization, we prefer a longitudinal incision to a transverse incision. Shallow traction sutures are placed in the edges of the pulmonary artery for facilitation of the operative field. Small retractors are placed in the right ventricle through this incision across the pulmonary valve.

Conduction System

The relationship between the VSD, pulmonary valve, and tricuspid valve is evaluated. This defect sits in the right ventricular outflow tract superior to the commissure between the anterior and septal leaflets of the tricuspid valve. The conduction system is remote from the inferior margin of the defect (see Fig. II-17-1).

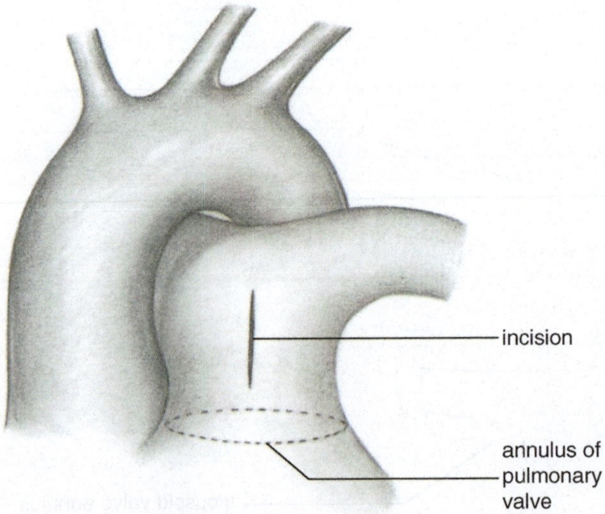

Fig. II-17-8. Operation view for doubly committed VSD. The pulmonary arteriotomy is placed far from the pulmonary valve and extended proximally with care to avoid damage to the valve

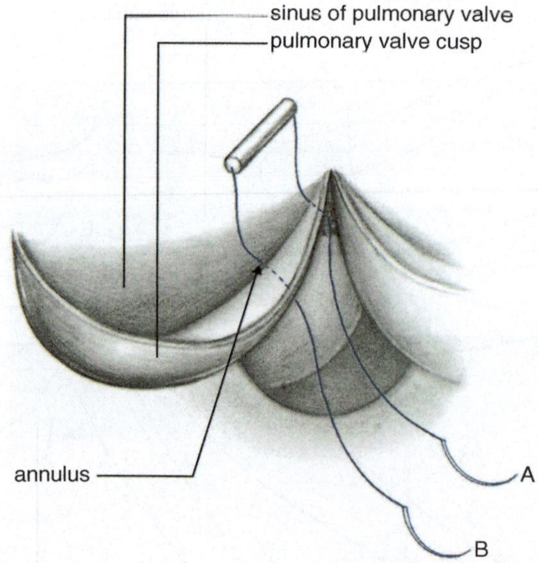

Fig. II-17-9. Doubly committed VSD closure: 1. Stitches are placed in the valve annulus, not the valve cusp itself

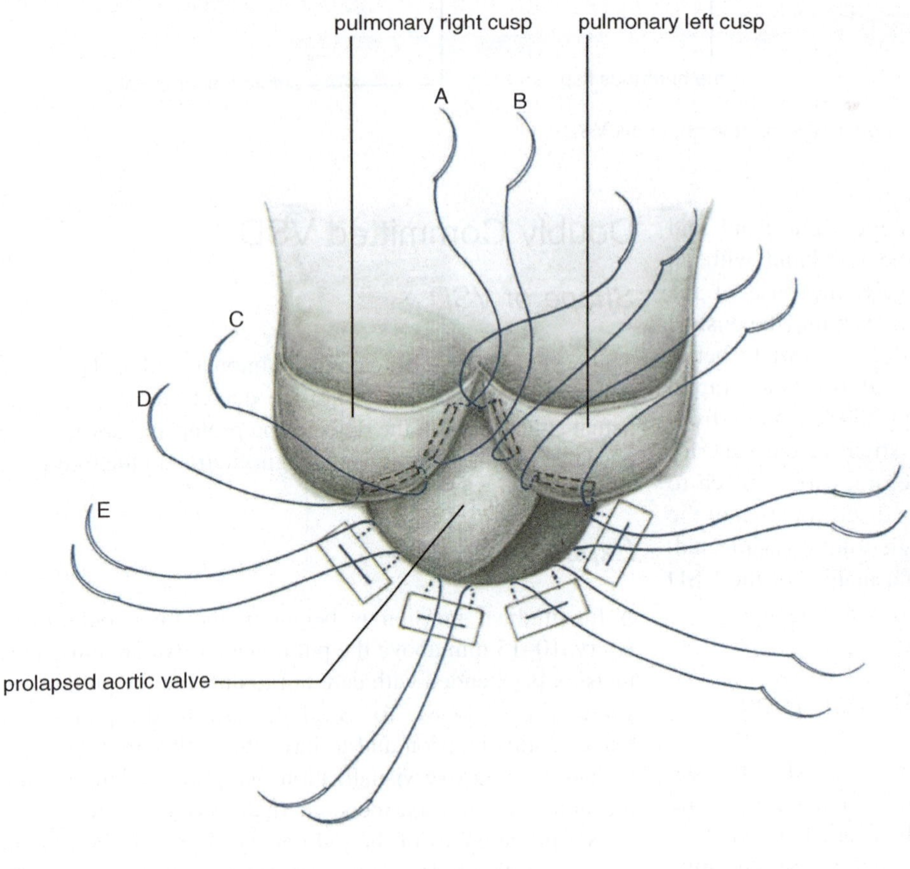

Fig. II-17-10. Doubly committed VSD closure: 2

Operative Procedure

An assistant retracts the right pulmonary cusp with forceps laterally and exposes the pulmonary valve annulus. A pledgetted mattress suture is placed in the pulmonary valve annulus from the pulmonary artery side to the right ventricle side toward the commissure between the right and left pulmonary valve cusps. It is important to put the stitch in the annulus, not the leaflet itself (Figs. II-17-9, II-17-10; stitch A). If this stitch is placed too deep, this might injure the left main coronary artery, which runs behind the proximal part of the sinotubular junction of the left pulmonary cusp. The next stitch is placed 3 mm from the first stitch at the pulmonary valve annulus (Figs. II-17-9, II-17-10; stitch B). These sutures are affixed to the "VSD drape." The following stitch is placed posteriorly 1 mm apart from the previous stitch (Fig. II-17-10; stitch C). The subsequent stitch is also placed 3 mm apart from the first stitch and 1.5 mm inferior from the pulmonary annulus (Fig. II-17-10; stitch D). Care is taken not to damage the prolapsing aortic valve cusp. A suture is placed in the left pulmonary valve annulus 1 mm apart from the first stitch. The next stitch is placed in the left valve annulus 3 mm from the initial stitch and affixed to the VSD drape.

Next, attention is turned to the inferior margin of the VSD. A pledgetted suture is placed in the right inferior margin 0.5 mm apart from the suture at the lowest right pulmonary valve annulus stitch (Fig. II-17-10; stitch E). A paired stitch is placed 4 mm from the VSD margin and brought out 3 mm from the first stitch. This suture is affixed to the drape as before. The size of the patch is about 3 mm larger than the defect. The sutures are brought through the patch, which is lowered into position. Finally, the sutures are carefully tied, paying attention to the pulmonary valve leaflets.

Muscular VSD

In this type of VSD, there are many shunts through the right ventricular trabeculations, and from the right ventricle clear visualization of whole margin of the VSD is difficult. It may be hard to obtain complete closure from the right ventricle. Therefore, VSD closure through the left ventriculotomy has sometimes been recommended. However, a left ventriculotomy in a small baby may compromise ventricular function, and so we prefer an approach through the right atrium using the technique of closure of many shunts between the trabeculation with patch closure or direct closure employing pledgetted mattress sutures. With this technique, complete closure is difficult. However, even after an incomplete closure, the left–right shunt decreases, the pulmonary artery pressure falls, weight gain is obtained, and in some cases the residual defect may close spontaneously (Fig. II-17-11).

For an apical muscular VSD, recently, Van Praagh et al. [7] and Tsang et al. [8] reported an approach through a small incision at the apex of the right ventricle. A small right ventriculotomy is made parallel to the anterior descending coronary artery, and the septomarginal trabeculation is pushed to the right. The VSD is closed between the septum and septomarginal trabeculation (Fig. II-17-12).

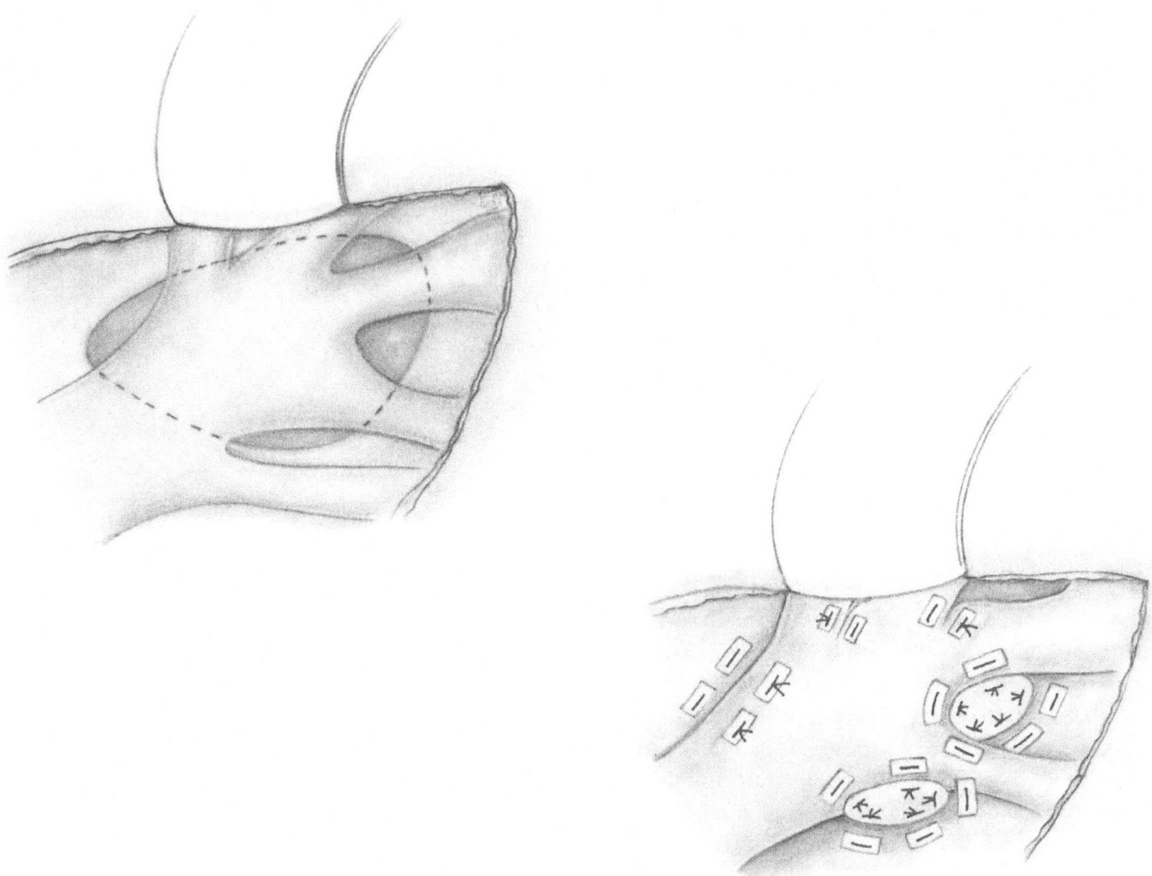

Fig. II-17-11. Transatrial muscular VSD closure

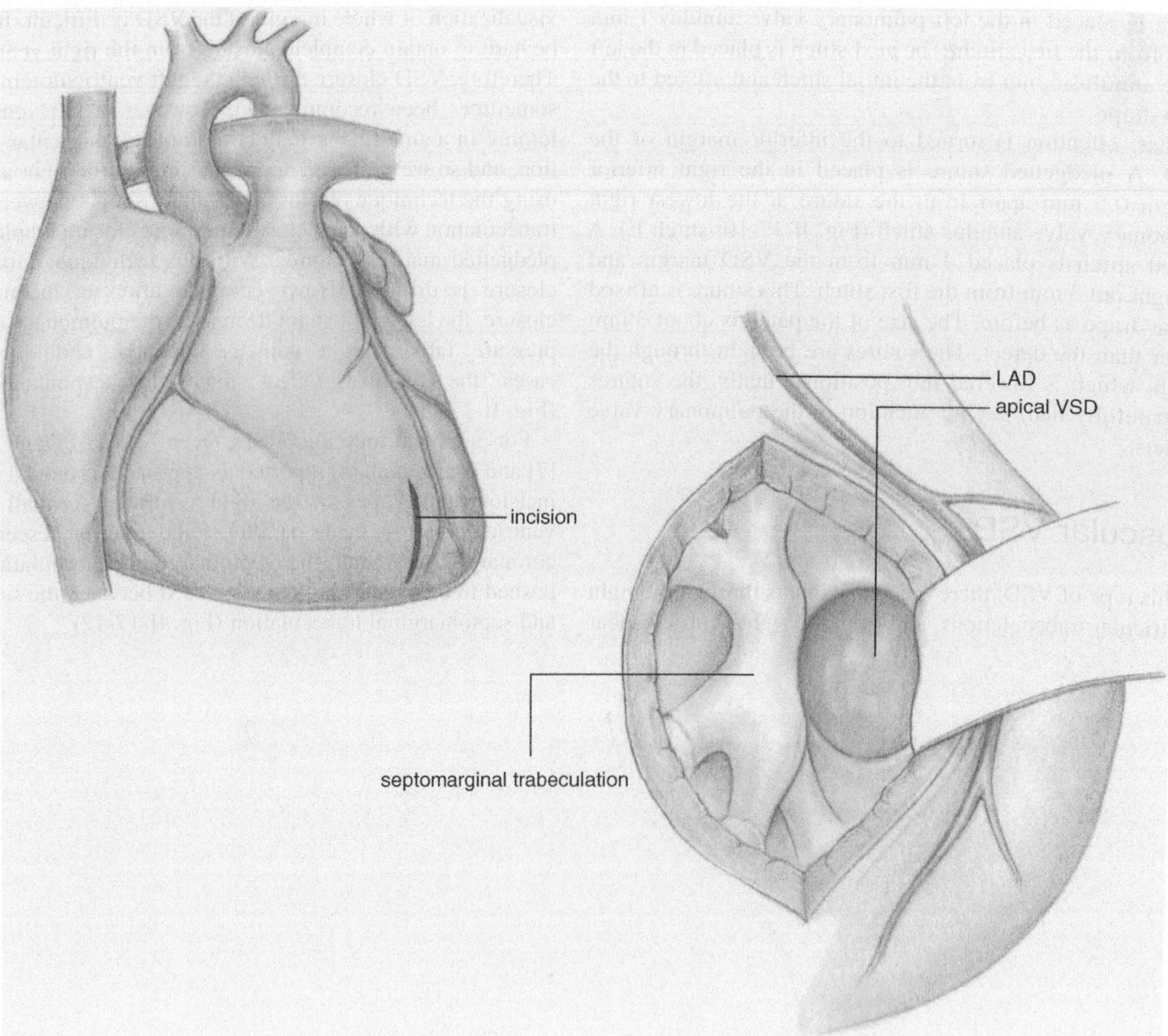

Fig. II-17-12. Right ventriculotomy for muscular VSD closure. *LAD*, left anterior descending artery

VSD with Membranous Septal Aneurysm

A membranous septum aneurysm does not usually originate from the membranous septum itself. In most cases, the remnant of membranous septum, redundant septal leaflet tissue, and the tricuspid valve chordae are fused and cover the VSD. A membranous septal aneurysm is made of contributions from all these structures. Simply closing the hole in the "aneurysm" may result in a residual shunt because in this condition there are often actually several holes. It is preferable to incise the "aneurysm sac" to clearly identify the margins of the original defect.

The opening of the sac is enlarged (Fig. II-17-13), and traction sutures are placed in each edge. An incision can be placed in the septal leaflet of the tricuspid valve toward the annulus of the tricuspid valve, to visualize the whole defect including margins to place the sutures for closure. Pledgetted mattress sutures are utilized to close the defect. The membranous flap, valve tissues, and fibrous tissue adhered to the VSD do not contain the conduction system and thus may be used for stitch placement if sufficiently strong. The aneurysmal tissue should not be used as a patch to close the defect because it is of uncertain strength.

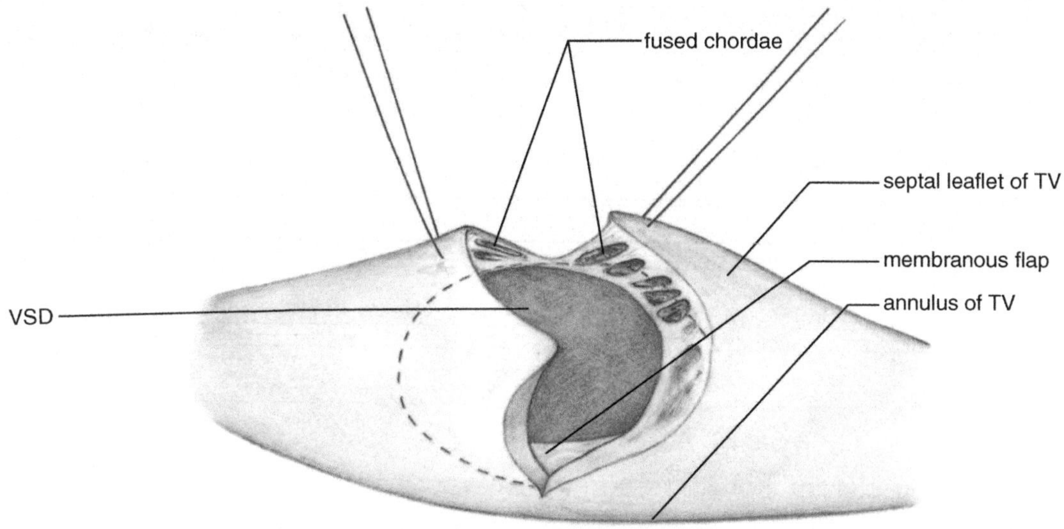

Fig. II-17-13. Membranous septal aneurysm. An incision is placed in the membranous septal aneurysm after traction suture placement. Usually the incision is made in the tricuspid valve (*TV*) leaflet itself perpendicular to the valve annulus

References

1. Soto B, Becker A, Moulaert AJ, et al (1980) Classification of ventricular septal defects. Br Heart J 43:332–343
2. Lincoln C, Jamieson S, Joseph M, et al (1977) Transatrial repair of ventricular septal defects with reference to their anatomic classification. J Thorac Cardiovasc Surg 74:183–190
3. Doty DB, McGoon DC (1983) Closure of perimembranous ventricular septal defect. J Thorac Cardiovasc Surg 85:781–790
4. Kurosawa H, Becker AE (1987) Atrioventricular conduction in congenital heart disease: In: Kurosawa H, Becker AE (eds) Surgical anatomy. Springer-Verlag, Tokyo
5. Yasui H, Takeda Y, Yamauchi S, et al (1977) The deleterious effects of surgically induced complete right bundle branch block on long-term follow-up results of closure of ventricular septal defect. J Thorac Cardiovasc Surg 74:210–217
6. Fukuda T, Suzuki T, Kashima I, et al (2002) Shallow stitching close to the rim of the ventricular septal defect eliminate injury to the right bundle branch. Ann Thorac Surg 74:550–555
7. Van Praagh S, Mayer JE Jr, Berman NB, et al (2002) Apical ventricular septal defects: follow-up concerning anatomic and surgical considerations. Ann Thorac Surg 73:48–56, discussion 56–57
8. Tsang VT, Hsia TY, Yates RW, et al (2002) Surgical repair of supposedly multiple defects within the apical part of the muscular ventricular septum. Ann Thorac Surg 73:58–62, discussion 62–63

II-18. Ruptured Aneurysm of the Sinus of Valsalva

In some patients, the wall of the sinus of Valsalva is abnormally thin and aortic diastolic pressure is sufficient to distort the sinus. The sinus may gradually become aneurysmal and rupture into an adjacent cardiac chamber, which causes acute volume overload. Before rupture occurs, the patient is usually asymptomatic. The aneurysm typically protrudes from the right coronary sinus into the right ventricle or right atrium, or from the noncoronary sinus into the right atrium. The fistula from the right coronary cusp toward the right ventricular outflow tract is the most common type, with or without a doubly committed ventricular septal defect (VSD) [1]. At operation, depending on the location of the rupture, a right atriotomy or pulmonary arteriotomy is chosen. If severe aortic valve prolapse or significant aortic valve regurgitation is present, an aortotomy is performed, and the aortic valve and Valsalva aneurysm are inspected from above and below. The fragile tissue is resected, and the fistula is closed via the right heart [2] or the aorta [3].

Rupture to the Right Ventricular Outflow Tract (Fig. II-18-1)

Through median sternotomy, with bicaval and ascending aortic cannulation, cardiopulmonary bypass is initiated. The ascending aorta is cross-clamped, and cardioplegic solution is injected. If cardioplegic solution cannot be infused adequately because of the size of the fistula, the main pulmonary artery is opened and the fistula is occluded digitally. If more than moderate aortic regurgitation is present, the ascending aorta is obliquely opened and cardioplegic solution is directly injected into the coronary orifices. Alternatively, retrograde cardioplegia can be delivered via the coronary sinus.

After cardioplegic arrest, the shape of the aneurysm and its relationship to adjacent structures are evaluated. The fragile tissue at the ruptured area is removed, and the defect is directly closed with fine monofilament suture (Fig. II-18-2, 3). When the tissue is particularly fragile, a felt strip is utilized to reinforce the closure. When the defect is large, and direct closure risks deformity of the aortic valve, a patch is used to close the defect. If a doubly committed VSD is present, pledgetted sutures are placed at the pulmonary valve annulus for the superior margin (Fig. II-18-4), and closure of VSD is performed as described in Chapter 17; the fistula is also closed. When aortic valve regurgitation is present, suspension of the aortic valve is performed. When aortic valve deformity is severe or the etiology of the aneurysm is infection, aortic valve replacement may be necessary [4].

Rupture to the Right Atrium (Fig. II-18-5)

After aortic cross-clamping, a right atriotomy is performed. The aneurysm and fistula exit site are identified. The fragile tissue is removed from the aneurysm, and the fistula is closed directly or with a patch. Care is taken to avoid damaging the atrioventricular node next to the membranous septum. The ascending aorta is opened, and the aortic sinus is repaired with direct closure or with a patch (Fig. II-18-6).

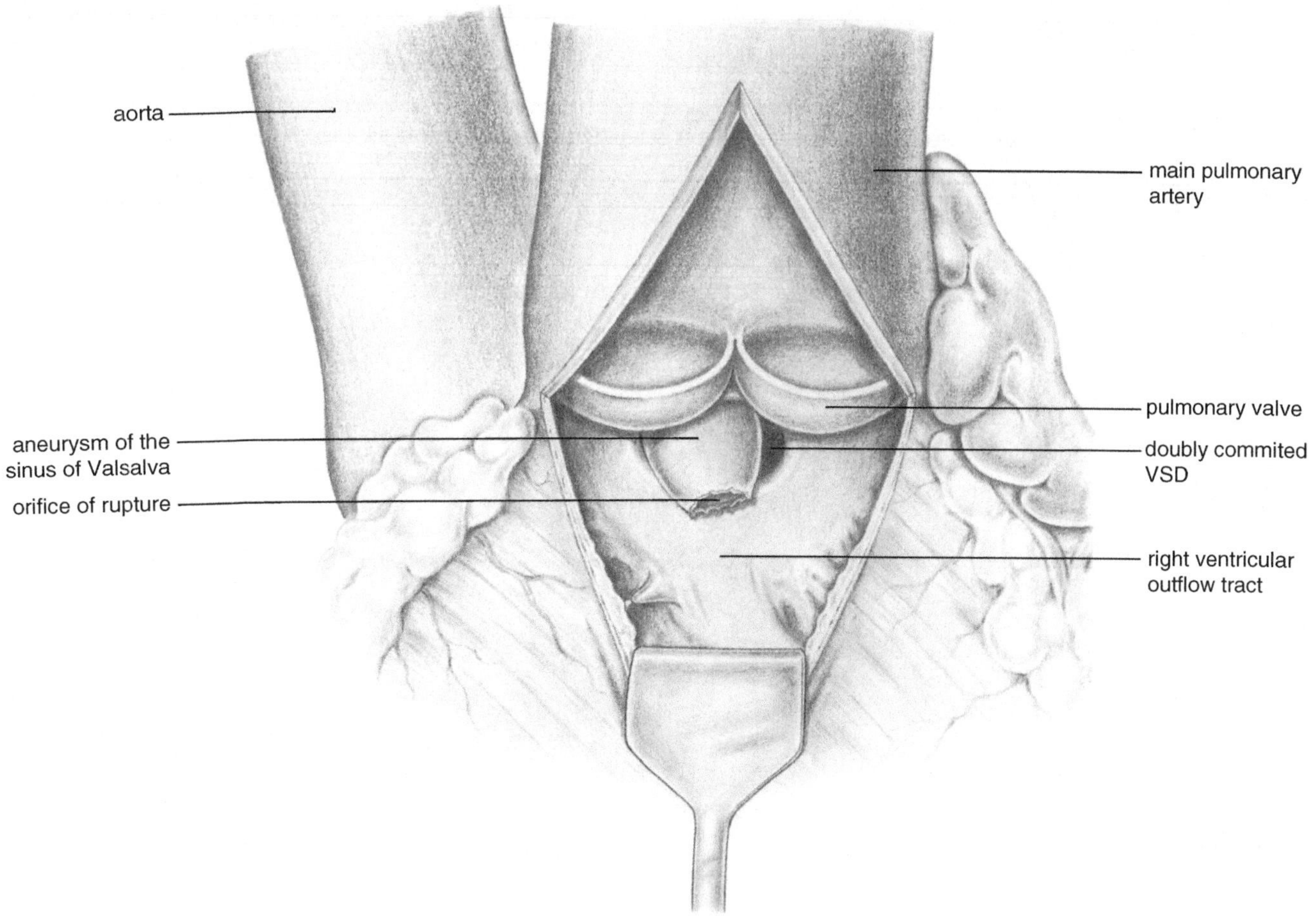

Fig. II-18-1. Ruptured aneurysm of the sinus of Valsalva into the right ventricular outflow tract (in the presence of doubly committed VSD)

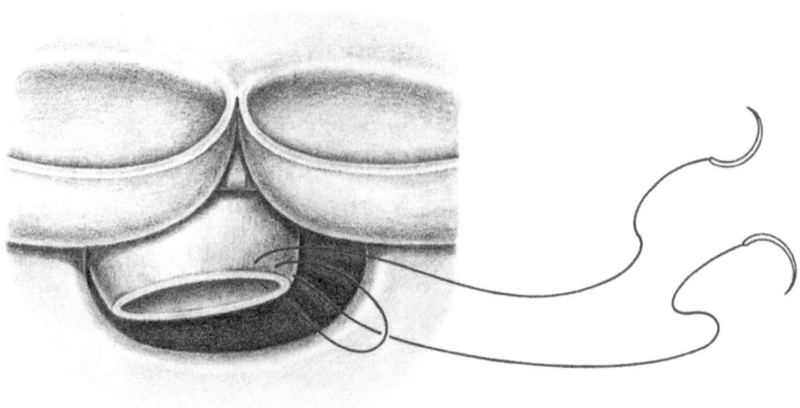

Fig. II-18-2. Closure of ruptured aneurysm of the sinus of Valsalva: 1

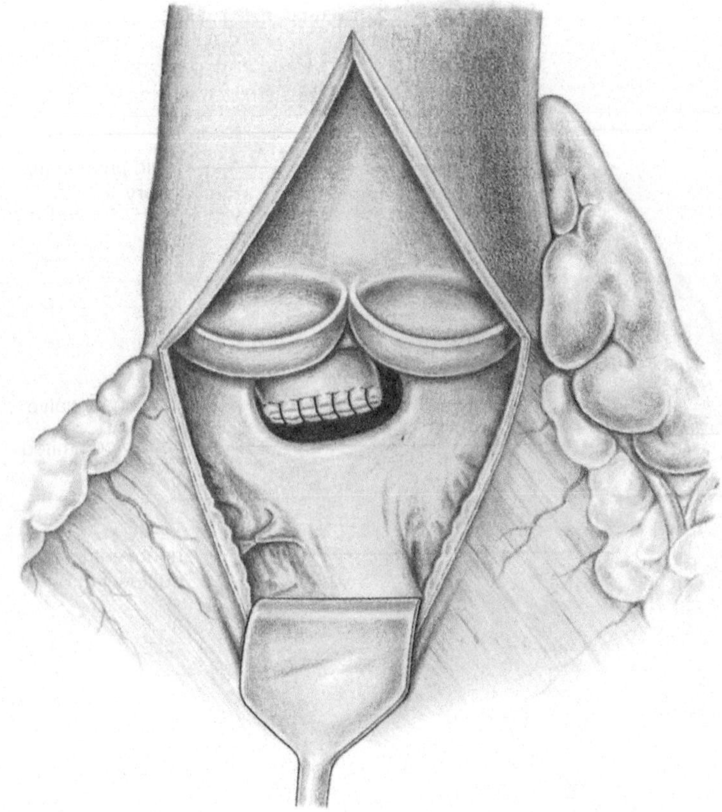

Fig. II-18-3. Closure of ruptured aneurysm of the sinus of Valsalva: 2

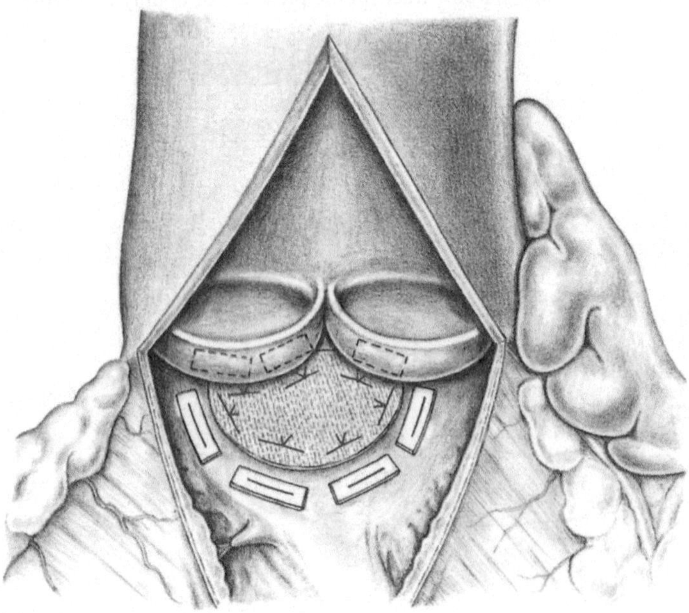

Fig. II-18-4. VSD closure (doubly committed VSD type)

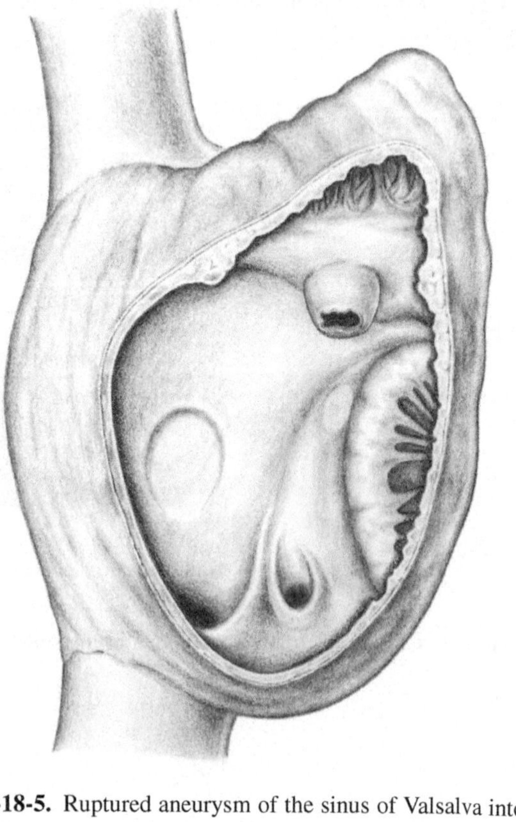

Fig. II-18-5. Ruptured aneurysm of the sinus of Valsalva into the right atrium

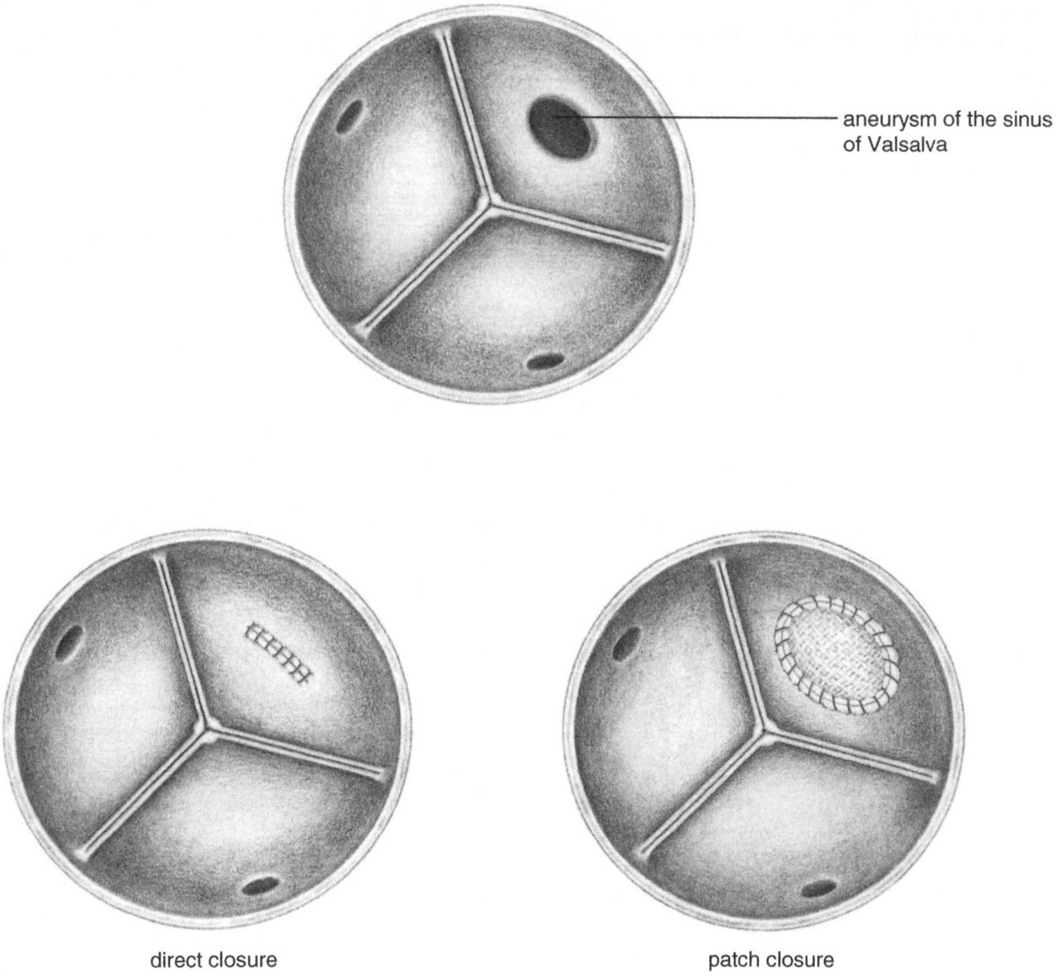

Fig. II-18-6. Fistula closure through the aorta

References

1. Sakakibara S, Konno S (1968) Congenital aneurysm of the sinus of Valsalva, associated with ventricular septal defect: anatomical aspects. Am Heart J 75:595–603
2. Burakovsky VI, Podsolkov VP, Sabirow BN (1988) Ruptured congenital aneurysm of the sinus of Valsalva. J Thorac Cardiovasc Surg 95:836–841
3. Hamid IA, Jothi M, Rajan S, et al (1994) Transaortic repair of ruptured aneurysm of sinus of Valsalva. J Thorac Cardiovasc Surg 107:1464–1468
4. Sugimoto T, Ogawa K, Asada T (1993) Surgical treatment of ruptured sinus of Valsalva aneurysm. Nippon Kyobu Geka Gakkai Zasshi 41:643–648

II-19. Mitral Stenosis

Congenital mitral valve stenosis is caused by malformation of one or more of several components of the mitral apparatus, including the annulus, leaflets, chordae, and papillary muscles.

Carpentier et al. [1,2] classified mitral valve stenosis into two groups according to papillary muscle anatomy. In the presence of normal papillary muscles, mechanisms of stenosis include papillary muscle commissural fusion, excess mitral valvar tissue, supravalvular mitral ring, and hypoplasia of the annulus. In the presence of abnormal papillary muscle, mechanisms include parachute mitral valve, hammock mitral valve, and absence of papillary muscle (Table II-19-1).

1. Papillary muscle commissure fusion: the commissure is fused and thickened. Papillary muscles are connected to the commissure directly without chordae.
2. Double mitral orifice: abnormal tissue between the chordae causes the mitral stenosis. Other parts of the mitral apparatus are usually normal.
3. Supravalvular ring: a fibrous circumferential rim is present above the mitral valve annulus and causes mitral stenosis.
4. Annular hypoplasia: the mitral valve annulus itself is underdeveloped; this often is seen in association with other causes of mitral valve stenosis.
5. Parachute mitral valve: all chordae are connected to a single papillary muscle. Because of limited space between the chordae, mitral stenosis is observed.
6. Hammock mitral valve: the commissure is fused, and many chordae are attached to the abnormally hypertrophic papillary muscle. This architecture causes mitral stenosis.
7. Absent papillary muscle: papillary muscles are absent, and many chordae are directly attached to the left ventricular wall. Because the space between the chordae is restricted, mitral stenosis is observed.

Because there is high pulmonary vein pressure secondary to mitral stenosis, clinical symptoms include respiratory distress manifest as tachypnea, retraction, and poor feeding. In severe cases, because of low cardiac syndrome, peripheral coldness and hepatomegaly are observed. Because there is no effective medical therapy, if the patient has severe heart failure, even if small, surgery should be considered. Valve replacement is often required, because subvalvular anomalies are involved and not amenable to repair. Occasionally balloon valvotomy can delay the need for surgery [3], which is helpful because an optimal small valve is not presently available. In Shone's anomaly [4] with multiple levels of left heart obstruction, including parachute mitral valve, subaortic stenosis, coarctation of the aorta, other lesions are approached first, and mitral valve surgery is performed later.

For preoperative evaluation, the mechanism of mitral stenosis should be investigated, with cardiac catheterization and transthoracic echocardiography. Transesophageal echocardiography (TEE) is most useful to examine the subvalvular apparatus. Mitral annulus size, possible valve implantation site, and relationship between the implantation site and pulmonary vein orifice are assessed [5].

Operative Procedure

In congenital mitral stenosis, subvalvular anomaly is usually present. Because the annulus is usually small, visualization of the operative field is typically suboptimal and mitral valvuloplasty is challenging. Potential surgical techniques are commissurotomy, papillary muscle division, chordal division, and supramitral ring resection. When the approach to the mitral valve is difficult, approach from the left ventricular apex has occasionally been used [6]. The heart is accessed via median sternotomy in the usual fashion.

Supravalvular Ring Resection

The mitral valve is inspected through the left atrium. Because of the obstructive supravalvular ring, the mitral valve is not seen. At the time of resection, care is taken to avoid damaging the mitral valve, especially the anterior leaflet. The mitral valve is usually normal, but occasionally the valve itself may be stenotic.

Commissurotomy

This procedure is performed in a patient with a fused commissure. The leaflets are usually thick. Retraction stitches are placed in the annulus at the commissures. These retraction stitches are placed on tension, and the commissures are fixed. The commissures are opened carefully with a fine scalpel. Subvalvular chordal tissue and the papillary muscles are inspected. If the subvalvular tissue is retracted with fusion, the chordae are cut sharply. When interventions on the commissure and chordae are not enough to create adequate mobility of the valve, papillary muscles are divided.

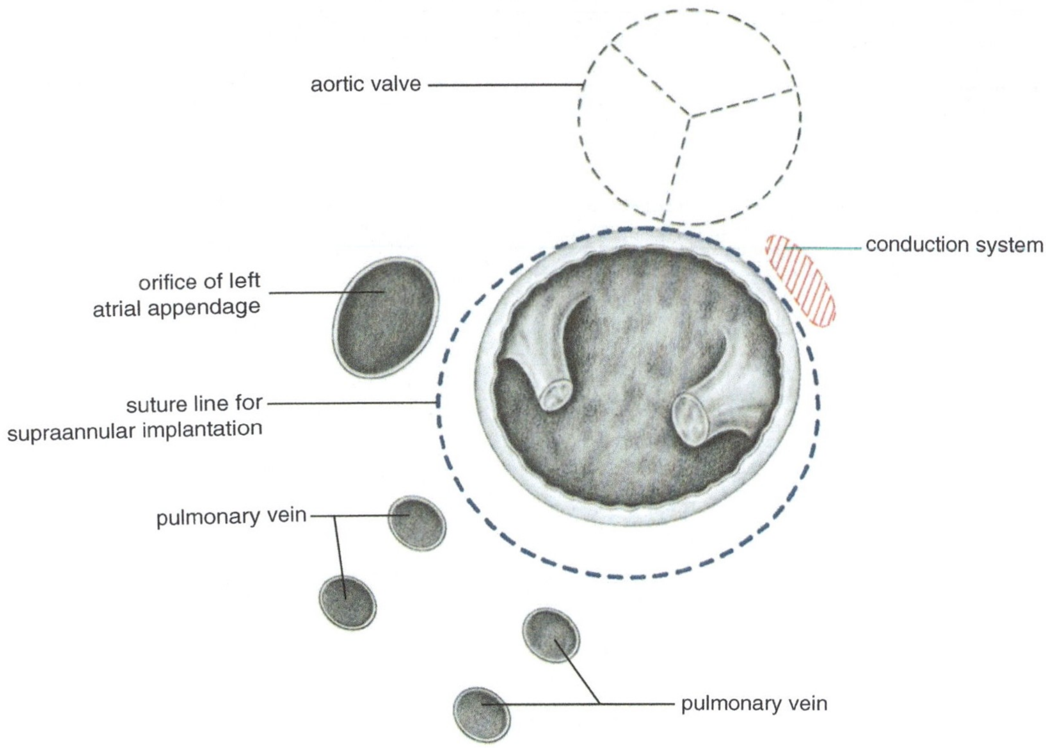

Fig. II-19-1. Mitral valve replacement

Table II-19-1. Carpentier classification of congenital mitral stenosis

Normal papillary muscles	Papillary muscle commissural fusion
	Excess valvar tissue
	Valvar ring
	Annular hypoplasia
Abnormal papillary muscles	Parachute mitral valve
	Hammock mitral valve
	Absent papillary muscle

Mechanical Valve Replacement, Supraannular Implantation (Fig. II-19-1)

If the valve annulus is small in infants, intraannular valve replacement is impossible and supraannular placement is necessary [5]. The Carbomedicus 16 mm (Sulzer Carbomedics Inc., Austin, TX, USA) has the smallest sewing cuff and is rotatable, so this valve has been our valve of choice [7,8]. Currently, similar small mechanical valves, the ATS Medical 16 mm (ATS Medical Inc., Minnedpolis, MI, USA) and St. Jude Medical 17 mm (St. Jude Medical Inc., St. Paul, MN, USA) regent mechanical valve are available. The native valve leaflets and subvalvular tissues are removed. If the middle of the anterior leaflet annulus is thought of as 12 o'clock, the aortic valve annulus and conducting system are located between 10 and 2 o'clock. Therefore, stitches are placed in the true annulus at this area. For the inferior suture line between 3 and 9 o'clock, stitches are placed 5–6 mm above the annulus in the left atrial wall. Pledgetted mattress sutures are used. The circumflex coronary artery runs from "7 to 10 o'clock," so care is taken to avoid putting the stitches too deep. In seating the valve, care is taken to avoid compromising pulmonary vein blood flow.

For all types of mitral surgery, at the time of left atrial closure using a running suture, the atrium is filled with blood. A vent is inserted through the suture line. After removal of the aortic clamp, de-airing is performed via the aortic root. After de-airing is complete, the vent is removed. At the separation from bypass, TEE is performed to evaluate the mitral valve function.

References

1. Carpentier A (1994) Congenital malformations of the mitral valve. In: Surgery for congenital heart defects, 2nd edn. Saunders, Philadelphia, pp 599–614
2. Carpentier A, Branchini B, Cour JC, et al (1976) Congenital malformation of the mitral valve in children. Pathology and surgical treatment J Thorac Cardiovasc Surg 72:854–866
3. Moore P, Adatia I, Spevak PJ, et al (1994) Severe congenital mitral stenosis in infants. Circulation 89:2099–2106
4. Shone JD, Sellers RD, Anderson RC, et al (1963) The developmental complex of "parachute mitral valve" supravalvular ring of left atrium, subaortic stenosis and coarctation of aorta. Am J Cardiol 11:714–725
5. Kadoba K, Jonas RA, Mayer JE, et al (1990) Mitral valve replacement in the first year of life. J Thorac Cardiovasc Surg 100:762–768
6. Barbero-Marcial M, Riso A, De Albuquerque AT, et al (1993) Left ventricular apical approach for the surgical treatment of congenital mitral stenosis. J Thorac Cardiovasc Surg 106:105–110
7. Masuda M, Kado H, Matsumoto T, et al (2000) Mitral valve replacement using bileaflet mechanical prosthetic valve in the first year of life. Jpn J Thorac Cardiovasc Surg 48:643–647
8. Masuda M, Kado H, Tatewaki H, et al (2004) Late results after mitral valve replacement with bileaflet mechanical prosthesis in children. Evaluation of prosthesis-patient mismatch. Ann Thorac Surg 77:913–917

II-20. Mitral Regurgitation: Artificial Chordae and Annuloplasty

Because the majority of patients with mild mitral valve regurgitation are asymptomatic and do not have cardiomegaly, these patients do not require surgery. With moderate to severe mitral valve regurgitation, some patients may develop heart failure and need to be treated with medications. If the patient responds well to medical treatment, the patient is followed, with particular attention paid to the amount of valve regurgitation and ventricular size. If there is persistent congestive heart failure, worsening regurgitation, or increasing ventricular size, surgery is indicated.

Operative Procedure

In children with mitral regurgitation, growth potential is of paramount concern in planning surgical treatment [1]. The surgical technique is determined according to the mechanism of regurgitation. The first technique to be discussed is mitral valvuloplasty using artificial chordae tendinea implantation, applicable to regurgitant valves with pathological elongation of native chordae.

The heart is accessed via median sternotomy, and cardiopulmonary bypass is instituted with bicaval and ascending aortic cannulation. After aortic cross-clamping, cardioplegic arrest is obtained. The mitral valve is accessed from the right side of the left atrium, through an incision parallel to the interatrial groove. The right-side left atrial approach provides good exposure because usually the depth of the chest is relatively shallow in children. If an atrial septal defect (ASD) is present, the trans-septal approach may be utilized. Traction sutures are placed on the left side of the edge of the atriotomy to hold the atriotomy open, and a Cooley retractor is applied if necessary. The mitral valve and subvalvular apparatus are inspected, and cold cardioplegic solution is injected into the left ventricle (LV) to evaluate the degree of regurgitation and prolapse of the mitral valve.

To create an artificial chorda, an expanded polytetrafluoroethylene (PTFE) suture is used. In children, determination of the length of the artificial chorda may be difficult, but this is facilitated using the following technique [2]. A double-armed suture is placed through the edge of the prolapsing anterior leaflet from the ventricular side to the atrial side. Both sutures are then placed 4–5 mm beneath the tip of the papillary muscle (Fig. II-20-1) and passed through a PTFE pledget. The suture is pulled up, bringing the leaflet down to the papillary muscle. The suture is then tied at the level of normal leaflet (Fig. II-20-2). Finally, the prolapsing leaflet is elevated, and the pledget is pushed down onto the papillary muscle, creating artificial chorda the same length as the normal chorda (Fig. II-20-3). If the prolapsing area is large, an additional chorda may be placed in a similar fashion.

To address mitral regurgitation caused by annular dilatation, the Kay–Reed annuloplasty technique [3] is useful. In this method, a 3-0 pledgetted mattress suture is placed 3–5 mm from the annulus, brought through the annulus at the commissure. The width of the mattress suture is about 3 mm. Care is taken to avoid placing the stitch in the leaflet itself. These stitches are placed through the posterior annulus according to the amount of plication needed and brought through a pledget (Fig. II-20-4). The amount of annular plication is determined using the Rowlatt criteria [4], as shown in a supplement at the end of this book. If the annular dilation is severe, this annuloplasty is performed at both commissures. Cold cardioplegic solution is injected into the ventricle again to confirm coaptation and mobility of the leaflet.

After the atrium is filled with blood, the atrial incision is closed using monofilament mattress and running suture. After separation from bypass, transesophageal echocardiography (TEE) is performed to evaluate the repair, including estimation of the amount of regurgitation and stenosis, as well as ventricular function. If significant regurgitation is still present, bypass is reinstituted, and additional valve repair or replacement is performed.

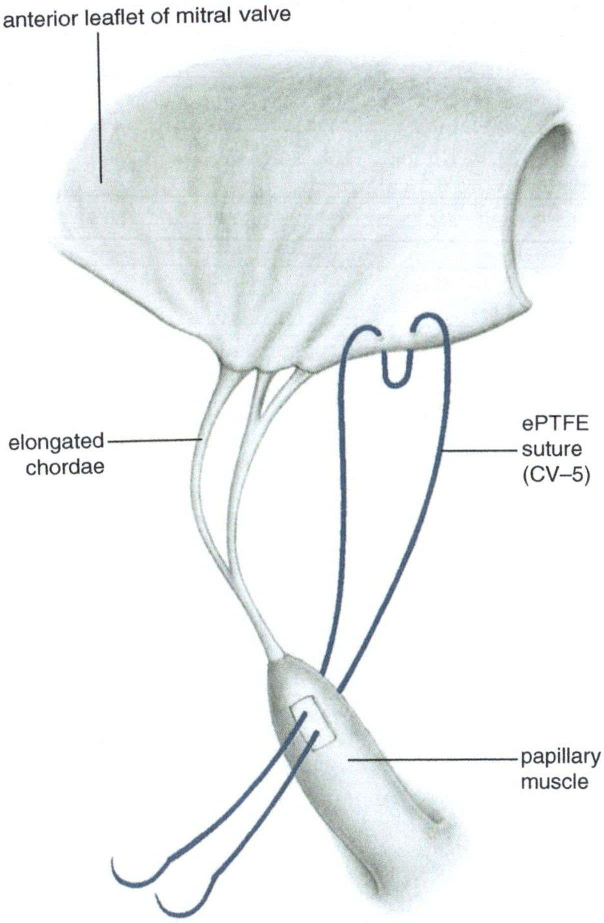

Fig. II-20-1. Placement of artificial chorda: stitch placement. A double-armed polytetrafluoroethylene (PTFE) suture is placed through the tip of the prolapsing anterior mitral valve leaflet from the ventricular side and placed 3–4 mm from the top of the papillary muscle. These stitches are placed through a free pledget of expanded PTFE (ePTFE)

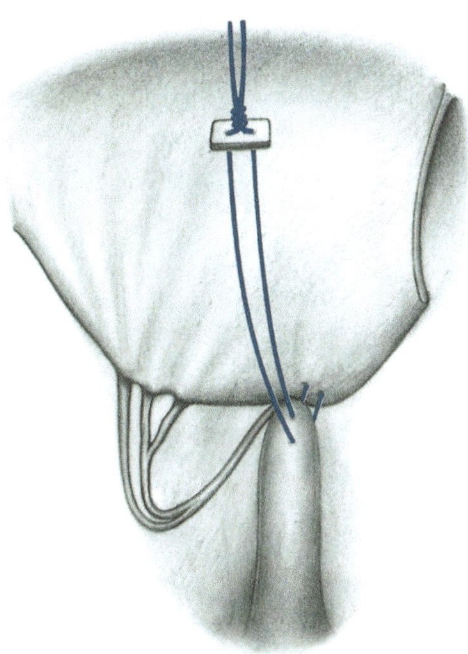

Fig. II-20-2. Placement of artificial chorda: tying sutures. The sutures are tightened to bring the leaflet edge down to the papillary muscle. The suture is tied at the level of the appositioning normal posterior leaflet

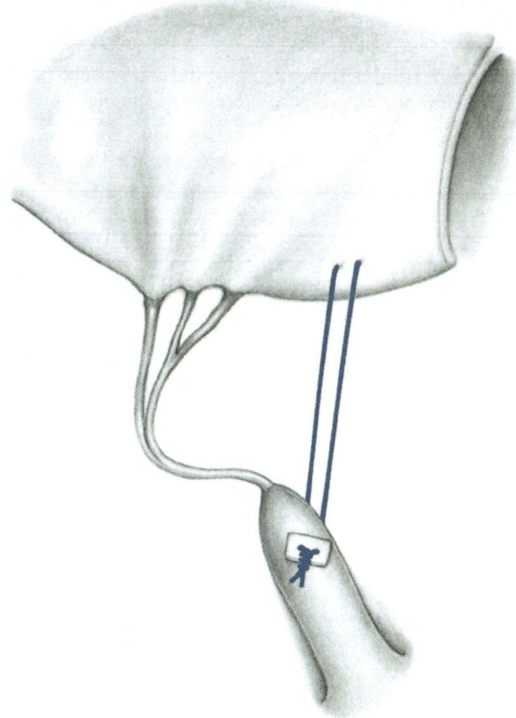

Fig. II-20-3. Placement of artificial chorda: completion of artificial chorda. By pushing the pledget down to the papillary muscle, the artificial chorda is completed. With this maneuver, a normal length for the artificial chorda is obtained

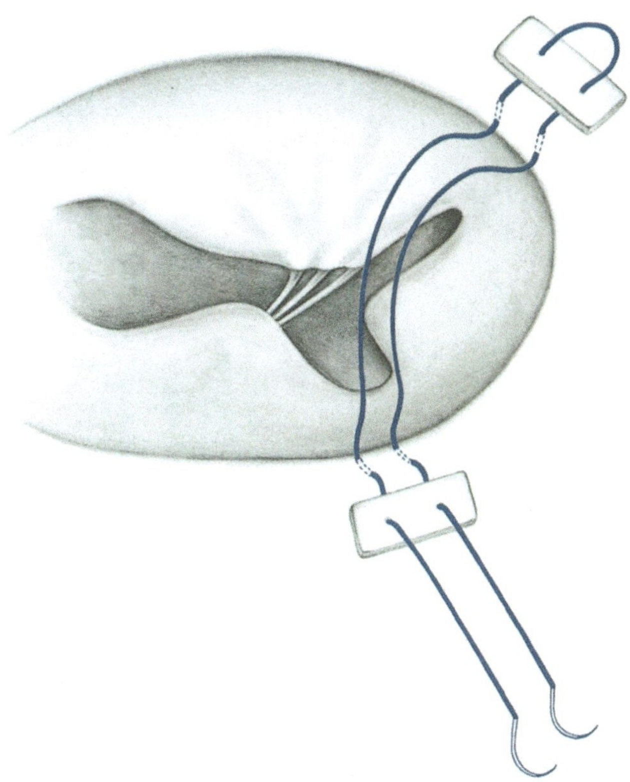

Fig. II-20-4. Annuloplasty. A pledgetted horizontal mattress suture is placed 3–5 mm from the annulus into the ventricular side and brought through the annulus at the commissure. These stitches are placed in the posterior annulus in parallel. These stitches should not be placed to the leaflet tissue itself. Tying the suture creates a measured annular plication

References

1. Masuda M, Kado H, Tatewaki H, et al (2004) Late results after mitral valve replacement with bileaflet mechanical prosthesis in children: evaluation of prosthesis-patient mismatch. Ann Thorac Surg 77:913–917
2. Matsumoto T, Kado H, Masuda M, et al (1999) Clinical results of mitral valve repair by reconstructing artificial chordae tendineae in children. J Thorac Cardiovasc Surg 118:94–98
3. Reed GE, Pooley RW, Moggio RA (1980) Durability of measured mitral annuloplasty: seventeen-year study. J Thorac Cardiovasc Surg 79:321–325
4. Rowlatt UF, Rimoldi HJA, Lev M (1963) The quantitative anatomy of normal child's heart. Pediatr Clin N Am 10:499–588

II-21. Tricuspid Regurgitation

Congenital tricuspid regurgitation is a rare disease. Etiologies of tricuspid valve regurgitation include Ebstein's anomaly, annular dilation, valve dysplasia, cleft at the leaflet, and Uhl's disease. Tricuspid valve regurgitation is often accompanied by other cardiac anomalies. In many patients with a large atrial septal defect, tricuspid regurgitation is observed. In the presence of a perimembranous ventricular septal defect, a left ventricle–right atrium (LV–RA) shunt is identified through a cleft in the septal leaflet of the tricuspid valve. After repair of tetralogy of Fallot or double-outlet right ventricle, tricuspid regurgitation is occasionally observed. In this chapter, surgical interventions for tricuspid regurgitation without Ebstein's anomaly or functional single ventricle are discussed.

Annuloplasty

A De Vega annuloplasty is most frequently applied tricuspid valve repair in children [1,2]. An annuloplasty ring is not usually used because of consideration of growth potential. After median sternotomy, cardiopulmonary bypass is instituted with ascending aortic and bicaval cannulation. Following ascending aortic cross-clamping and cardioplegic arrest, the RA is opened obliquely. Retraction sutures are placed on the edges of the atriotomy. The tricuspid valve leaflets, annulus, and subvalvular apparatus are carefully evaluated.

A tape is placed around the main pulmonary artery (PA) before testing for tricuspid regurgitation. Cold saline is injected into the right ventricle, and regurgitation is inspected. To avoid deformity of the tricuspid valve, retractors are not used for visualization during testing; only traction sutures are used to facilitate visualization of the valve. The location of the conduction system is identified, according to the positions of the triangle of Koch and the membranous part of the atrioventricular septum. A pledgetted double-armed suture is begun from the commissure between the anterior and septal leaflets. Sufficient depth bites are taken by elevating the endocardium with forceps. Too-shallow bites may tear the tissue, and bites that are too deep may damage the aortic valve or the right coronary artery. The leaflet will tear if the stitch is placed in the leaflet itself, so stitches should only be placed in the annulus. The assistant holds a retractor with one hand and follows the suture with the other hand. A stitch is placed every 3–4 mm, and stitching is finished in front of the coronary sinus. The other arm of the stitch is placed slightly outward from the first stitch, in atrial muscle, with care not to catch the first stitch (Fig. II-21-1). A Hegar dilator or valve sizer is used to check the size of the annulus, with a goal for annulus size of 80%–90% of the Rowlatt normal value, as shown in a supplement at the end of this book. The stitch is tied over a pledget (Fig. II-21-2).

Kay et al. [3] reported an annuloplasty technique performed only at the base of the posterior leaflet, in effect creating a bileaflet valve (Figs. II-21-3, II-21-4). A double-armed pledgetted suture is used. One arm of the suture is placed in the anteroposterior commissure and the posteroseptal commissure. The other arm of the suture is then placed 3 mm from the first suture, and the stitch is tied over a pledget. Occasionally, two pairs of suture are used.

In the majority of cases secondary to an LV–RA shunt, tricuspid regurgitation is significantly diminished after ventricular septal defect (VSD) closure. In unusual cases, cleft closure and commissuroplasty of the anteroseptal commissure is performed with two or three interrupted sutures when tricuspid valve deformity is severe secondary to a prior LV–RA shunt and there is residual significant regurgitation.

Tricuspid Valve Replacement

Tricuspid valve replacement is required when an adequate repair is not possible. Tissue valves are typically selected because of the risk of thrombogenesis [4]. Valve leaflets and the subvalvular apparatus are not removed, to preserve right ventricular function. Care is taken to avoid compromising the prosthetic valve function by the native valve tissue. Pledgetted mattress sutures are placed in the annulus from the RA toward the RV. At the atrioventricular (AV) node, sutures are placed in the tricuspid valve leaflet itself. However, in Ebstein's anomaly, sutures are not placed in the leaflet and are instead placed in the atrial wall superior to the coronary sinus. This method results in the coronary sinus being on the ventricular aspect of the valve. Another approach is to place the sutures in the ventricular septum inferior to the His bundle to avoid conducting system damage.

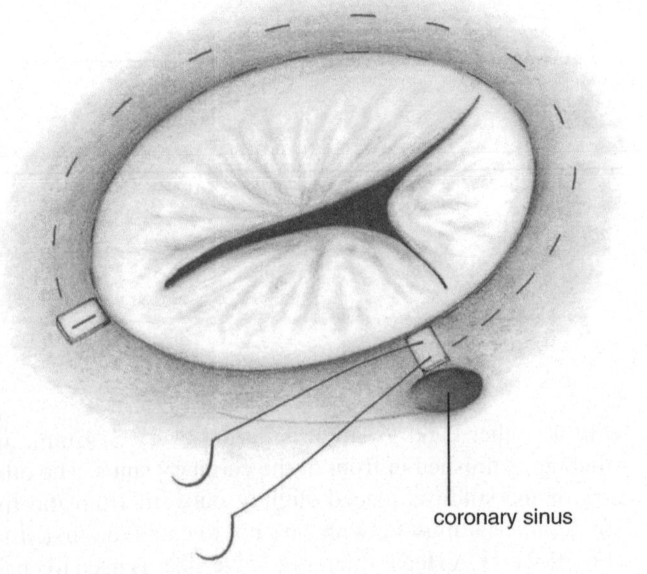

Fig. II-21-1. De Vega annuloplasty: stitch placement. The annuloplasty stitch is started at the commissure between the anterior and septal leaflet of the tricuspid valve and finished anterior to the coronary sinus

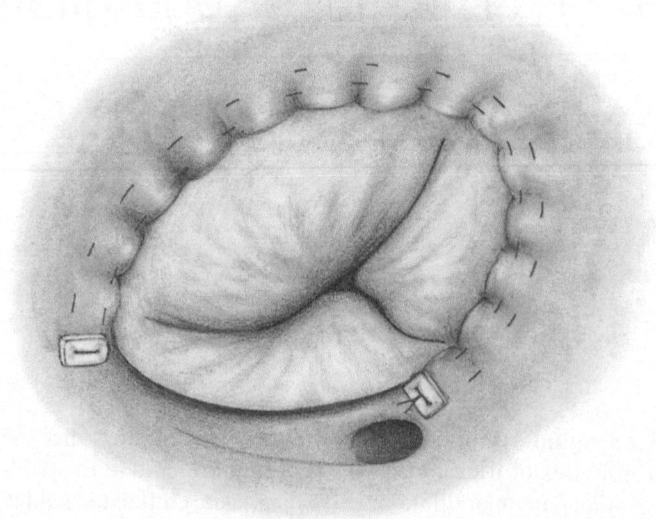

Fig. II-21-2. De Vega annuloplasty: completion of annuloplasty

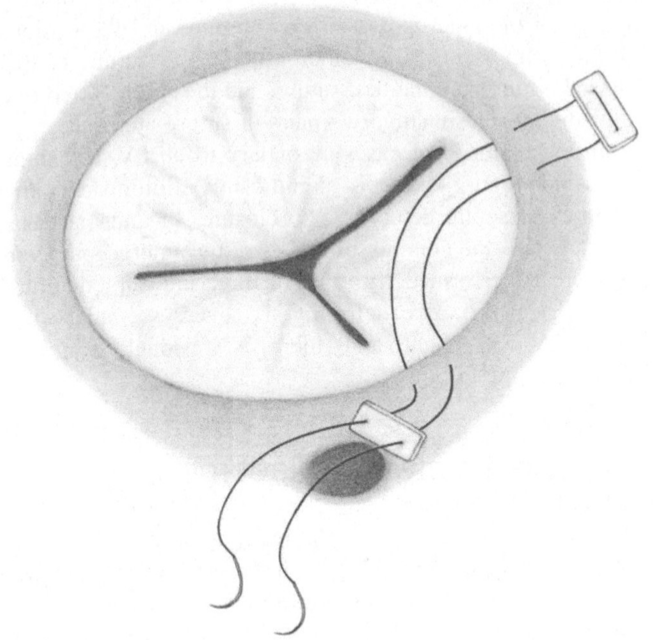

Fig. II-21-3. Kay annuloplasty

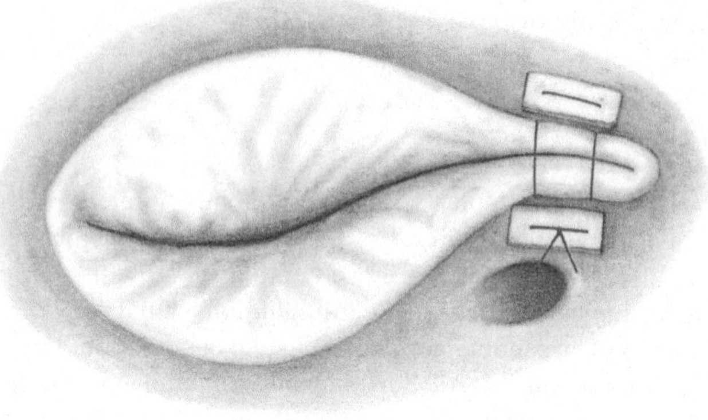

Fig. II-21-4. Bicuspidization. Annuloplasty is performed in the posterior leaflet by converting three leaflet valve into two leaflet valve

References

1. Kanter KR, Doelling NR, Fyfe DA, et al (2001) DeVega tricuspid annuloplasty for tricuspid regurgitation in children. Ann Thorac Surg 72:1344–1348
2. De Vega NG (1972) La anuloplastia selective, regulable y permanente. Rev Esp Cardiol 25:555–556
3. Kay JH, Mendez AM, Zubiate P (1976) A further look at tricuspid annuloplasty. Ann Thorac Surg 22:498–500
4. Kawachi Y, Tominaga R, Tokunaga K (1992) Excellent durability of the Hancock porcine bioprosthesis in the tricuspid position. A sixteen year follow-up study. J Thorac Cardiovasc Surg 104:1561–1566

II-22. Ebstein's Anomaly: Carpentier Procedure and Danielson Procedure

Anatomical Properties (Fig. II-22-1)

Ebstein's anomaly comprises 0.5% of all congenital heart disease and is thus a very rare defect. The septal and posterior leaflets of the tricuspid valve are displaced toward the apex of the heart and plastered to the ventricular wall. Depending on the degree of the valvar deformity and dysfunction, patients develop a wide spectrum of clinical conditions. Coexistent cardiac problems are also common: 40%–60% of patients have atrial septal defects, and 5%–10% have Wolff–Parkinson–White syndrome. A commonly used classification scheme was developed by Carpentier [1]. In type A, the anterior leaflet is large and mobile, and there is no subpulmonary stenosis. Displacement of the septal and posterior leaflets is moderate. In type B, chordae of the anterior leaflet attaches to the right ventricular wall, and anterior leaflet movement is restricted. There is subpulmonary stenosis. Displacement of the septal and posterior leaflets is severe. In type C, the leaflets are sacular and attach to the ventricular wall. They have no movement. The right ventricle has a giant atrialized portion. The right ventricular outflow tract has a tiny opening.

Surgical Indication

Marked cardiomegaly, severe tricuspid regurgitation, and cyanosis are observed in the symptomatic neonate. In the presence of patent ductus arteriosus, the pulmonary valve may be functionally atretic. Surgical intervention for the neonate with Ebstein's anomaly remains challenging. In neonates, the Starnes procedure [2], consisting of closure of the tricuspid valve with a patch to create tricuspid atresia, has had some success. Many patients are asymptomatic in infancy but may later develop symptoms of dyspnea or exercise intolerance.

Indications for surgery include severe desaturation caused by right–left shunt through an atrial septal defect, congestive heart failure, and severe arrhythmias. Early surgical intervention has recently been recommended when the patient becomes symptomatic with dyspnea. Previously, the Hardy procedure [3] has been performed with suboptimal results. More recently, several newer, more successful approaches including tricuspid annuloplasty, tricuspid valve replacement, the Danielson procedure [4], and the Carpentier procedure [5] have been employed. If the right ventricle has a small volume capacity and poor function, valve repair or replacement alone will likely not be successful, and concomitant bidirectional cavopulmonary anastomosis (one-and-a-half ventricular repair) or the Fontan procedure will be indicated [6].

Carpentier Procedure

This procedure includes the following interventions: (1) the anterior and posterior leaflets are detached from the annulus; (2) the atrialized ventricle is plicated; (3) the detached leaflets are advanced clockwise and reattached to the normal annulus; and (4) a tricuspid annuloplasty ring is placed.

Before the chest opening, the anatomy of the right ventricle and tricuspid valve is evaluated with transesophageal echocardiography. The degree of displacement of the septal and posterior leaflets, anterior leaflet size and mobility, functional right ventricle size, right ventricle free wall thickness, and contractility of the right ventricle are examined. The Carpentier approach is indicated when the anterior leaflet is large enough and right ventricular function is normal.

Cardiopulmonary bypass is started with bicaval and ascending aortic cannulation, and cardioplegic cardiac arrest is obtained. The right atrium (RA) is opened, and the tricuspid valve is carefully inspected, taking note of the true tricuspid valve annulus, coronary sinus, tendon of Todaro, membranous septum, and atrialized ventricle (Fig. II-22-2: dotted line shows ventricular septum).

When the septal leaflet is severely displaced, the whole triangle composed of the coronary sinus, membranous septum, and commissure between the septal and posterior leaflets is located in the ventricular septum. Two-thirds of the anterior leaflet is detached from the annulus. Accessory chordae are divided and freed from the ventricular wall to improve mobility of the leaflet, leaving true chordae that attach to the leaflet edge intact (Fig. II-22-3). The area of plication of the atrialized ventricle is between the detached line of the posterior leaflets and the adjacent septal wall of the displaced septal leaflet (Fig. II-22-4). A series of 3-0 pledgetted mattress sutures are used for plication of the atrialized ventricle up to the inferior margin of the coronary sinus.

At the atrial side, a running suture is used for plication of the atrium (Figs. II-22-4, II-22-5). Care is taken to avoid damaging the posterior descending coronary artery, which runs along the epicardial surface, because the atrialized ven-

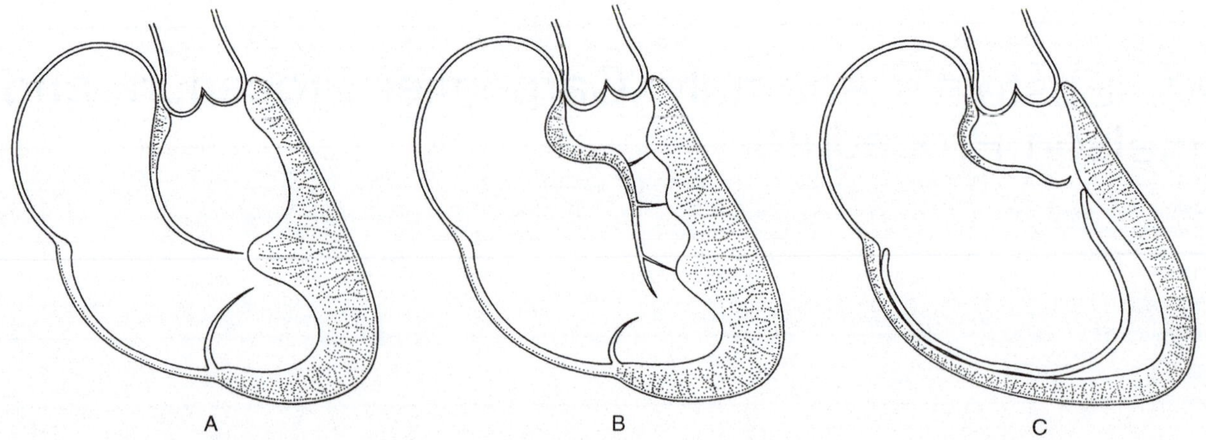

Fig. II-22-1. Classification of Ebstein's anomaly

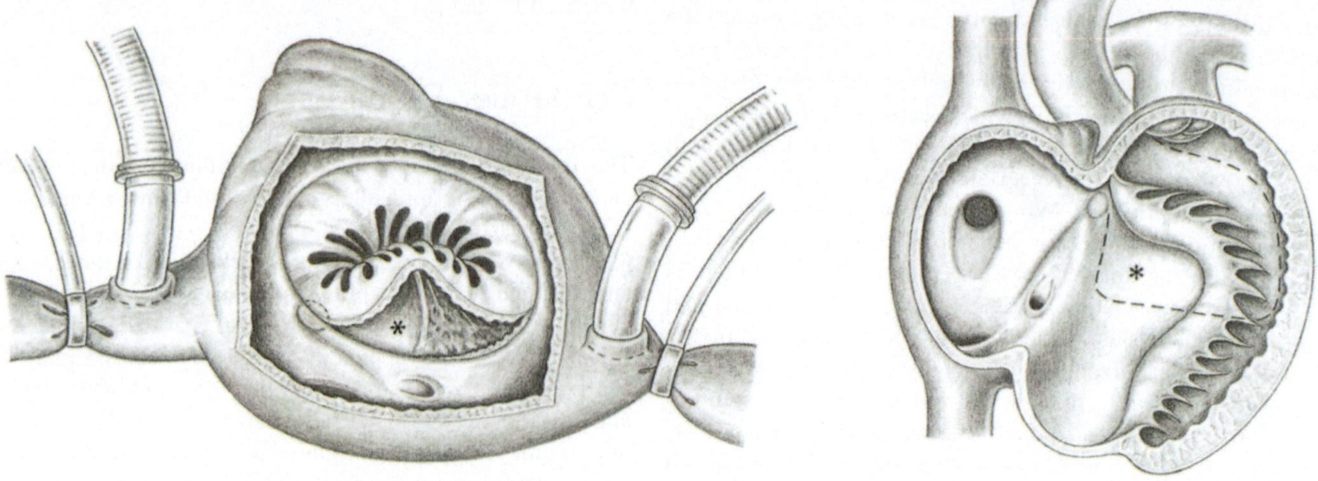

Fig. II-22-2. Carpentier procedure: appearance of the tricuspid valve. *Ventricular septum; --- (*dotted line*), position of the left ventricle

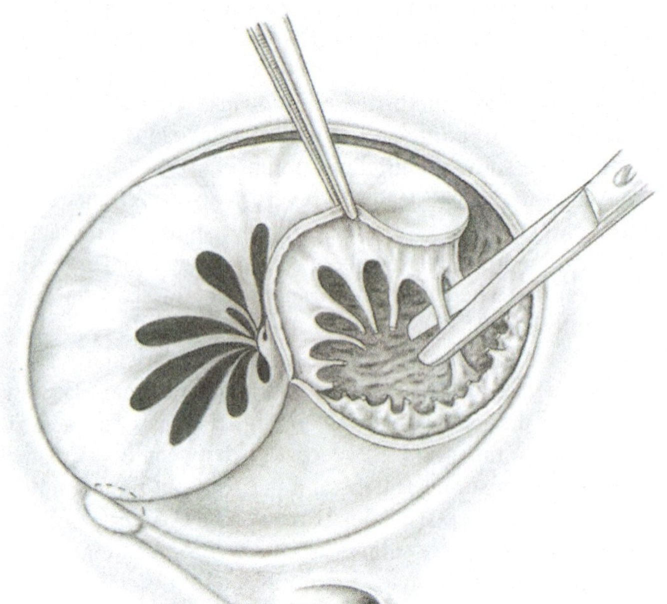

Fig. II-22-3. Carpentier procedure: detachment of the anterior and posterior leaflets and mobilization

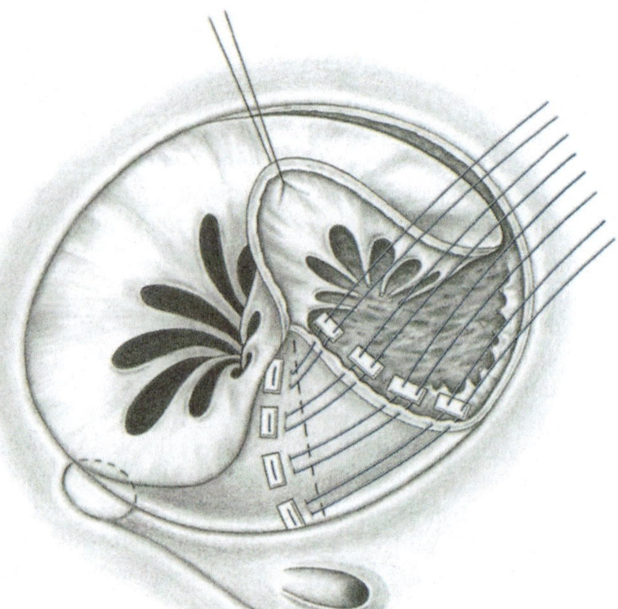

Fig. II-22-4. Carpentier procedure: plication of atrialized ventricle. The *dotted line* indicates position of posterior descending coronary artery

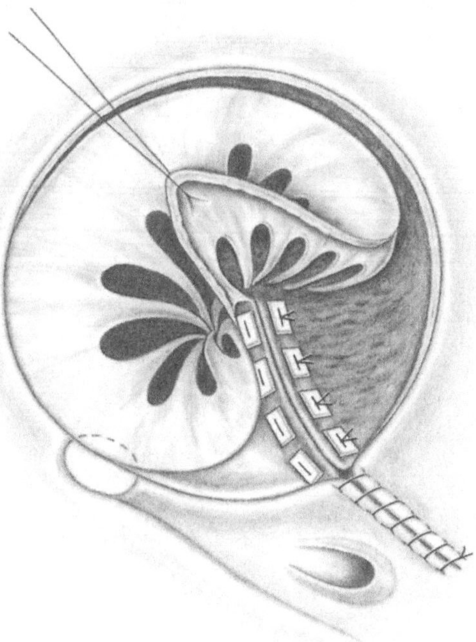

Fig. II-22-5. Carpentier procedure: plication of the right atrium

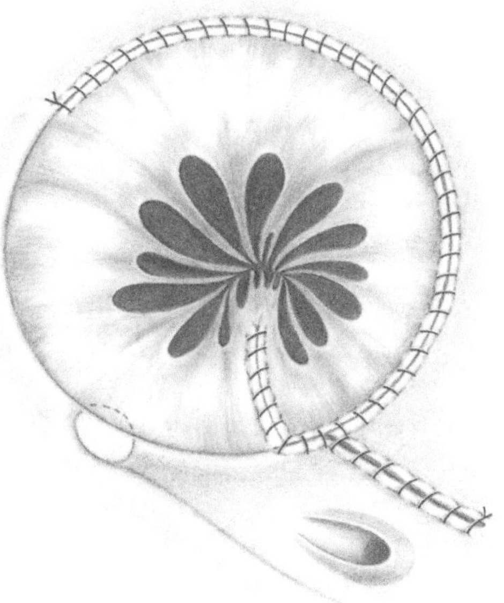

Fig. II-22-6. Carpentier procedure: reattachment of anterior and posterior leaflets

tricular wall is very thin. The position of the posterior descending coronary artery is shown in Fig. II-22-4 with a dotted line. The detached anterior and posterior leaflets are then reattached to the true annulus. Both leaflets are advanced clockwise and used to cover the whole annulus using a 5-0 monofilament running suture. With these procedures of the longitudinal plication and elevation of the tricuspid valve annulus, bicuspidization is accomplished (Fig. II-22-6). Valve competence is assessed by injecting saline into the right ventricle. Finally, the annulus is reinforced with a ring. In patients older than 15 years of age, a Carpentier ring, Duran ring, or polytetrafluoroethylene (PTFE) strip are

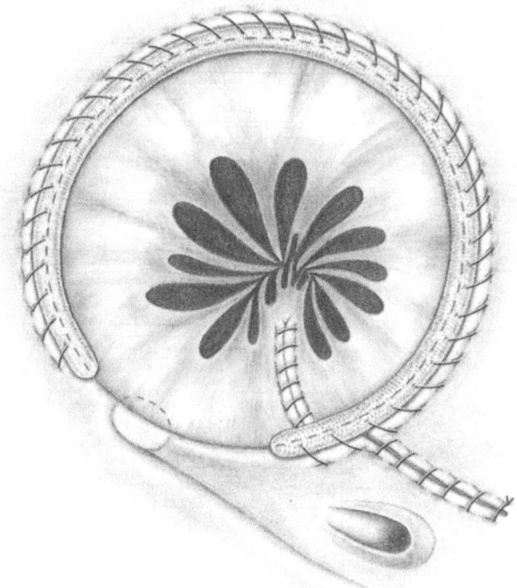

Fig. II-22-7. Carpentier procedure: ring placement on the annulus

used. In smaller children, an autologous pericardial strip is used (Fig. II-22-7). The size of the annulus after plication should be 80%–90% of the normal value by Rowlatt et al., as shown in the supplement at the end of this book.

Modified Carpentier Procedure [7]

In patients with severe displacement of the septal leaflet, it may be difficult to cover the whole tricuspid valve orifice with the anterior and posterior leaflets. In these situations, the plastered septal leaflet is peeled off from the ventricular septum with some supporting chordate. The previously detached posterior leaflet and this septal leaflet are combined, and a new leaflet is created. True chordae of the anterior and posterior leaflets are preserved, and accessory chordae are divided to improve movement. The composite leaflet (septal and posterior leaflets) is placed 2 mm below the true annulus (Fig. II-22-8).

Danielson Procedure

The Danielson procedure is a modification of the Hardy procedure, with suspension of displaced leaflet and annular plication at the posterior leaflet. Plication of the atrialized right ventricle (RV) is performed by transverse plication with suspension of the anterior and posterior leaflets to the true annulus and longitudinal plication by posterior leaflet annuloplasty. In the Hardy procedure, the valve suspension is performed along the whole annulus, whereas in the Danielson procedure valve suspension is performed in the annulus of the anterior and posterior leaflets, but not in the annulus of the septal leaflet. An annuloplasty suture is placed along the posterior leaflet of the tricuspid valve (Fig. II-22-9). With this technique a functional single leaflet valve (monocuspidization) is created.

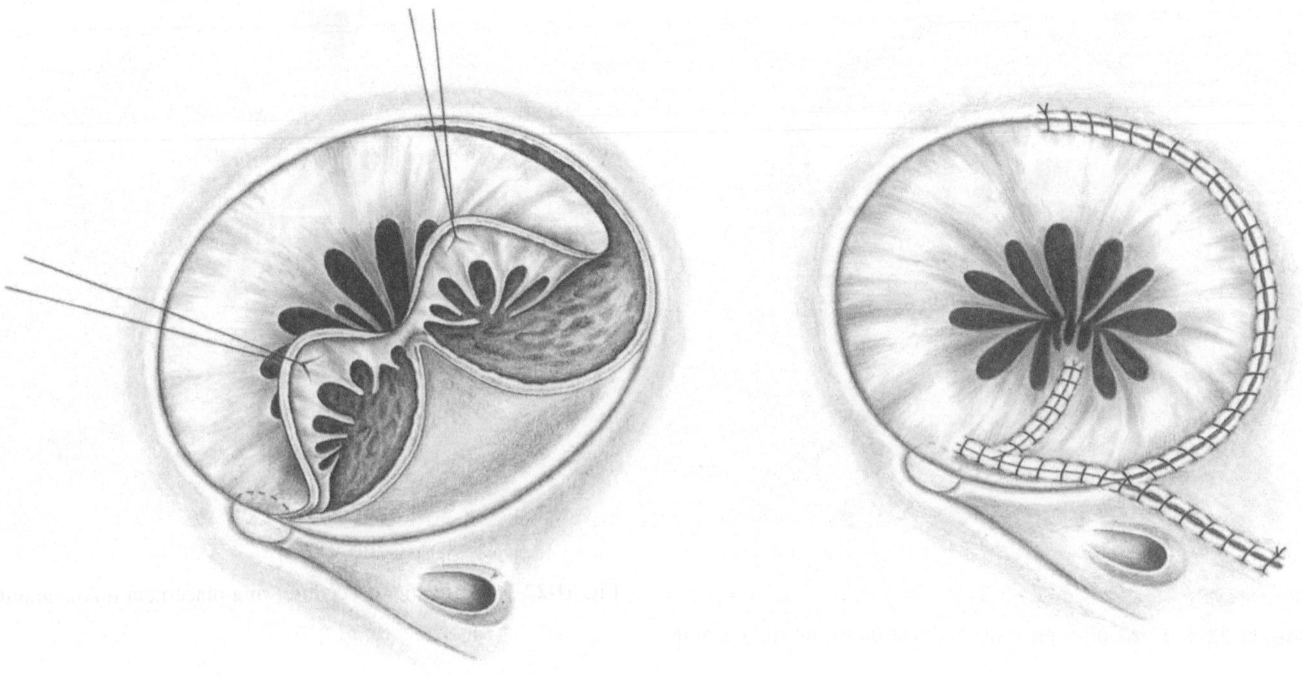

Fig. II-22-8. Modified Carpentier procedure (Nagata procedure)

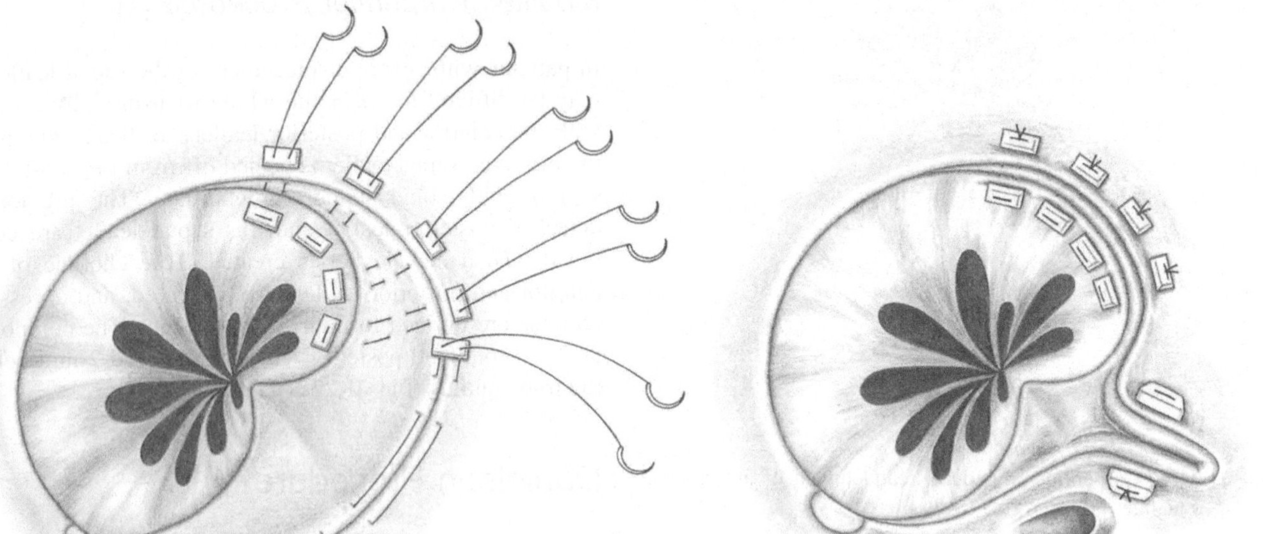

Fig. II-22-9. Danielson procedure

References

1. Stark J, de Leval M (1994) Malformation of the tricuspid valve and Ebstein's anomaly. Surgery for congenital heart defect, 2nd edn. Saunders, Philadelphia, pp 615–622
2. Starnes VA, Pitlick PT, Bernstein D, et al (1991) Ebstein's anomaly appearing in the neonate. A new surgical approach. J Thorac Cardiovasc Surg 101:1082–1087
3. Hardy KL, May IA, Webster CA, et al (1964) Ebstein's anomaly: a functional concept and successful definitive repair. J Thorac Cardiovasc Surg 48:927–940
4. Danielson GK, Driscoll DJ, Mair DD, et al (1992) Operative treatment of Ebstein's anomaly. J Thorac Cardiovasc Surg 104:1195–1202
5. Carpentier A, Chauvaud S, Macé L, et al (1988) A new reconstructive operation for Ebstein's anomaly of the tricuspid valve. J Thorac Cardiovasc Surg 96:92–101
6. Chauvaud S, Fuzellier JF, Berrebi A, et al (1998) Bi-directional cavopulmonary shunt associated with ventriculo and valvuloplasty in Ebstein's anomaly: benefits in high risk patients. Eur J Cardiothorac Surg 13:514–519
7. Kaneko Y, Okabe H, Nagata N, et al (1998) Repair of septal and posterior tricuspid leaflets in Ebstein's anomaly. J Card Surg 13:229–235

II-23. Truncus Arteriosus: Rastelli Procedure, Lecompte Maneuver, Barbero–Marcial Procedure, and Mee Procedure

Truncus arteriosus is one of the major cardiac defects that require surgical intervention in the neonatal or early infant period. This disease is relatively rare. Edwards defined this condition as a common trunk that derives blood flow from both ventricles and carries blood to the aorta, coronary arteries, and pulmonary arteries.

Collett and Edwards [1] classified this disease into four groups (Fig. II-23-1). In type I, the trunk gives rise to the ascending aorta and a short main pulmonary artery. In type II, the branch pulmonary arteries arise separately, but in close proximity, from the trunk. In type III, the origins of the pulmonary arteries are widely separated, arising from the lateral sides of the trunk. In type IV, the pulmonary arteries do not arise from the trunk. This type is now more commonly termed pulmonary atresia with ventricular septal defect (VSD). (This entity is discussed in Chapter 25.)

Surgical Indication

If the patient has not developed Eisenmenger syndrome, surgery is indicated, although results are much worse if there is high pulmonary vascular resistance, more than 8 Wood units. Complete repair should be performed at less than 6 months of age, even if medical treatment is apparently effective.

Complete Repair

For this disease, currently there are three types of operative procedure named for their proponents: the Rastelli [2], Lecompte [3], and Barbero-Marcial [4] procedures. In all, the ventricular septal defect is closed; the procedures differ in the means of establishing right-ventricle-to-pulmonary-artery (RV–PA) continuity. Historically, the Rastelli procedure was the first successful operation, described in 1967. As an RV–PA conduit, a Hancock valved conduit has been used. Cryopreserved homograft valves have also been used for the RV–PA conduit, and better surgical results have been reported. Recently, bovine jugular vein conduit has also been employed. All conduits will become stenotic because of both structural deterioration and patient growth, and conduit replacement is therefore inevitable. To avoid initial conduit placement, the Lecompte [3] and Barbero-Marcial [4] procedures, which create RV–PA continuity without a conduit, were reported in 1982 and 1990, respectively.

For all types of truncus repair, the initial approach is similar. The heart is accessed via median sternotomy. Branch PAs are dissected and encircled with tapes before cardiopulmonary bypass (CPB). This dissection is very important and is advanced to each hilum to improve the mobility of the PAs, for the Lecompte or Barbero-Marcial procedure. Ascending aortic and bicaval cannulation is performed. Because surgical manipulation of the common trunk is required, the aortic cannula is placed far distal in the ascending aorta or in the aortic arch. As soon as bypass is initiated, tapes on the PAs are snared down to avoid runoff into the pulmonary bed. The ascending aorta is cross-clamped as distally as possible, and cardiac arrest is obtained with cardioplegic solution administration.

Rastelli Procedure

The trunk is opened along a planned excision line (Fig. II-23-2 ①, ②), and the orifices of the PAs and the coronary arteries are identified from the interior of the trunk. The PAs are carefully excised from the trunk. In types II and III, the PA is excised with the posterior wall of the ascending aorta (Fig. II-23-2 ②), and the defect of the ascending aorta is closed directly or using a patch. A longitudinal incision is made in the anterior wall of the right ventricle beneath the truncal valve. Care is taken to avoid damaging the truncal valve, and it may be helpful to plan this incision before closing the defect in the truncal wall while the truncal valve is visualized. Keeping a distance from the coronary arteries, the edges of the ventriculotomy incision are excised to create a spindle-shaped ventriculotomy. Retractors are inserted into this ventriculotomy site, through which the VSD is inspected. A muscle band between the posteroinferior margin of the VSD and the tricuspid valve annulus is often observed, defining this as a muscular defect. It is safe to put stitches in this muscle band (Fig. II-23-3 ①). The ventricular septal defect (VSD) is closed using a patch with interrupted or running suture technique. When the VSD is small and development of left ventricular outflow tract (LVOT) obstruction after surgery is a concern, the VSD is enlarged anterosuperiorly, by excising a wedge of septal muscle (Fig. II-23-3 ②). The atrial septal defect (ASD) or patent foramen ovale (PFO) is closed, de-airing is completed, and the aortic cross-clamp is released. For an RV–PA conduit, a 12-mm Hancock valved conduit is used in neonates. The orifice of the PA is closed with an autologous

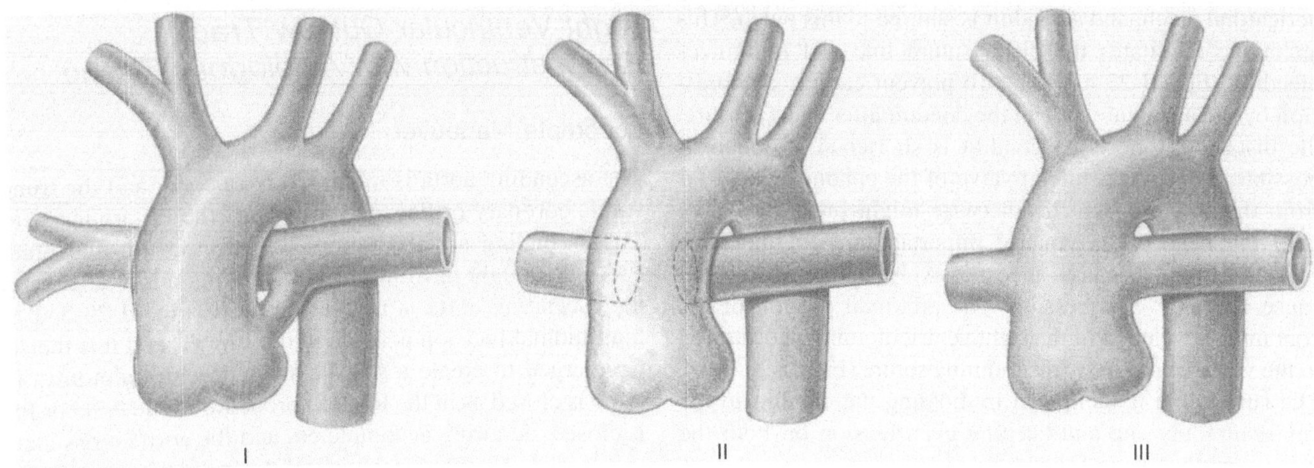

Fig. II-23-1. Collett and Edward classification

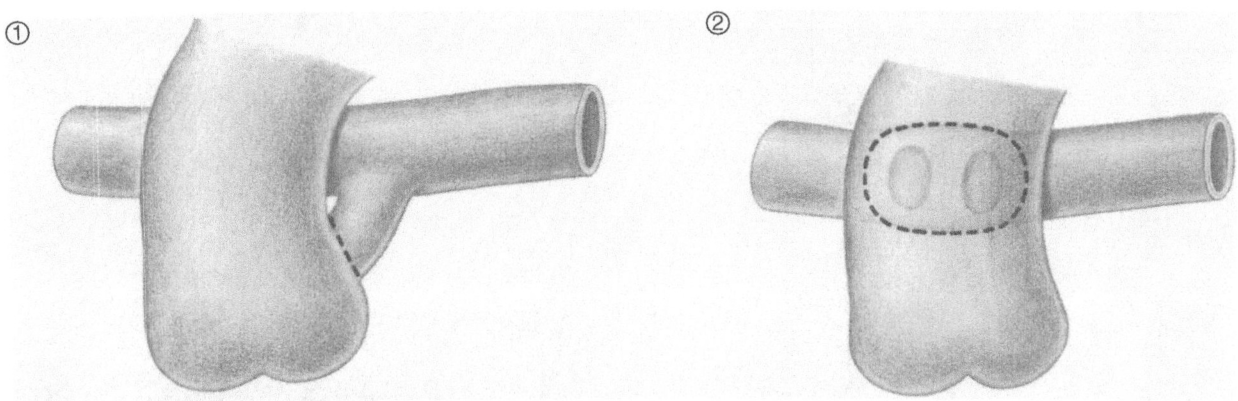

Fig. II-23-2. Rastelli procedure: removal of branch pulmonary arteries

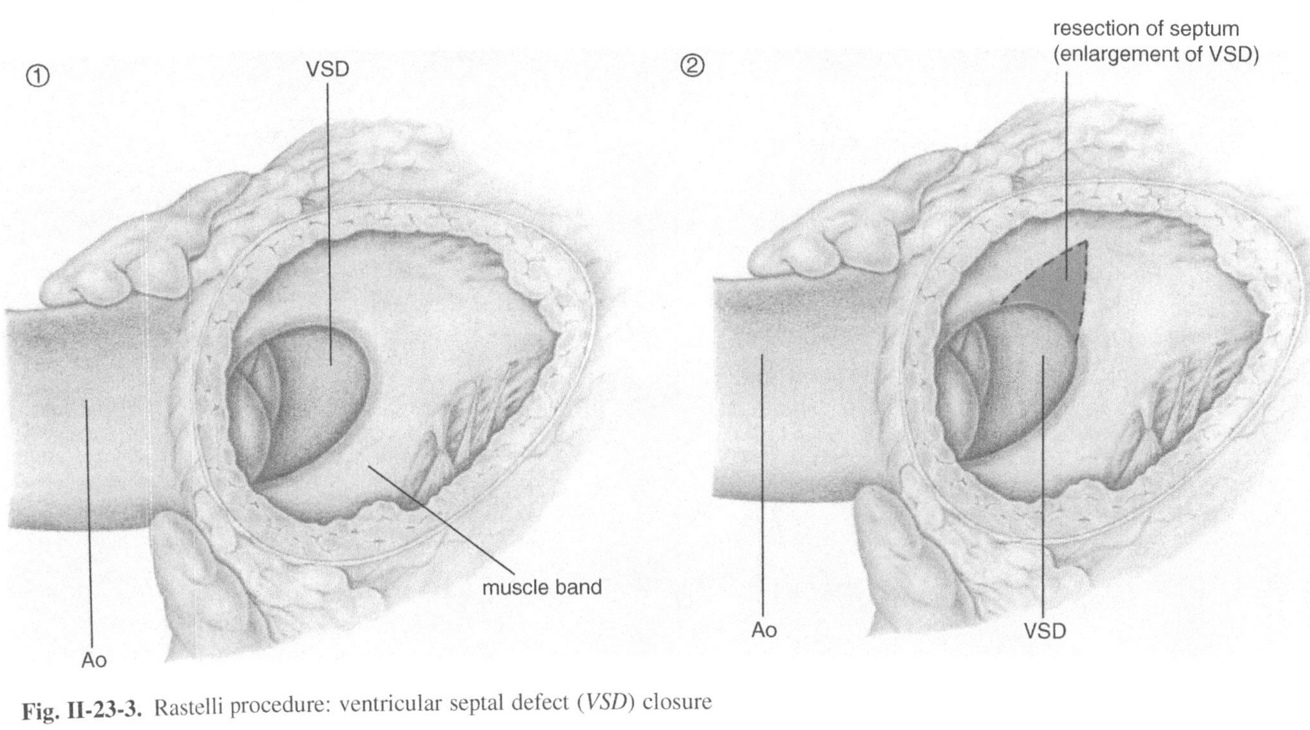

Fig. II-23-3. Rastelli procedure: ventricular septal defect (*VSD*) closure

pericardial patch, and a conduit is sutured to this patch. This technique facilitates the distal suture line and minimizes bleeding (Fig. II-23-4 ①, ②). To prevent cardiac compression by the artificial valve in the conduit after chest closure, the distal portion of the conduit is shortened as much as possible. Thus, the artificial valve of the conduit is kept far from the sternum, which otherwise might press the valve onto the heart. It is equally important not to undersize conduit length, because an excessively short conduit can cause coronary compression. The proximal portion of the conduit is beveled to fit the right ventriculotomy and sutured to the ventriculotomy with a running suture (Fig. II-23-4 ③). The suture line is facilitated by holding the conduit to the ventriculotomy site and keeping even tension on both the suture and the edge of the muscle.

Right Ventricular Outflow Tract Reconstruction with Autologous Tissue

Lecompte Maneuver

The ascending aorta is transversely opened, and the truncal valve, coronary orifice, and origins of the PA are inspected. The ascending aorta is completely transected, and branch PAs are brought in front of the ascending aorta, after which the ascending aorta is re-anastomosed (Fig. II-23-5 ①). A longitudinal incision is made in the RVOT, and this incision is enlarged to create a spindle-shaped ventriculotomy. The VSD is closed as in the Rastelli procedure. The ASD or PFO is closed, de-airing is completed, and the aortic cross-clamp is released. The posterior wall of the pulmonary confluence

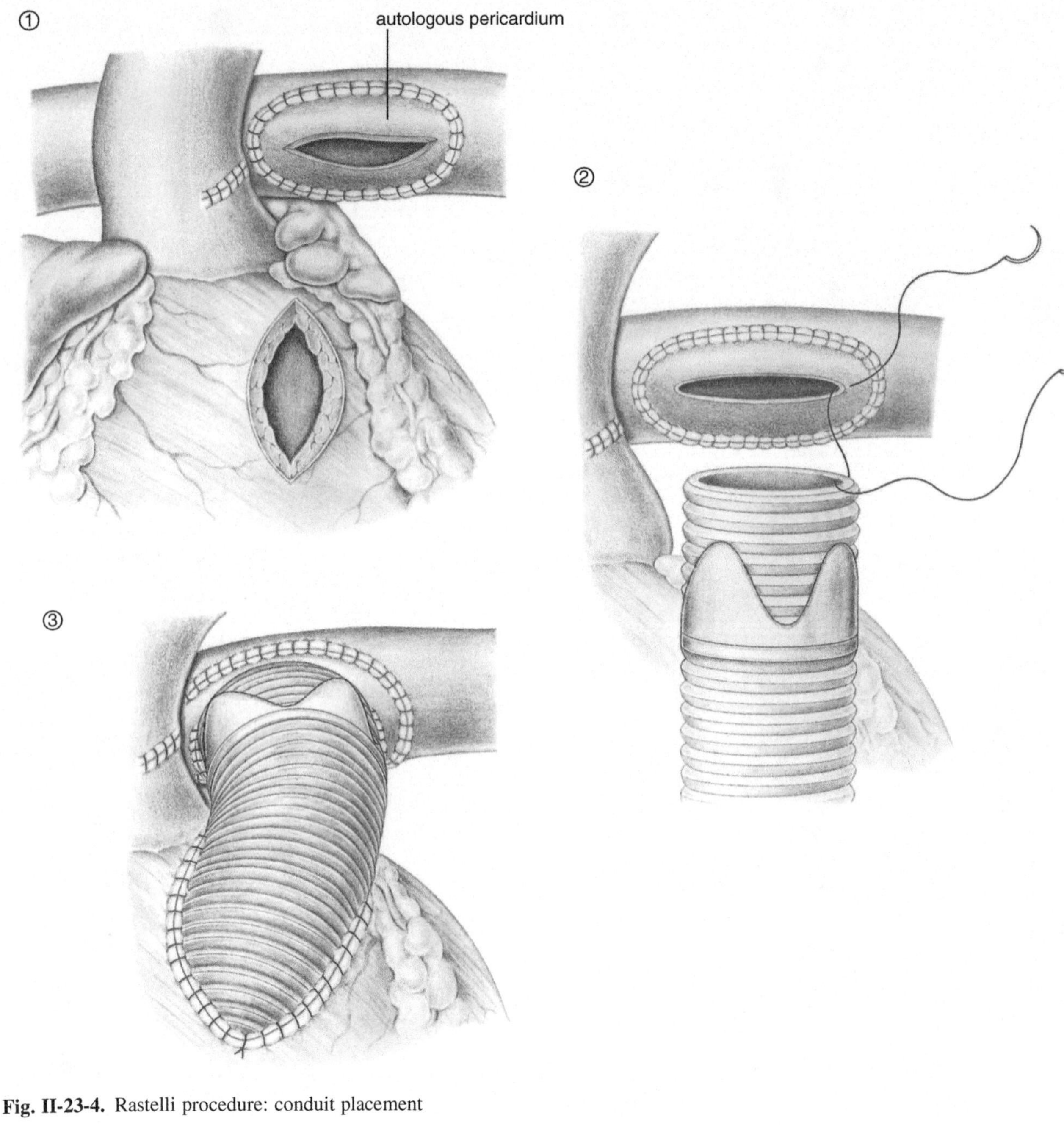

Fig. II-23-4. Rastelli procedure: conduit placement

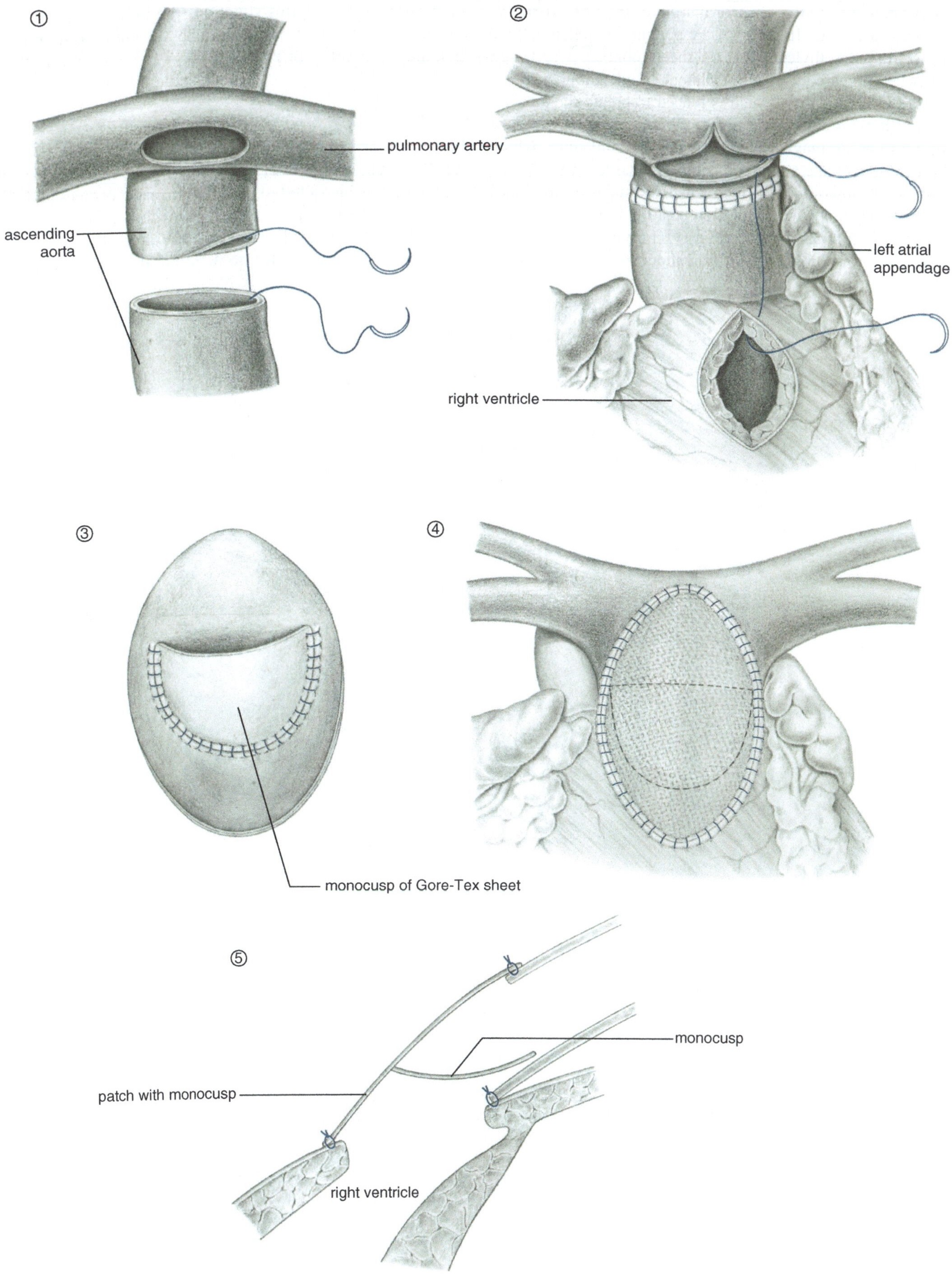

Fig. II-23-5. Lecompte maneuver

is anastomosed to the superior margin of the right ventriculotomy site (Fig. II-23-5 ②). A pericardial patch with a polytetrafluoroethylene (PTFE) sheet monocusp (0.1 mm thick) is prepared. After attachment of the monocusp, an autologous pericardial patch is placed to create the anterior part of RV–PA continuity (Fig. II-23-5 ③, ④). Currently, we prefer to use Yamagishi's patch with a bulging sinus, which is proven to create a more physiological vortex flow [5]. To improve coaptation of the monocusp, the superior margin of the monocusp is placed at a high position opposite the posterior wall of the PA (Fig. II-23-5 ⑤). In type I, the main PA may reach to the RVOT directly without translocation of the pulmonary artery. In this situation, the branch PAs are dissected out to the first-order branches to improve mobilization and to avoid right PA stenosis.

Barbero-Marcial Procedure

For type I, an oblique incision is made from the base of the left PA to the left sinus of Valsalva, and the interior surface of the trunk is inspected to identify coronary orifices and the orifice of the right pulmonary artery. At the side of the trunk, a PTFE patch is placed to separate the ascending aorta and main PA segment (Fig. II-23-6 ①, ②) in the same way as an

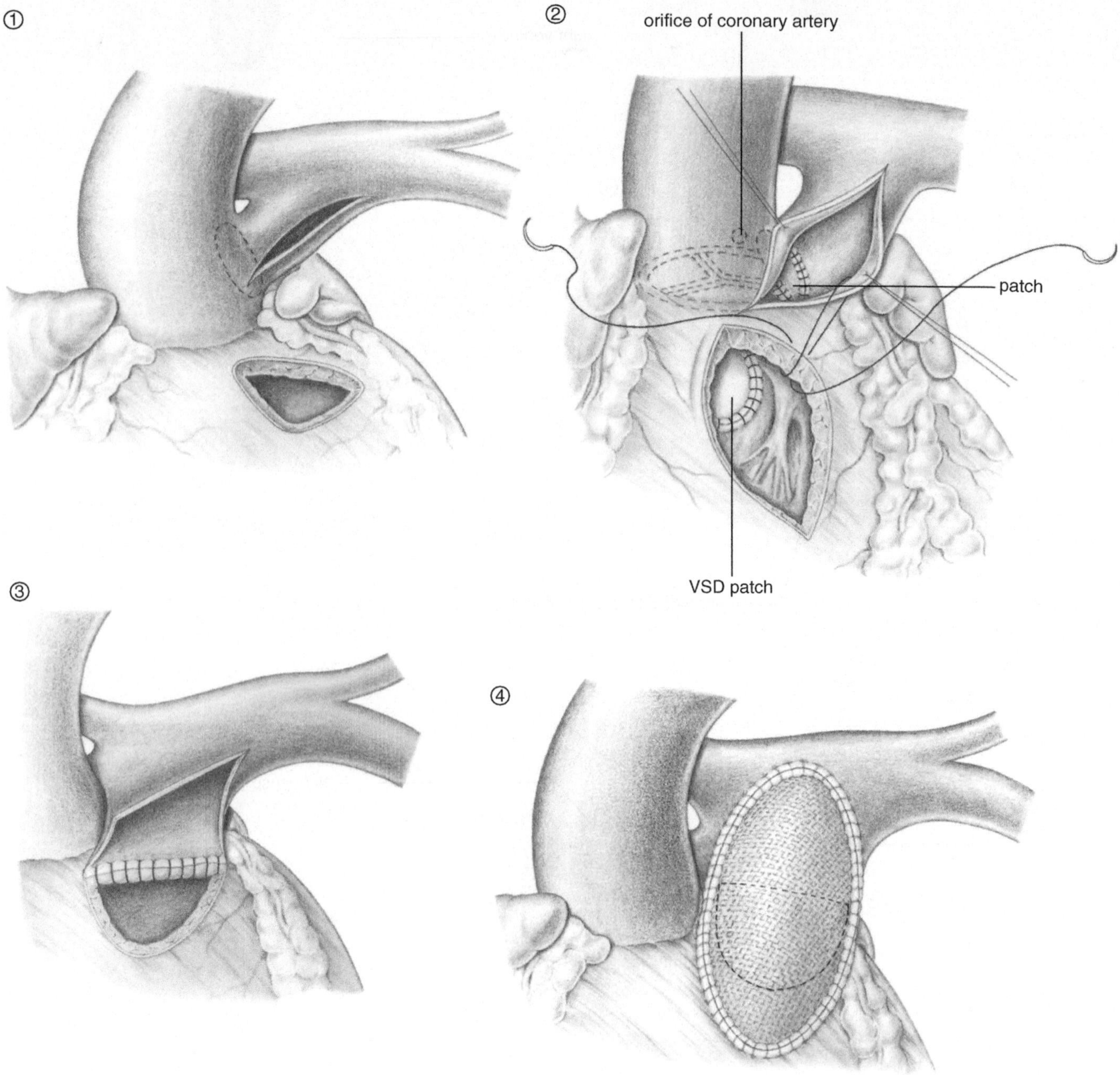

Fig. II-23-6. Barbero-Marcial procedure

aortopulmonary window is closed. This patch is placed to avoid compromise of the pulmonary channel. A ventriculotomy is made in the RV beneath the left sinus of Valsalva, and this ventriculotomy is enlarged inferiorly and leftward. Muscular trabeculations are removed, and the VSD is closed as mentioned previously. After closing ASD or PFO, deairing is completed, and the aortic cross-clamp is released. The superior margin of the ventriculotomy and the inferior edge of the pulmonary arteriotomy are anastomosed, and this becomes the posterior wall of the RVOT (Fig. II-23-6 ③). To complete the anterior wall, an autologous pericardial patch with a PTFE monocusp is used as in the Lecompte procedure (Fig. II-23-6 ④). Barbero-Marcial and colleagues have also reported a technique using the left atrial appendage to construct the posterior wall between the ventriculotomy and pulmonary artery for type II. We believe that the Lecompte procedure is more applicable for types II and III.

Surgery for Truncal Valve Regurgitation

Mee Procedure

In truncus arteriosus, the truncal valve may be a quadricuspid valve with severe regurgitation. Imamura et al. [6] reported a technique to address this by "tricuspidization" of the quadricuspid valve. The smallest valve cusp with its sinus of Valsalva is removed, and the truncal wall is closed. A new commissure is thus created, and a commissuroplasty stitch is placed with good results [7] (Fig. II-23-7 ①, ②, ③).

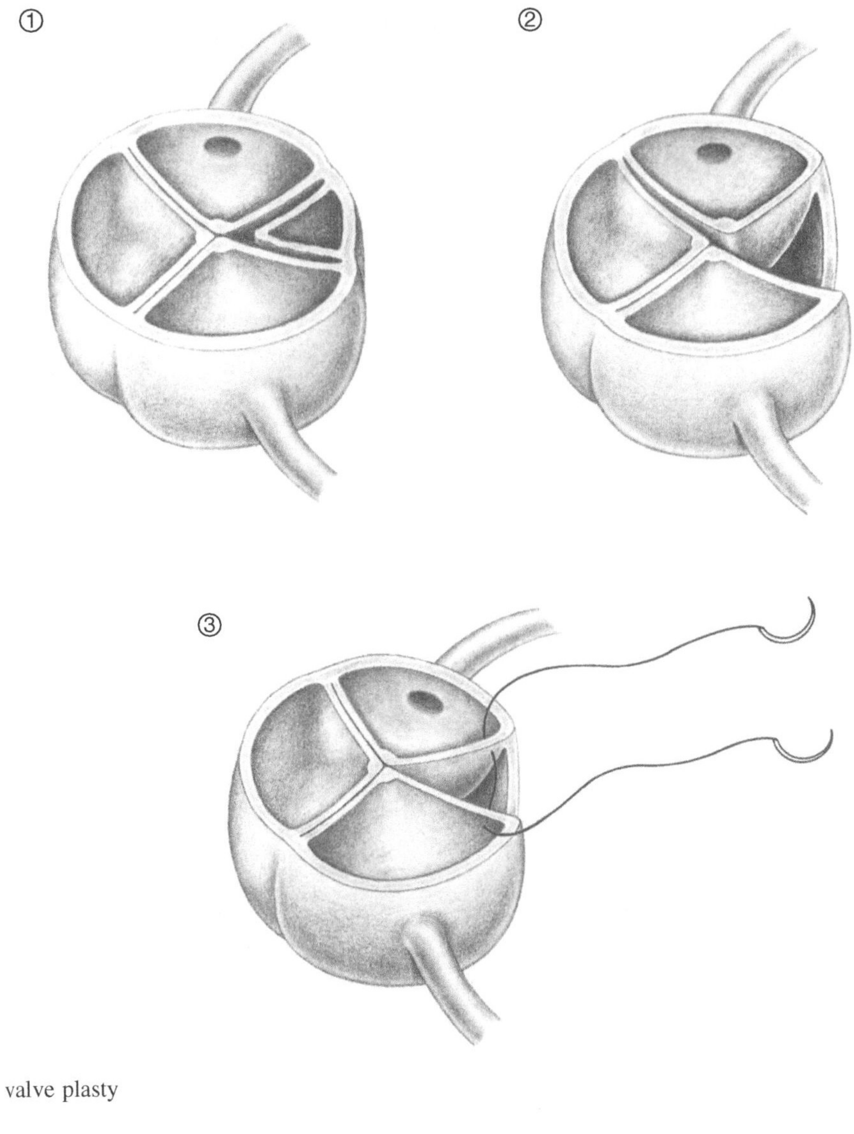

Fig. II-23-7. Truncal valve plasty

References

1. Collett RW, Edwards JE (1949) Persistent truncus arteriosus: a classification according to anatomic type. Surg Clin North Am 29:1245–1270
2. McGoon DC, Rastelli GC, Ongley PA (1968) An operation for correction of the truncus arteriosus. JAMA 205:69–73
3. Lecompte Y, Neveux JY, Leca F, et al (1982) Reconstruction of pulmonary outflow tract without prosthetic conduit. J Thorac Cardiovasc Surg 84:727–733
4. Barbero-Marcial M, Riso A, Atik E, et al (1990) A technique for correction of truncus arteriosus types I and II without extracardiac conduits. J Thorac Cardiovasc Surg 99:364–369
5. Miyazaki T, Yamagishi M, Nakashima A, et al (2007) Expanded polytetrafluoroethylene valved conduit and patch with bulging sinuses in right ventricular outflow tract reconstruction. J Thorac Cardiovasc Surg 134:327–332
6. Imamura M, Drummond-Webb JJ, Sarris GE, et al (1999) Improving early and intermediate results of truncus arteriosus repair: a new technique of truncal valve repair. Ann Thorac Surg 67:1142–1146
7. Chiu IS, Wu SJ, Chen MR, et al (2002) Anatomic relationship of the coronary orifice and truncal valve in truncus arteriosus and their surgical implication. J Thorac Cardiovasc Surg 123:350–352

II-24. Anomalous Origin of the Right Pulmonary Artery from the Ascending Aorta

Anomalous origin of the right pulmonary artery (PA) from the ascending aorta is a very rare congenital cardiac defect in which the right PA derives blood supply from systemic circulation and the left PA receives the entirety of the systemic venous blood. Heart failure develops in early infancy consequent to increased pulmonary blood flow, with progression of pulmonary hypertension. Prognosis is poor without surgery.

This disease is classified into proximal and distal types [1–4] (Fig. II-24-1). Many patients with this disease develop cardiorespiratory failure soon after birth, and as such, early surgery is necessary. Complete repair is recommended before 6 months of age, especially in the proximal type, as pulmonary vascular obstructive disease may develop rapidly [5].

In the distal type, ductal tissue at the origin of the right PA may become stenotic, and congestive heart failure may diminish secondary to the banding effect of this ductal tissue. Stenosis of the origin of the right PA progresses, and complete occlusion may preclude repair. Therefore, to prevent right PA hypoplasia, early surgery should be performed [6].

For repair of the abnormal right PA, a direct anastomosis or, rarely, a graft interposition technique is utilized. With direct anastomosis, future growth can be expected. Vascular graft interposition risks graft stenosis or occlusion by intimal hyperplasia or thrombosis. The decision to use interposition grafting is based on extreme distance between the main and right PAs. In the neonate or infant, the PA can usually be mobilized well, and direct anastomosis is usually possible.

Direct Anastomosis

The heart is accessed via median sternotomy. When the patient is hemodynamically unstable, a tape is placed around the right PA and snared. With this maneuver, systemic blood pressure is improved and stable hemodynamics is obtained (Fig. II-24-2 ①). The right PA is fully dissected to the hilum. The ascending aorta is separated from the main PA. Dissection is advanced further to the ductus arteriosus and to the left PA at the level of the hilum. During this dissection, the area behind the aorta is fully dissected to obtain sufficient space for right PA growth and avoid postoperative right PA stenosis. A patent ductus arteriosus is often present, and this is doubly ligated and divided. This division facilitates mobilization of the main PA.

Anastomosis is occasionally possible without cardiopulmonary bypass (CPB), if stable hemodynamics is maintained with retraction and side-clamping of the great vessels. In neonates, however, anastomosis employing bypass is more typically used. Ascending aortic and bicaval cannulation is instituted. A left-sided vent catheter is inserted from the base of the right upper pulmonary vein. Ascending aortic cannulation is placed at the base of the brachiocephalic artery or even on the aortic arch. When intracardiac anomalies are not present, the following procedure is performed with a beating heart. A side-clamp is placed on the ascending aorta at the base of the right PA and the right PA is transected. The ascending aorta is closed with a double running monofilament suture (Fig. II-24-2 ②). Next, the right PA is brought behind the ascending aorta. An incision is made in the right side of the main PA, and the right PA is anastomosed with a running suture technique (Fig. II-24-2 ③).

Graft Interposition

In the distal type, graft interposition is frequently used. To allow for the growth of the patient, a graft as large as possible should be chosen. The graft route may be placed in either the anatomic or extra-anatomic position. In the anatomic or extra-anatomic position, the graft is placed posterior or anterior to the ascending aorta, respectively. If a large vascular graft is used, the anatomic route might be difficult, and the extra-anatomic route is necessary. In the extra-anatomic route, the graft may be placed distally at the base of the brachiocephalic artery to avoid compression of the graft by the sternum (Fig. II-24-3).

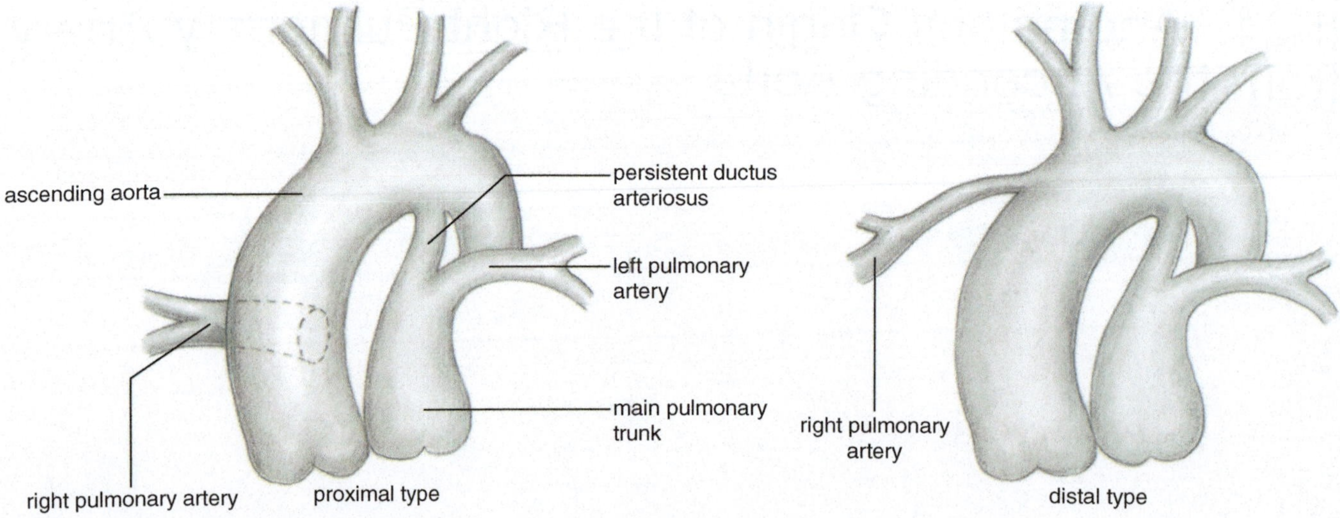

Fig. II-24-1. Classification of anomalous origin of the right pulmonary artery from the ascending aorta

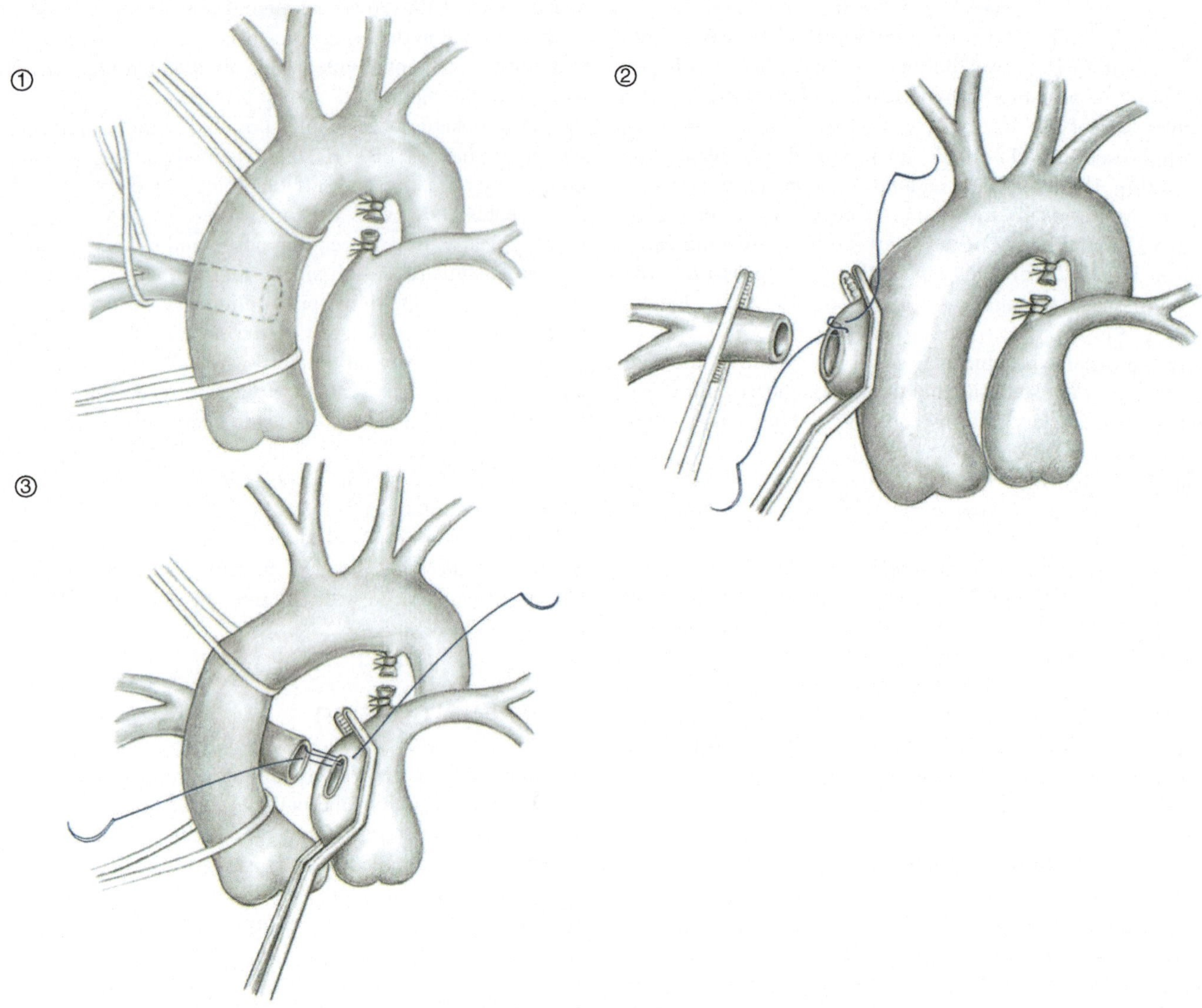

Fig. II-24-2. Direct anastomosis. The ascending aorta and the proximal aortic arch are fully dissected. Dissection behind the ascending aorta is necessary to prevent postoperative pulmonary artery (PA) stenosis

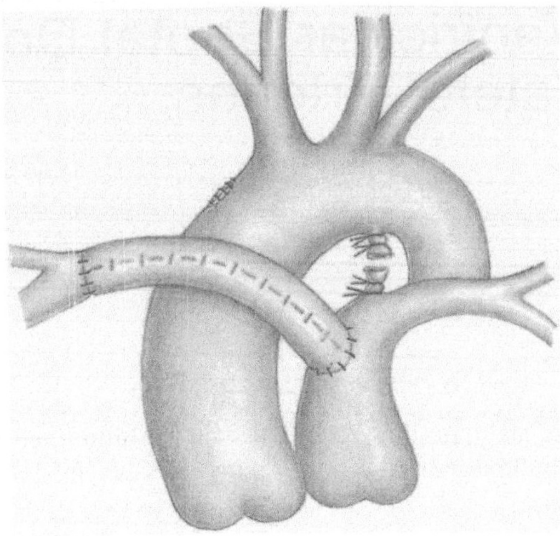

Fig. II-24-3. Graft interposition

References

1. Cucci CE, Doyle EF, Lewis EW (1964) Absence of a primary division of the pulmonary trunk. An ontogenic theory. Circulation 29:124–131
2. Schneiderman LJ (1958) Isolated congenital absence of the right pulmonary artery: a caution as to its diagnosis and a proposal for its embryogenesis. Report of a case with review. Am Heart J 55:772–780
3. Odell JE, Smith JC (1963) Right pulmonary artery arising from ascending aorta. Am J Dis Child 105:53–62
4. Wagenvoort CA, Neufeld H, Birge RF, et al (1961) Origin of right pulmonary artery from ascending aorta. Circulation 23:84–90
5. Yamaki S, Suzuki Y, Ishizawa E, et al (1983) Isolated aortic origin of right pulmonary artery: report of a case with special reference to pulmonary vascular disease in the left and right lungs. Chest 83:575–578
6. Nakamura Y, Yasui H, Kado H, et al (1991) Anomalous origin of the right pulmonary artery from the ascending aorta. Ann Thorac Surg 52:1285–1291

II-25. Pulmonary Atresia with Ventricular Septal Defect and Major Aortopulmonary Collateral Arteries (MAPCAs)

This disease is an extremely heterogeneous and complex congenital heart disease characterized by a highly variable pulmonary blood supply and arborization abnormalities. Each patient has a different clinical presentation and course, determined by the number, size, origin, route, and structure of major aortopulmonary collateral arteries (MAPCAs). One collateral artery supplies blood to one or to multiple lung segments and occasionally supplies blood to the bilateral lung field. Some pulmonary segments are hypoperfused while other segments are hyperperfused, leading to pulmonary hypertension. The difficulty of surgical treatment of this disease is dependent on the diversity of pulmonary blood flow. Previously, a patient with this disease was thought not to be a candidate for surgical treatment. In 1980, Haworth and colleagues [1] reported unifocalization of MAPCAs, and subsequently the surgical approach was expanded [2–5]. Multiple teams reported obtaining growth of the pulmonary arteries (PAs) by staged unifocalization and performing complete repair. Only approximately one-half of patients may have a complete repair through the staged approach. At the time of presentation, some patients fail to become a candidate for any type of unifocalization approach. Therefore, the final rate of successful complete repair for all patients with this disease will be less than 50%.

The target of surgical intervention for this disease is obtaining low right ventricular pressure after complete repair. Right ventricular pressure after repair depends on pulmonary vascular resistance. A decrease in pulmonary vascular resistance is the main goal of treatment for this defect. To create a PA without stenosis and to combine as many as pulmonary segments as possible are important goals. Peripheral PA growth should be considered, and as such, foreign material should be avoided and autologous material should be chosen to reconstruct the PA. In this chapter, several techniques of unifocalization to obtain low pulmonary vascular resistance are discussed.

Approach to MAPCAs

Multistage Unifocalization

Each lung field is serially accessed via thoracotomy with the side with the least chance for hypoxia preferentially chosen for first intervention. During dissection of MAPCAs, the aorta and the airway of the bronchus are used as landmarks [3]. When unifocalized vessels are needed to be brought to the mediastinum, the space between the hilum and phrenic nerve is dissected, and unifocalized vessels are brought to this space.

One-Stage Unifocalization

Delaying of surgical intervention causes poor vascular growth of some pulmonary arterial segments or pulmonary vascular obstructive disease. In this situation, low pulmonary vascular resistance is difficult to obtain after surgery. Another approach is performing bilateral unifocalization in one stage via median sternotomy in early infancy before development of pulmonary vascular obstructive disease occurs [6–9]. In the majority of cases the ventricular septal defect (VSD) is simultaneously closed. Between the SVC and ascending aorta, the posterior pericardium is dissected, and trachea, carina, and descending aorta are accessed. MAPCAs from the descending aorta are identified (Fig. II-25-1). MAPCAs are located anterior or posterior to the bronchus. If possible, unifocalization should be performed before cardiopulmonary bypass (CPB) with care not to cause hypoxemia [10].

Direct Anastomosis of Own Tissue

1. End-to-side anastomosis (Fig. II-25-2 ①). Between the MAPCA and true PA or the MAPCA and MAPCA, this technique is utilized to create as large an anastomosis as possible [11,12].
2. Side-to-side anastomosis is shown in Fig. II-25-2 ②.
3. Aortic button (Fig. II-25-3 ①,②). When multiple collateral arteries arise from the small segment of the aorta, the origins of the collaterals are removed together. Several collaterals are transferred to the PA in one button.
4. Untypical technique (Fig. II-25-4 ①,②,③). To obtain a large anastomosis between the peripheral PA and central PA, this technique is used. Two or three MAPCAs are gathered together, and one large anastomosis is created.

Material of Patch

Autologous Pericardium

Autologous pericardium is used as a central PA in a roll or as a patch to the peripheral PA (Fig. II-25-4 ④,⑤).

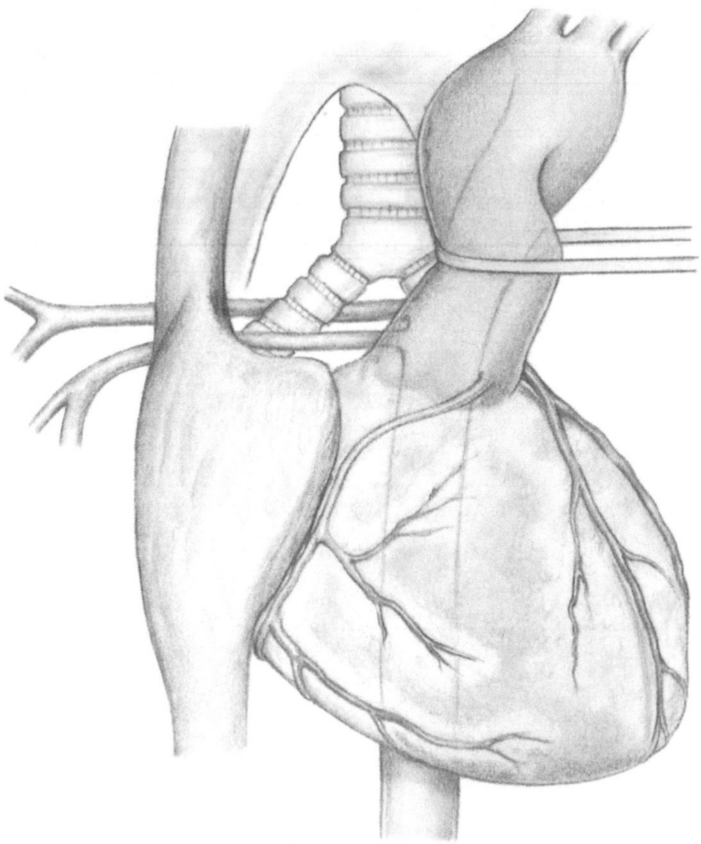

Fig. II-25-1. One-stage unifocalization. The space between the ascending aorta and the superior vena cava (SVC) is dissected. The pericardium above the left atrium is opened. The connective tissue around the carina is dissected. The descending aorta and major aortopulmonary collateral arteries (MAPCAs) from the descending aorta are identified. The MAPCAs can be anterior and posterior to the bronchus

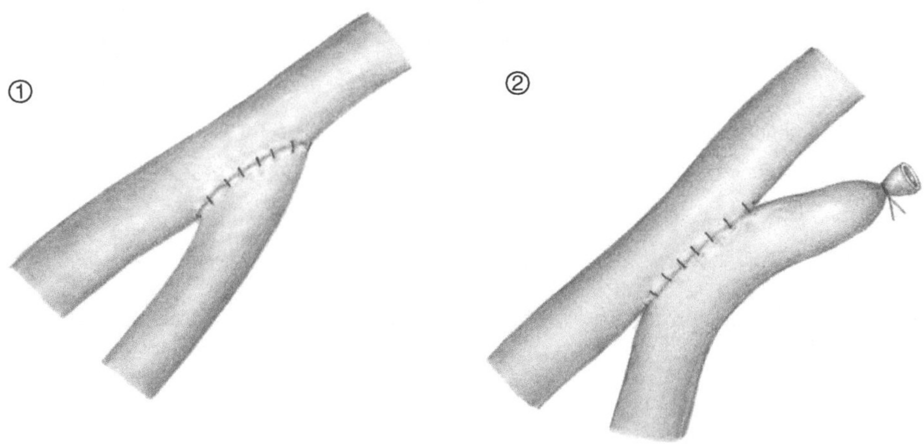

Fig. II-25-2. Anastomosis technique. ① End-to-side technique: this technique is used to create anastomosis between MAPCA and MAPCA or between an MAPCA and true pulmonary artery (PA). ② Side-to-side technique

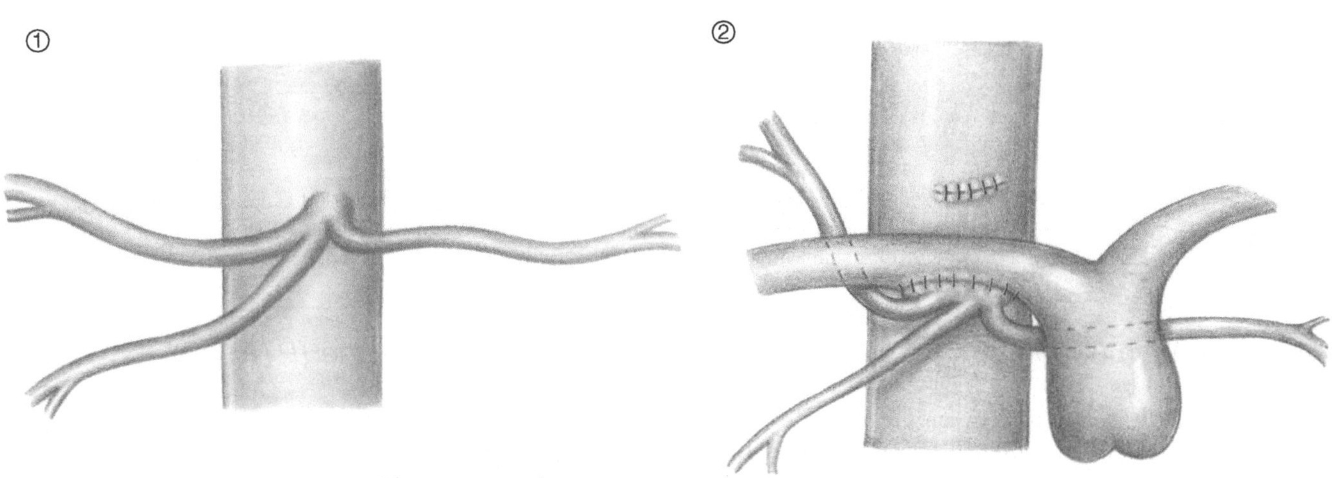

Fig. II-25-3. Aortic button. When several MAPCAs arise from the same location at the descending aorta ①, the aortic wall is removed and reimplantated to the true PA ②

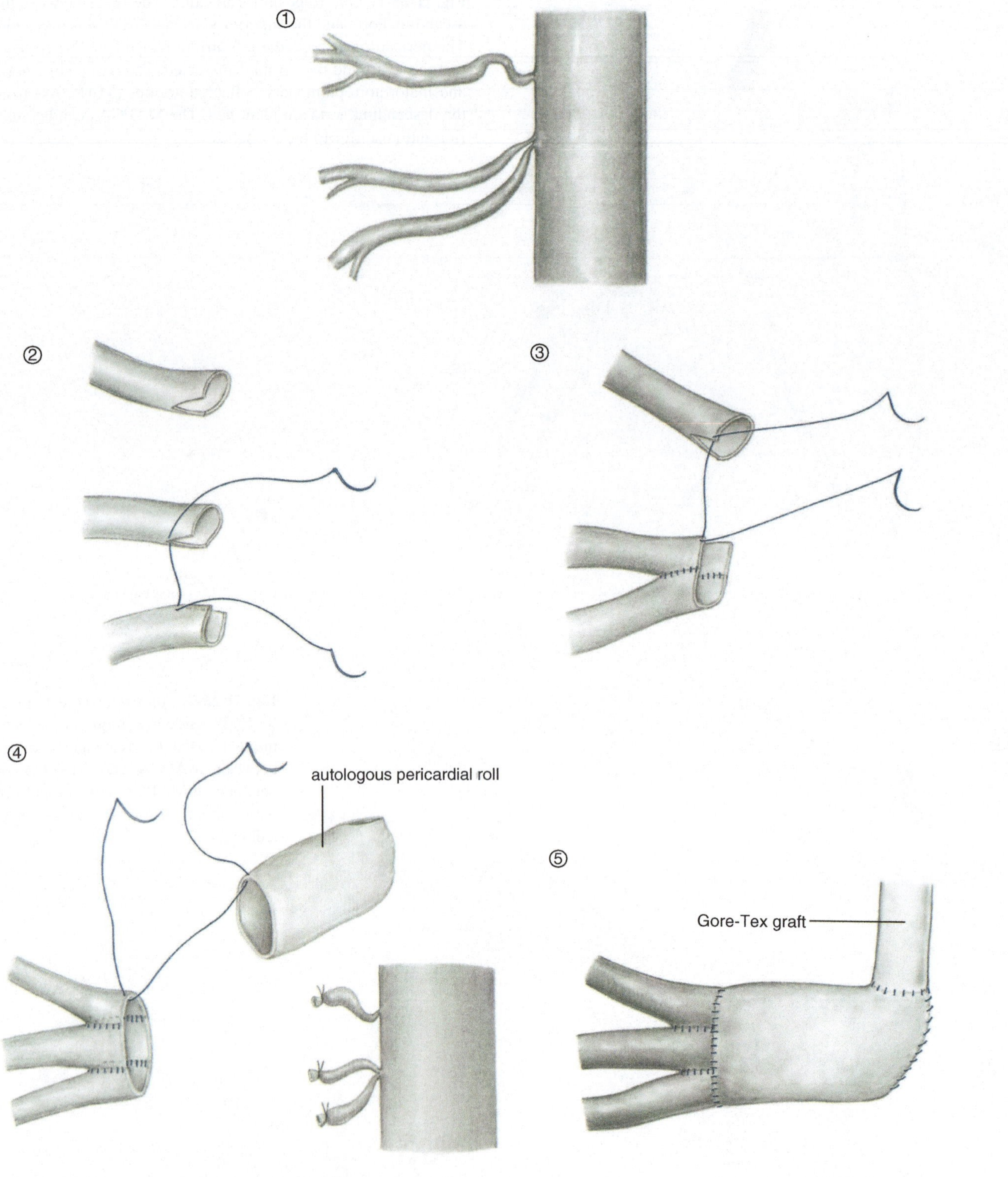

Fig. II-25-4. Special technique of unifocalization. This technique is applied between the peripheral and central PA to obtain the large central PA. Two to three MAPCAs are combined to create a large anastomosis site. When the central PA is missing, an autologous pericardial roll is created, and a systemic-to-PA shunt is placed

Azygous Vein (Fig. II-25-5)

When a distance is present between the PA and collateral, the azygous vein is interposed between two vessels. For peripheral PA or collateral artery stenosis, this vein is used as patch material because of growth potential [13].

Polytetrafluoroethylene (PTFE)

PTFE is frequently used for the Blalock–Taussig shunt (Fig. II-25-4 ⑤). Choice of this material should be avoided for peripheral PA. When an alternative material is not available, this material is used as a patch.

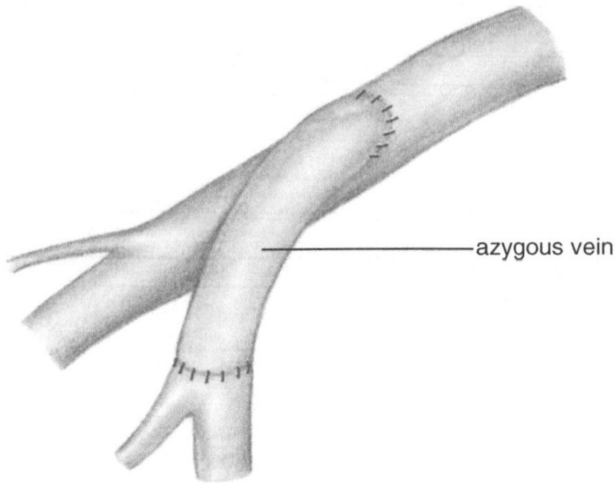

Fig. II-25-5. Use of the azygous vein. In the presence of a significant distance between the true PA and MAPCA, the azygous vein can be used as an interposition graft. Also, the azygous vein can be used as a patch material

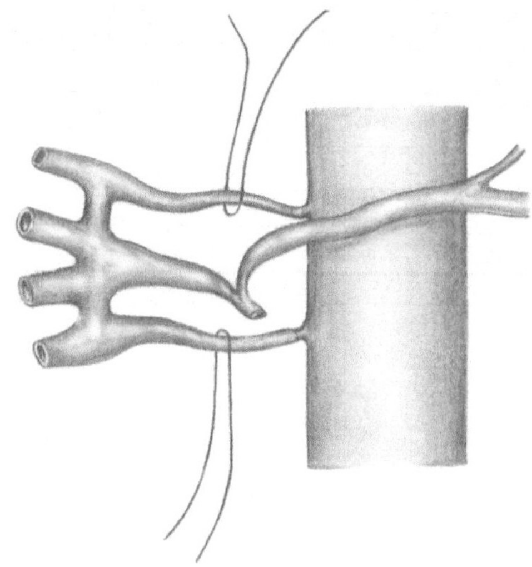

Fig. II-25-6. Simple ligation. When one of the lung segments is perfused by both the large native PA and a small MAPCA, this MAPCA can be ligated. If the MAPCA itself is very small, the area of perfusion by this MAPCA seems tiny, and the effect of unifocalization seems to be insignificant, this MAPCA may be simply ligated

Simple Ligation (Fig. II-25-6)

When the lung has a dual supply, the MAPCA can be ligated. If the area of perfusion by the MAPCA is small and MAPCA itself is tiny, and the effect of unifocalization is thought to be minimal, simple ligation with or without shunt placement is performed.

References

1. Haworth SG, Macartney FJ (1980) Growth and development of pulmonary circulation in pulmonary atresia, ventricular septal defect and major aortopulmonary collateral arteries. Br Heart J 44:14–24
2. Puga FJ, Leoni FE, Julsrud PR, et al (1989) Complete repair of pulmonary atresia, ventricular septal defect and severe peripheral arborization abnormalities of the central pulmonary arteries. Experience with preliminary unifocalization procedures in 38 patients. J Thorac Cardiovasc Surg 98:1018–1029
3. Sawatari K, Imai Y, Kurosawa H, et al (1989) Staged operation for pulmonary atresia and ventricular septal defect with major aortopulmonary collateral arteries. New technique for complete unifocalization. J Thorac Cardiovasc Surg 98:738–750
4. Yagihara T, Yamamoto F, Nishigaki K, et al (1996) Unifocalization for pulmonary atresia with ventricular septal defect and major aortopulmonary collateral arteries. J Thorac Cardiovasc Surg 112:392–402
5. Iyer KS, Mee RBB (1991) Staged repair of pulmonary atresia with ventricular septal defect and major systemic to pulmonary artery collaterals. Ann Thorac Surg 51:65–72
6. McElhinney DB, Reddy VM, Hanley FL (1998) Tetralogy of Fallot with major aortopulmonary collaterals: early total repair. Pediatr Cardiol 19:289–296
7. Reddy VM, Liddicoat JR, Hanley FL (1995) Midline one-stage complete unifocalization and repair of pulmonary atresia with ventricular septal defect and major aortopulmonary collaterals. J Thorac Cardiovasc Surg 109:832–845
8. Reddy VM, Petrossian E, McElhinney DB, et al (1997) One stage complete unifocalization in infants: when should the ventricular septal defect be closed? J Thorac Cardiovasc Surg 113:858–866
9. Lofland GK (2000) The management of pulmonary atresia, ventricular septal defect and multiple aortopulmonary collateral arteries by definitive single stage repair in early infancy. Eur J Cardiovasc Surg 18:480–486
10. Mignosa C, Comas JV, Kitayama H, et al (1996) Avoiding hypoxemia during unifocalization. Ann Thorac Surg 61:715–717
11. Watterson KG, Wilkinson JL, Karl TR, et al (1991) Very small pulmonary arteries: central end-to-side shunt. Ann Thorac Surg 52:1132–1137
12. Fraser CD, Latson LA, Mee RBB (1995) Surgical repair of severe bilateral branch pulmonary artery stenosis. Ann Thorac Surg 59:738–740
13. Iyer KS, Varma M, Mee RBB (1989) Use of azygos vein as interposition graft for surgical unifocalization of pulmonary blood supply. Ann Thorac Surg 48:776–778

II-26. Tetralogy of Fallot

All patients with tetralogy of Fallot require surgery. Whether to proceed to complete repair or whether to begin with shunt placement is determined based on the development of the branch pulmonary arteries (PAs). An initial systemic-to-pulmonary shunt has historically been placed when branch PA growth is poor. However, currently, complete repair is possible for even rather small PA (PA index, 100–150 mm^2/m^2), and a shunt can be avoided. Even if an initial shunt is employed, complete repair is performed relatively shortly thereafter [1]. In our center, to decrease the psychological burden to the child and family of multiple hospitalizations, a preliminary shunt operation has been performed less frequently.

Infantile Repair

The timing of complete repair has evolved to younger ages, and is based primarily on symptoms. If the patient has a hypercyanotic spell or severe cyanosis, complete repair is performed in infancy if the PAs are well developed. Our current practice is repair at around 4 to 9 months of age.

Complete Repair with Preservation of Pulmonary Valve [2]

Pulmonary valve preservation is pursued because long-standing pulmonary valve insufficiency impairs right ventricular function [2]. In 1992, Dr. Yasui and colleagues proposed the pulmonary preservation approach at complete repair of tetralogy of Fallot. In their approach, the pulmonary valve area (PVA) was measured with preoperative angiography. If the PVA is more than 1.8 cm^2/m^2, the pulmonary valve can be preserved. Even if the PVA is less than 1.8 cm^2/m^2, but the valve leaflet is thin, mobile, and not calcified, and the PVA is more than 1.4 cm^2/m^2 after commissurotomy, the pulmonary valve may still be preserved. Using these criteria, in 117 of 148 patients (80%), the pulmonary valve was preserved. To evaluate growth of the pulmonary valve, a catheterization study was performed in 54 patients with small preoperative PVA less than 1.8 cm^2/m^2 late after surgery. A lower right ventricle/left ventricle (RV/LV) systolic pressure ratio was seen in late follow-up compared to soon after surgery. Growth of the preserved pulmonary valve was confirmed. Pulmonary valve regurgitation in the valve-preserved group was much less compared to the group with a transannular patch. In patients who were younger at time of their complete repair, the dysmorphism of the valve tissue was less, and the preservation rate was high. Because the growth potential of the pulmonary valve after surgery was significantly higher if the patient was young at surgery, early complete repair was recommended.

This policy of pulmonary valve preservation is applied to a transatrial and transpulmonary approach [3–5]. Although the transatrial and transpulmonary approach increases the chance of opening the pulmonary valve annulus when compared to that of complete repair with pulmonary valve preservation, by minimizing application of a right ventriculotomy such as 2–4 mm in length, postoperative pulmonary valve insufficiency can be reduced. An incision at the pulmonary annulus decreases postoperative residual pulmonary stenosis. In patients with a hypoplastic pulmonary annulus, this approach might create ideal postoperative conditions of mild pulmonary stenosis and mild pulmonary insufficiency. When valve deformity is mild, even in the presence of a hypoplastic pulmonary valve annulus, growth of the valve itself is expected, and complete repair with pulmonary valve preservation could suggest that the much shorter right ventriculotomy could be safely applied.

Transatrial and Transpulmonary Approach

Surgical techniques that preserve right ventricular function by limiting any right ventriculotomy have significantly contributed to improved surgical results for tetralogy of Fallot [3–7]. In this section, the transatrial and transpulmonary approach is discussed.

Transatrial and Transpulmonary Approach

The trans-right atrial and transpulmonary approach minimizes right ventriculotomy and optimizes postoperative ventricular function. In this approach, the maximum ventriculotomy is 1 cm. From the right atrium, through the tricuspid valve, right ventricular outflow tract (RVOT) muscle is resected. The muscle beneath the pulmonary valve is excised from above, via a pulmonary arteriotomy. Pulmonary valve function and right ventricular function are preserved with this approach. The ventricular septal defect (VSD) is closed through the right atriotomy.

If there is a previously placed Blalock–Taussig (BT) shunt, the vascular graft is dissected and silk strings are placed around the graft. After initiation of bypass the graft is doubly ligated and divided, and each end is oversewn with monofilament suture. Next, the main PA is opened longitudinally, and diameters of the branch PAs are assessed with a calibrated dilator. When an appropriate-sized dilator [8] cannot be passed without resistance, the branch PAs are opened longitudinally, and an autologous pericardial patch is placed later. The ascending aorta is cross-clamped, and cardioplegic solution is injected to the aortic root. The RA is opened, and a vent tube is inserted through the patent foramen ovale to vent the left side of the heart.

Right Ventricular Outflow Tract Muscle Resection

To perform the RVOT muscle resection accurately, exposure of the operative field is most important [9]. The assistant holds two small retractors placed in the tricuspid valve annulus. The left hand retracts toward the pulmonary valve while the right hand retracts toward the surgeon. The forces of the right and left hand retractors create a rectangular opening (Fig. II-26-1). The retractors have different-sized hooks at each end (Fig. II-26-2). The left-hand retractor with a larger blade is pulled toward the pulmonary artery, and the right-hand retractor with a smaller blade is pulled toward the surgeon. With good visualization of the operative field, the position and size of the VSD are checked. An obtusely angled fluted coronary sinus sucker is held by the second assistant and is placed at the posterior surface of the RVOT, applying pressure posteriorly and inferiorly. With two retractors and this sucker, three-point traction improves visualization of the RVOT. The RVOT is inspected from the right atrium (RA). Scissors are utilized to cut from the junction of infundibular septum, ventriculoinfundibular fold, and septoparietal insertion toward the PA. Care is taken to keep the blades of the scissors parallel to the ascending aorta. Deep muscle resection should not be performed in this area through the tricuspid valve, as muscle resection beneath the pulmonary valve can be more easily performed through the PA. The resection is advanced clockwise in the right ventricular free wall. Only the inner-layer muscle is resected. Care is taken to avoid creating a perforation in the ventricular free wall. It is important to identify the outer and inner layer of the muscle and to excise only the inner layer (Fig. II-26-3). The inner layer muscle is loose, and the outer layer muscle is compact. After muscle excision, the VSD is closed through the RA.

VSD Closure

In tetralogy of Fallot, 75% of patients have a perimembranous, outlet-type VSD [10,11]. The VSD is bordered by the tricuspid valve annulus, the aortic valve annulus, and ventricular muscle (Fig. II-26-4). Through the RA, the VSD is closed using a patch, with interrupted or running suture technique. The former technique is more commonly used. With an interrupted technique, a stitch is first placed to the membranous septum, then stitches are placed clockwise. Alternatively, the sutures are placed counterclockwise. For VSD closure in tetralogy of Fallot, visualization of the ven-

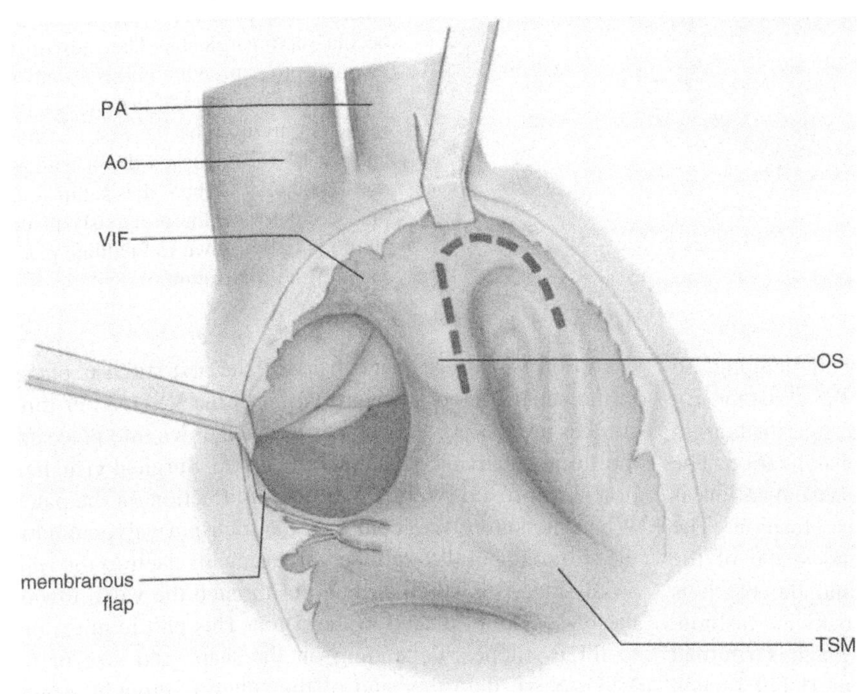

Fig. II-26-1. Exposure of right ventricular outflow tract (RVOT). Two small retractors placed through the tricuspid valve improve exposure. One larger blade of the retractor is pulled anteriorly toward the RVOT. The other, smaller blade of the retractor is pulled rightward toward the surgeon. Care is taken to create a rectangular opening by appropriately directed retractor tension. The area shown by the *dotted line* is incised with scissors. The inner layer of the muscle is excised toward the pulmonary valve. *PA*, pulmonary artery; *Ao*, aorta; *VIF*, ventriculoinfundibular fold; *OS*, outlet septum; *TSM*, trabecula septomarginalis

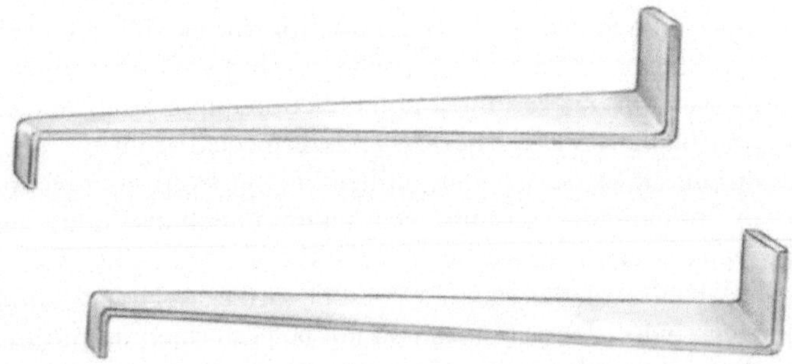

Fig. II-26-2. Retractors for exposure of ventricular septal defect (VSD) margin. The retractor has two different-sized blades

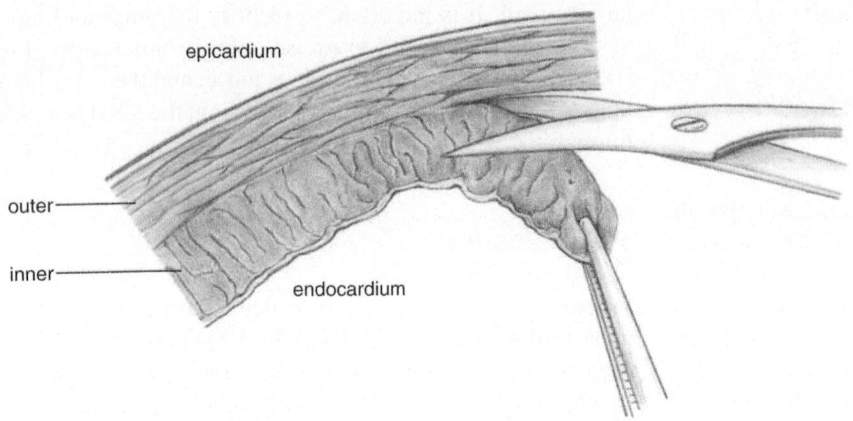

Fig. II-26-3. Structure of right ventricular free wall. The key concept to resect the muscle safely is to identify the two-layer structures of the right ventricular free wall. The inner and outer layers have a looser and a more compact structure, respectively. During muscle resection, resection should be limited to the inner, less compact layer, to prevent perforation of the ventricular wall

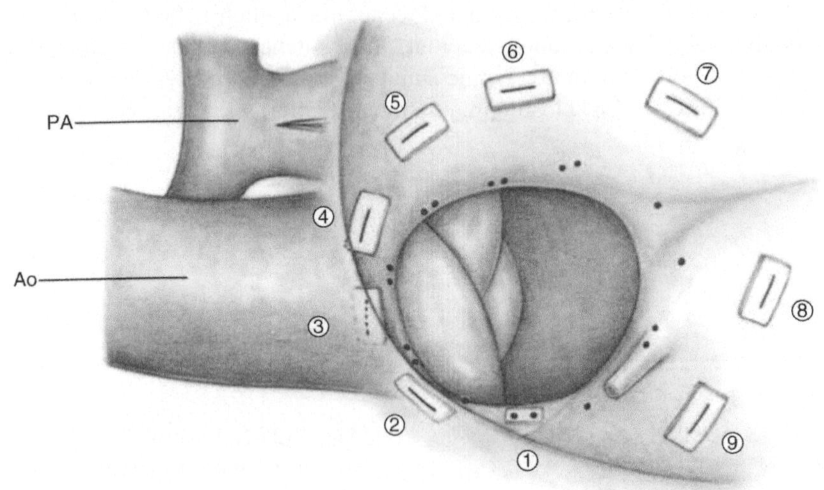

Fig. II-26-4. VSD closure with interrupted sutures. The VSD is bordered by the membranous flap, tricuspid valve annulus, aortic valve annulus, ventricular muscle of infundibular septum, and the anterior and posterior branches of trabecula septomarginalis. The most difficult areas to expose are points ③ and ④. To facilitate exposure of these areas, two retractors are used by the first assistant, and the RVOT is pushed down with the aortic annulus. When the sutures are placed clockwise, the previously placed suture is pulled down to facilitate placement of the next suture

triculoinfundibular fold (VIF) is technically challenging. To expose the VIF, two retractors are used by the assistant. By pushing the RVOT over the aortic root, the superior margin of the VSD is pulled down to obtain better visualization. The previous suture is pulled down to improve visualization as well, when suturing in a counterclockwise fashion. The patch is trimmed according to the size and shape of the defect. Sutures are placed in the patch, and the patch is pushed into place. Sutures are tied in a clockwise fashion. When using a running suture technique, the patch is trimmed first (Fig. II-26-5). A polytetrafluoroethylene (PTFE) patch is chosen because it is not friable. The first stitch is placed in the superior and anterior margin of the VSD. After three stitches are placed, the patch is lowered down into place and the suture is advanced counterclockwise. Surgical visualization is improved by gentle downward traction on the patch. When the suture line comes to the tricuspid valve annulus, the suture is put through the valve annulus itself to the right atrial side. This stitch is then put through the valve toward the RV side and placed to the patch. This part requires one to three stitches, depending on the shape and size of the VSD. Next, the other end of the suture is brought around

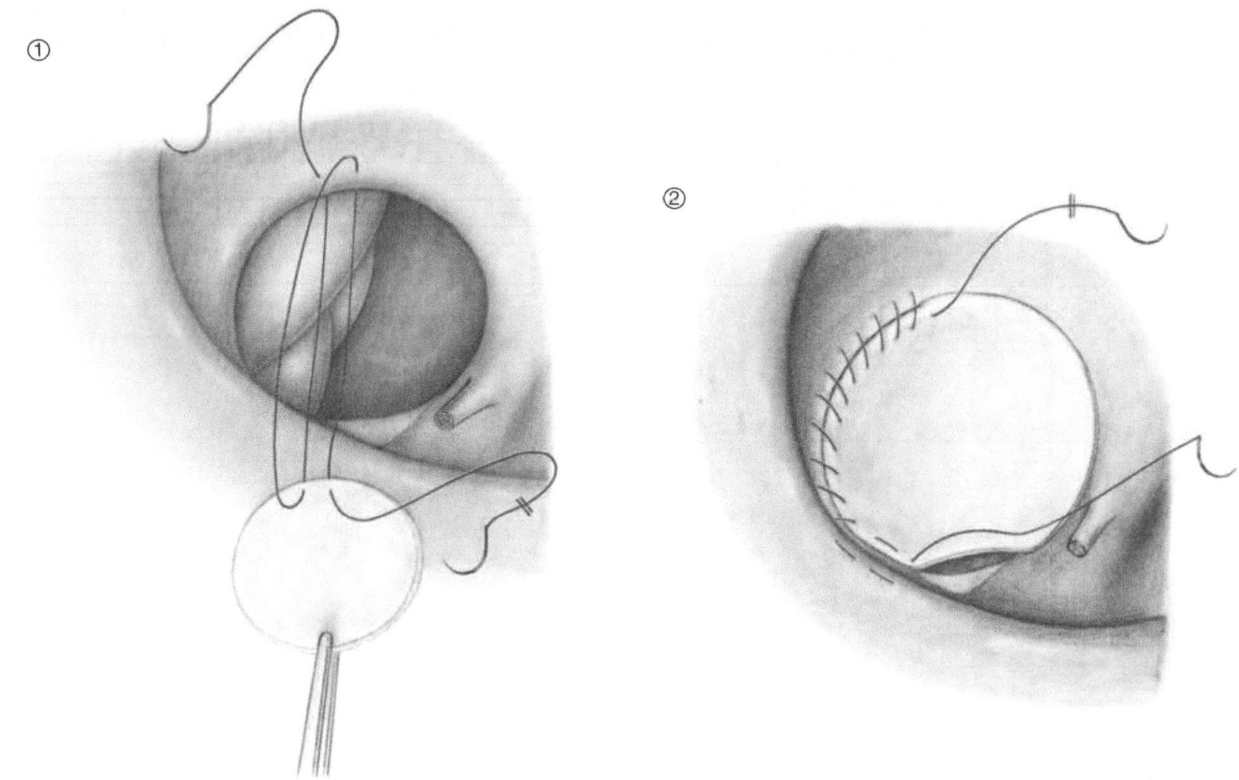

Fig. II-26-5. VSD closure with running suture. After evaluation of the shape and size of the VSD, a patch is cut and trimmed. To avoid fraying of the margin of the patch, polytetrafluoroethylene (PTFE) is used. Suturing is commenced from the anterior and superior margin of the defect ①. After three stitches are placed, the patch is lowered into place. The suture is carried counterclockwise along the infundibular septum and aortic valve. Mild traction on the patch downward helps expose the margin of the defect. This arm of the suture is brought to the right atrium at the tricuspid annulus. The suture is then placed from the annulus and to the patch. The extent of this horizontal mattress suturing along the tricuspid valve depends on the shape of the ventricular infundibular fold. The other end of the suture is brought clockwise inferiorly ②

clockwise. In the location of the right bundle of the conduction system, slightly wider advancement is used to minimize injury to the conduction system. Complete elimination of right bundle branch block is, however, impossible. At the membranous region, stitches are placed in the same place as the interrupted suture technique. Finally, the suture ends are tied on the patch side. One of the advantages of a running suture technique is a shorter VSD closure time. Another merit of the running suture technique is decreased chance of long-term tricuspid valve dysfunction, as pledgets are not used at the tricuspid site and good tricuspid valve movement is preserved. With either technique, the patch is checked to find loose points or "dog ears" of the patch.

Right Ventricular Outflow Tract Reconstruction

Pulmonary valvotomy and RVOT muscle resection are performed via a pulmonary arteriotomy. This muscle resection is effectively carried out in the area just next to the aortic root (Fig. II-26-6). Two retractors are used to visualize the right ventricular outflow tract. The desired-sized dilators are used to measure the RVOT. The incision at the main PA could be carried down to the pulmonary annulus, if still inadequate (less than normal value from the Rowlatt's nomogram [8], which is shown in the Supplement (Fig. II-26-7). It should be emphasized that relying on intraoperative probing with dilators, however, might be misleading because a dilator larger than the real size can pass through easily in a relaxed heart during cardioplegic arrest. The measurement with dilators is thus one of the indices when determining the optimal size of the pulmonary annulus and the RVOT. Direct visualization is also important, especially when the RVOT is checked. The incision at the RVOT is kept as short as possible. In many cases, a 2- to 3-mm incision is sufficient. With a longitudinal incision at the inside of the free wall portion of the outflow tract, enlargement of the outflow tract is obtained. After intervention on the RVOT, the patent foramen ovale (PFO) or atrial septal defect (ASD) is closed. De-airing is accomplished, and the aortic cross-clamp is released. Any further repair of RVOT is performed with a beating heart.

Both relief of stenosis and minimization of regurgitation need to be obtained for the repair of the RVOT. Significant pulmonary valve regurgitation may develop when an exten-

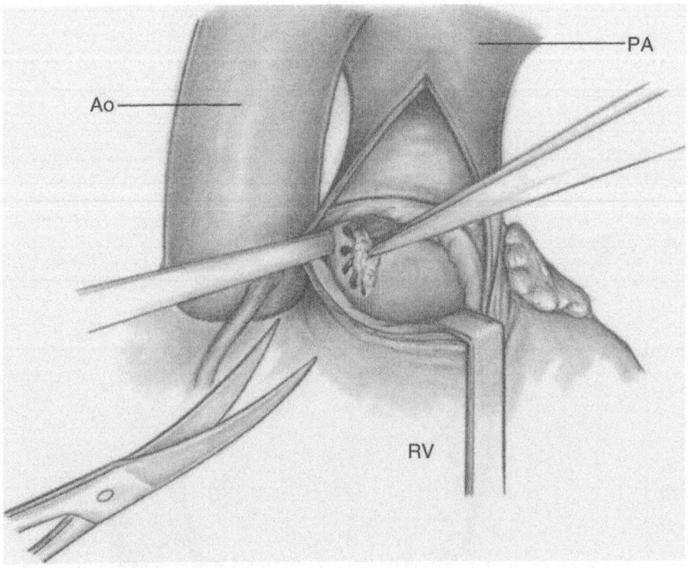

Fig. II-26-6. Transpulmonary subpulmonary RVOT muscle resection. After pulmonary valve commissurotomy, muscle resection is performed beneath the pulmonary valve. The muscle resection can be performed effectively at the right side of the RVOT through this approach. *Ao*, aorta; *RV*, right ventricle

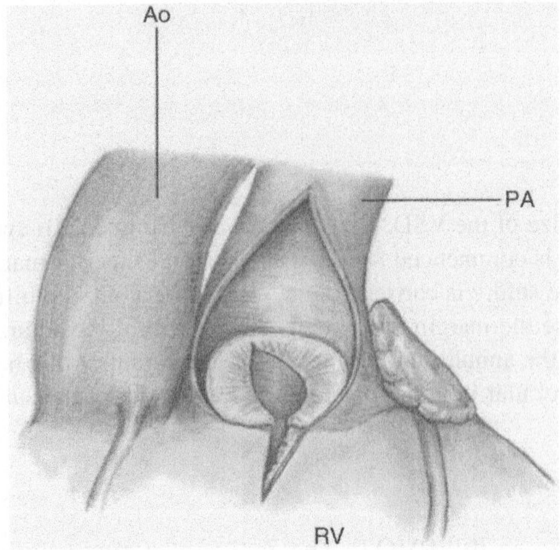

Fig. II-26-7. Incision through the annulus. When the annulus is smaller than normal size, an incision is placed through the annulus of the pulmonary valve. Ventriculotomy is kept minimal. In the majority of cases, the length of this ventriculotomy is 2–3 mm

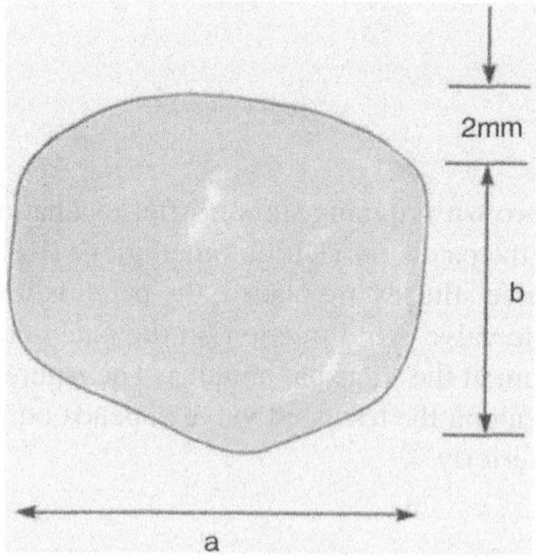

Fig. II-26-8. Shape of the monocusp. The monocusp is fashioned from a PTFE sheet (0.1 mm thickness). The width of the cusp is tailored to allow apposition against the posterior wall of the native main pulmonary artery (a). The height is determined according to the length of the ventriculotomy (b)

sive ventriculotomy or a large patch at the valve annulus are used. In the transatrial and transpulmonary approach, the ventriculotomy is usually minimal and severe pulmonary regurgitation is rare. If needed in a patient with severely hypoplastic annulus, a monocusp is used to reduce regurgitation. As the material for a monocusp, a PTFE membrane (0.1-mm PTFE sheet) is used; the shape of the monocusp is shown in Fig. II-26-8. The width of the cusp is fashioned to fit against the posterior pulmonary wall in diastole. With apposition between native pulmonary valve tissue and the monocusp, regurgitation is reduced. The superior ends of the monocusp are placed 2–3 mm higher than the native pulmonary valve annulus. The height of the monocusp is determined based on the length of the ventriculotomy. Stitches are placed only in the epicardium (not full thickness) as the proximal portion of the monocusp is secured at the ventriculotomy site. By suturing the monocusp and the anterior free wall patch separately, the monocusp can be placed more exactly. The monocusp is implanted first, and then the free wall patch is placed (Fig. II-26-9). In the presence of branch PA stenosis, a longitudinal incision is made beyond the stenosis site, and an autologous pericardial patch is placed (Fig. II-26-10). It is important to carry the incision far enough distally without any tension and to use a patch fitting to the PA. A sufficiently long incision on the stenotic PA and a proper trimming of the patch will provide adequate relief of the stenosis. The suture is started at the most distal part of the pulmonary artery and brought proximally. Cardiopulmonary bypass is weaned and discontinued. Separation from bypass is straightforward so long as there is no significant residual VSD or RVOT obstruction.

171

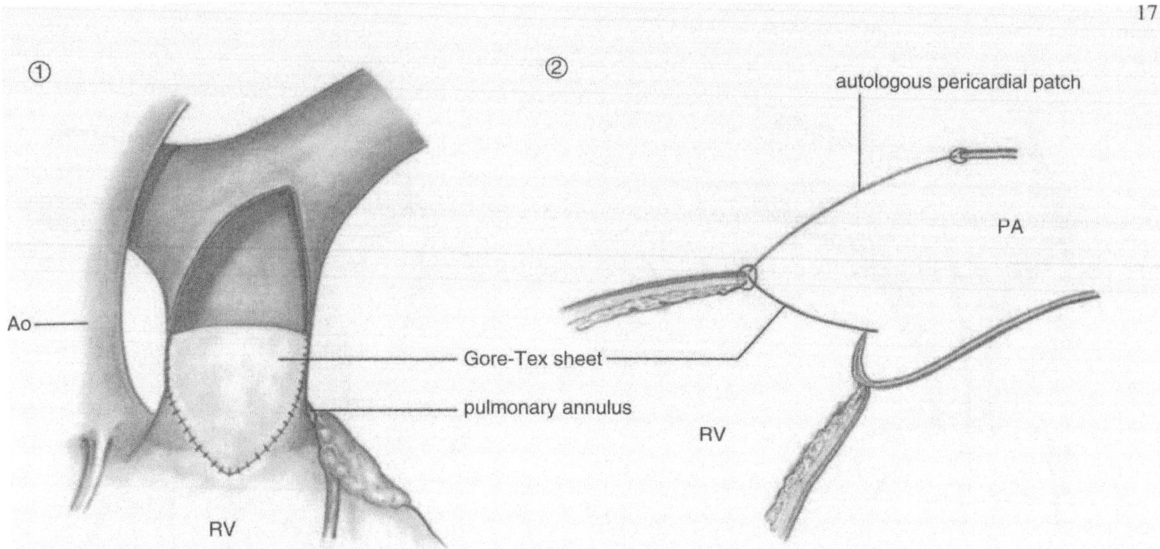

Fig. II-26-9. Monocusp patch placement. The distal ends of the monocusp are sutured 2–3 mm superior to the original pulmonary valve cusp site ①. Suturing to the epicardial surface of the free wall of right ventriculotomy site, as opposed to the whole thickness of the ventriculotomy, helps minimize the ventriculotomy. A free wall patch of autologous pericardium is sutured later ②

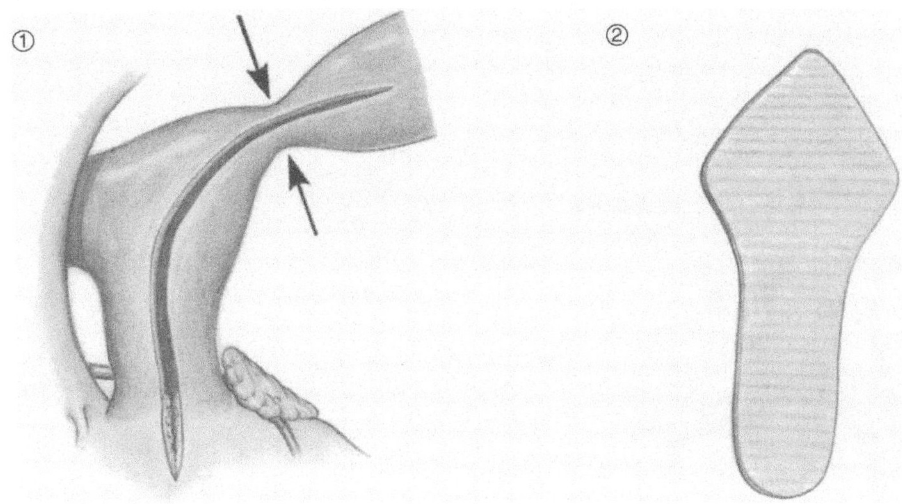

Fig. II-26-10. Relief of branch pulmonary artery stenosis. In the presence of branch pulmonary artery stenosis, an incision is placed far beyond the stenosis (①). An autologous pericardial patch, cut according to the stenosis, is sutured to the branch pulmonary artery (②)

Special Type of RVOT Reconstruction

Tetralogy of Fallot with Pulmonary Atresia

The main PA is anastomosed to the ventriculotomy site, and a new posterior RVOT is created, if the distance between the main PA and RVOT is short. This approach provides autologous tissue continuity. The branch PAs are fully mobilized to improve mobilization. The main PA is opened longitudinally, and this incision is carried onto the RVOT. The inferior end of the main PA is anastomosed to the superior end of the ventriculotomy site with several interrupted sutures to create posterior RVOT–PA continuity (Fig. II-26-11). The length of ventriculotomy is typically more than 1 cm but is minimized. For reconstruction of the anterior wall of RVOT, a monocusp patch is placed. Currently, we prefer to use a PTFE monocusp patch with a bulging sinus (Yamagishi valve) [12]. If the distance between the main PA and the RVOT is so long as to preclude direct anastomosis, the PA is placed anteriorly to the ascending aorta (Lecompte maneuver).

Absent Pulmonary Valve Syndrome (Fig. II-26-12)

In absent pulmonary valve syndrome, the pulmonary valve annulus is hypoplastic and the branch PA is extremely dilated. Incisions are made at the main and branch PAs, as shown in Fig. II-26-12, and portions of the branch pulmonary arterial wall are removed. As a result, the diameters of the branch PAs are decreased and compression of the airway is reduced. A right ventriculotomy is created at the outflow tract, and a monocusp is placed. The flap-shaped main PA is pulled down to the ventriculotomy site. This inferior and anterior traction on the PA decreases the pressure on the airway, which can be confirmed by bronchoscopy. To

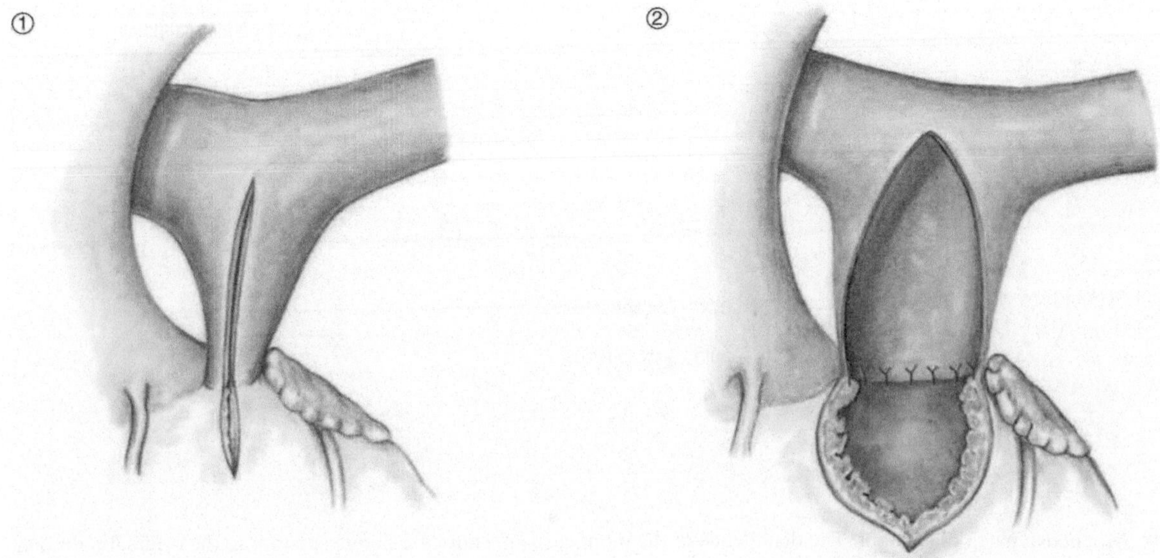

Fig. II-26-11. RVOT reconstruction in the presence of pulmonary atresia ①. When the distance between RVOT and main PA is short, the main PA is directly anastomosed to the superior margin of the ventriculotomy site to create autologous tissue continuity ②. The branch PAs are mobilized to reduce tension. The length of the ventriculotomy is usually longer than 1 cm, but is kept as short as possible and minimized

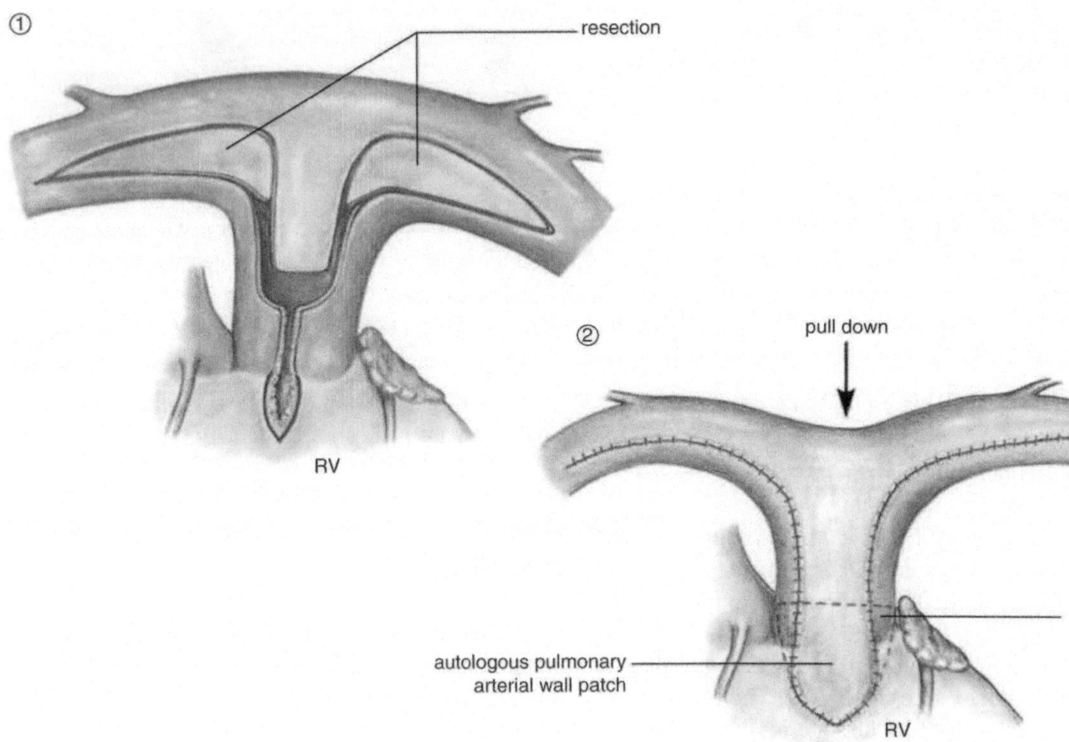

Fig. II-26-12. Reconstruction of pulmonary valve and right ventricular outflow tract in absent pulmonary valve syndrome. ① In absent pulmonary valve syndrome the pulmonary valve annulus is hypoplastic and the branch pulmonary arteries are markedly dilated. The anterior aspects of the branch pulmonary arteries are resected. ② The RVOT is opened longitudinally. The main PA flap is pulled down as a patch to the RVOT to enlarge the outflow tract. This downward traction creates an arteriopexy effect and decreases pressure to the airway

improve the arteriopexy effect, the posterior walls of the branch pulmonary arteries are not dissected.

Long-Term Outcomes and Future Trends for TOF Repair

The combination of a ventriculotomy and free pulmonary insufficiency, both associated with the transannular patch, is implicated in the deterioration of right ventricular function and the development of arrhythmias after repair of tetralogy of Fallot. The transatrial-transpulmonary approach has been believed to avoid these long-term complications by the minimum ventriculotomy and the limited use of transannular patch on RVOT [4]. Recent study using magnetic resonance imaging has shown, however, even in patients after optimal repair by a transatrial-transpulmonary approach at a young age, that right ventricular function and exercise tolerance are impaired at mid- to late follow-up in tetralogy of Fallot although the clinical condition appears well preserved [13]. Considering these long-term outcomes of right ventricular function, pulmonary valve-sparing strategy [14] or pulmonary valve cusp augmentation [15,16] has been currently spotlighted at complete repair of tetralogy of Fallot (TOF) to reduce the incidence of pulmonary regurgitation and maintain right ventricular function in the long term. These strategies, in fact, had been already reported in 1981 [6] and 1992 [2]. Yasui et al. revealed a pulmonary valve-sparing strategy in which 80% of their patients underwent complete repair of TOF with preserving the native pulmonary annulus intact and showed excellent results [2]. The important residual pressure gradient across a small pulmonary annulus can decrease in the midterm period in that the growth potential for pulmonary annulus in tetralogy of Fallot has been demonstrated. Kawashima et al. reported techniques of repair of the pulmonary valve in corrective surgery in TOF and showed excellent early results of right ventricular function [6]. Currently, pulmonary valve repair techniques have become more elegant and used as an approach toward valve repair with the concomitant minimum transannular patch enlargement of RVOT to reduce the pulmonary regurgitation as well as residual stenosis. Sung et al. augmented the anterior pulmonary cusp by using PTFE membrane [15]. Anagnostopoulos et al. also reported pulmonary cusp augmentation repair technique and used a triangular patch of glutalaldehyde-preserved autologous pericardium [16]. We prefer to use the patient's own azygos vein patch for the more elegant technique of pulmonary cusp augmentation, expecting its growth potential in the long term. The long-term outcomes of these approaches remain to be determined, although the short-term outcomes have been proved excellent.

References

1. Touati GD, Vouhé PR, Amodeo A, et al (1990) Primary repair of tetralogy of Fallot in infancy. J Thorac Cardiovasc Surg 99:396–403
2. Yasui H, Nakamura Y, Kado H, et al (1992) Preservation of the pulmonary valve during intracardiac repair of tetralogy of Fallot. J Cardiovasc Surg 33:545–553
3. Hudspeth AS, Cordell AR, Johnston FR, et al (1963) Transatrial approach to total correction of tetralogy of Fallot. Circulation 27:796–800
4. Karl TR, Sano S, Pornviliwan S, et al (1992) Tetralogy of Fallot: favorable outcome of nonneonatal transatrial, transpulmonary repair. Ann Thorac Surg 54:903–907
5. Brizard CPR, Mas C, Sohn YS, et al (1998) Transatrial-transpulmonary tetralogy of Fallot repair is effective in the presence of anomalous coronary arteries. J Thorac Cardiovasc Surg 116:770–779
6. Kawashima Y, Kitamura S, Nakano S, et al (1981) Corrective surgery for tetralogy of Fallot without or with minimal right ventriculotomy and with repair of the pulmonary valve. Circulation 64:II-147–II153
7. Kurosawa H, Morita K, Yamagishi M, et al (1998) Conotruncal repair for tetralogy of Fallot: midterm results. J Thorac Cardiovasc Surg 115:351–360
8. Rowlatt UF, Rimoldi HJA, Lev M (1963) The quantitative anatomy of the normal child's heart. Pediatr Clin N Am 10:499–588
9. Asou T, Rachmat J (2001) Slicing technique of the RV outflow tract in transatrial-transpulmonary repair for tetralogy of Fallot. J Cardiovasc Surg 42:639–642
10. Kurosawa H, Becker AE (1987) Tetralogy of Fallot. Atrioventricular conduction in congenital heart disease. In: Kurosawa H, Becker AE (eds) Surgical anatomy. Springer-Verlag, Tokyo, pp 97–144
11. Kurosawa H, Imai Y(1988) Surgical anatomy of the atrioventricular conduction bundle in tetralogy of Fallot. J Thorac Cardiovasc Surg 95:586–591
12. Miyazaki T, Yamagishi M, Nakashima A, et al (2007) Expanded polytetrafluoroethylene valved conduit and patch with bulging sinuses in right ventricular outflow tract reconstruction. J Thorac Cardiovasc Surg 134:327–332
13. Van den Berg J, Hop WC, Strengers JLM, et al (2007) Clinical condition at mid-to-late follow-up after transatrial-transpulmonary repair of tetralogy of Fallot. J Thorac Cardiovasc Surg 133:470–477
14. Stewart RD, Backer CL, Young L, et al (2005) Tetralogy of Fallot: results of a pulmonary valve-sparing strategy. Ann Thorac Surg 80:1431–1439
15. Sung SC, Kim S, Woo JS, et al (2003) Pulmonic valve annular enlargement with valve repair in tetralogy of Fallot. Ann Thorac Surg 75:303–305
16. Anagnostopoulos P, Azakie A, Natarajan S, et al (2007) Pulmonary valve cusp augmentation with autologous pericardium may improve early outcome for tetralogy of Fallot. J Thorac Cardiovasc Surg 133:640–647

II-27A. Transposition of the Great Arteries: Senning Procedure

The Senning [1] and Mustard [2] procedures are called the atrial switch operation and were the standard surgical procedures for transposition of the great arteries before the introduction of the arterial switch operation, which has become the surgical procedure of choice. The Senning procedure is now applied as part of a double switch operation for congenitally corrected transposition of great arteries. In the presence of an abnormal coronary pattern, this procedure still may be applied in d-transposition. The Senning procedure is believed to be technically difficult in the presence of apicocaval juxtaposition. Both atrial switch procedures share the potential complications of systemic venous stenosis, pulmonary vein stenosis, and late supraventricular tachyarrhythmias.

Cardiopulmonary Bypass

Venous cannulae are inserted high in the superior vena cava and low in the inferior vena cava.

Atrial Incision

After cardioplegic arrest, a right atriotomy is performed. The first incision is started from the base of the right atrial appendage, 10 mm anterior to the sulcus terminalis, and is advanced inferiorly parallel to the sulcus terminalis (Fig. II-27A-1) [3]. During this incision, the interior of the right atrium is inspected and the incision terminated approximately 5 mm from the crista terminalis. As this incision is carried down, the incision is close to the sulcus terminalis. From the superior point, the incision is carried anteriorly to create an L-shaped incision line. The interior trabeculations are removed. With the right atriotomy, two flaps are created.

The space between the interatrial groove and the right atriotomy becomes a flap separating systemic and pulmonary venous pathways (posterior flap). The right atrial wall anterior to the incision becomes a flap creating a pulmonary venous pathway (anterior flap). Care is taken to create a wide posterior flap because a narrow posterior flap may cause systemic venous obstruction. The interatrial groove is dissected, and a second incision is placed between the right atrium and right pulmonary veins (Fig. II-27A-2). This incision should not be extended beyond the pulmonary veins.

Septal Flap Suturing

Next, a septal flap is created (Fig. II-27A-3). A foramen ovale is closed, if present. In the case of a large atrial septal defect, it is closed with a patch. An incision is placed anterior to the fossa ovalis. It is extended to the upper margin of the right upper pulmonary vein orifice superiorly and the lower margin of the right lower pulmonary vein orifice inferiorly. This septal flap is sutured inside the left atrium, creating the posterior wall of the systemic venous tunnel. The suture is started anterior to the midpoint between the left upper and lower pulmonary veins and carried around the pulmonary vein orifices (Fig. II-27A-4). A double-armed monofilament running suture is used, and the suture lines are completed when the inferior and superior boundaries of the septal incision are reached (Fig. II-27A-5).

Creation of Systemic Venous Route

To complete the systemic venous route, a running suture is started at the inferior end of the right atriotomy. It is important to create a wide pathway (Fig. II-27A-6), as the inferior margin of the posterior flap is sutured to the crista terminalis. If a well-developed Eustachian valve is present, the suture is placed to this tissue. The suture line is advanced toward the posterior margin of the coronary sinus. A Hegar dilator is used as a stent during this portion of the suturing as this area is prone to stenosis. The superior portion of the posterior flap is sutured to the right atrial wall anterior to the crista terminalis toward the right atrial appendage to avoid stenosis. As this suture line is constructed, a Hegar dilator is used to stent the superior limb of the pathway. After this suture line is completed, tapes on both cavae are released, and adequacy of the venous pathway dimension is confirmed.

Pulmonary Vein Pathway Construction

The anterior flap is used to cover the right atrium and the pulmonary vein route is completed. To avoid damage to the sinus node, the suture line is placed superior or inferior to the node [4]. The suture is started from the end of the right atriotomy incision. Figure II-27A-7 shows a suture line avoiding the sinus node inferiorly and posteriorly. Increased

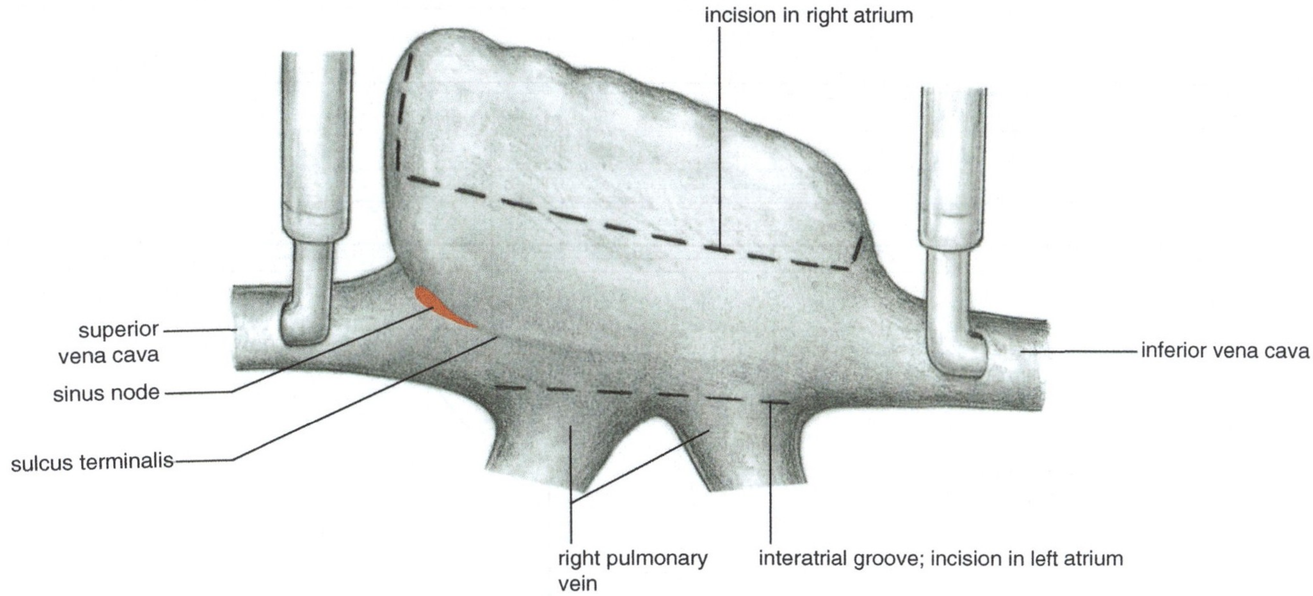

Fig. II-27A-1. Right and left atrial incision lines. The first incision is placed to the base of the right atrial appendage 10 mm anterior to the sulcus terminalis. The incision is carried inferiorly parallel to the sulcus terminalis. The superior end is extended anteriorly to create an L-shape toward the appendage. Any large trabeculations are excised from the flap

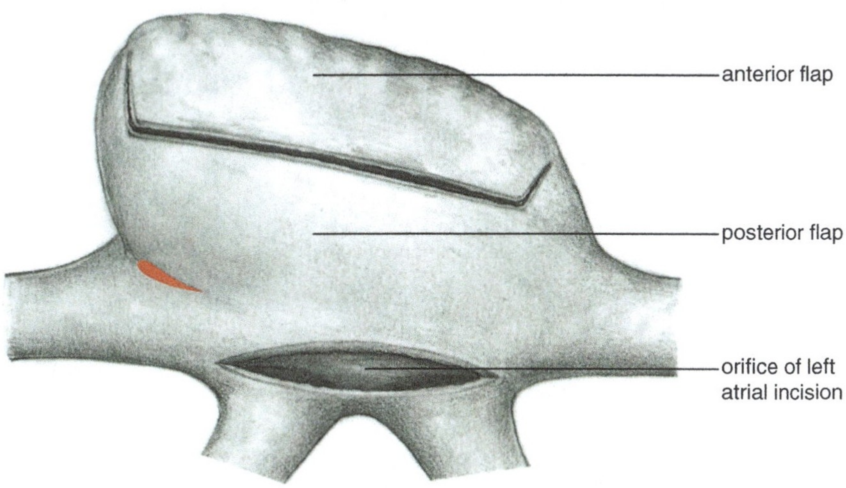

Fig. II-27A-2. Left atrial incision. After development of the interatrial groove, the left atrial incision is placed. The incision should not extend beyond the width of the upper and lower pulmonary veins

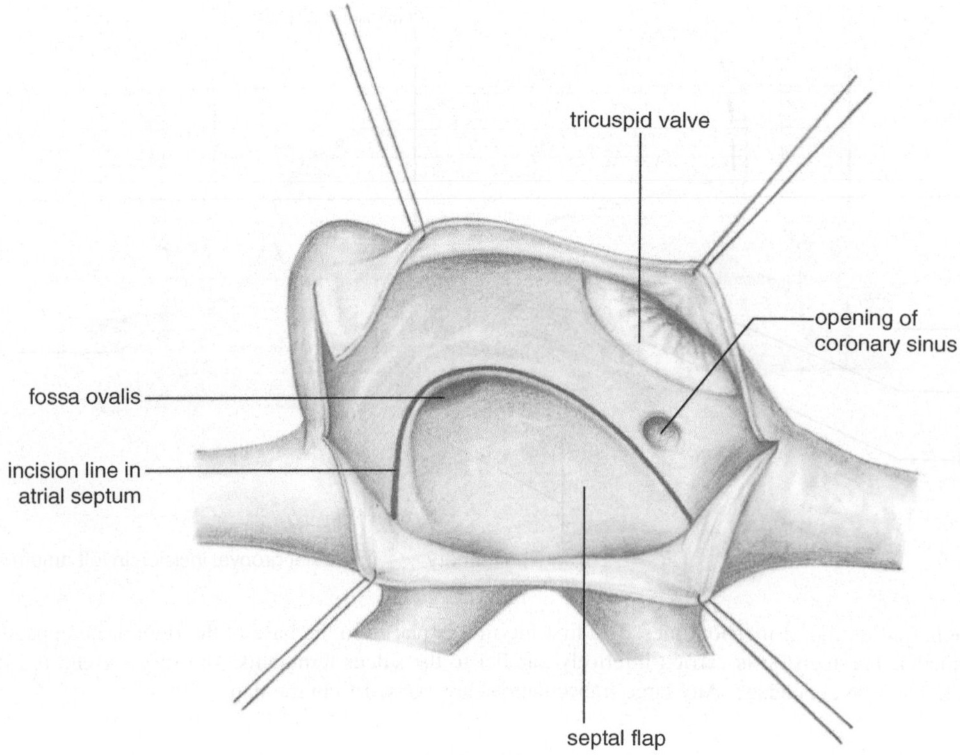

Fig. II-27A-3. Septal flap creation. A patent foramen ovale, if present, is closed directly or using a patch. The septal incision is placed anterior to the fossa ovalis. The superior incision is carried toward the superior margin of the right upper pulmonary vein orifice. The inferior incision is brought to the inferior margin of the right lower pulmonary vein orifice

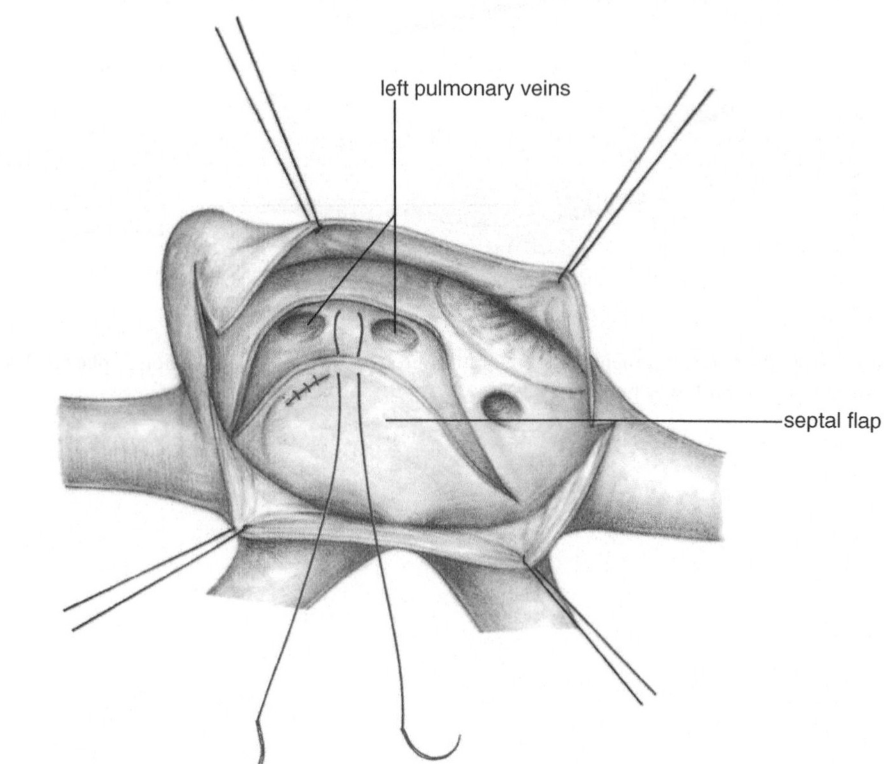

Fig. II-27A-4. Start of septal flap suture. The suture line is started anterior to a point midway between the left superior and inferior pulmonary vein orifices

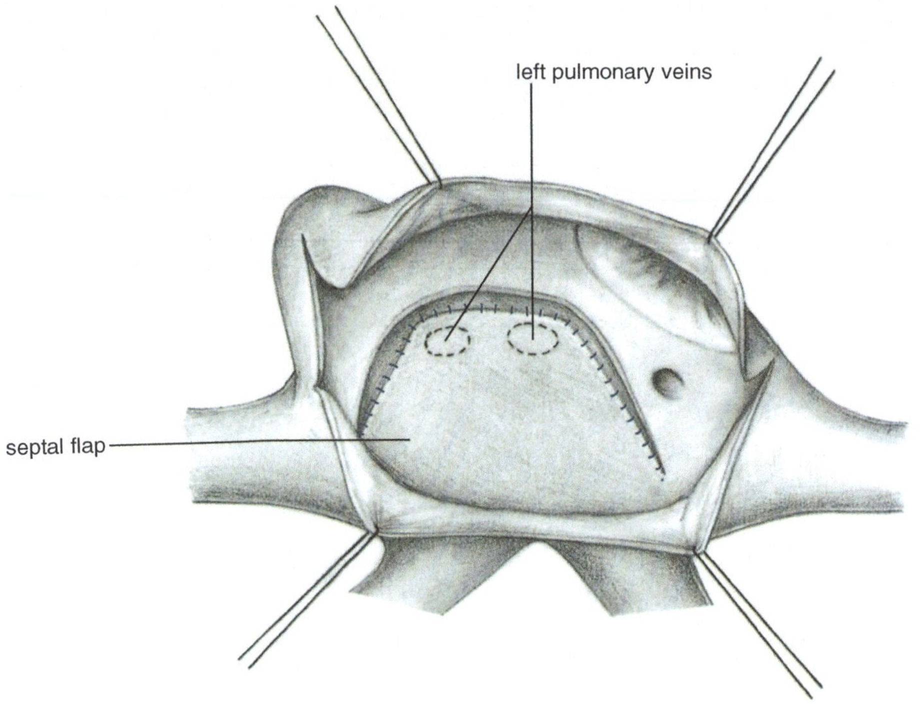

Fig. II-27A-5. Suture of septal flap. For the superior suture line, the edge of the septal flap is carried to the superior margin of the upper pulmonary vein. For the inferior suture line, the inferior margin of the lower pulmonary vein is used

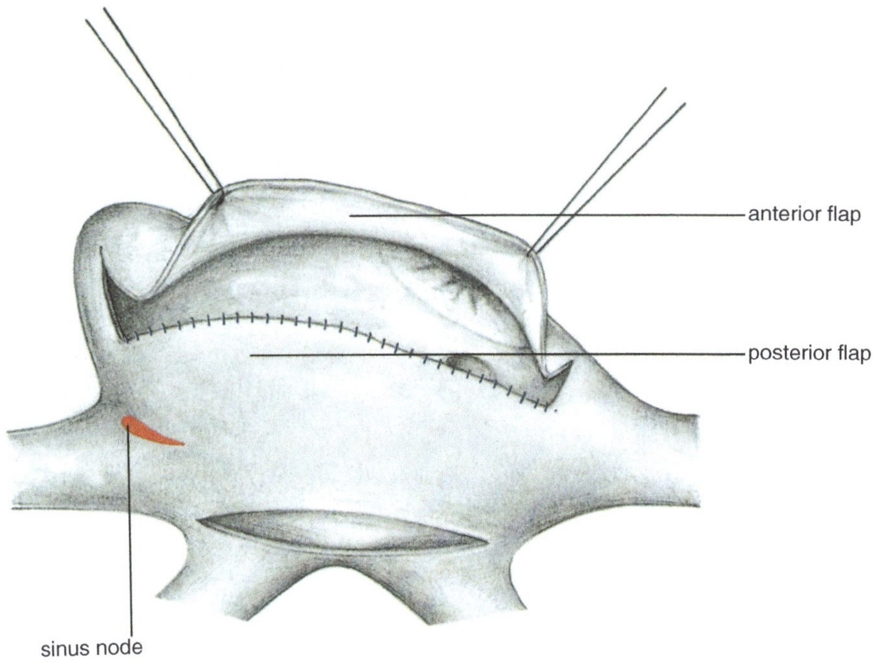

Fig. II-27A-6. Systemic venous pathway completion. The posterior flap is sutured from the inferior vena cava to the posterior margin of the coronary sinus. The superior end of the posterior flap is sutured superior to the crista terminalis close to the right atrial appendage. A Hegar dilator is used as a stent to prevent narrowing of each caval orifice

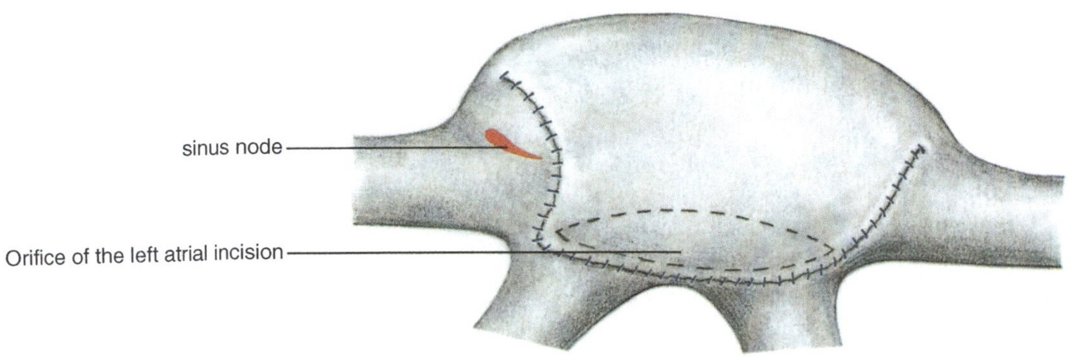

Fig. II-27A-7. Pulmonary venous pathway completion. The anterior wall of the pulmonary venous pathway is completed with the anterior flap. Around the sinus node, the suture line is placed inferiorly to avoid injury to the node

suture line tension on the pulmonary venous pathway may cause stenosis. When the superior suture line reaches the superior end of the left atriotomy, the inferior suture line is begun and brought up superiorly to complete the pulmonary venous channel.

References

1. Senning A (1959) Surgical correction of transposition of the great vessels. Surgery (St. Louis) 45:966–980
2. Mustard WT (1964) Successful two-stage correction of transposition of the great vessels. Surgery (St. Louis) 55:469–472
3. Pacifico AD (1994) Concordant transposition: Senning operation. In: Surgery for congenital heart defects, 2nd edn. Saunders, Philadelphia, p 457–466
4. Kirklin JW, Barratt-Boyes BG (1993) Complete transposition of the great arteries. Cardiac surgery, 2nd edn. Churchill Livingstone, New York, p 1383–1467

II-27B. Transposition of the Great Arteries: Mustard Procedure

In contradistinction to the Senning procedure, a foreign material is used in the Mustard procedure to separate the systemic and pulmonary venous pathways. Because foreign material is utilized, there is no restriction in the size of the patch. However, a disproportionately large patch may compromise the systemic or pulmonary venous pathway. Therefore, choosing the shape and size of the patch is both challenging and vitally important [1]. A simple rectangular-shaped patch known as the Toronto patch [2] has been used by some groups.

An alternative trouser-shaped patch [3] is discussed here. Although autologous pericardium is usually used as patch material, a xenopericardial or polytetrafluoroethylene (PTFE) patch may be necessary if the native tissue is not suitable for reoperations.

Cardiopulmonary Bypass

The technique of cardiopulmonary bypass is the same as for the Senning procedure.

Harvesting Pericardium

A generously sized piece of native pericardium is harvested and cleared of all connecting tissue.

Atriotomy and Removal of Atrial Septum

After cardioplegic arrest, a right atriotomy is performed. This incision may be parallel to the interatrial groove or obliquely oriented. Here, the latter technique of an oblique atrial incision is discussed. The incision is begun at the base of the right atrial appendage and advanced to a point between the superior and inferior pulmonary veins (Fig. II-27B-1). If the incision is curved caudally, the sinus node is protected and visualization of the atrium is improved. The atrial septum is fully resected (Fig. II-27B-2). Of particular importance is full excision of the superior septum to minimize late superior vena caval stenosis. If the septal excision causes an atrial perforation, the intima is approximated with monofilament suture. The coronary sinus is incised about 10 mm (Fig. II-27B-3).

Trimming of an Intraatrial Patch

The shape of the trouser-shaped patch (Fig. II-27B-4) is based on the following principles. For the systemic venous pathway, more than half the circumference of the pathway is constructed with atrial tissue and less than half is composed of patch material. The width of the leg portion of the patch is half the circumference of the vena cavae. The angle created by the two legs is approximately 30°. The legs are left long initially and later trimmed.

Suturing of Patch

Patch placement is started anterior to the left pulmonary vein orifices (Fig. II-27B-5). To maintain a smooth surface in the pulmonary venous pathway, the rough side of the pericardium is placed superiorly. The larger curvature of the patch is sutured toward the superior vena cava posteriorly (point A → point B) (Fig. II-27B-6). A smaller curvature is placed anteriorly and brought to the superior end of the atrial septum, joining the posterior suture line at the superior caval orifice. At the crista terminalis, shallow suture bites are used. Care is taken to avoid placing the suture line too close to the superior caval orifice to avoid stenosis. At the sinus node, small suture bites are taken to avoid injury. Next, the suture line around the inferior vena cava is placed (point E → point D). At the coronary sinus, a flap of cut-back coronary sinus wall is used to protect the conduction system. With this suture line, the coronary sinus drains to the functional left atrium. Then, the suture line carried to the crista terminalis and the inferior vena cava orifice.

For the smaller curvature suturing, a U-stitch is placed at point C of the middle anterior portion of the atrial septum. From this point, the lesser curvature is sutured to the remnant of the atrial septum, superiorly joining the posterior suture line. To avoid superior vena caval stenosis, a Hegar sizer is used as a stent intermittently, and the patch is trimmed. In a similar fashion, the inferior suture line is placed around the inferior caval orifice over a Hegar sizer. After patch placement, the tapes on the cavae are loosened and the patch is distended. In the presence of redundancy or stenosis, plication or patch augmentation is performed.

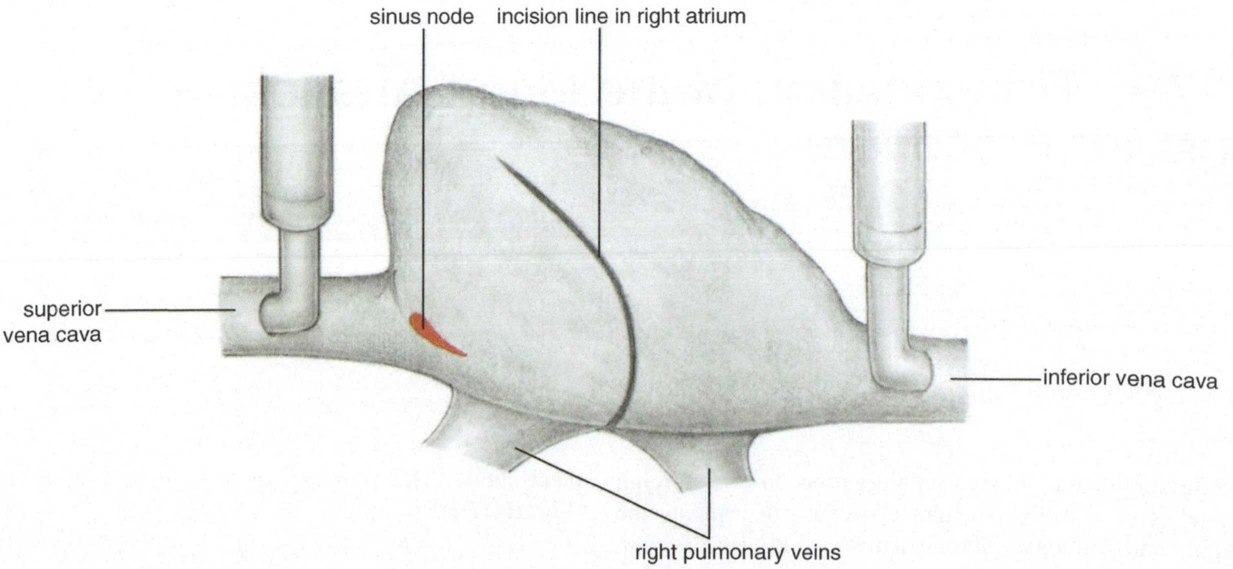

Fig. II-27B-1. Right atriotomy. A transverse incision is placed from the right atrial appendage to the midpoint between the upper and lower pulmonary veins

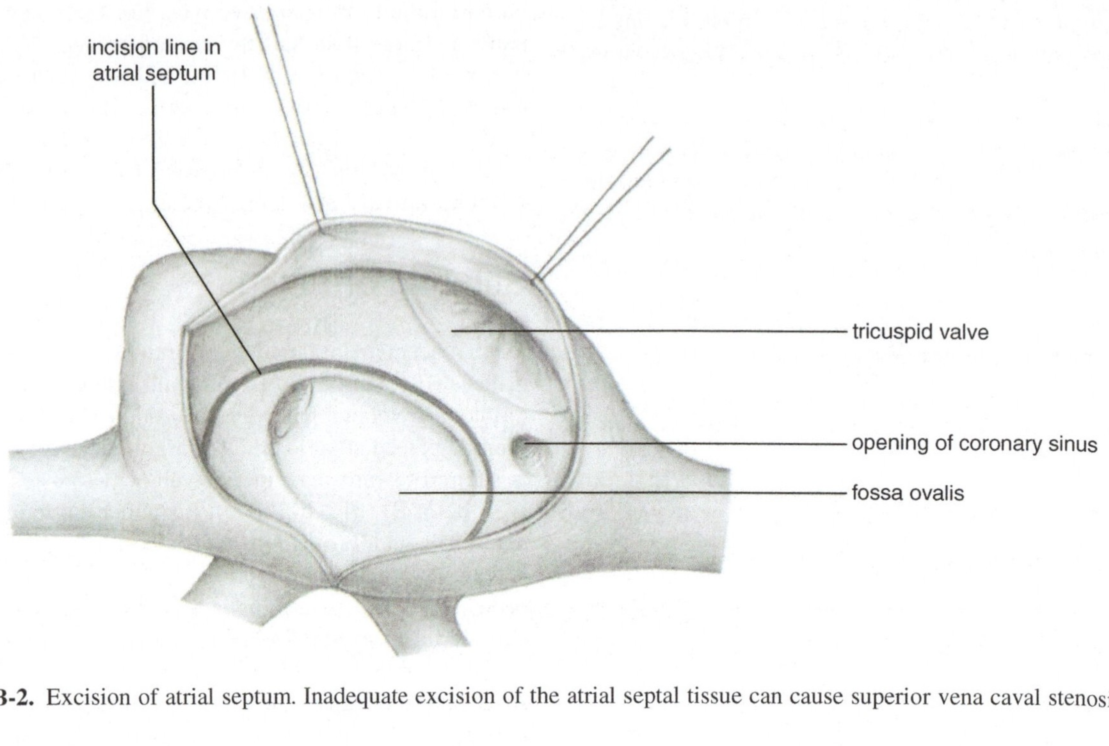

Fig. II-27B-2. Excision of atrial septum. Inadequate excision of the atrial septal tissue can cause superior vena caval stenosis

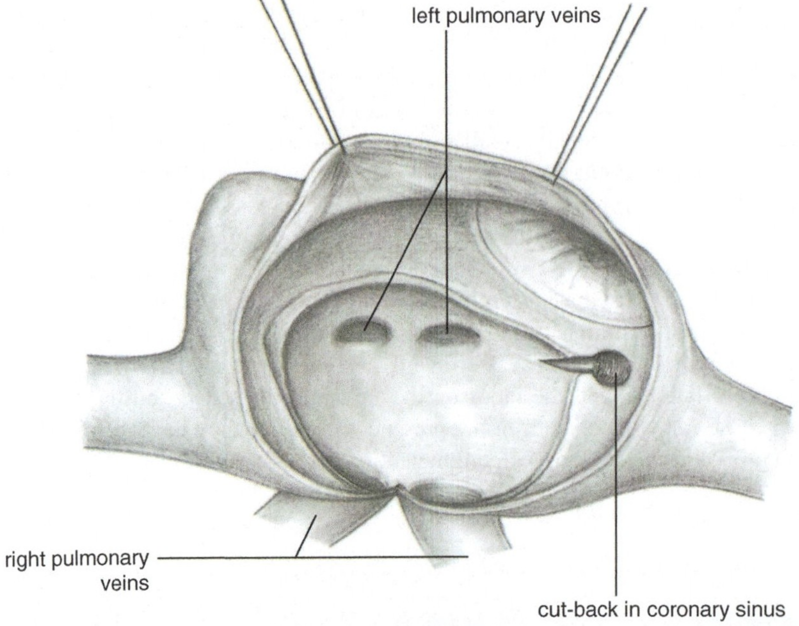

Fig. II-27B-3. After excision of atrial septum. The coronary sinus is enlarged by a cut-back incision

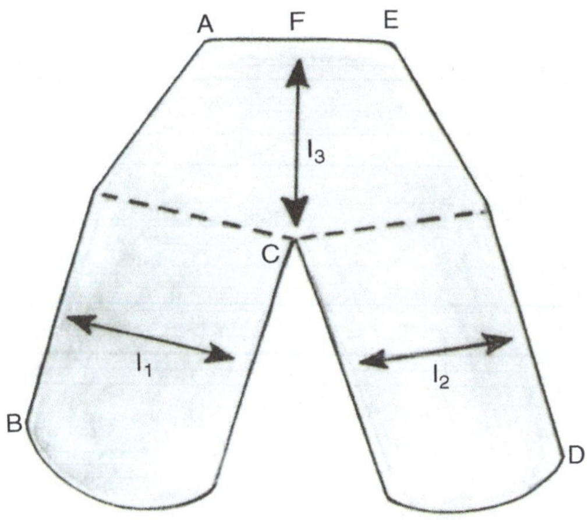

Fig. II-27B-4. Trouser-shaped patch. l_1 and l_2 are half the circumference of the superior and inferior vena cavae, respectively; l_3 is the average of l_1 and l_2. The angle between the legs is approximately 30°

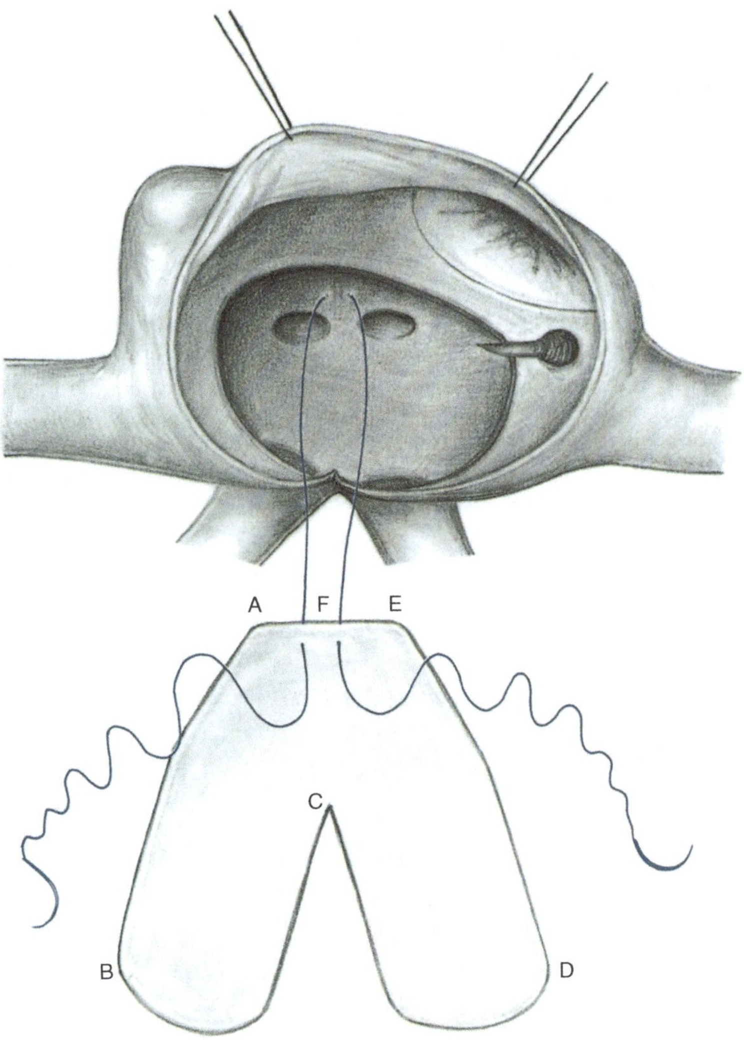

Fig. II-27B-5. Trouser-shaped patch placement: 1. Patch placement is started anterior to the midpoint between the left upper and lower pulmonary vein orifices. Point *F* (see Fig. II-27B-4) is turned to this starting point

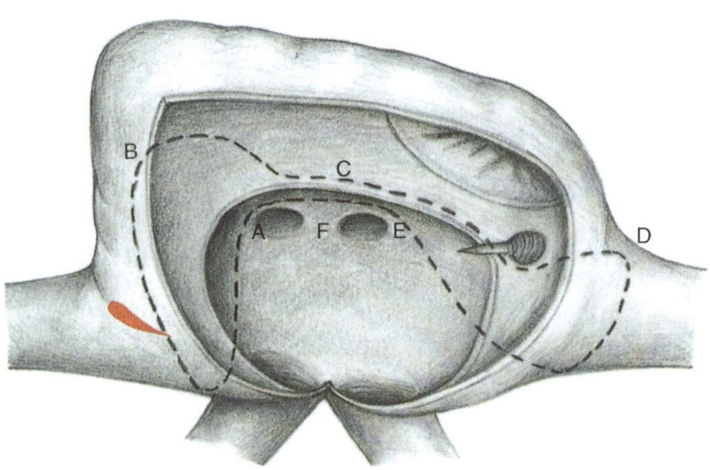

Fig. II-27B-6. Trouser-shaped patch placement: 2. The *dashed line* shows suture line placement. Points *A–F* correspond to points on the patch (Fig. II-27B-4)

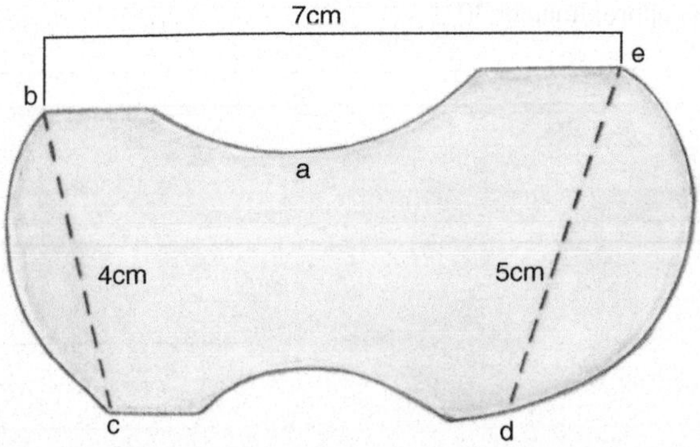

Fig. **II-27B-7.** Toronto patch. The patch has a reverse trapezoid shape and the middle portion is slightly narrowed. The size of the patch corresponds to the size of the patient. The patch illustrated is for a patient weighing 10 kg

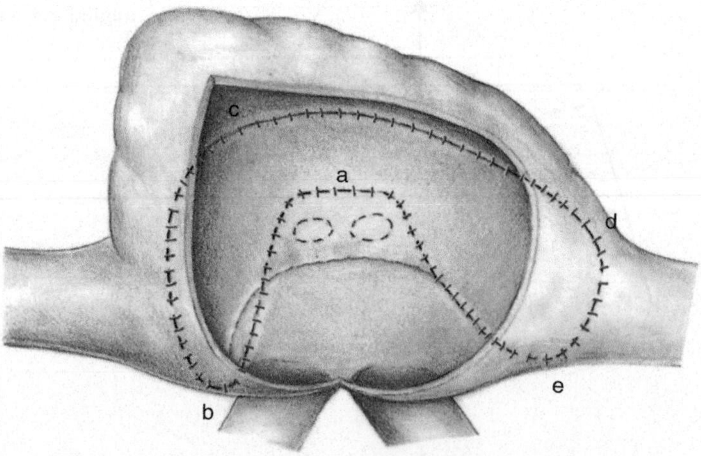

Fig. II-27B-8. Completion of the Toronto patch placement. Points *a–e* are joined to the corresponding points shown in Fig. II-27B-7

Pulmonary Venous Pathway

The right atriotomy is closed directly or with an autologous or xenograft patch, completing the pulmonary venous pathway.

Toronto Patch

A reverse trapezoid-shaped patch is used. The midportion narrows slightly (Figs. II-27B-7, II-27B-8). The suture technique is similar to that for the trouser-shaped patch.

References

1. Mustard WT, Keith JD, Trusler GA, et al (1964) The surgical management of transposition of the great vessels. J Thorac Cardiovasc Surg 48:953–958
2. Trusler GA, Williams WG, Izukawa T, et al (1980) Current results with the Mustard operation in isolated transposition of the great arteries. J Thorac Cardiovasc Surg 80:381–389
3. Stark J (1994) Concordant transposition: Mustard operation. In: Surgery for congenital heart defects, 2nd edn. Churchill, Livingston, New York, p 447–456

II-27C. Transposition of the Great Arteries: Arterial Switch Operation

In transposition of the great arteries (TGA), the aorta arises from the right ventricle and is located anterior and to the right. The pulmonary artery (PA) arises from the left ventricle and is located posterior and to the left. In the arterial switch operation, the aorta and PA are switched, and coronary arteries are transferred to the posteriorly located great vessel [1]. One classification of the coronary artery pattern in TGA is the Shaher classification [2] (Fig. II-27C-1). It is important to avoid kinking of the transferred coronary arteries or compression by the neo-PA. The introduction of the Lecompte maneuver [3] has reduced the incidence of such complications. In Shaher type 5, coronary translocation is very difficult. To avoid branch PA stenosis late after surgery [4–6], several techniques are utilized, including autologous pericardial patch placement and direct anastomosis in neo-PA reconstruction [7].

Operative Procedure

Before cardiopulmonary bypass, the aorta and PAs are dissected completely: the aorta is dissected up to the arch, and the PAs are mobilized out to each hilum including the first branches (Fig. II-27C-2). Tapes are applied to each branch PA and are later used to retract and mobilize branch PAs. Proposed coronary translocation sites are marked on the posterior great vessel using fine monofilament sutures, after careful inspection of the coronary anatomy. The aortic cannula is inserted into the base of the brachiocephalic artery. Bicaval venous cannulation is employed. After initiation of cardiopulmonary bypass, the ductus arteriosus is ligated and divided. Further dissection of the branch PA is accomplished after division of the duct. A cardioplegia needle is inserted 5 mm above the sinotubular junction, and this will be the site of aortic transection. After application of the aortic cross-clamp, cardioplegic solution is injected.

After cardiac arrest, a right atriotomy is performed, and a vent catheter is inserted into the left atrium across the atrial septum. The cardioplegia needle is removed and the aorta carefully transected. After visualization of the aortic valve and coronary artery orifices, this transection is completed posteriorly. Following aortic transection, the right coronary button is excised (Fig. II-27C-3). With fine-tip scissors, an incision is started from the aortic wall down the sinus of Valsalva, while viewing the sinus of Valsalva from the interior. A 1-mm cuff of aortic wall is left adjacent to the valve leaflet attachment site. A U-shaped or teardrop-shaped coronary button is created. The tissue around the coronary arteries is carefully dissected with scissors and diathermy. The coronary button is further dissected a few millimeters and mobilized. The left coronary button is created in a similar fashion. Cardioplegic solution is infused directly into the coronary ostia using a small feeding tube. A traction suture is placed on the anterior wall of proximal ascending aorta and pulled inferiorly. The connective tissue between the aorta and main PA is dissected. The main PA is transected just proximal to its branching point. To obtain a larger branch PA portion, this incision is made obliquely to give a longer posterior wall of the PA. A small hole is created to the previously marked site with a knife and enlarged with a 4-mm punch. This position is above the sinotubular junction. Care is taken to avoid coronary kinking and deformity of the sinus. Translocation of the coronary artery is started from the left side. Absorbable fine monofilament suture is used (Fig. II-27C-4). Any redundant part of the button is excised during anastomosis. A small feeding tube is inserted into the coronary orifices, and cardioplegic solution is injected to confirm the absence of any kinking. The right coronary artery is translocated in a similar way. If a trap-door technique [6] is utilized, the coronary buttons are harvested in a U shape. A J-shaped incision is created in the proximal main PA, and the coronary button is anastomosed (Fig. II-27C-5). Care is taken to avoid extending the J-incision beyond the sinotubular junction [4]. As shown in Fig. II-27C-5, the superior edges of the button and PA are partially sutured, and the trap-door anastomosis is completed.

After coronary translocation, the Lecompte maneuver, transferring the distal ascending aorta behind the pulmonary artery bifurcation, is performed. The pulmonary confluence is pulled anteriorly and the distal ascending aorta is brought beneath the PA. Another clamp is placed on the ascending aorta proximal to the first clamp and branch PAs. The right side of the ascending aortic curvature is left longer, and now this part is trimmed, pulling the aorta downward posteriorly. To avoid compression of the PA by the ascending aorta, occasionally the ascending aorta is shortened even more. The proximal main PA and distal ascending aorta are anastomosed using fine monofilament suture. The diameter of the main PA is larger than that of the distal ascending aorta, and each bite is adjusted accordingly. If the diameter differ-

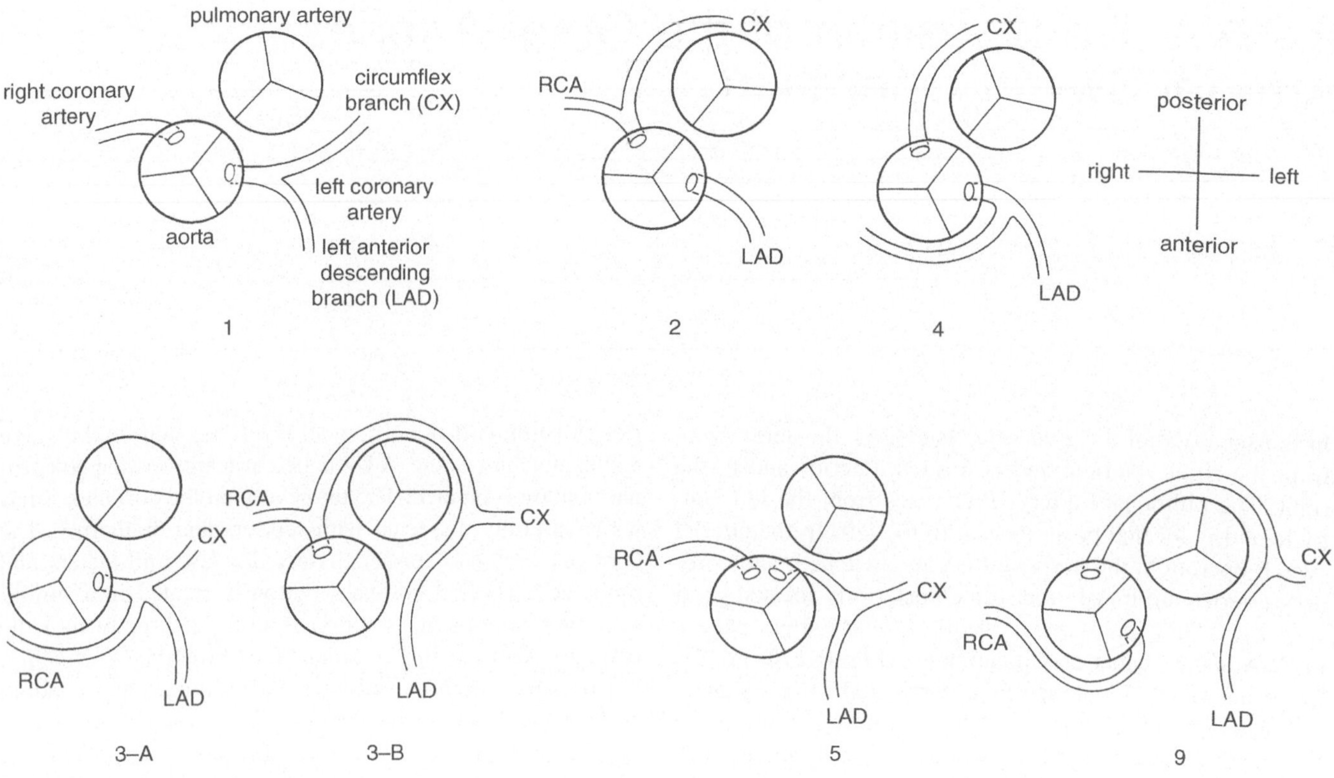

Fig. II-27C-1. Shaher classification. *RCA*, right coronary artery; *PA*, pulmonary artery; *CX*, circumflex branch; *LCA*, left coronary artery; *LAD*, left anterior descending branch

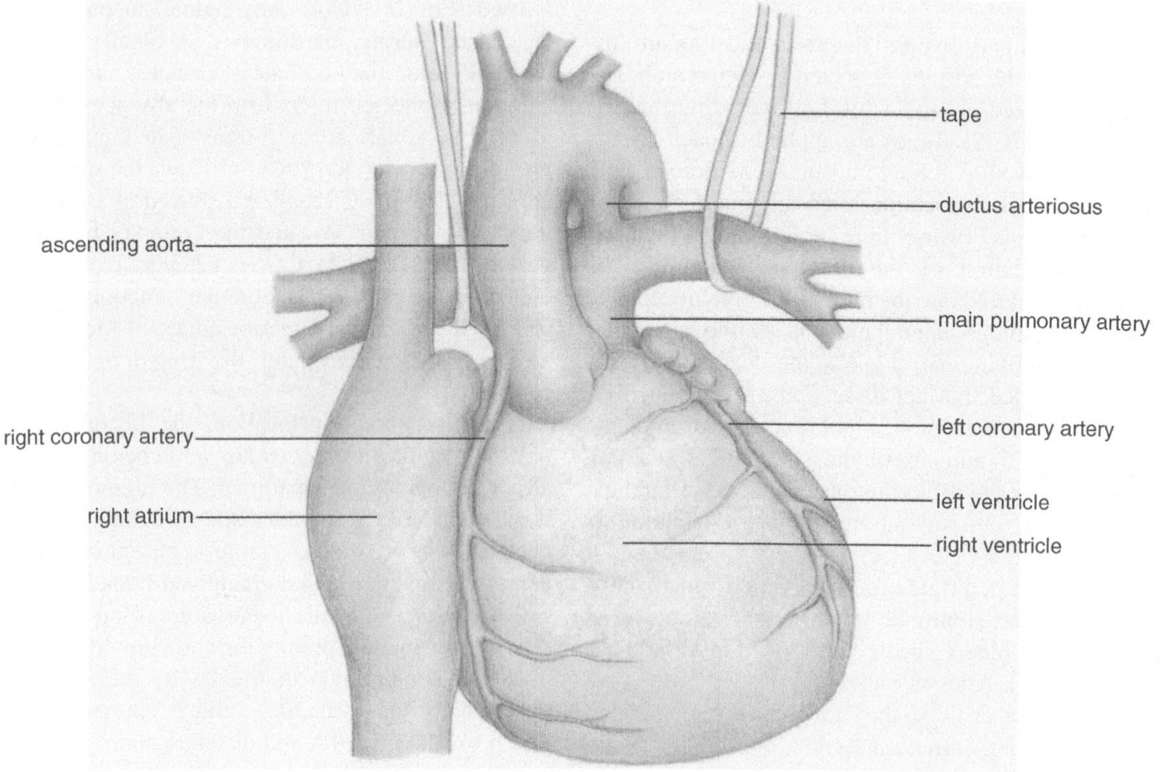

Fig. II-27C-2. Anatomy of transposition of the great arteries. Tapes are placed around the branch pulmonary arteries (PAs), which are dissected out to the origin of the upper branch

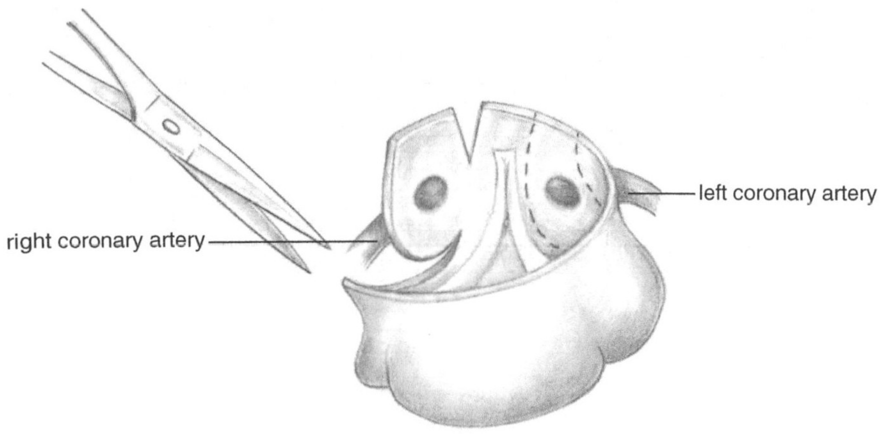

Fig. II-27C-3. Creation of the coronary buttons. The right coronary button is excised first. This removal is accomplished while viewed from the inside of the sinus of Valsalva

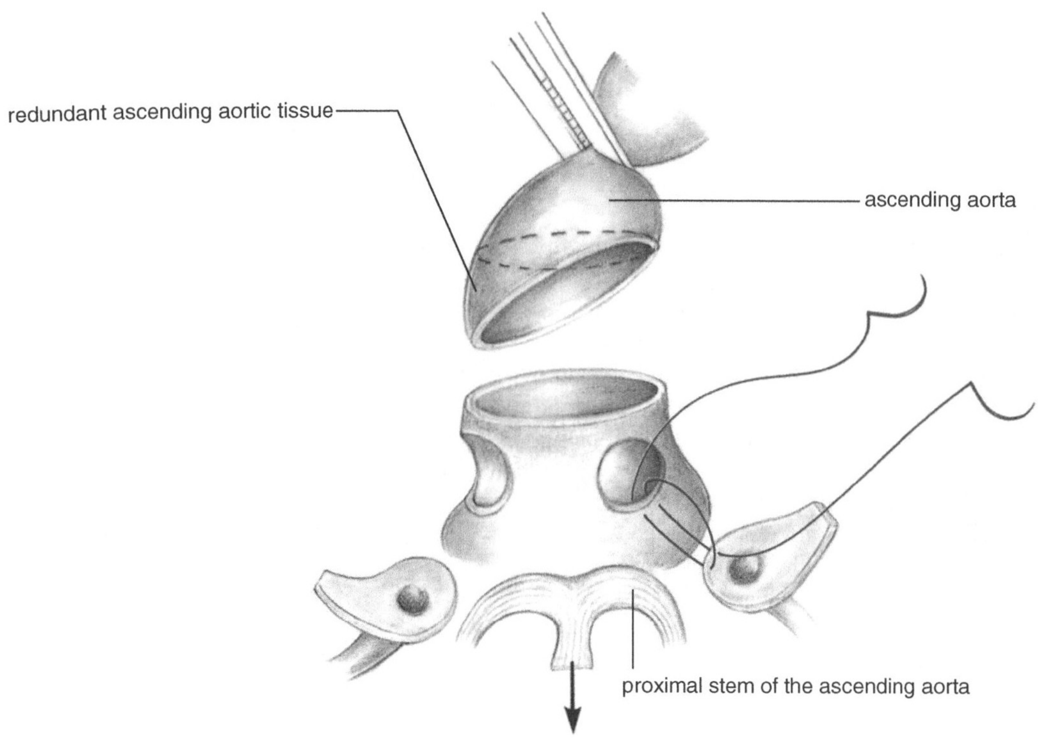

Fig. II-27C-4. Suturing of the coronary button. Holes are created above the sinotubular junction with a coronary punch. The anastomosis is started from the left side

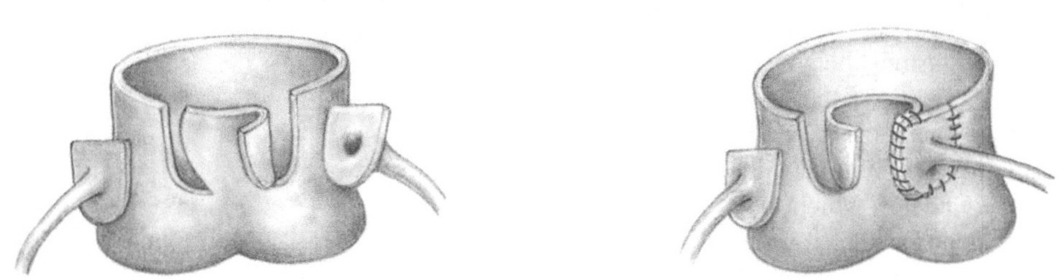

Fig. II-27C-5. Coronary translocation by trap-door technique. A J-shaped incision is placed in the proximal pulmonary artery, and coronary buttons are anastomosed with the trap-door technique. The J-incision should not extend into the Valsalva sinus

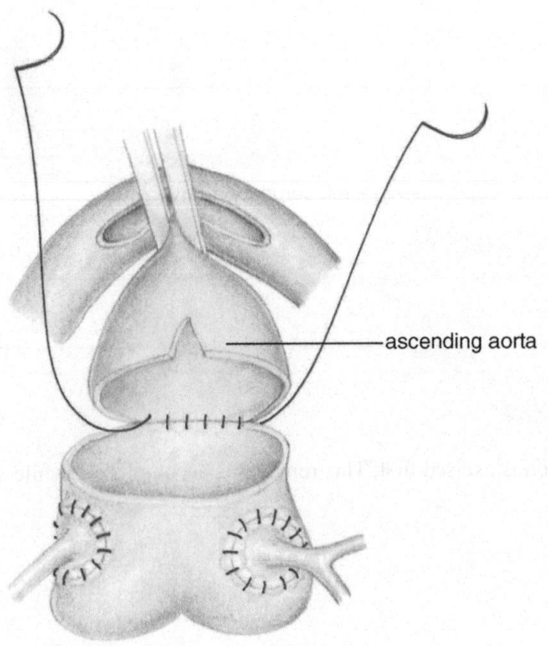

Fig. II-27C-6. Aortic reconstruction. Excessive aortic tissue is removed, and the anterior surface of the aortic wall is longitudinally cut to create a longer suture line

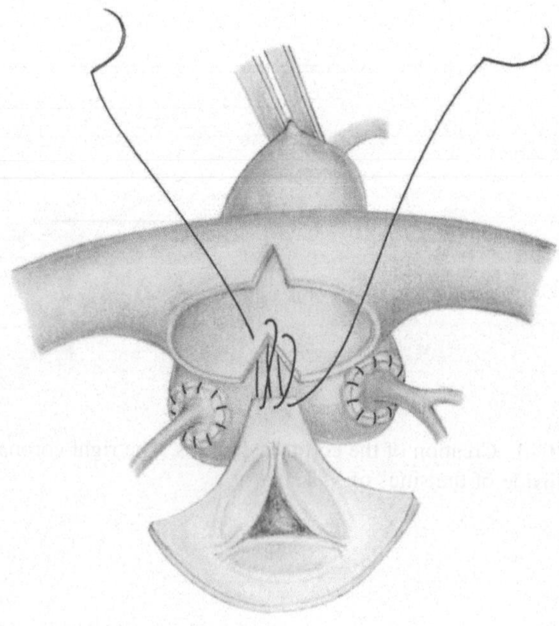

Fig. II-27C-7. Pulmonary reconstruction: 1. The posterior wall of the distal pulmonary artery is opened longitudinally to fit the proximal ascending aorta

ence is large, the distal ascending aorta is cut longitudinally (Fig. II-27C-6).

After coronary translocation and neo-aortic reconstruction, the aortic cross-clamp is loosened and bleeding is checked. The branch PAs are pulled down and a clamp is placed distal to the branch PAs. The cardioplegia needle is inserted into the ascending aorta and cardioplegia solution is infused. The pulmonary confluence is pulled down, and the length of the left PA is checked. The potential for compression of the coronary arteries is checked. Applicability of the Pacifico procedure (direct anastomosis between the distal main PA and the proximal ascending aorta) is also checked. If there is a concern about tension, an autologous pericardial patch can be placed to reconstitute the sinus from which the coronaries were harvested.

In the Pacifico procedure, proximal ascending aortic tissue above the commissure between the removed coronary buttons is excised. A counter-incision is placed in the posterior wall of the distal main PA. An anastomosis is begun, aligning this cut-back site at the commissure with absorbable monofilament running suture (Fig. II-27C-7). The suture is carried into the sinus defects. The anterior suture line is not completed at this stage (Fig. II-27C-8).

A vent tube in the left atrium though the patent foramen ovale (PFO) is removed. The tip of the double-lumen central line through the vein is brought into the left atrium via the PFO. With this technique, the left and right atrial pressures are measured with one catheter, which may reduce the risk of bleeding at the time of catheter removal. After PFO closure, the aortic cross-clamp is removed. Blood is allowed to vent from the unclosed main PA portion, thus avoiding ventricular distension. After cardiac function is recovered, the main PA is closed, and separation from cardiopulmonary bypass is instituted (Fig. II-27C-9). Hemostasis is ensured and temporary pacing wires are placed. The chest is closed in the usual fashion.

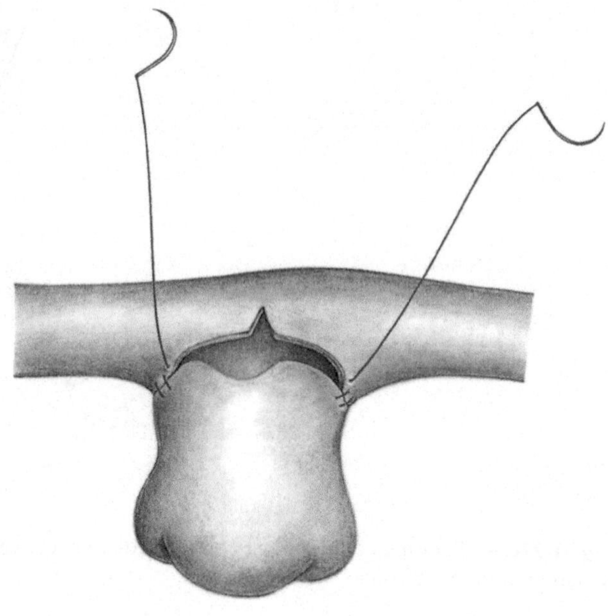

Fig. II-27C-8. Pulmonary reconstruction: 2. The anterior surface of the distal pulmonary artery (PA) is cut to fit the size of the proximal neo-PA. The anterior suture line is completed after removal of the aortic clamp. This opening works as a PA vent. After recovery of ventricular function, the anterior suture line is closed

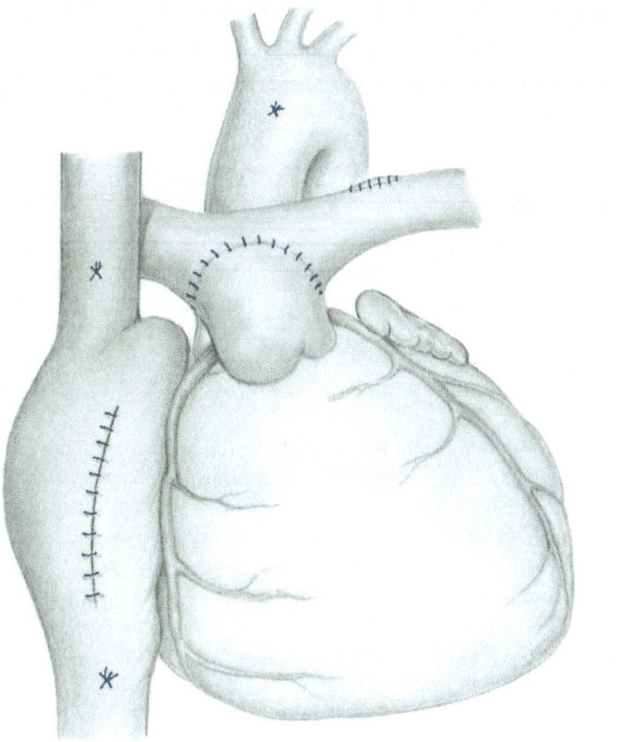

Fig. II-27C-9. Completion of arterial switch operation (ASO). The coronary arteries are translocated to the posterior neo-aorta

Other Techniques

An intramural coronary is considered very difficult to transfer. In such an intramural coronary, a coronary button creation performed in the regular fashion will cause damage to the coronary arteries. It is important to identify the course of the coronary artery from the interior in all cases. In the presence of the intramural coronary artery, a small orifice of the coronary artery is often observed, and the Mee procedure [5,8] is utilized. A portion of the internal aortic wall is carefully excised. Care is taken to avoid perforating the aortic wall, and two coronary buttons are created (Fig. II-27C-10). In the case of an intramural coronary artery that courses behind the commissure, this commissure is shaved off from the aortic wall. The coronary button excision site is repaired with a patch, and the previously detached commissure is resuspended by suturing it to the patch. The coronary buttons are transferred to the main pulmonary artery in the regular way.

The Imai procedure is used when, in Shaher type 5, a coronary button is not created (Fig. II-27C-11). The aortic wall above the coronary orifices is excised in a U shape. The facing part of the anterior wall of the proximal main PA is cut in a similar U shape fashion. These two vascular walls are sewn together. The noncoronary aortic sinus is used to

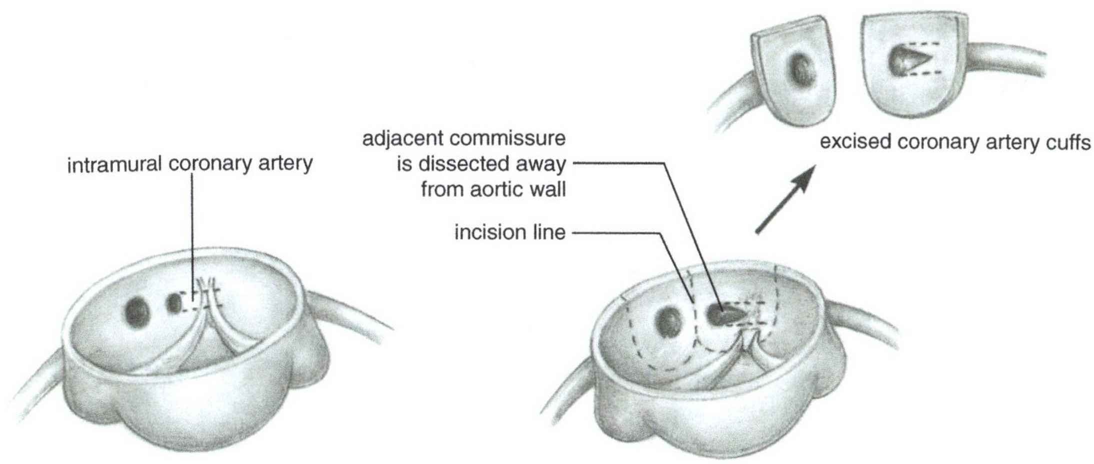

Fig. II-27C-10. Mee technique to create coronary buttons. The aortic commissure is detached from the aortic wall, and the intramural coronary artery is unroofed

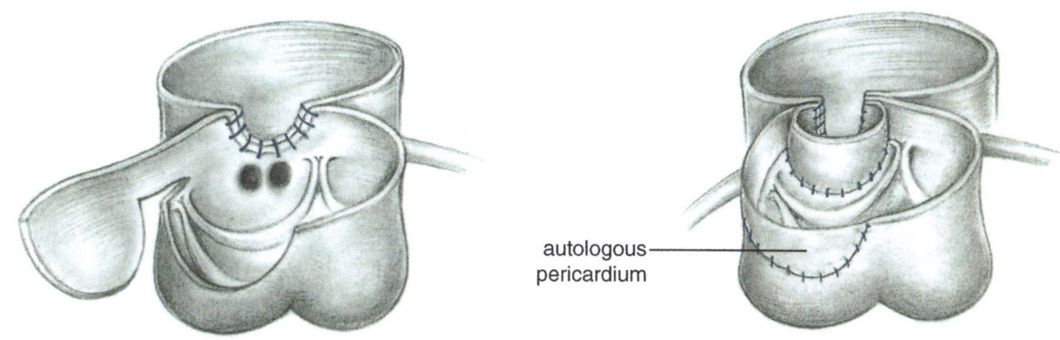

Fig. II-27C-11. Imai procedure for intramural coronary artery (Shaher type 5): 1. The aortic wall above the coronary orifices is excised in a U shape. The adjacent pulmonary wall is also excised in a U shape. These edges are joined. The adjacent positioned sinus wall is used as a flap to cover the coronary orifices

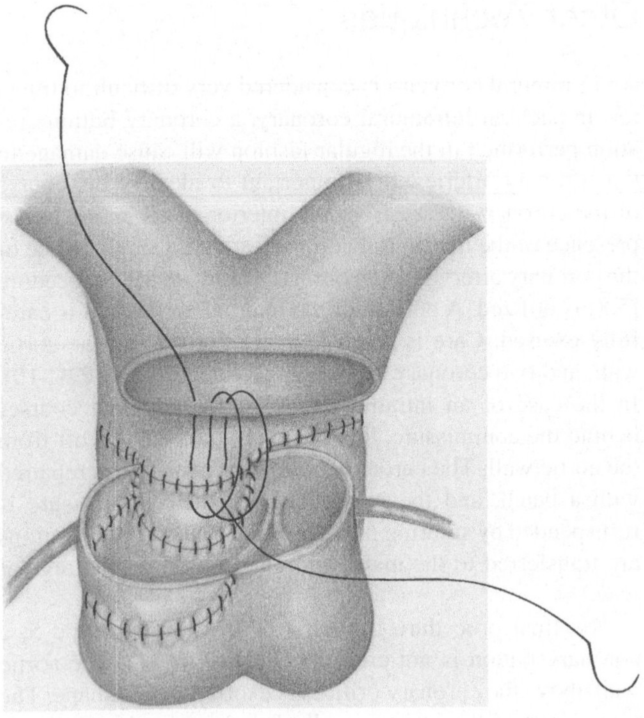

Fig. II-27C-12. Imai procedure for intramural coronary artery (Shaher type 5): 2. After neo-aortic reconstruction, the neo-pulmonary artery is reconstructed

create a D-shaped flap covering these coronary orifices while maintaining continuity at the commissure site. This flap is brought over the coronary orifices and sewn to the aortic wall with running suture. The noncoronary sinus defect is repaired with a patch. The superior wall of the flap is used as aortic wall, and the neo-aorta is reconstructed. The reconstruction of the neo-pulmonary artery is shown in Fig. II-27C-12.

References

1. Jatene AD, Fontes VF, Paulista PP, et al (1976) Anatomic correction of transposition of the great vessels. J Thorac Cardiovasc Surg 72:364–370
2. Shaher RM, Puddu GC (1966) Coronary arterial anatomy in complete transposition of the great vessels. Am J Cardiol 17:355–361
3. Lecompte Y, Zannini L, Hazan E, et al (1981) Anatomic correction of transposition of the great arteries. J Thorac Cardiovasc Surg 82:629–631
4. Yasui H, Yonenaga K, Kado H, et al (1992) Arterial switch operation for transposition of the great arteries: surgical techniques to avoid complications. J Cardiovasc Surg 33:511–517
5. Imoto Y, Yasui H, Tominaga R, et al (1996) Arterial switch operation in transposition of the great arteries. Ann Thorac Cardiovasc Surg 2:117–122
6. Mee RBB (1994) The arterial switch operation. In: Surgery for congenital heart defect, 2nd edn. Saunders, Philadelphia, pp 483–500
7. Pacifico AD, Stewart RW, Bargeron LM (1983) Repair of transposition of the great arteries with ventricular septal defect by an arterial switch operation. Circulation 68(suppl II):49–55
8. Asou T, Karl TR, Pawade A, et al (1994) Arterial switch: translocation of the intramural coronary artery. Ann Thorac Surg 57:461–465

II-28. Congenitally Corrected Transposition of the Great Arteries—De Leval Procedure, Transaortic Closure of VSD, Transtricuspid Closure of VSD, Double-Switch Operation [Mustard or Senning Procedure + Arterial Switch Operation with Closure of VSD or Rastelli Procedure (REV Procedure)]

Anatomical Properties

Congenitally corrected transposition is a heart defect with atrioventricular and ventriculoatrial discordances. According to the visceral–atrial relationship, there are normal situs (SLL; situs solitus, l-loop, l-malposition) and inverse situs (IDD; situs inversus, d-loop, d-malposition). In the SLL type, the ventricles rotate counterclockwise and the apex of the heart is located in the midline or on the right side (dextrocardia). The ventricular septum stays upright, and the right-sided atrium is located behind the morphological left ventricle (LV); this is called apicocaval juxtaposition (Fig. II-28-1). In the presence of pulmonary stenosis or pulmonary atresia, the free wall of the right atrium is often small. The morphological tricuspid valve is often regurgitant and may be dysplastic or Ebstein like. Usually the morphological mitral valve is normal, although straddling of the chordae or a cleft is observed occasionally. The ventricular septal defect (VSD) is usually perimembranous or subpulmonary but is occasionally doubly committed [1]. The conduction system is located in an unusual position.

If there is a perimembranous VSD in the SLL type, the bundle arises from an anterior node, courses anterior to the pulmonary valve annulus, and descends along the anterior VSD margin, giving rise to the right bundle at the surface of the morphological LV side of the ventricular septum [2].

In the presence of a straddling mitral valve or IDD-type anatomy, a posterior node is present, and there may also be an anterior node [3,4]. In many patients the coronary pattern is a mirror image to Shaher I type in transposition of the great arteries (TGA). (See Fig. II-27C-1 in Chapter 27C.)

Surgical Indication and Operative Procedure

Functionally, blood flows as follows: right atrium → morphological LV → pulmonary artery (PA) → left atrium (LA) → morphological right ventricle (RV) → aorta (Ao), and in the absence of intracardiac shunts, the patient may be asymptomatic. However, many patients have surgical indications resulting from intracardiac anomalies such as VSD, pulmonary stenosis (PS), or atrial septal defect (ASD). Previously, so-called "classic" repairs consisting of simple VSD closure or PS repair were performed. However, late systemic ventricle dysfunction or systemic atrioventricular (AV) valve regurgitation may be seen after classic repair because the systemic circulation is maintained by a morphological RV [5]. Therefore, more recently, the "double-switch operation" (DSO), assigning the morphological LV to the systemic circulation, has been introduced, although long-term results are not yet available [6,7]. In DSO, two levels of switch are instituted for two levels of discordance (Fig. II-28-2). For AV discordance, an intraatrial switch procedure (the Senning or Mustard procedure), and for VA discordance, the arterial switch operation (ASO) or Rastelli procedure or REV (réparation à l'étage ventriculaire) are performed (Fig. II-28-2). The indication for DSO is controversial because DSO is a much more extensive undertaking than classic repair, and long-term results of atrial switch procedure for d-TGA are less than optimal. In our center, in the absence of morphological RV dysfunction or severe tricuspid valve (TV) regurgitation, classic repair remains the surgical treatment of choice. The surgical strategy for DSO is as follows.

Without Pulmonary Stenosis

An atrial switch plus ASO procedure is performed. In the presence of a large VSD, pulmonary artery banding (PAB) is performed in infancy and DSO is performed after the age of 1 year. When the patient does not have a VSD, or the VSD is small and the morphological LV pressure is low, LV training by PAB is initiated early in infancy. After elevation of LV pressure (LV/RV > 0.9), DSO is performed.

With Pulmonary Stenosis

Atrial switch plus Rastelli procedure (see Fig. II-28-2) is performed. The choice of atrial switch by the Mustard or Senning procedure is determined by the size of the right atrial free wall. If the atrial wall is large, the Senning procedure is chosen. When the atrial free wall is small because of dextroversion, the Mustard procedure is preferred owing to the increased difficulty of the Senning procedure in this setting.

Classic Procedure

Cardiopulmonary bypass is initiated with ascending aortic and bicaval cannulation. After aortic cross-clamping, a right atriotomy is performed. In SLL type congenitally corrected TGA with PS, the apex is located to the right. The RA is found behind the morphological left ventricle, and the free wall of the right atrium is often small. The anterior node is located anterior to the fibrous continuity between the pulmonary valve and the mitral valve, and careful exposure of the operative field with retractors is necessary. The coronary sinus, fossa ovalis, mitral valve, papillary muscle, and VSD are identified (Fig. II-28-3). At this stage, the approach for repair of the VSD is decided. Trans-right atrial or transaortic approaches are the standard approaches to the VSD. When marked dextroversion is present, a trans-left atrial approach can be used.

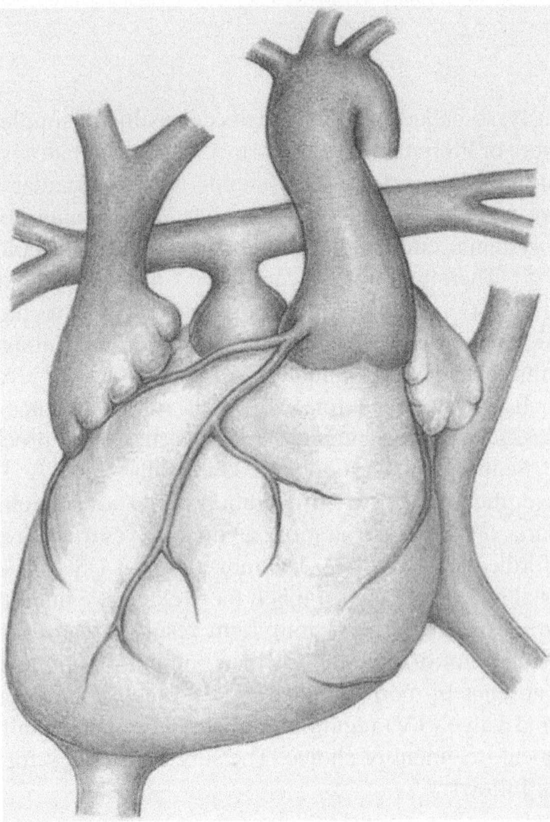

Fig. II-28-1. Anatomy of apicocaval juxtaposition. Pulmonary stenosis is often present in patients with apicocaval juxtaposition

Transmitral VSD Closure (de Leval Procedure) [8]

A pledgetted mattress suture is placed at the midportion of the base of the septal leaflet. This suture is retracted, and the whole VSD is visualized. In a membranous-type VSD, from the anterior node the bundle courses anterior to the pulmonary valve annulus and reaches the endocardium of the morphological LV. It then gives rise to the right bundle branch at the anterior margin of the VSD. To avoid damage to the conduction system, at the superior and anterior margin of the VSD, pledgetted sutures are placed from the morphological RV side 2–3 mm from the VSD margin (Fig. II-28-4). Other sutures are placed to the VSD margin on the morphological LV side and mitral valve annulus. The sutures from the morphological RV are brought to the patch. The patch is pushed down, and sutures are tied. The rest of the sutures are then brought to the patch and tied.

Transaortic VSD Closure (Fig. II-28-5)

A longitudinal incision is made at the ascending aorta, and the VSD is visualized with care to protect the aortic valve. Mattress pledgetted sutures are placed around the whole VSD margin. Given that the conduction system is located at the anterior margin of the morphological LV side, damage does not occur provided the sutures are not placed too deeply.

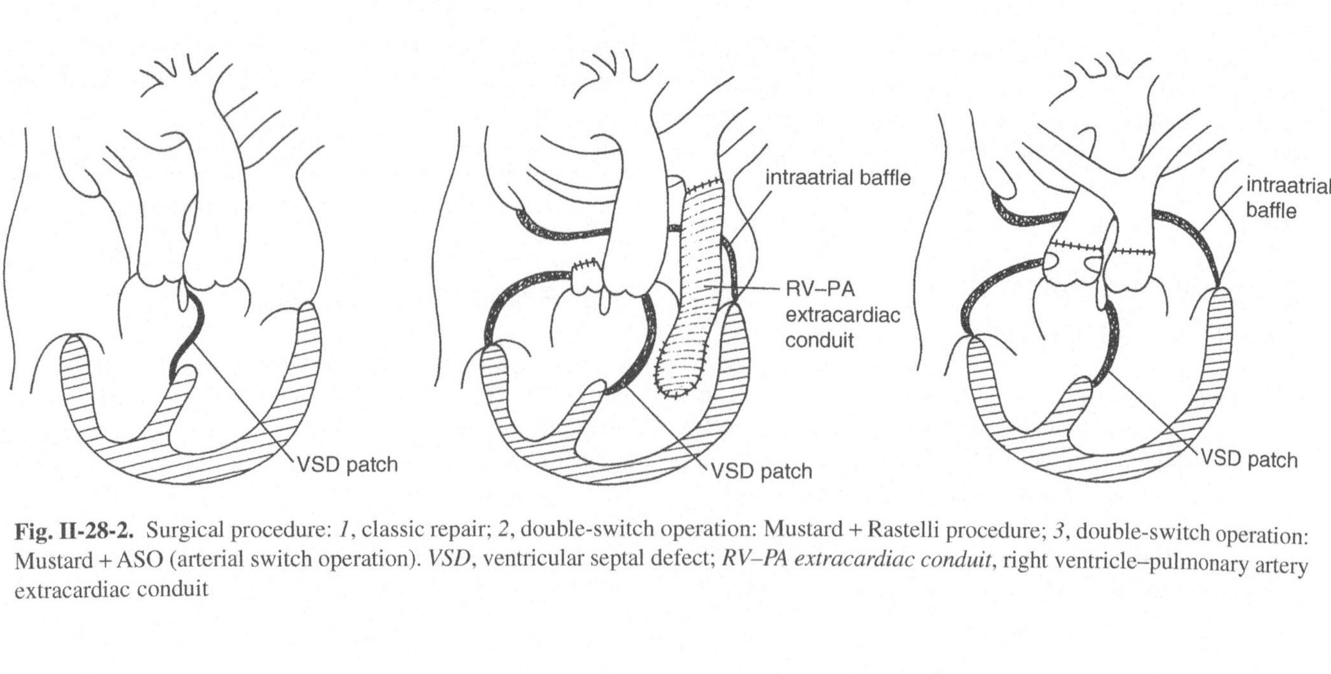

Fig. II-28-2. Surgical procedure: *1*, classic repair; *2*, double-switch operation: Mustard + Rastelli procedure; *3*, double-switch operation: Mustard + ASO (arterial switch operation). *VSD*, ventricular septal defect; *RV–PA extracardiac conduit*, right ventricle–pulmonary artery extracardiac conduit

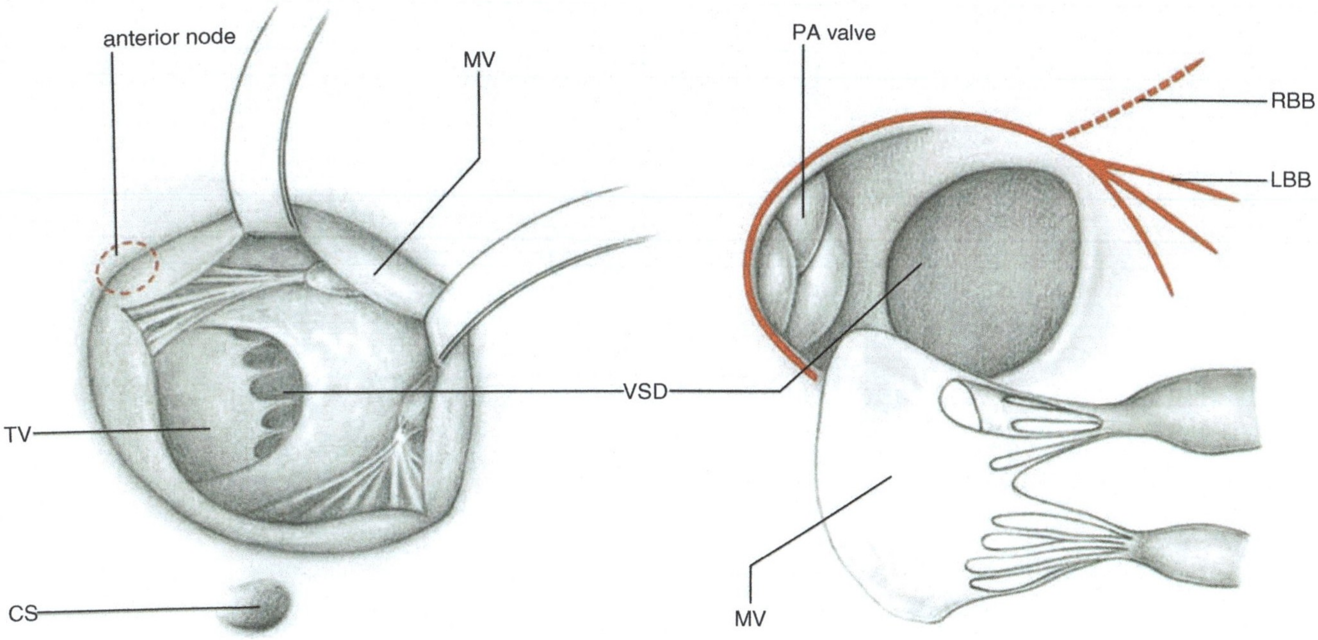

Fig. II-28-3. Location of the conduction system viewing through the right atrium and mitral valve. *TV*, tricuspid valve; *MV*, mitral valve; *CS*, coronary sinus; *VSD*, ventricular septal defect; *PA valve*, pulmonary artery valve; *RBB*, right bundle branch; *LBB*, left bundle branch

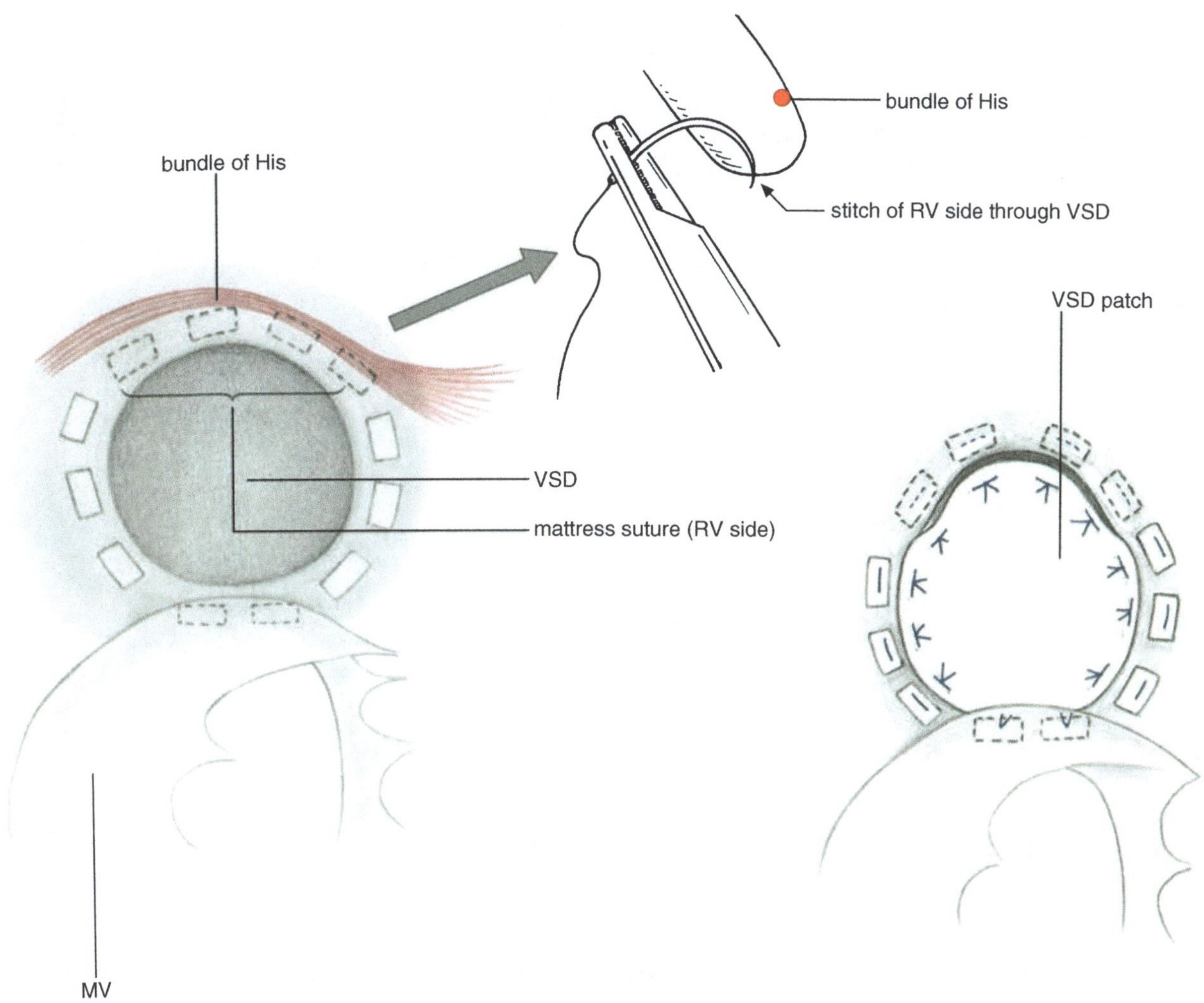

Fig. II-28-4. VSD closure through the mitral valve (de Leval approach). *VSD*, ventricular septal defect; *MV*, mitral valve

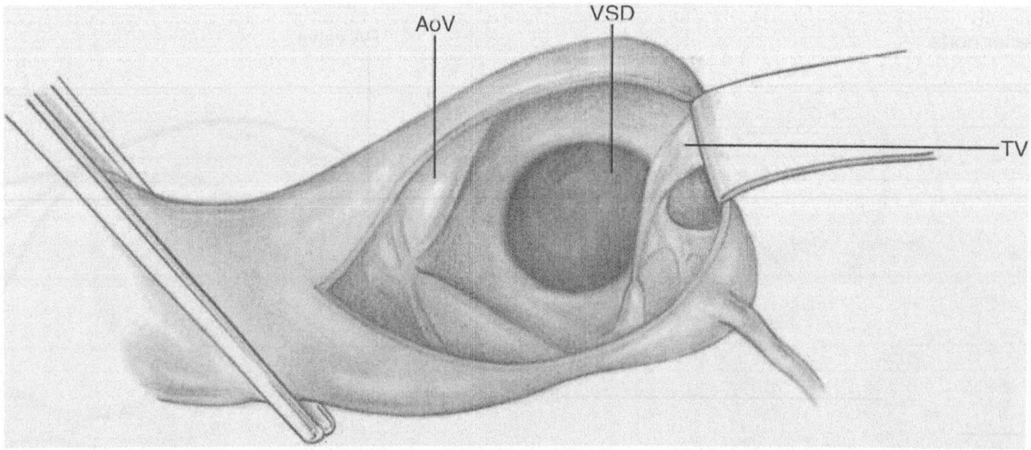

Fig. II-28-5. VSD closure through the aortic valve. *AoV*, aortic valve; *VSD*, ventricular septal defect; *TV*, tricuspid valve

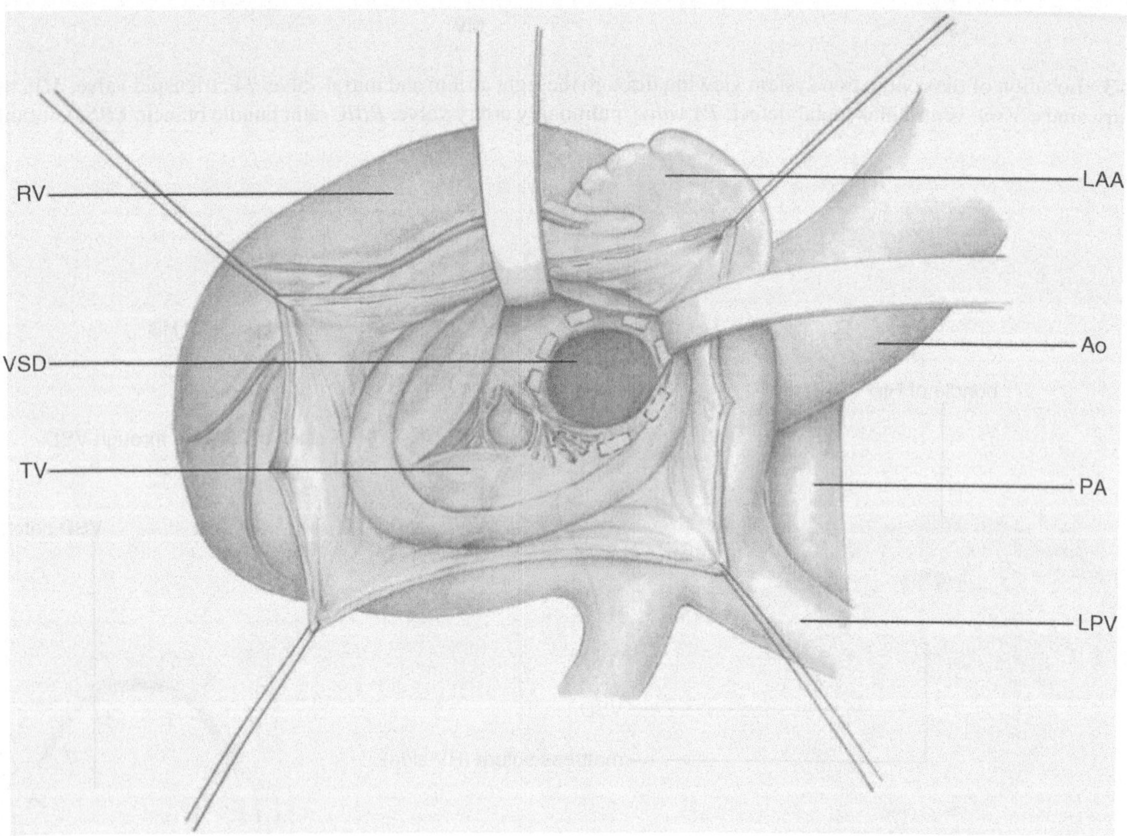

Fig. II-28-6. VSD closure through the tricuspid valve. *RV*, right ventricle; *LAA*, left atrial appendage; *LPV*, left pulmonary vein

Transtricuspid VSD Closure (Fig. II-28-6)

In the presence of marked dextroversion of the apex, the left atrium can be placed anterior and the VSD exposed through the tricuspid valve. This approach has the benefit of facilitating avoidance of conduction system damage. It is, however, important to preserve TV function, as the morphological RV will be the systemic ventricle. The stitches are not placed in the septal leaflet of the tricuspid valve. Instead, sutures are placed in the membranous flap at the inferior margin.

LV–PA Conduit Placement

At the apex of the LV, a ventriculotomy is made parallel to the anterior descending coronary artery. To determine the ventriculotomy site, a finger is placed through the right atrium and the position of the papillary muscles is checked. The ventriculotomy is performed distal to the base of the papillary muscles (Fig. II-28-7). Muscle trabeculations are partially removed from the LV, and an orifice of the ventricle is enlarged. For the conduit, a valved prosthesis or non-

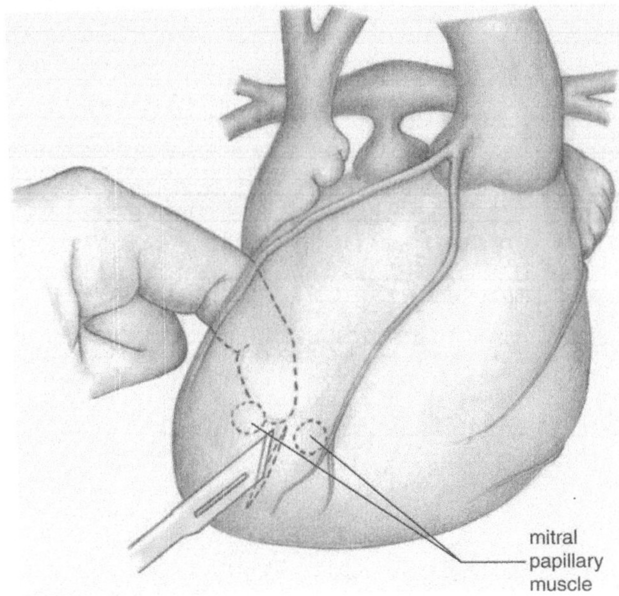

Fig. II-28-7. LV-PA conduit placement: ventriculotomy. Ventriculotomy is placed between the anterior and posterior papillary muscles

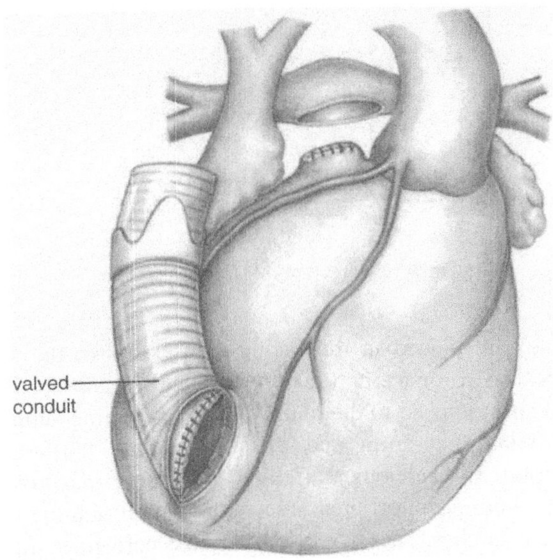

Fig. II-28-8. LV-PA conduit placement: conduit suture

valved vascular graft is used. When compression of the conduit by the sternum is a concern, a longer conduit is used to fit inside the right hemithorax (Fig. II-28-8).

Double-Switch Operation

Mustard + ASO + VSD Closure

Via median sternotomy, the heart is exposed. Before bypass, both great vessels are dissected. The pulmonary arteries are

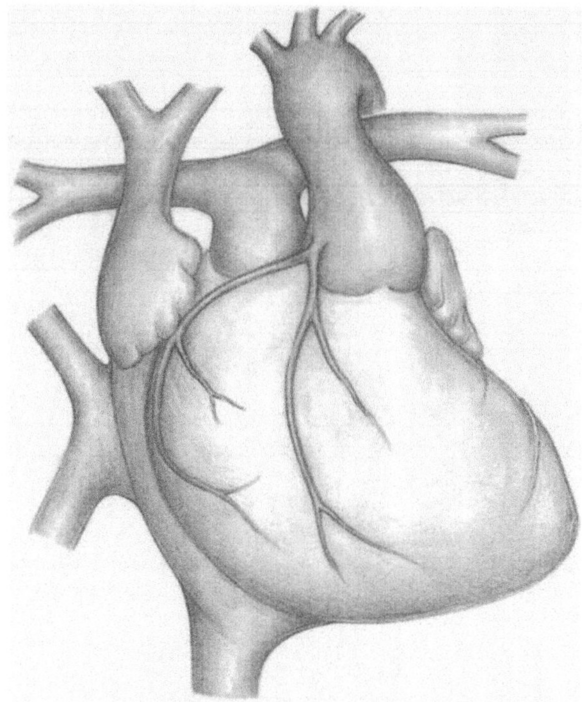

Fig. II-28-9. Congenitally corrected transposition of the great arteries (c-TGA) (S, L, L). VSD (+), PS (pulmonary stenosis) (−)

dissected to the hilum, and the ligamentum is divided. In patients with SLL type, with high pulmonary blood flow, the apex of the heart is often located on the left side (Fig. II-28-9).

When the Mustard procedure is utilized for an atrial switch, an autologous pericardial patch is harvested. If this patch is not available, a xenopericardium or polytetrafluoroethylene (PTFE) patch is used. Cardiopulmonary bypass is initiated with high ascending aortic and bicaval cannulation.

Mustard Procedure

After cardiac arrest, an oblique right atriotomy is performed from the base of the right atrial appendage (Fig. II-28-10 ①). The atrial septum is removed, and the posterior portion and edges of the excised septum are repaired with monofilament suture. The septum at the superior margin is thoroughly removed to avoid superior vena cava (SVC) stenosis (Fig. II-28-10 ②). At the inferior margin, the coronary sinus is cut back and coronary sinus blood is redirected to the functional RA. In this anatomy the right atrial volume is small, so this atriotomy is extended beyond the crista terminalis and down to the point between the upper and lower right pulmonary veins (Fig. II-28-10 ③). The shape of the patch is trapezoid. The distance between points B and F correlates to the distance between the SVC and inferior vena cava (IVC). The suture line is started at the point anterior to the left pulmonary vein orifices (point A). The patch point A comes to this starting point. The suture is advanced superiorly toward point B, which is at the crista terminalis. At this

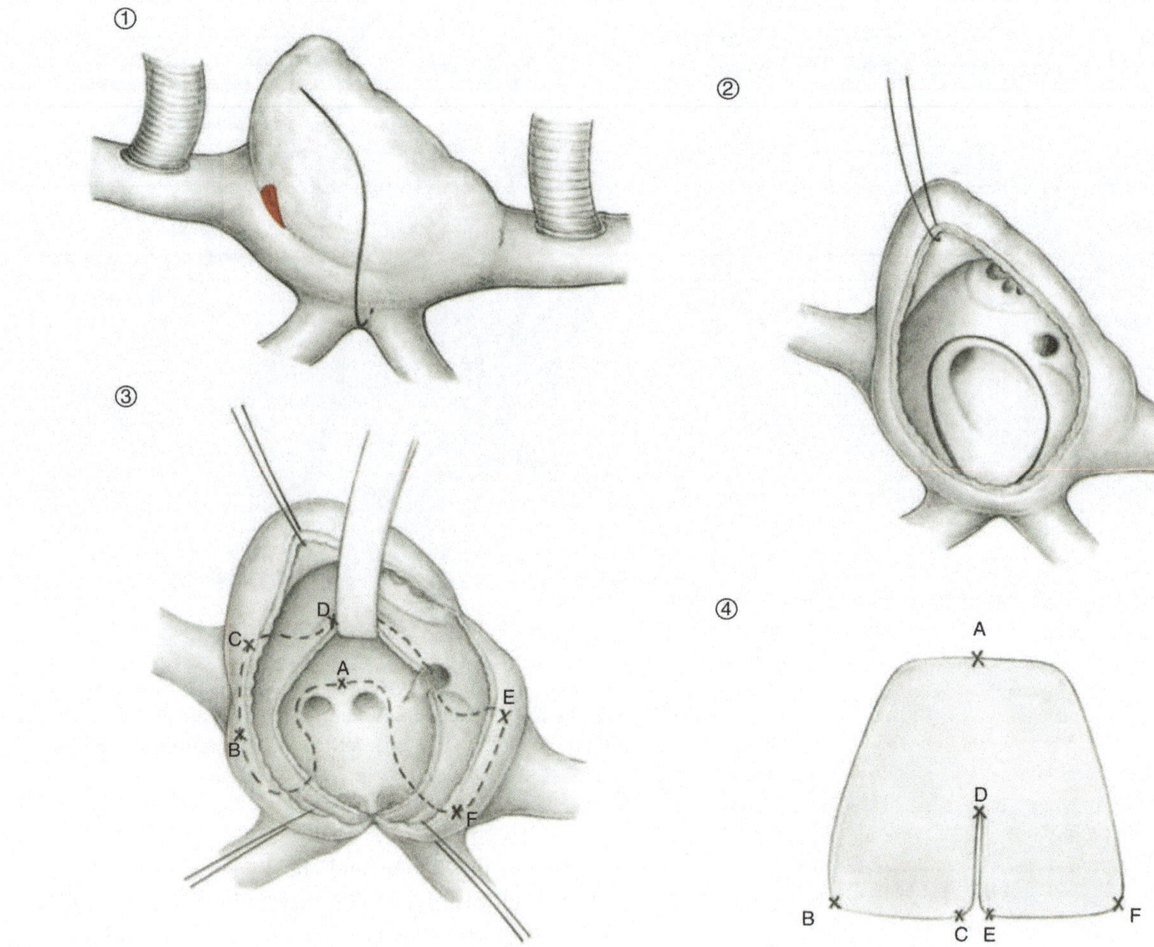

Fig. II-28-10. Mustard procedure. *A–E*, points on patch for placement

stage an incision is made to the patch toward point D to adjust the suture line. The distance from point B to point D (Fig. II-28-10 ④) joins to the most anterior point of the atrial septum. The distance from point D to point F (Fig. II-28-10 ④) is from the IVC orifice to point D of the atrial septum (Fig. II-28-10 ③). The orifice of the coronary sinus is cut back. In type SLL, the conduction system originates from the anterior AV node and runs anterior to the pulmonary valve annulus, and it is thus safe to use the anterior part of this incised coronary sinus wall for the suture. Before finishing this suture line, a Hegar dilator is applied to check the size of systemic venous channels. The right atriotomy is closed directly or with a patch to obtain an unobstructed pulmonary venous pathway.

Arterial Switch Operation (ASO)

The surgical technique of the ASO is basically the same as that of d-TGA. The ascending aorta is transected several millimeters distal to the sinotubular (ST) junction. Coronary buttons are created from the ascending aorta. The main PA is transected at its bifurcation. J-shaped incisions (trap-door technique) are placed in the facing sinuses above the ST junction. The coronary buttons are trimmed to appropriate size and anastomosed to the main PA with a running suture. The proximal neo-aorta and distal ascending aorta are anastomosed to each other after the Lecompte maneuver. Coronary button donor sites are repaired with autologous pericardial patches. The PA reconstruction is performed after removal of the aortic cross-clamp following VSD closure (Fig. II-28-11).

VSD Closure

VSD closure during ASO can be performed through the aortic valve. We often prefer the transmorphological RV approach because the aortic valve is occasionally small, limiting exposure (Fig. II-28-12). When marked dextroversion is present, the transtricuspid approach is also reasonable. Regardless of approach, mattress pledgetted sutures are used to close the defect. In the SLL type, the conduction system is located at the anterosuperior margin of the morphological LV surface, and so in this area stitches should not be placed too deep.

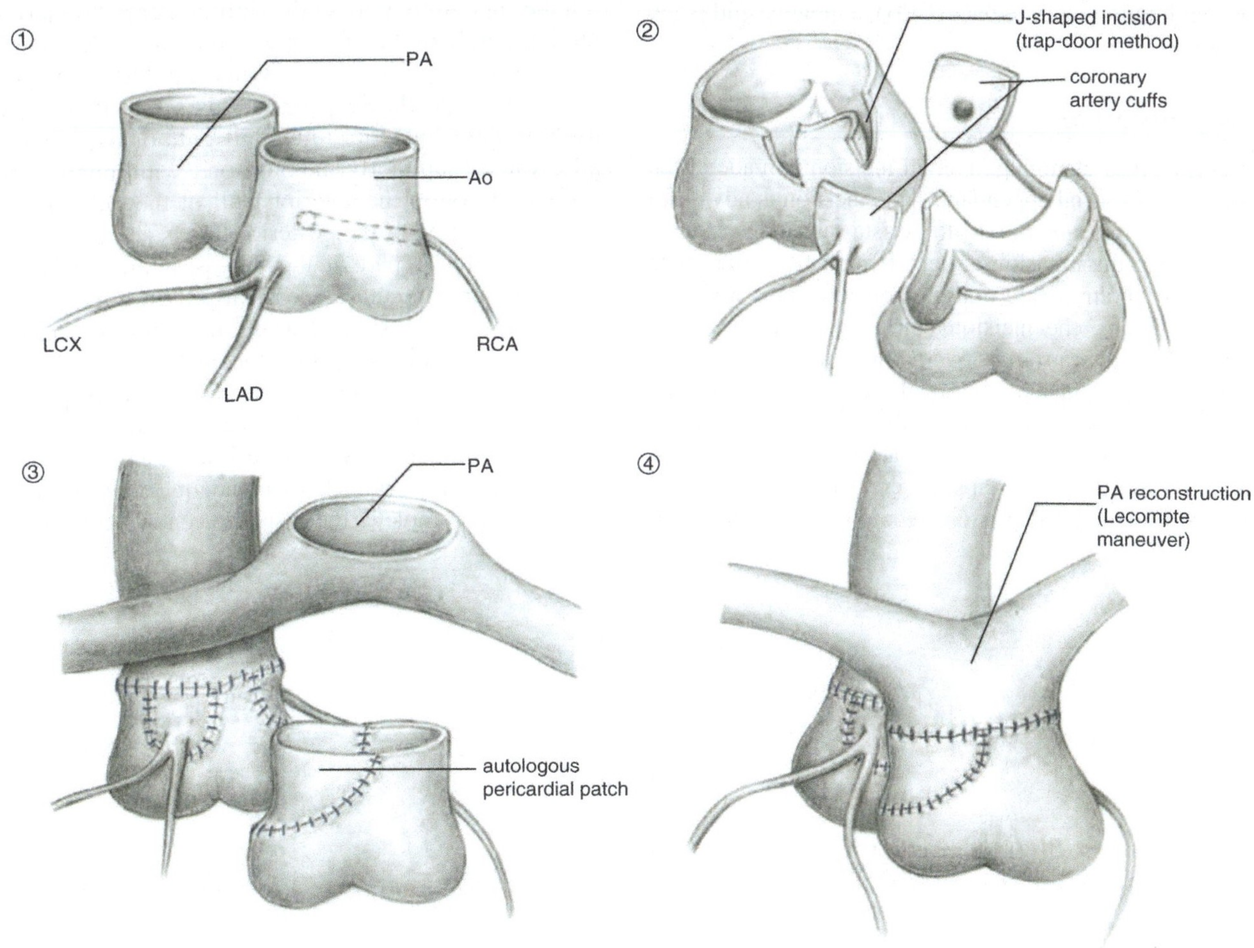

Fig. II-28-11. Arterial switch operation. *LCX*, left circumflex branch; *LAD*, left anterior descending branch; *RCA*, right coronary artery

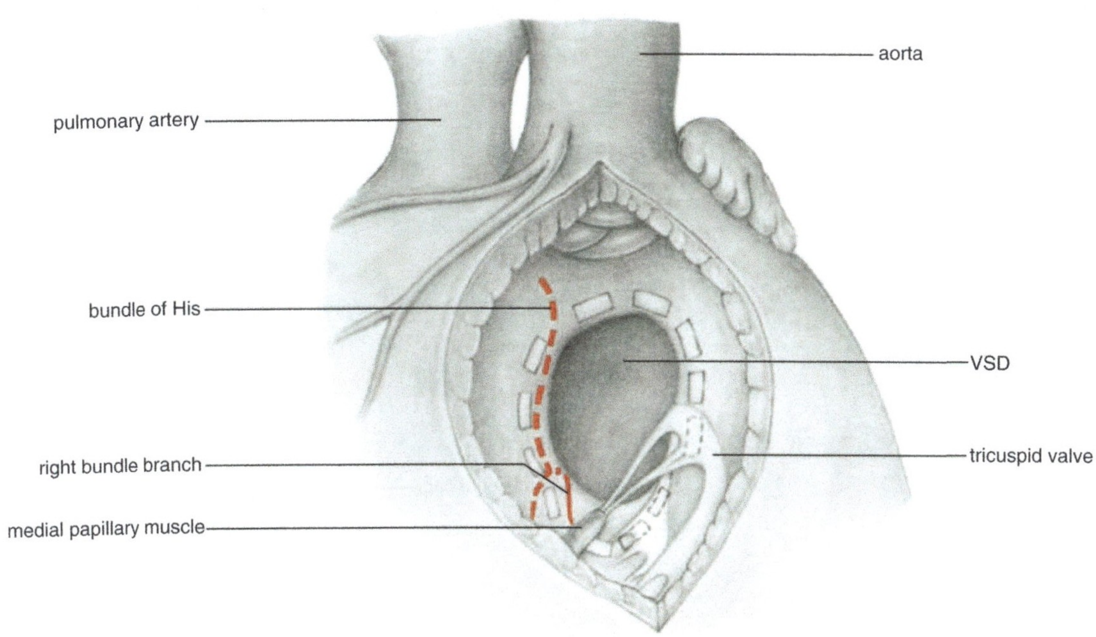

Fig. II-28-12. VSD closure from right ventriculotomy

Senning Procedure + REV Procedure

Before cardiopulmonary bypass (CPB), a monocuspid patch is prepared.

Senning Procedure

After aortic cross-clamping, a small incision is made at the base of the right atrial appendage. This incision is advanced inferiorly 5–6 mm anterior to the crista terminalis. At the superior point, this incision is kept 10 mm from the crista terminalis to obtain a safe margin from the sinus node. At the inferior point, the incision comes close to the crista terminalis. The interatrial groove is dissected. The incision is made to the LA at the edge of the RA. The size of the incision should not extend beyond the orifices of the superior and inferior right pulmonary veins. With these incisions, the anterior and posterior flaps are created (Fig. II-28-13). Next, the atrial septal flap is created. When a small patent foramen ovale is present, this is directly closed. The atrial septum is incised to create a septal flap at the line created with the superior margin of the right upper pulmonary vein–anterior margin of the fossa ovalis and inferior margin of the right lower pulmonary vein. When the ASD is large, it is closed with a patch. Suturing of this septal flap to the left atrium is started anterior to the left pulmonary vein orifices and advanced superiorly and inferiorly with running sutures. This flap becomes the anterior wall of the pulmonary vein pathway. Suturing of the posterior flap is started at the IVC. The most inferior part of the flap is sutured to the crista terminalis, and this suture line is carried toward the posterior flap of the coronary sinus. During this suturing, Hegar dilators are placed to check that the orifice of the systemic venous pathway is sufficient. The most superior part of the flap is sutured to the base of the right atrial appendage and the crista terminalis. This suture line is advanced parallel to the atrial septum with checking adequacy of the orifice of the SVC; this completes the systemic venous pathway. Then,

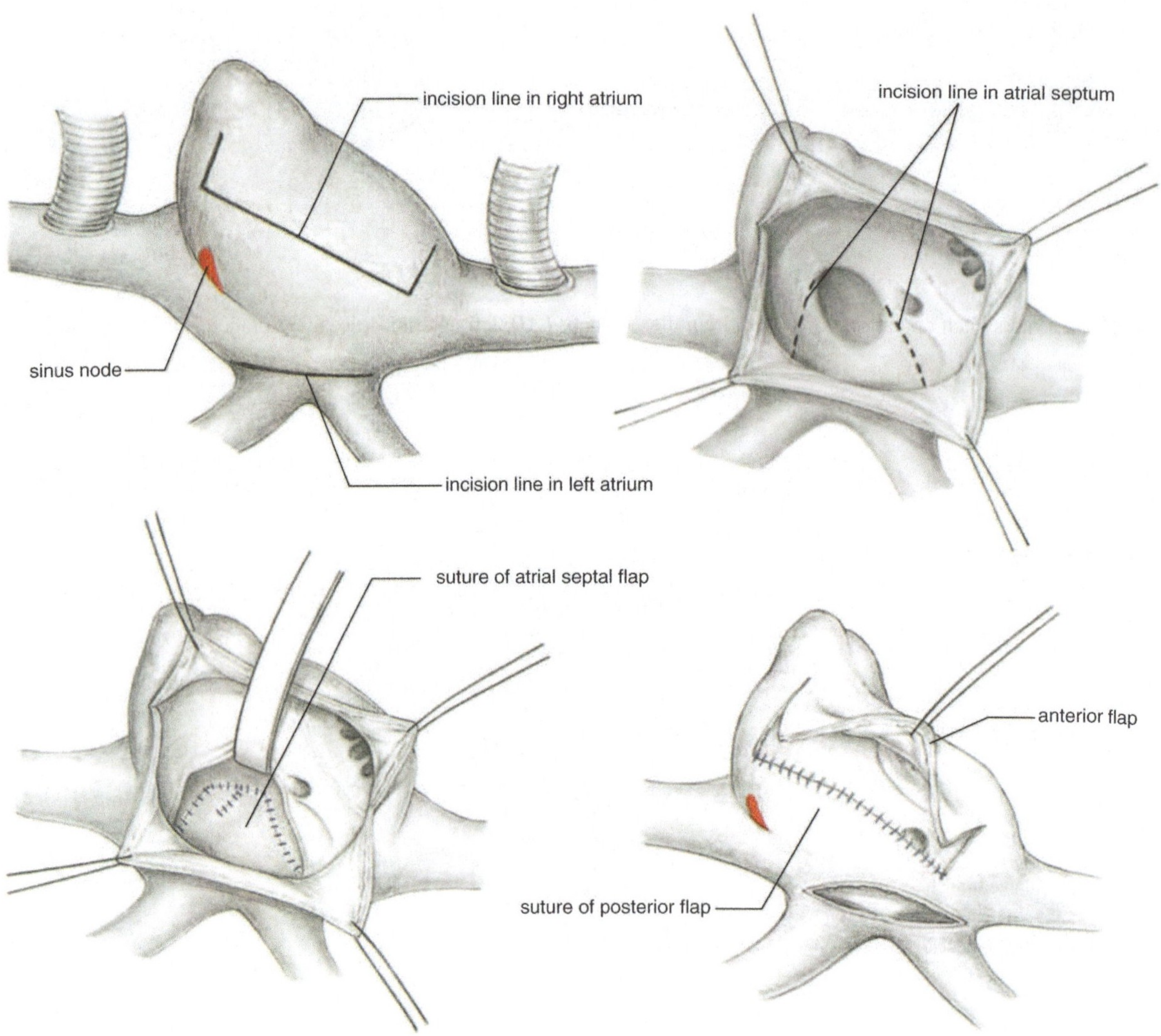

Fig. II-28-13. Senning procedure: septal flap and posterior flap suturing

with the anterior flap the pulmonary vein pathway is created. To reduce tension on the suture line, an L-shaped incision is made at both ends of the anterior flap. The ends of the longitudinal incision of the flap reach each end of the left atrial incision. The suture line is located posterior to the sinus node (Fig. II-28-14).

VSD Closure

A 15- to 20-mm right ventriculotomy is made in the anterior wall of the right ventricle, beginning 10 mm from the aortic valve annulus. Trabeculations in the right ventriculotomy site are removed. The VSD, the TV, the aortic valve annulus, the medial papillary muscle, and the relationship between the inferior margin of the VSD and TV are inspected. To create the pathway from the VSD to the aortic valve, pledgetted mattress sutures are used to perform rerouting with a PTFE patch (Fig. II-28-15). When VSD enlargement is necessary, the conus of the morphological RV may be partially excised.

REV Procedure [9]

The ascending aorta is transected 15–20 mm above the ST junction. It is important to preserve as much main PA as possible for the REV procedure. The main PA is transected

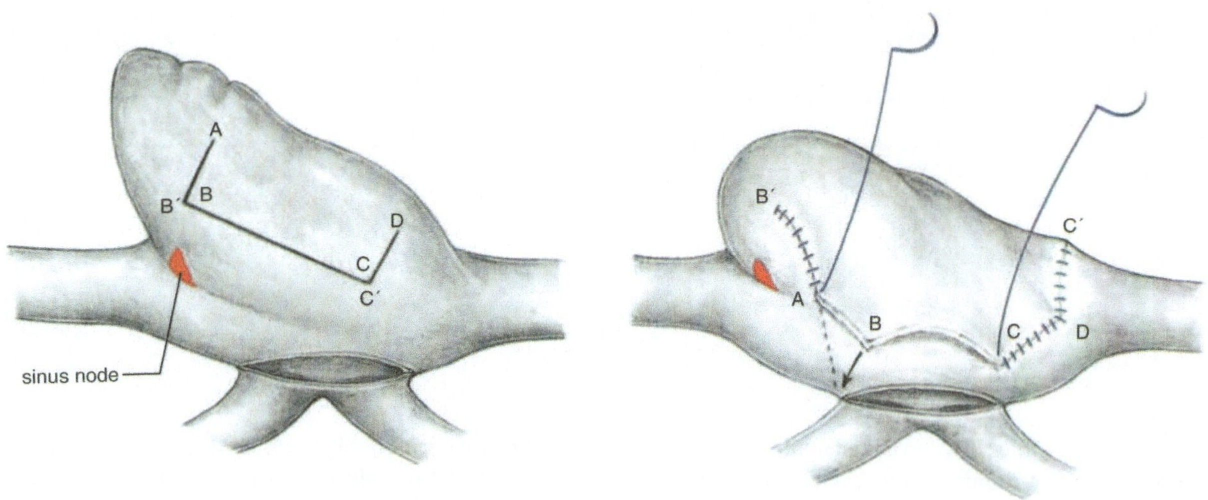

Fig. II-28-14. Senning procedure: anterior flap suturing

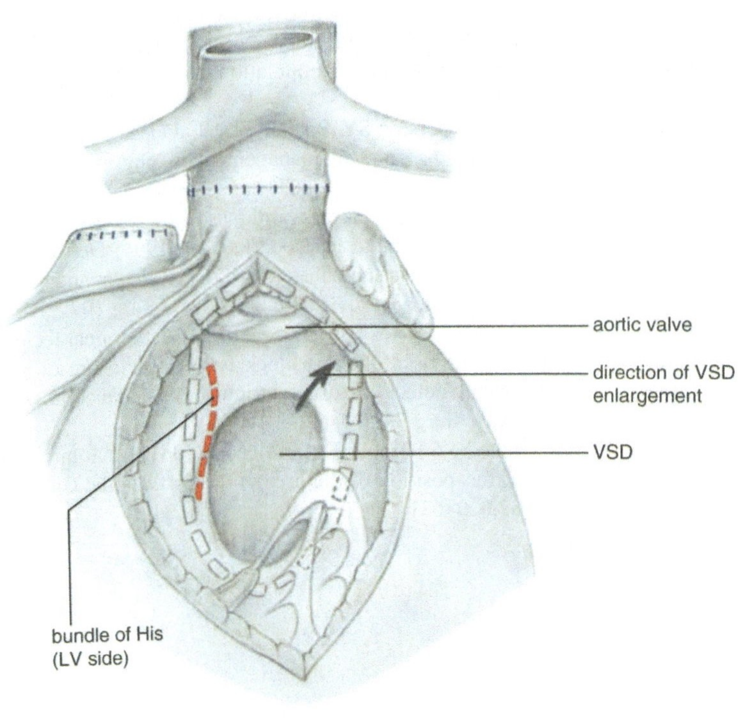

Fig. II-28-15. VSD closure in REV (réparation à l'étage ventriculaire) with Senning procedure

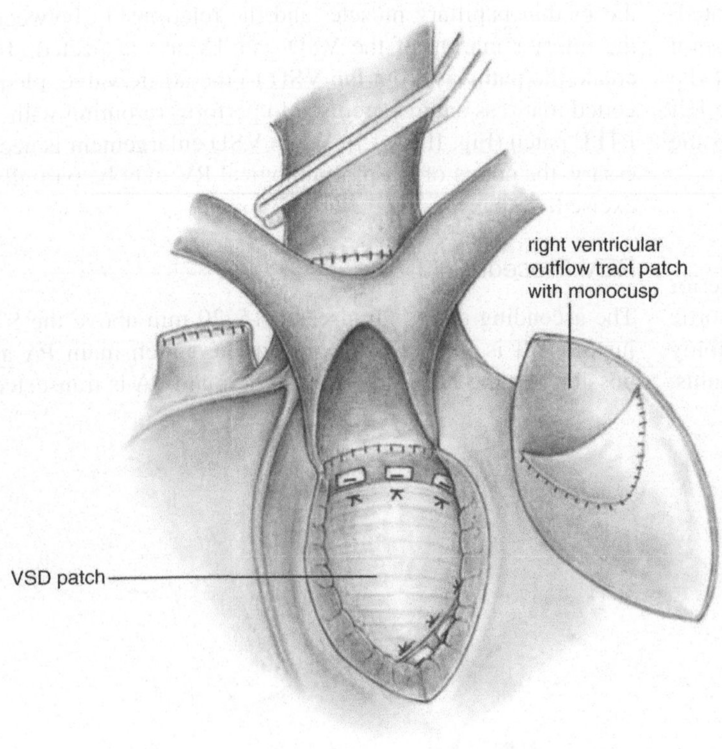

Fig. II-28-16. Right ventricular outflow tract (RVOT) reconstruction in REV procedure

as proximal as possible. The proximal main PA is closed using a double-layer running suture. The branch PAs are dissected at the hilum and brought in front of the ascending aorta (Fig. II-28-16). When the branch PAs are markedly stretched, 5–6 mm of ascending aorta is excised to reduce its length, and the ascending aorta is reanastomosed. When the branch PAs are large enough, in older patients, the branch PAs are transected, brought anterior to the ascending aorta, and reanastomosed. After removing the aortic clamp, the distal main PA and right ventriculotomy site are anastomosed with a double-layer monofilament suture, and this becomes the posterior wall of the RVOT. A monocuspid patch is placed to create the anterior wall of the right ventricular outflow tract.

References

1. Allwork SP, Bentall RH, Becker AE, et al (1976) Congenitally corrected transposition of the great arteries; morphologic study of 32 cases. Am J Cardiol 38:910–923
2. Anderson RH, Becker AE, Arnold R, et al (1974) The conducting tissue in congenitally corrected transposition. Circulation 50:911–923
3. Dick M II, Van Praagh R, Rudd M, et al (1977) Electrophysiologic delineation of the specialized atrioventricular conduction system in two patients with corrected transposition of the great arteries in situs inversus (IDD). Circulation 55:896–900
4. Becker AE, Ho SY, Caruso G, et al (1980) Straddling right atrioventricular valves in atrioventricular discordance. Circulation 61:1133–1141
5. Biliciler-Denktas G, Feldt RH, Connolly HM, et al (2001) Early and late results of operations for defects associated with corrected transposition and other anomalies with atrioventricular discordance in a pediatric population. J Thorac Cardiovasc Surg 122:234–241
6. Ilbawi MN, DeLeon SY, Backer CL, et al (1990) An alternative approach to the surgical management of physiologically corrected transposition with ventricular septal defect and pulmonary stenosis or atresia. J Thorac Cardiovasc Surg 100:410–415
7. Yagihara T, Kishimoto H, Isobe F, et al (1994) Double switch operation in cardiac anomalies with atrioventricular and ventriculoarterial discordance. J Thorac Cardiovasc Surg 107:351–358
8. de Leval MR, Bastos P, Stark J, et al (1979) Surgical technique to reduce the risks of heart block following closure of ventricular septal defect in atrioventricular discordance. J Thorac Cardiovasc Surg 78:515–526
9. Lecompte Y, Zannini L, Hazan E, et al (1981) Anatomic correction of transposition of the great arteries. J Thorac Cardiovasc Surg 82:629–631

II-29. Double-Outlet Right Ventricle—Kawashima Procedure, Patric–McGoon Procedure, Arterial Switch Operation + Intraventricular Re-routing, Primary Repair for False Taussig–Bing Malformation with Type B IAA

Anatomical Properties

Double-outlet right ventricle (DORV) is diagnosed whenever more than half of the circumference of both arterial valves is connected to the morphological right ventricle [1]. The definition by Kirklin and Lev et al. that more than 50% of both great vessels arise from the right ventricle is generally accepted and differentiates the condition from tetralogy of Fallot [2]. This disease is usually classified into four groups based on the location of the ventricular septal defect (VSD): subaortic, subpulmonary, doubly committed, and noncommitted type (Fig. II-29-1). In the subaortic type, the VSD is typically a perimembranous-outlet type, and the physiology mimics either a simple VSD or tetralogy of Fallot. DORV with subpulmonary VSD is also known as the Taussig–Bing anomaly. According to the relationship of the great arteries, this is classified into original Taussig–Bing and false Taussig–Bing [3] (Fig. II-29-2). Anatomic features of each anomaly are described in Table II-29-1. In doubly committed-type DORV, the VSD is adjacent to both aortic and pulmonary valves and the shape of the VSD is similar to that of a total conus defect. In noncommitted-type VSD, a perimembranous inlet-type VSD is typically present. For biventricular repair, the type of VSD, relationship of the great arteries, the presence of pulmonary stenosis or subaortic stenosis, and associated cardiac anomalies must be evaluated to plan an appropriate surgical procedure.

Subaortic VSD

In the absence of pulmonary stenosis (PS), hemodynamics are similar to those in patients with a typical perimembranous VSD. Surgical treatment is single-stage repair of VSD closure, or, in unusual cases, two-stage repair with initial pulmonary artery banding before complete repair (VSD closure). If pulmonary stenosis is present, the surgical treatment is similar to that of tetralogy of Fallot.

The heart is accessed via median sternotomy. Bypass is established with ascending aortic and bicaval cannulation. After aortic cross-clamping, a right atriotomy is performed and right ventricular structures are inspected, including the VSD, the trabecula septomarginalis, and the position and shape of the infundibular septum. It is important in creating a baffle from the left ventricle to the aorta to avoid left ventricular outlet tract (LVOT) obstruction. If the VSD is small, the anterosuperior margin of the ventriculoinfundibular fold and the infundibular septum are resected. The baffle is created from a polytetrafluoroethylene (PTFE) tube graft and secured with pledgetted mattress sutures (Fig. II-29-3).

Doubly Committed VSD

The surgical procedure varies depending on the extension of the VSD toward the pulmonary or aortic valve. In most cases the depth (superior–inferior distance) of the VSD is shallow, and subarterial stenosis tends to occur after repair. Therefore, two-stage repair is often recommended in symptomatic small infants. The baffle is occasionally placed via the right atrium or main pulmonary artery, but often a right ventriculotomy is required for baffle placement. The ventriculotomy may be a longitudinal incision below the great artery to which the VSD extends or may be a transverse incision below both vessels. For baffle placement, care is taken to avoid compromising the right ventricular outflow tract (RVOT) as well as the LVOT. A PTFE tube graft is tailored to create a baffle and is sutured with pledgetted mattress stitches. In the absence of a conal septum, sutures are placed through the pulmonary valve. If the baffle may cause RVOT obstruction, an additional patch is placed to augment the right ventricular free wall (Fig. II-29-4).

Noncommitted VSD

In patients with DORV and a noncommitted VSD, a large RV volume is required for biventricular repair, because the distance between the aortic valve and superior margin of the VSD is long and a large baffle is required. If the VSD is small, it may be enlarged at the anterosuperior margin. Even if the VSD is large enough, in the presence of a straddling atrioventricular (AV) valve or subaortic stenosis, biventricular repair may not be feasible. In this situation, a single ventricle pathway should be considered. Therefore, surgery is ideally performed in late infancy.

For a biventricular repair, an intraventricular baffle is placed through the right atrium in most cases. First, the VSD is aggressively enlarged at the superior margin to at least the normal aortic valve size. A tailored PTFE tube graft is recommended for a baffle, secured with pledgetted mattress sutures. If a straddling tricuspid valve is present, the papillary muscle is divided at its base and sutured to the baffle (Fig. II-29-5).

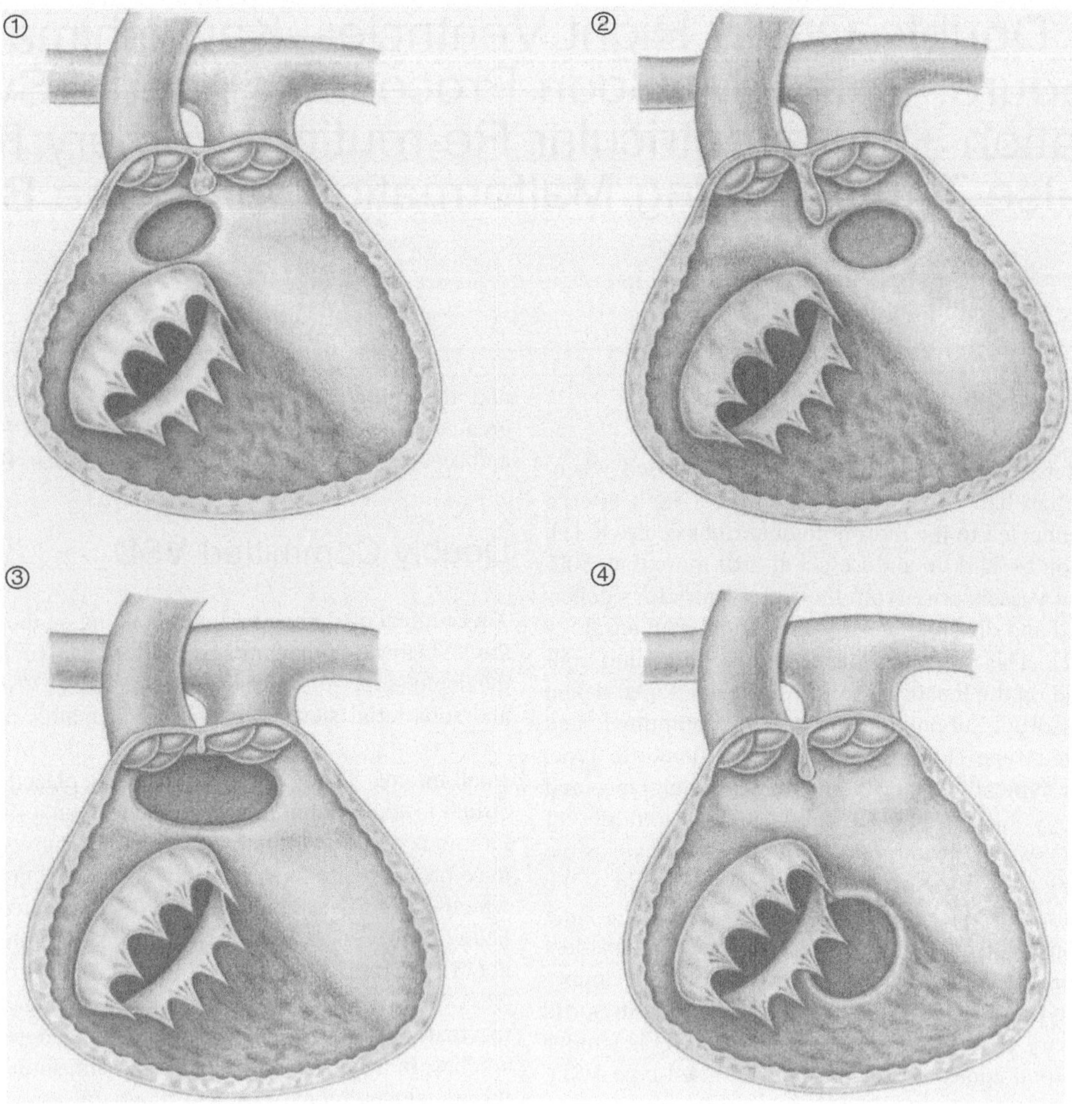

Fig. II-29-1. Classification of double-outlet right ventricle (DORV): ①, subaortic type; ②, subpulmonary type; ③, doubly committed type; ④, noncommitted or remote type

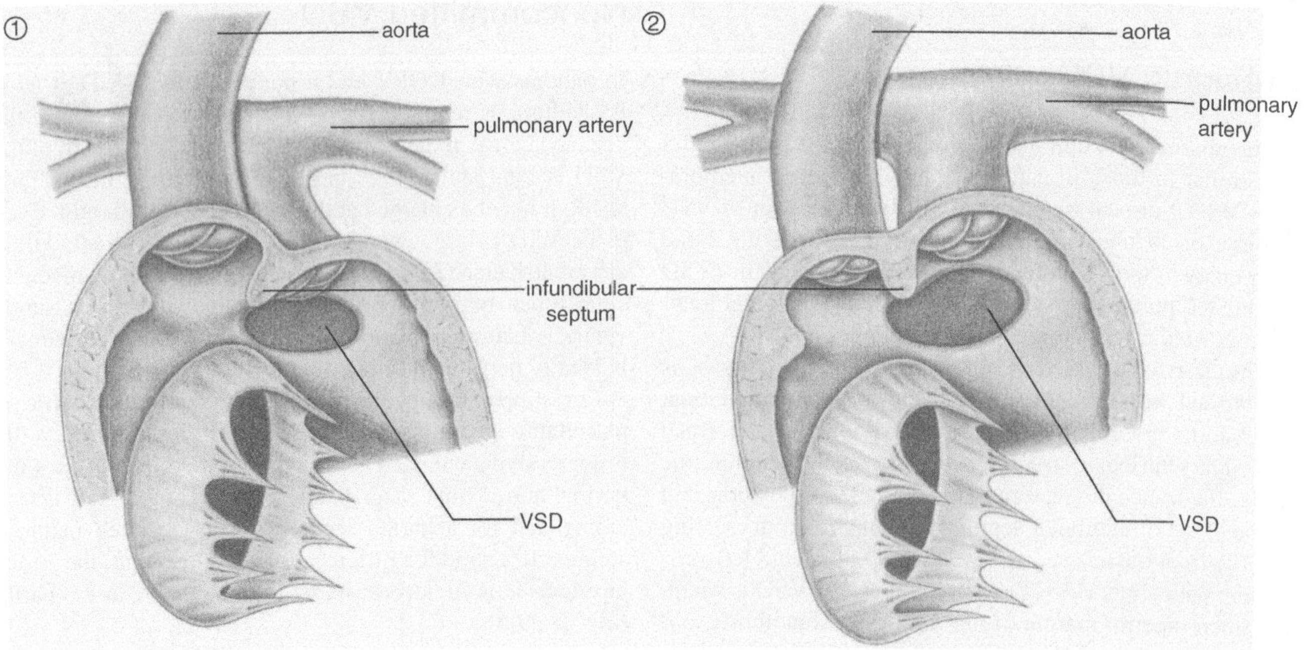

Fig. II-29-2. Classification of subpulmonary ventricular septal defect (*VSD*): ①, false Taussig–Bing anomaly; ②, original Taussig–Bing anomaly

Table II-29-1. Anatomical features of false Taussig–Bing anomaly and original Taussig–Bing anomaly

Anatomical properties	False Taussig–Bing	Original Taussig–Bing
Great vessel relationship	Anterior-posterior Aorta anterior-rightward	Side by side Aorta posterior-rightward
Coronary type	LAD+Cx-sinus 1, RCA-sinus 2 LAD-sinus 1, Cx+RCA-sinus 2	LAD+RCA-sinus 1, Cx-sinus 2 RCA-sinus 1, LAD+Cx-sinus 2
Infundibular septum extension	Tricuspid side VIF	Mitral side VIF
Alignment of infundibular septum and ventricular septum	Good	Poor
Subaortic stenosis/aortic arch anomaly	Often	Often

LAD, left anterior descending branch; Cx, circumflex branch; RCA, right coronary artery; VIF, ventriculoinfundibular fold

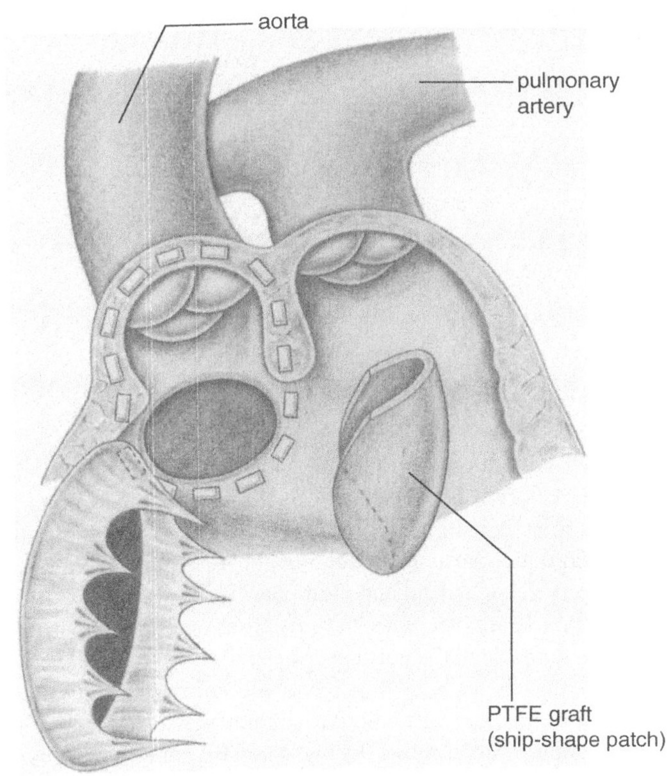

Fig. II-29-3. Subaortic VSD. *PTFE*, polytetrafluoroethylene

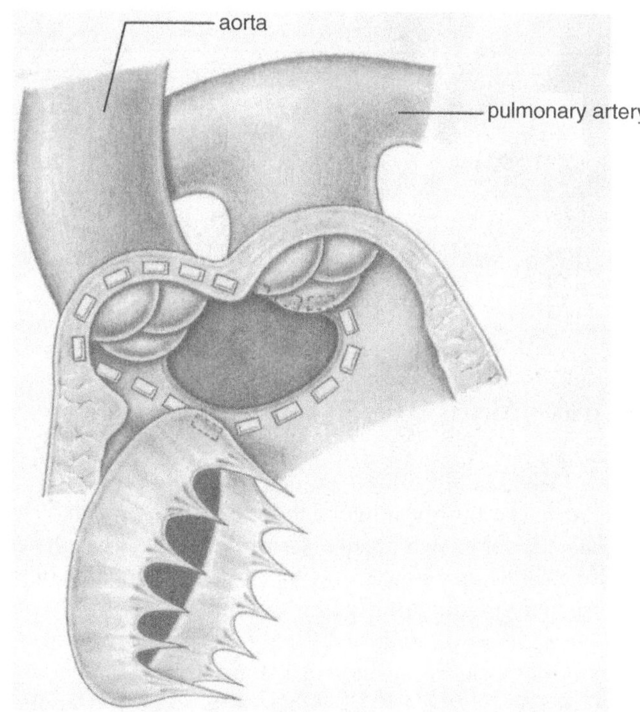

Fig. II-29-4. Doubly committed VSD

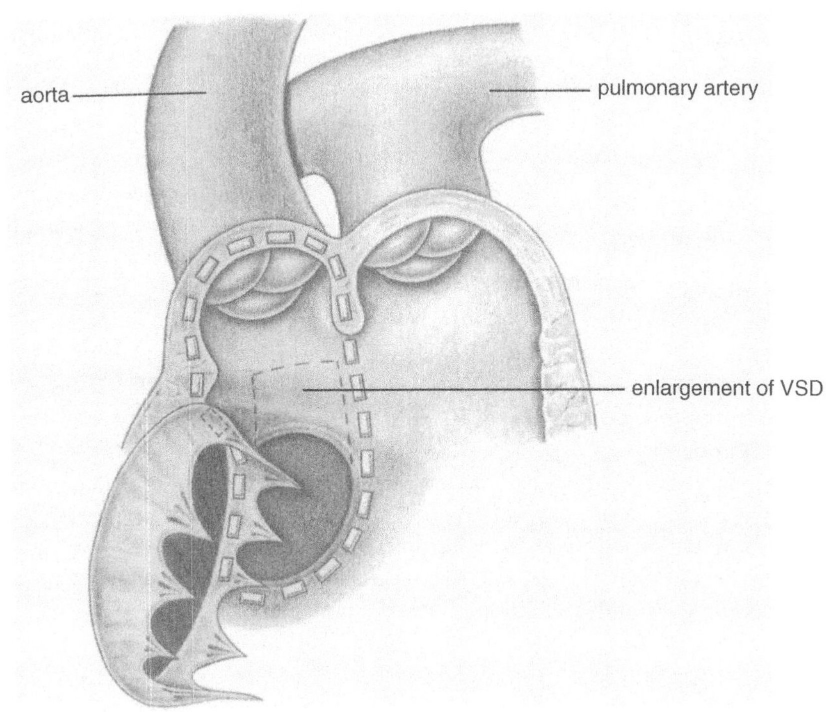

Fig. II-29-5. Noncommitted VSD

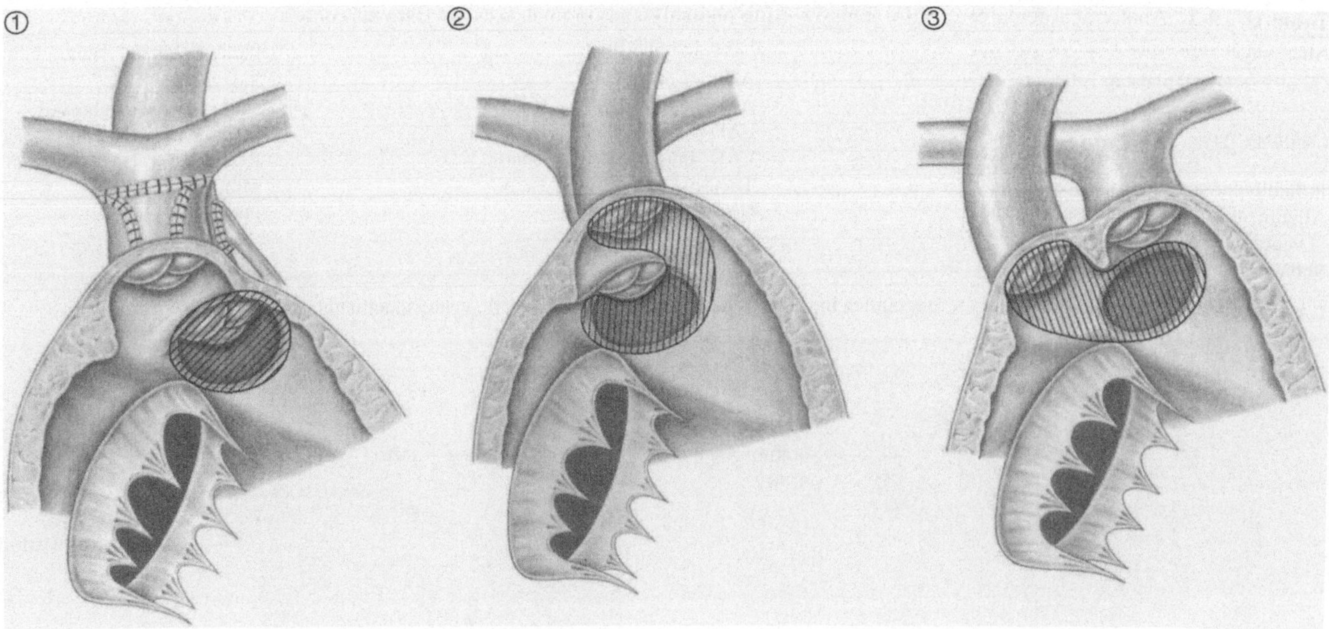

Fig. II-29-6. Subpulmonary VSD: ①, arterial switch operation; ②, Patrick–McGoon procedure; ③, Kawashima procedure

Subpulmonary VSD

For a false Taussig–Bing type of DORV, the physiology is similar to the transposition of the great arteries with VSD, and an arterial switch operation with VSD closure is generally the surgical treatment of choice [4]. Occasionally, intraventricular rerouting (the Kawashima procedure [5]) may be employed as an alternative. If the great vessel relationship is anterior–posterior position or L-transposition, and a large VSD is present, the Patrick–McGoon procedure is applied [6]. In patients with original Taussig–Bing anomaly, either the arterial switch or the Kawashima procedure is applied. If the great vessel relationship is side by side and the distance between the tricuspid valve and pulmonary valve is larger than the annulus of the normal aortic valve, the Kawashima procedure can be applied (Fig. II-29-6).

Kawashima Procedure

This procedure is an intraventricular rerouting used for the original Taussig–Bing anomaly. Median sternotomy is performed, and bypass is instituted with ascending aortic and bicaval cannulation. After aortic cross-clamping, a right atriotomy is performed. Intra-right ventricular structures including the VSD, septal trabeculation, and infundibular septum are inspected. If these structures are not seen well through the right atrium, the right ventricle is evaluated through a pulmonary arteriotomy. Based on these evaluations, the method of rerouting is determined. Occasionally the baffle in the right ventricle is placed through the right atrium, but more commonly a right ventriculotomy is required. The site of right ventriculotomy is determined based on the coronary anatomy with attention to the size and location of the conus branch. A transverse subarterial incision or a subpulmonary longitudinal incision is chosen (Fig. II-29-7). In applying this technique, particular attention must be paid to the distance between tricuspid and pulmonary valves, because after repair this space becomes the posterior wall channel from the left ventricle to the aorta inside the right ventricle. Therefore, it must be at least the size of the normal aortic valve. To ensure this, the infundibular septum is excised as much as possible to enlarge the LVOT. A PTFE tube graft is tailored to create a baffle. One-third of the circumference is constructed with autologous tissue (Fig. II-29-8). Occasionally, VSD enlargement is not required. However, if enlargement is necessary, this is performed at the anterosuperior margin. If the distance between the tricuspid and pulmonary valves is small, the baffle is attached to the posterior wall of the pulmonary artery to obtain sufficient outflow tract diameter (Fig. II-29-9). The anterior free wall of the right ventricle will usually require an augmentation patch, which may cross the pulmonary annulus and require a monocusp valve. If the papillary muscle of the tricuspid valve is attached to the infundibular septum, this papillary muscle should be detached and transferred to the baffle [7] (Fig. II-29-10).

Arterial Switch Operation (ASO) for False Taussig–Bing Anomaly

In this section, the surgical approach for a patient with transposition of the great vessels (TGA)-type DORV and type B interrupted aortic arch (IAA) is described (Fig. II-29-11). Arch reconstruction with direct anastomosis and ASO are performed simultaneously.

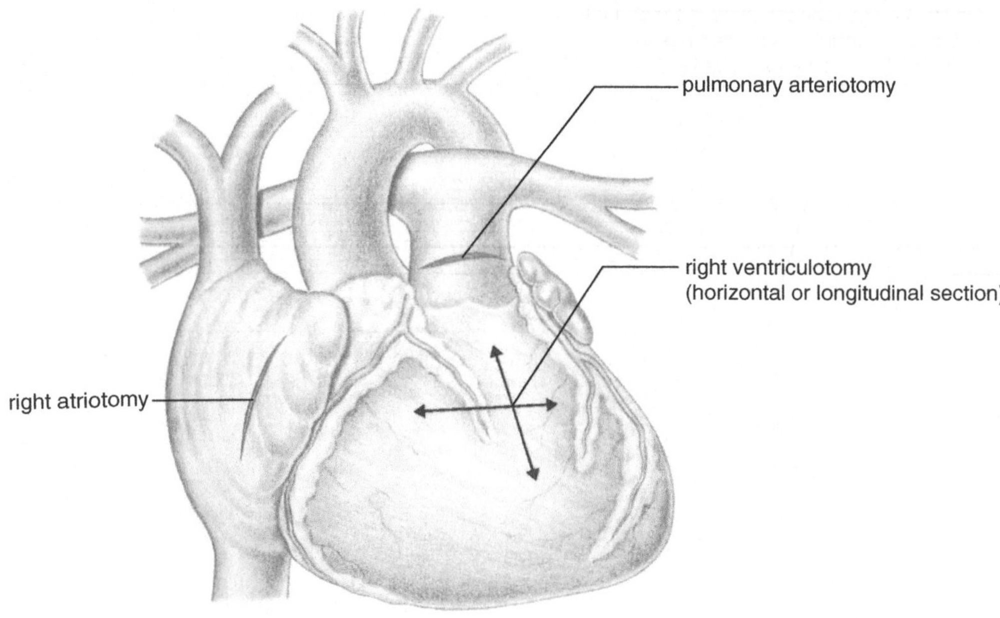

Fig. II-29-7. Kawashima procedure: ventriculotomy

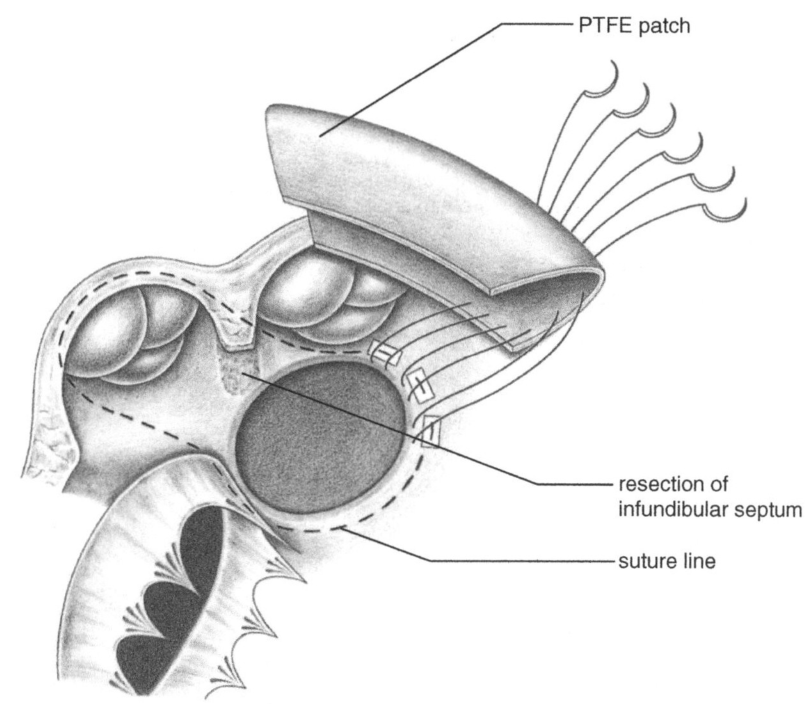

Fig. II-29-8. Kawashima procedure: patch placement

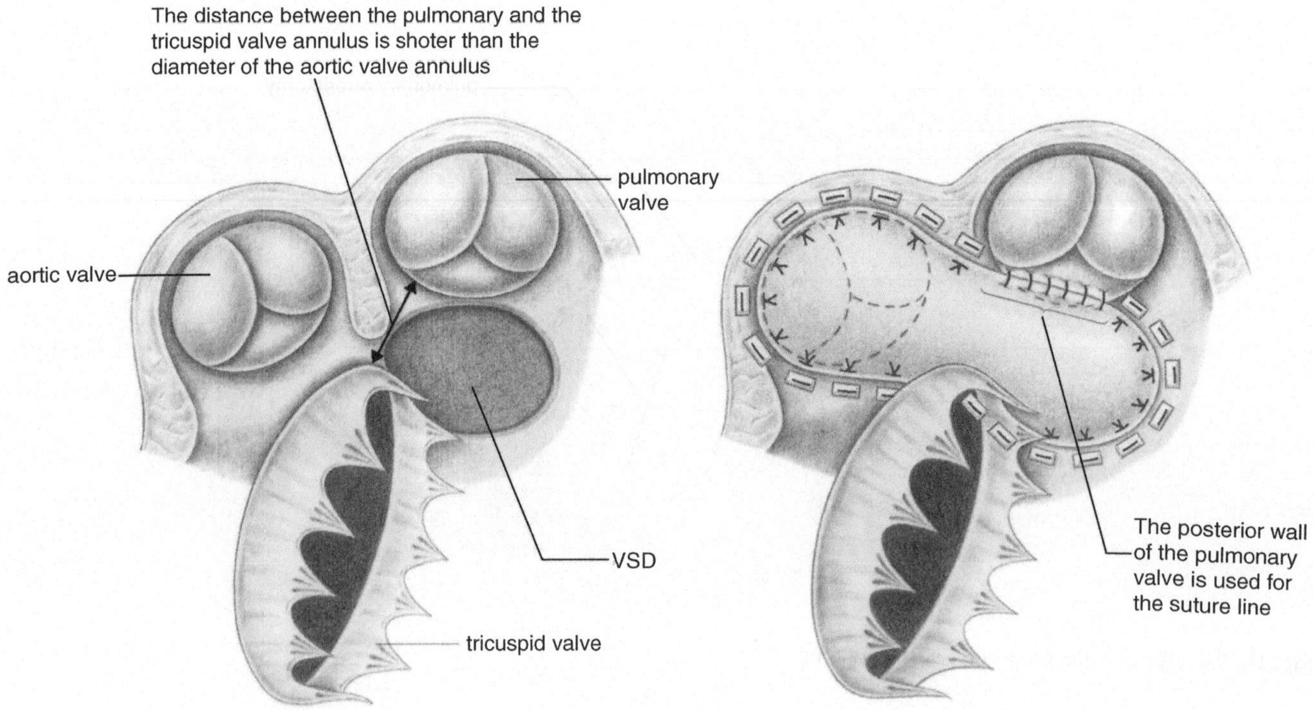

Fig. II-29-9. Kawashima procedure: narrow distance between the pulmonary valve and the tricuspid valve (less than diameter of aortic valve annulus)

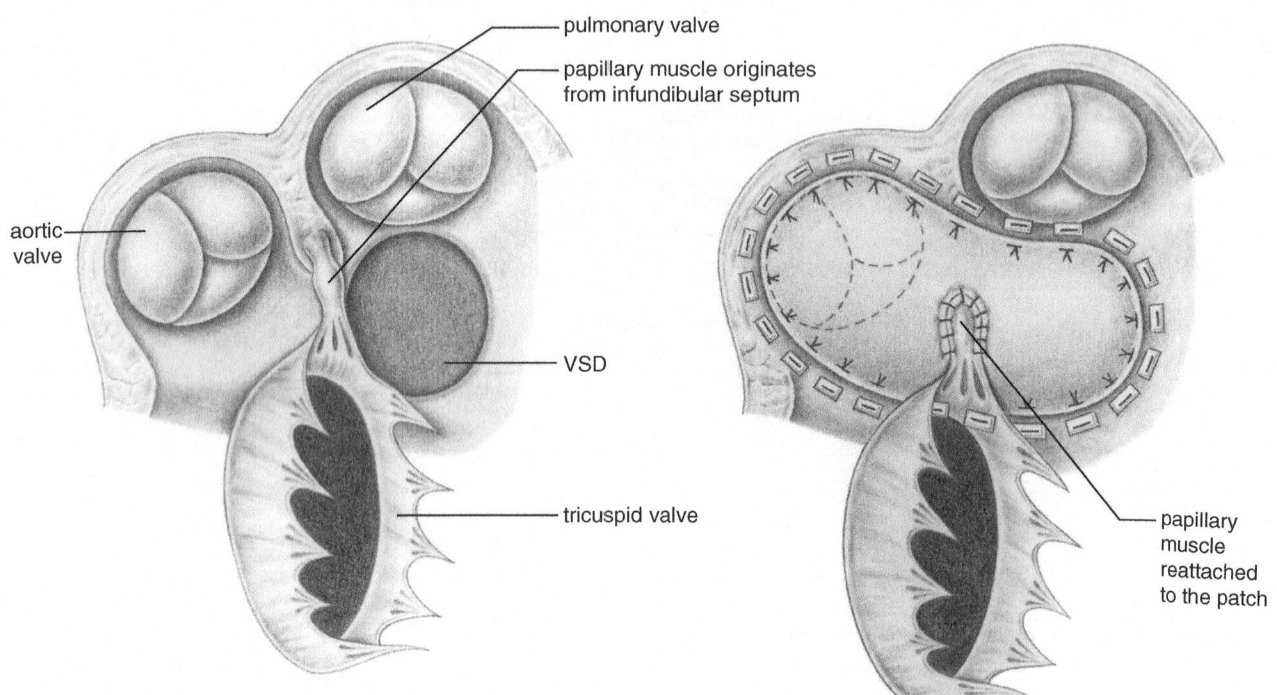

Fig. II-29-10. Kawashima procedure: require reattachment of papillary muscle

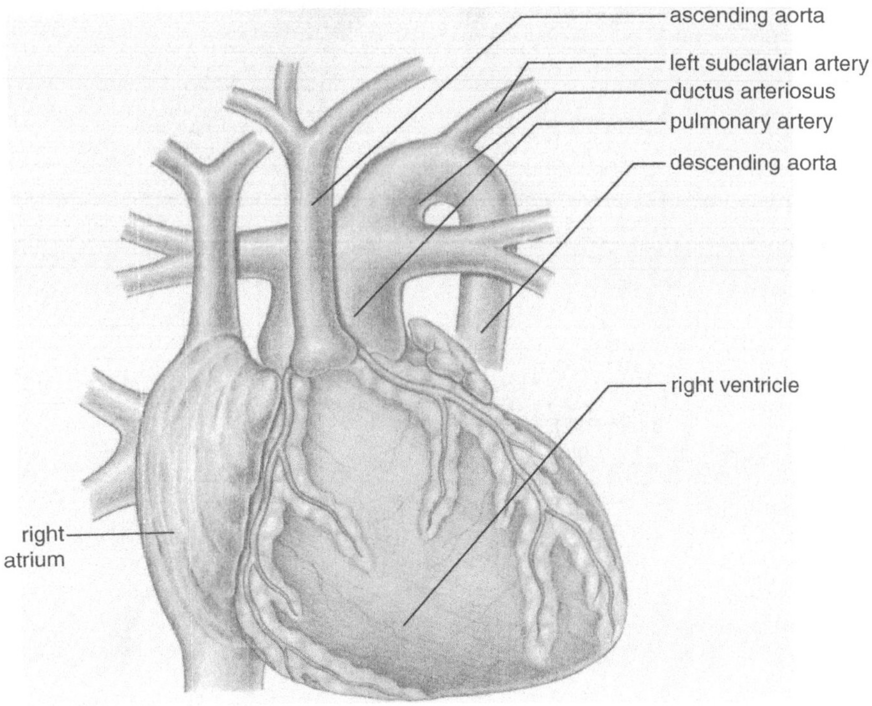

Fig. II-29-11. Double-outlet right ventricle (DORV) with type B interrupted aortic arch

Cardiopulmonary Bypass (CPB)

With brachiocephalic artery and descending aortic cannulation, cardiopulmonary bypass without circulatory arrest is utilized [8]. A median sternotomy is performed, and an 8 Fr. straight arterial cannula is inserted into a 3-mm PTFE tube anastomosed to the brachiocephalic artery. This cannula is used to perfuse the upper body. A right-angle arterial cannula (2.1 mm) is inserted into the descending aorta above the diaphragm to perfuse the lower body (Fig. II-29-12). Both cannulae are joined with a Y-connector, and bicaval cannulae are connected to the bypass circuit. Mild hypothermic CPB is instituted [rectal temperature of 31°C, 2.8 l/min/body surface area (BSA)] (Fig. II-29-12). With this technique, circulatory arrest is completely avoided.

ASO

Following ductal ligation, the ascending aorta is cross-clamped and transected 5 mm above the sinotubular junction. The main pulmonary artery is transected obliquely just proximal to its bifurcation. The right side of the main pulmonary artery is shorter and the left side is longer. In this anomaly, the ascending aorta is small, and care is taken to avoid damaging the aortic valve cusp during coronary button creation. The coronary buttons are transferred to the main pulmonary artery above the sinotubular junction (Fig. II-29-13).

Aortic Reconstruction

If the discrepancy between the distal ascending aorta and proximal main pulmonary artery is large, a patch is placed to augment the distal ascending aorta (Fig. II-29-14). More recently, aortic reconstruction without patch material has been employed. In this procedure, the aortic arch, ascending aorta, and descending aorta are anastomosed directly (Fig. II-29-14). After division of the duct, all ductal tissue is excised. The pulmonary confluence is brought in front of the reconstructed ascending aorta (Lecompte maneuver). If the ductal tissue is present at the base of the left subclavian artery, the left subclavian artery is ligated and divided.

Intraventricular Rerouting

When aortic valve stenosis and subaortic stenosis are present, RVOT repair is required combined with an ASO. Intraventricular rerouting is performed through a right ventriculotomy. A longitudinal incision is placed in the RVOT, and a rerouting patch is placed from the inferior margin of intraventricular foramen to the neo-aortic valve (Fig. II-29-15). Enlargement of intraventricular foramen is rarely necessary.

Right Ventricular Outflow Tract Reconstruction

If the original aortic valve is small (less than 2.0 cm^2/m^2 BSA), or is a bicuspid valve, a transannular patch may be necessary. After removal of the aortic clamp, the anterior commissure is longitudinally opened, and the annulus is enlarged while the heart is beating. Any obstructive muscle is resected to relieve neo-subpulmonary stenosis. Neo-pulmonary sinus defects (coronary button sites) are repaired with an autologous pericardial patch. A patch with a 0.1-mm-thick PTFE monocusp is placed to augment the anterior wall of the RVOT (Fig. II-29-16).

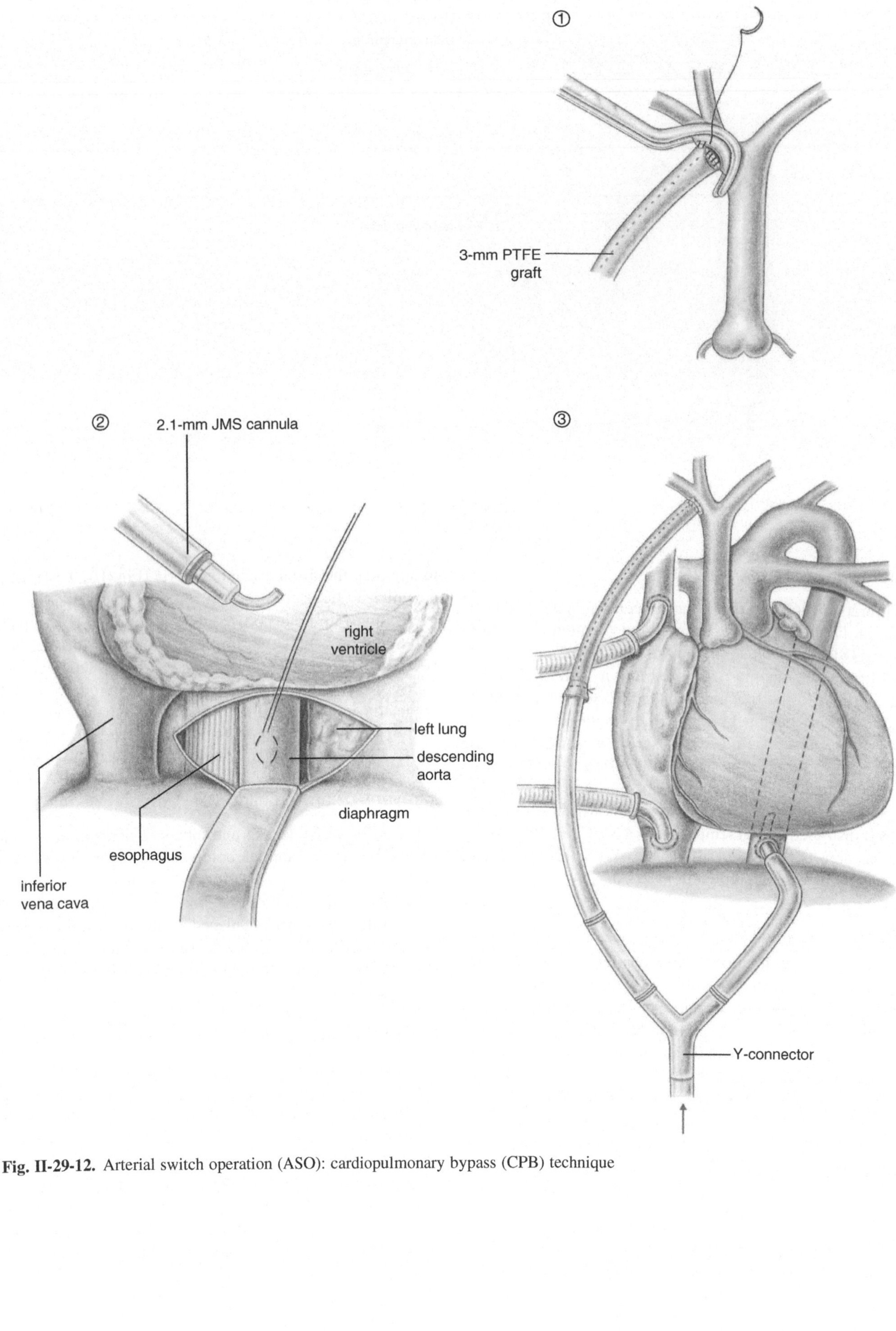

Fig. II-29-12. Arterial switch operation (ASO): cardiopulmonary bypass (CPB) technique

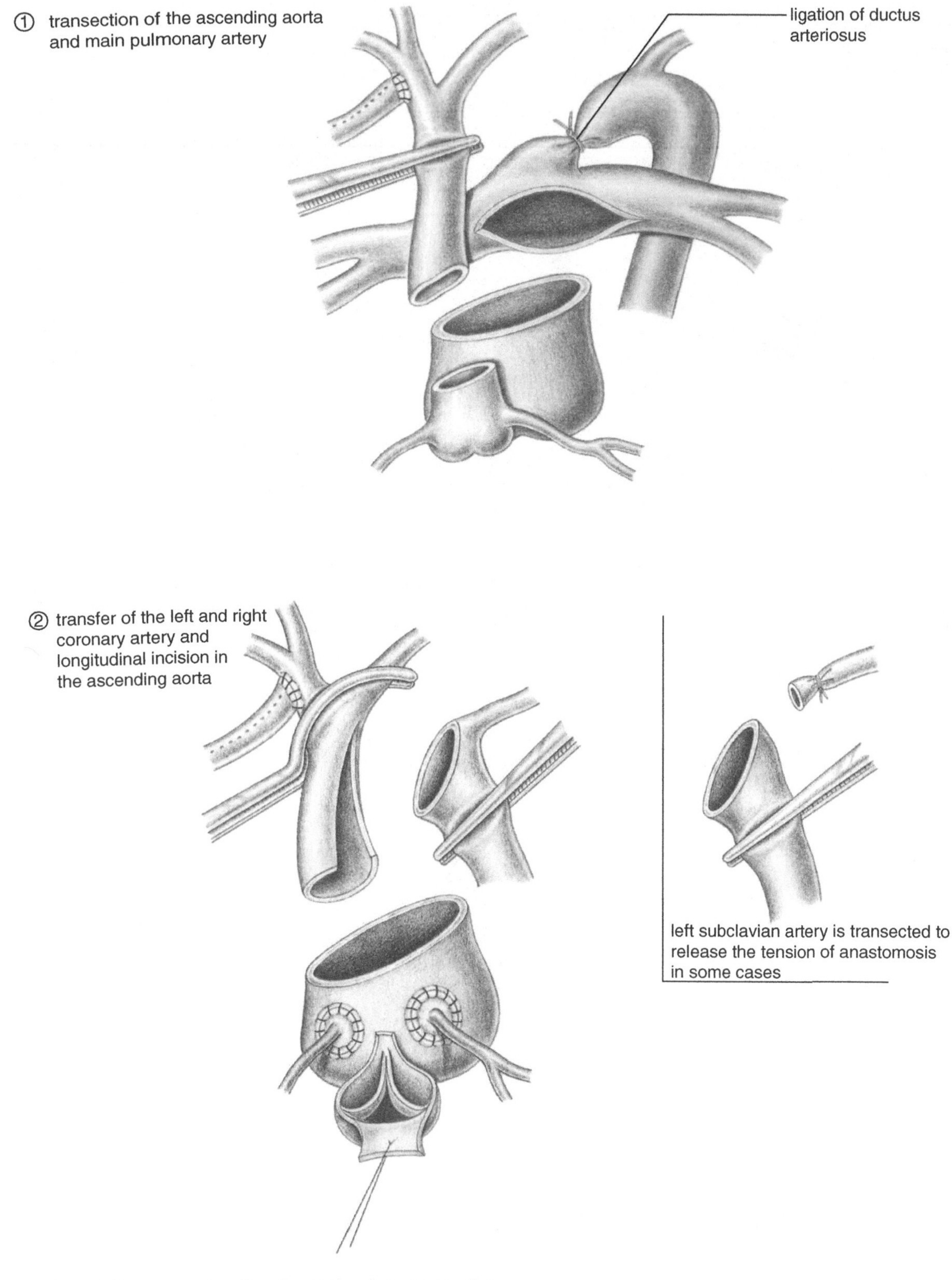

Fig. II-29-13. ASO: coronary translocation and arch reconstruction

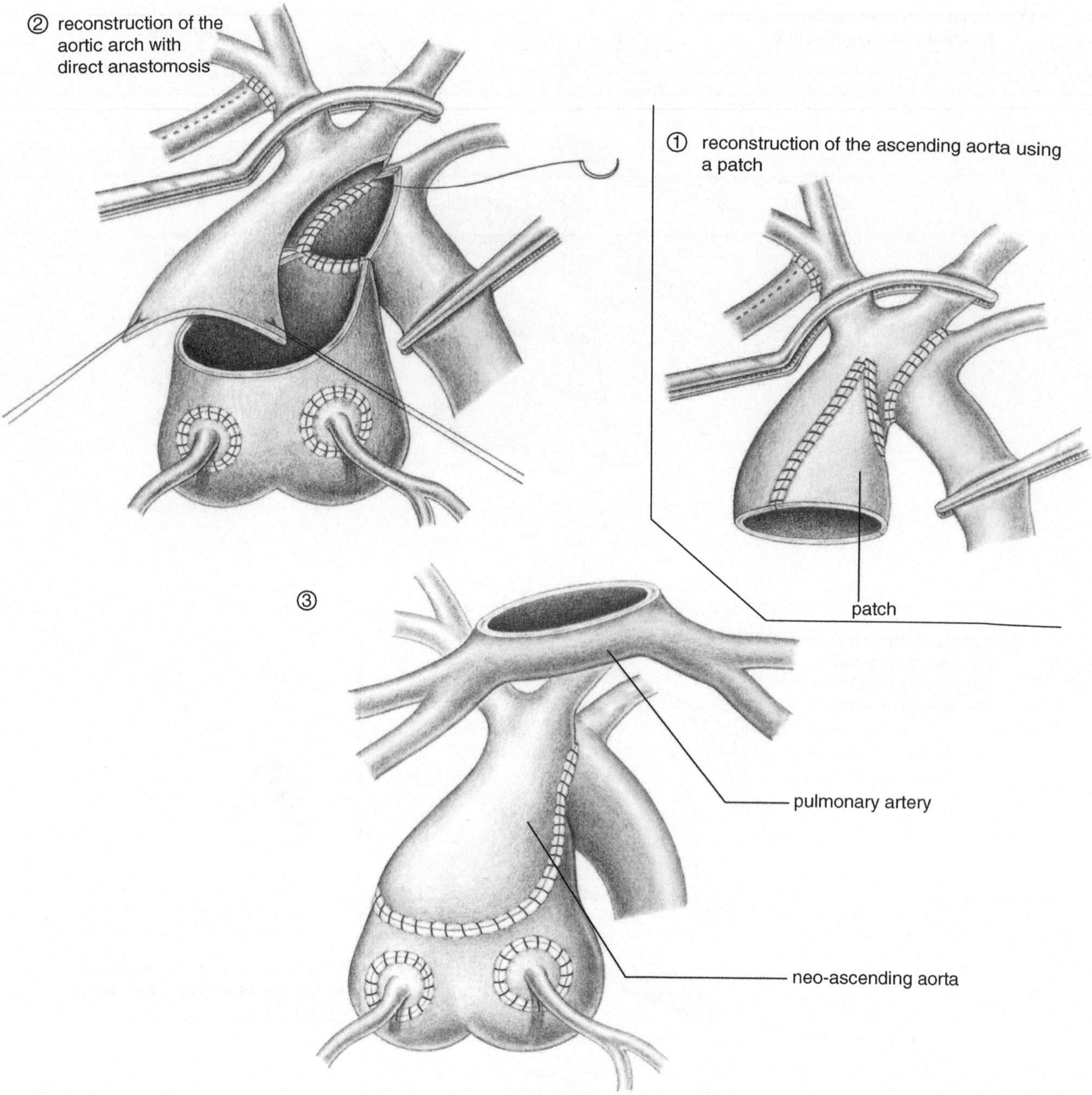

Fig. II-29-14. ASO: arch reconstruction

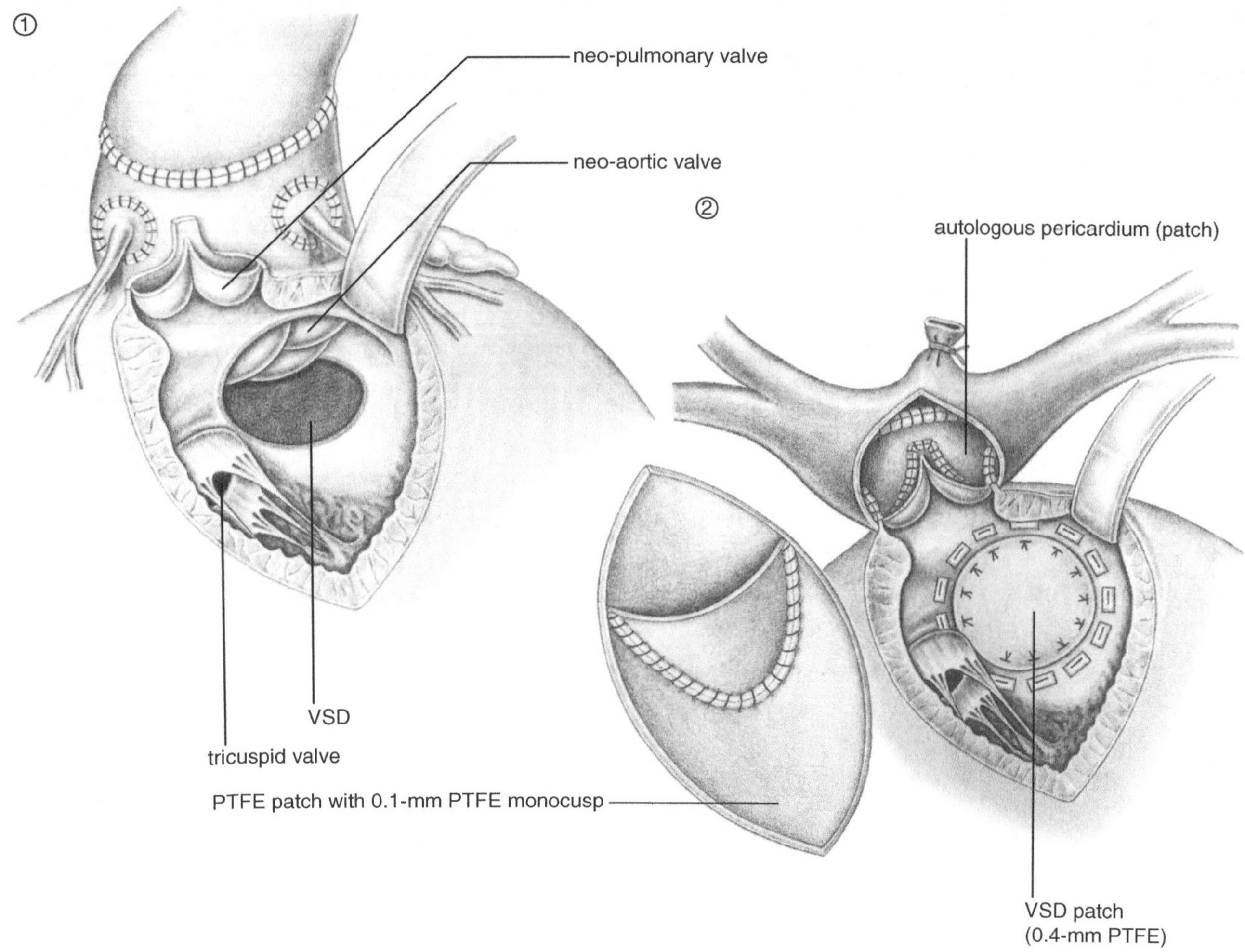

Fig. II-29-15. ASO: intraventricular rerouting

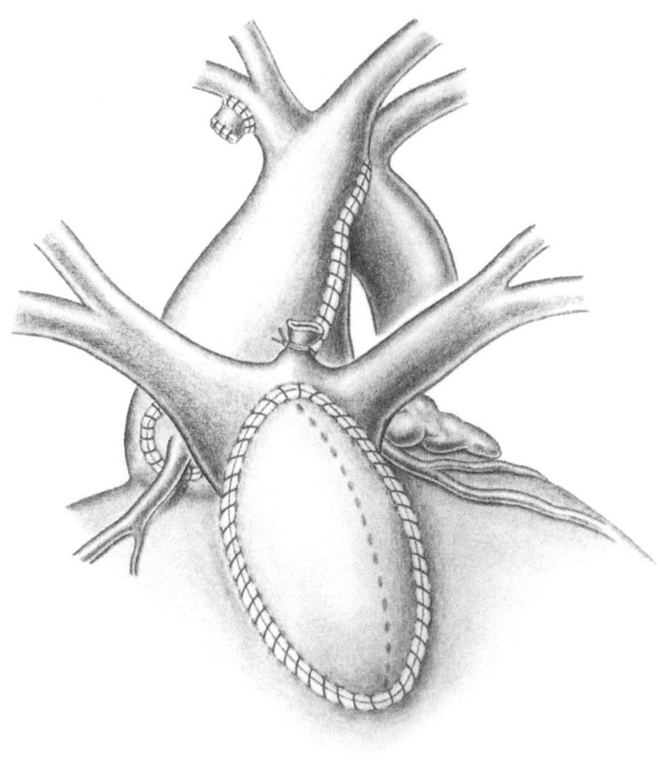

Fig. II-29-16. ASO: right ventricular outflow tract (RVOT) reconstruction. *PTFE*, polytetrafluoroethylene

References

1. Tynan MJ, Becker AE, Macartney FJ, et al (1979) Nomenclature and classification of congenital heart disease. Br Heart J 41:544–553
2. Lev M, Bharati S, Meng CC, et al (1972) A concept of double outlet right ventricle. J Thorac Cardiovasc Surg 64:271–281
3. Kurosawa H, Van Mierop LHS (1986) Surgical anatomy of the infundibular septum in transposition of the great arteries with ventricular septal defect. J Thorac Cardiovasc Surg 91: 123–132
4. Brawn WJ, Mee RB (1988) Early results for anatomic correction of transposition of the great arteries and for double-outlet right ventricle with subpulmonary ventricular septal defect. J Thorac Cardiovasc Surg 95:230–238
5. Kawashima Y, Fujita T, Miyamoto T, et al (1971) Intraventricular rerouting of blood for the correction of Taussig–Bing malformation. J Thorac Cardiovasc Surg 62:825–829
6. Patrick DL, McGoon DC (1968) An operation for double-outlet right ventricle with transposition of the great arteries. J Cardiovasc Surg (Torino) 9:537–542
7. Kawashima Y, Matsuda H, Yagihara T, et al (1993) Intraventricular repair for Taussig–Bing anomaly. J Thorac Cardiovasc Surg 105:591–596
8. Imoto Y, Kado H, Shiokawa Y, et al (1999) Norwood procedure without circulatory arrest. Ann Thorac Surg 68:559–561

II-30. Tricuspid Atresia: Bidirectional Cavopulmonary Anastomosis (Bidirectional Glenn Procedure)

Tricuspid atresia is classified into the following three groups according to the great vessel relationship:

1. Normally related great vessels (concordant ventriculoarterial connection)
2. Transposition of great vessels (discordant ventriculoarterial connection)
3. Double-outlet right ventricle or persistent truncus arteriosus

Pulmonary blood flow is determined by the sizes of the ventricular septal defect (VSD) and the infundibulum. Each group is subdivided into three groups: (A) pulmonary atresia, (B) pulmonary stenosis, and (C) without pulmonary stenosis (Fig. II-30-1).

All types of patients are managed toward ultimate Fontan physiology, but the operative strategy varies by anatomic classification. If an appropriate degree of pulmonary stenosis is present, no preliminary surgery is needed in the neonatal period. In patients with pulmonary atresia, a systemic-to-pulmonary shunt is placed in the neonatal period. In the absence of pulmonary stenosis, pulmonary artery banding is required. In the presence of transposition of the great vessels without pulmonary stenosis, aortic arch obstruction is often present, and the Norwood procedure is required. Bidirectional cavopulmonary anastomosis (BCPA) is discussed in this chapter.

Indication for Bidirectional Cavopulmonary Anastomosis (BCPA)

In all patients with a functional single ventricle, BCPA is indicated because staged progression to Fontan completion has better results as compared to single-stage total cavopulmonary connection [1]. In contrast to the hemi-Fontan procedure [2], BCPA does not require aortic cross-clamping and complex suture lines. If extracardiac Fontan completion is performed, the benefits of hemi-Fontan procedure of usage of the superior vena cava orifice for Fontan pathway are lost. Thus, hemi-Fontan operations are appropriate only for patients for whom a lateral tunnel Fontan is planned.

Surgical indications are carefully evaluated in very young infants or patients with pulmonary venous obstruction, because severe desaturation or pulmonary hypertension may occur after BCPA. After the age of 3 months, BCPA can be performed with reasonably low risk. Mild hypoplasia of the pulmonary artery does not contraindicate BCPA so long as the pulmonary vascular resistance is low. The lower limit of the size of the pulmonary artery required for successful BCPA is controversial. From our experience, a pulmonary artery index more than 100 (see supplement) is sufficient to perform BCPA. Pulmonary vascular resistance lower than 2 Wood units·m^2 is considered desirable. Preoperative pulmonary artery pressure should be assessed in conjunction with systemic-to-pulmonary blood flow ratio (Qp/Qs). If the PA pressure is greater than 20 mmHg, BCPA surgery construction is unlikely to be successful, unless the Qp/Qs is high. From the perspective of ventricular function, ejection fraction of less than 30% or atrial pressure higher than 10 mmHg is a relative contraindication to BCPA.

Operative Procedure

The heart is accessed via median sternotomy. Before bypass, the superior vena cava and the right pulmonary artery are fully dissected. The superior vena cava is dissected fully up to the jugular vein, including the innominate vein, to improve mobilization. The azygous vein is doubly ligated and divided (Fig. II-30-2). A right-angle venous cannula is inserted directly into the superior vena cava.

A second right-angle venous cannula is inserted into the inferior vena cava. If aortic cross-clamping is not necessary, the tip of the inferior vena cava cannula can be directed toward the right atrium. High-flow mildly hypothermic cardiopulmonary bypass is initiated. A tape around the superior vena cava is snugged up, and a vascular clamp is applied to the superior vena cava as close as possible to the right atrium with care taken to avoid compromising sinus node blood flow. After clamp placement, attention is paid to the electrocardiogram for a time to be certain the node has not been compromised. The superior vena cava is then divided 1 mm above the clamp site. The right atrial side is oversewn with double-layer running suture (Fig. II-30-3). If total cavopulmonary connection with an extracardiac conduit is planned as the surgical procedure for Fontan completion, stitches are tied after the clamp is released without worrying about a purse-string effect at the superior vena cava end. The tied sutures are held with a rubber-shod clamp and pulled caudally. The anterior and superior aspects of the right pulmonary artery are opened longitudinally. The surgeon holds the superior edge and the assistant holds the inferior edge. An incision is made with a sharp knife and is extended with Pott's scissors. To the leftward end of this incision, care is

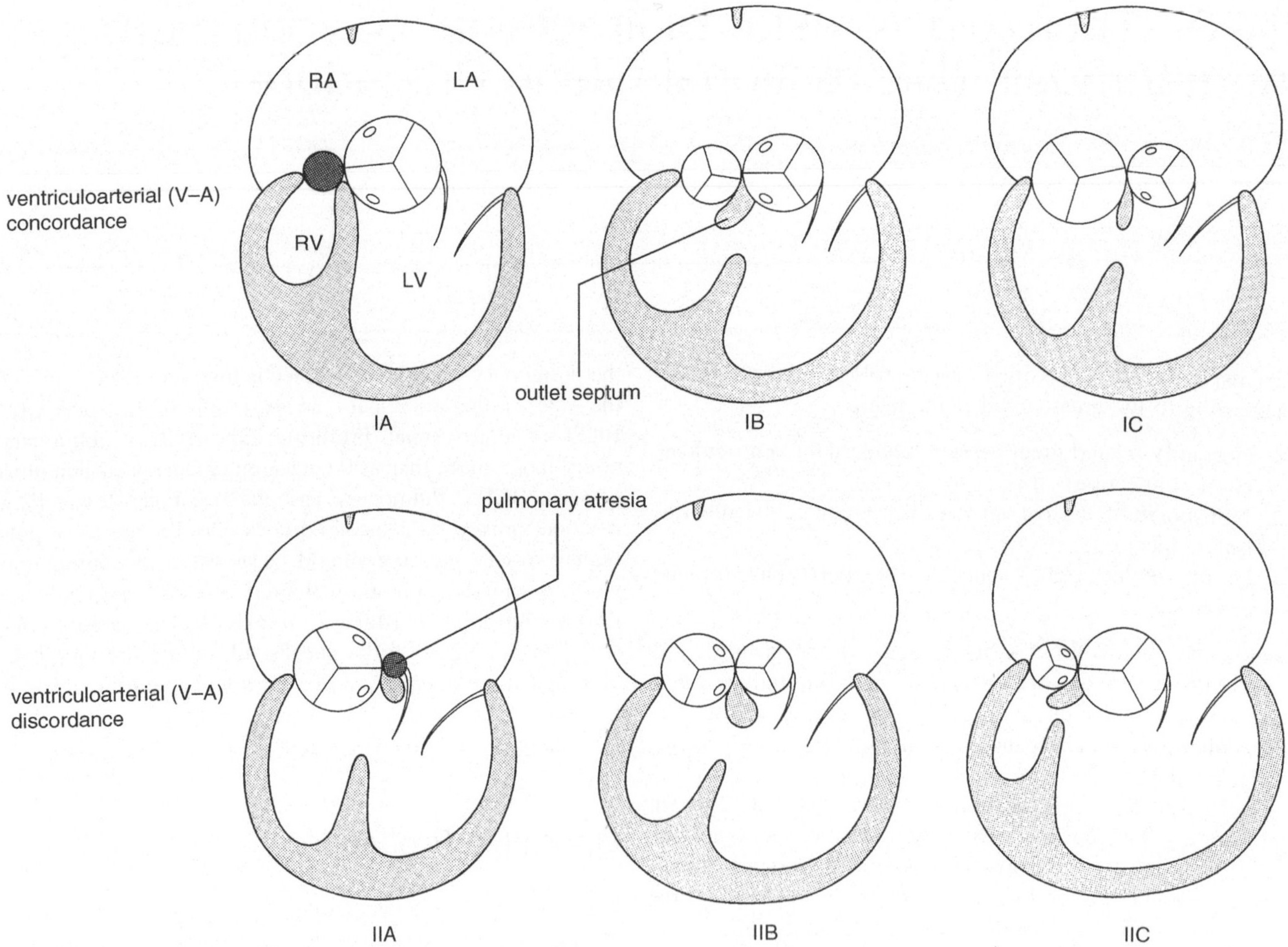

Fig. II-30-1. Classification of tricuspid atresia

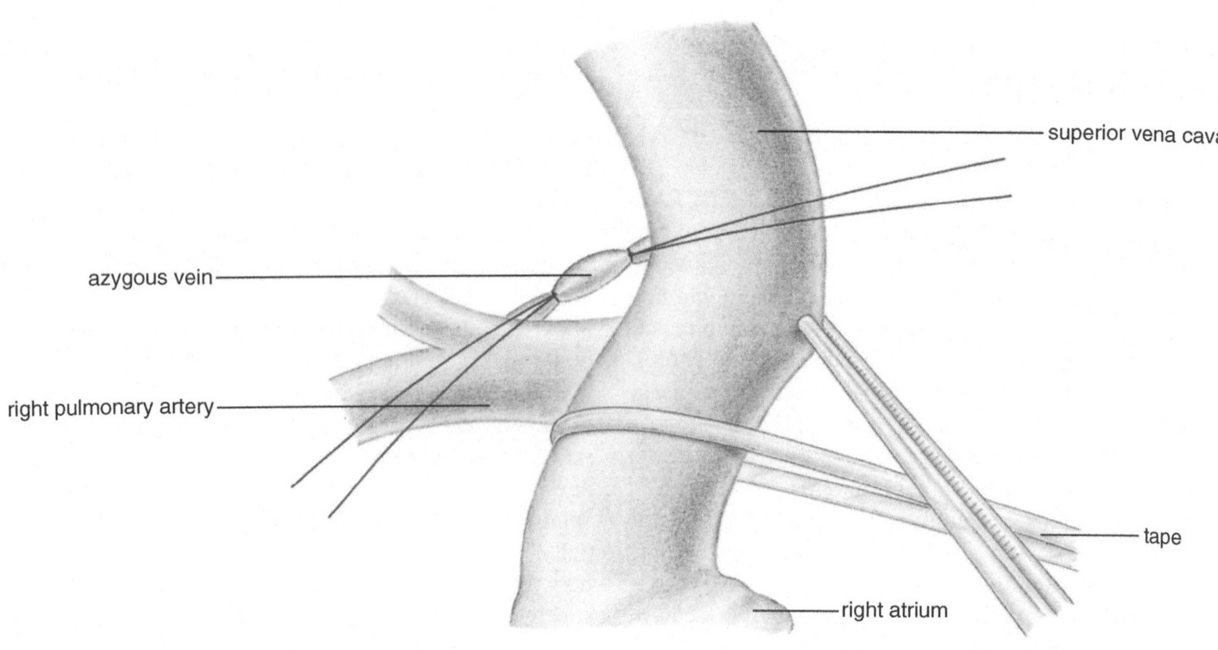

Fig. II-30-2. Ligation of the azygous vein

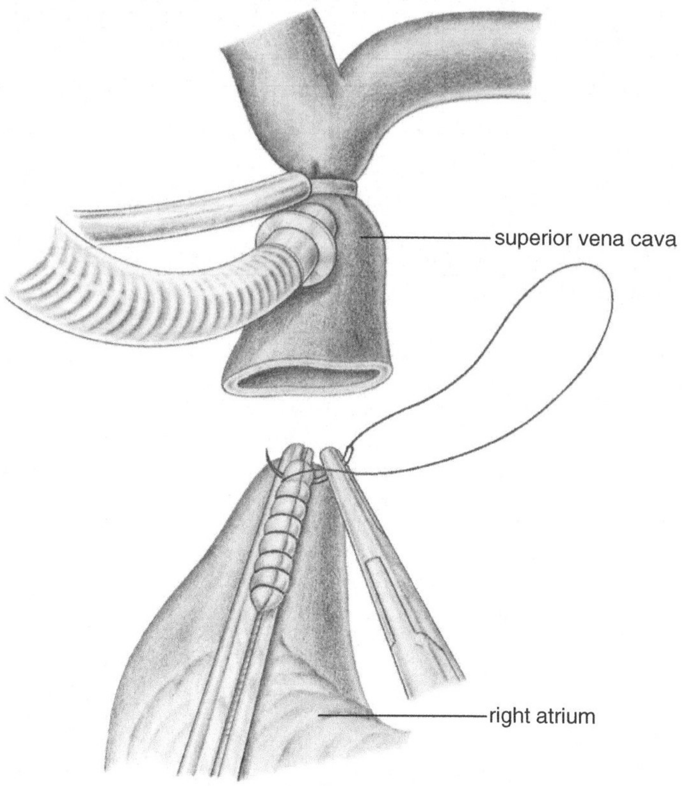

Fig. II-30-3. Closure of the proximal superior vena cava

taken to avoid compression by the ascending aorta. A stay suture is placed on the inferior edge of the pulmonary arteriotomy. The assistant holds the superior vena cava venous cannula with the right hand and relieves tension on the suture line by pushing caudally. The suture line is started at the middle of the posterior wall with care taken to avoid twisting the anastomosis (Fig. II-30-4). Alternatively, the suture line can be initiated at the left end of the arteriotomy. The assistant follows the suture with the left hand with appropriate tension to avoid a purse-string effect. At each end, great care is taken to avoid tearing the pulmonary artery, which is usually very thin walled (Figs. II-30-5, II-30-6). In the presence of a size mismatch, the anterior surface of the superior vena cava is cut longitudinally (Fig. II-30-5). Interrupted sutures are used to fashion the anterior suture line. Alternatively, if a continuous suture technique is used, an air knot is made (Fig. II-30-6). In the presence of a left superior vena cava, the surgical technique is similar. The anastomosis site is located deep, and the anastomosis is more technically difficult, as the left pulmonary artery is located posteroinferior to the aorta. The anastomosis is initiated from the left end of the arteriotomy.

If distortion of the pulmonary artery is not present after a modified Blalock–Taussig (BT) shunt, the shunt is simply divided and the anastomosis site is created on the pulmonary artery separate from the shunt site. In the presence of shunt-related pulmonary artery stenosis, the shunt tube is removed completely from the pulmonary artery. If severe stenosis is present, an untreated autologous pericardial patch is placed.

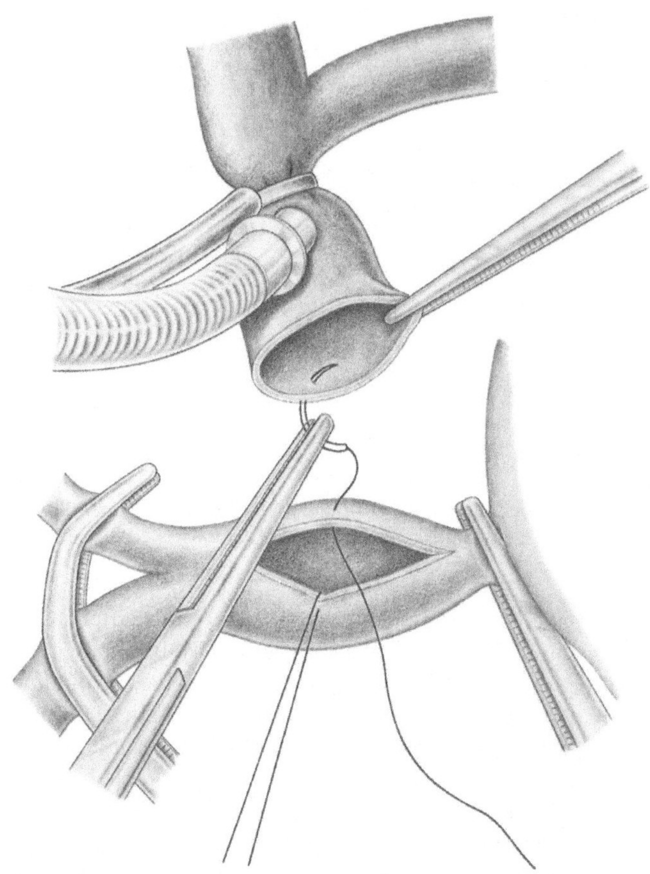

Fig. II-30-4. Initiation of the superior vena cava–right pulmonary artery anastomosis

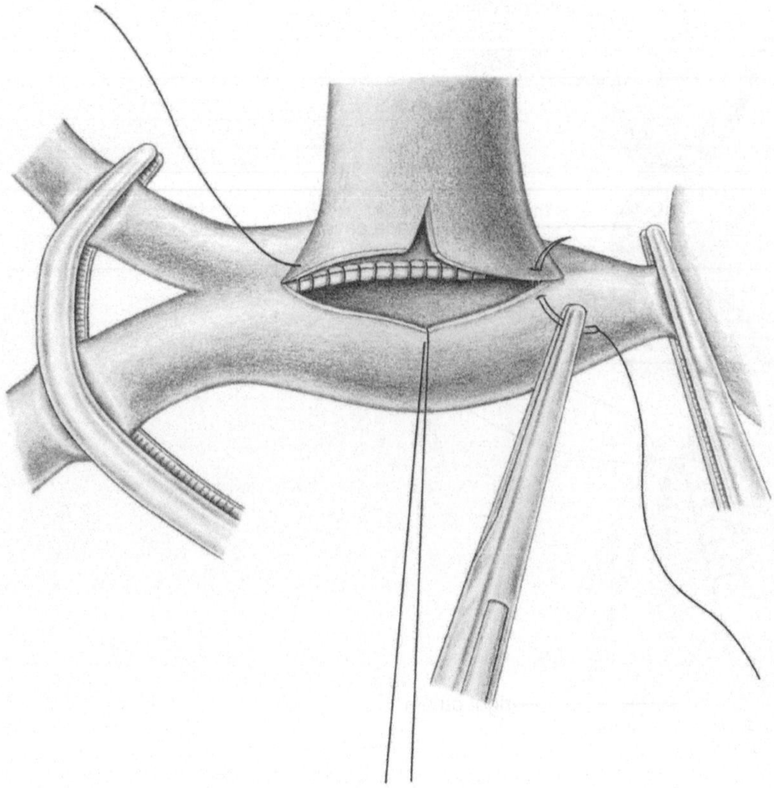

Fig. II-30-5. Enlargement of the superior vena cava

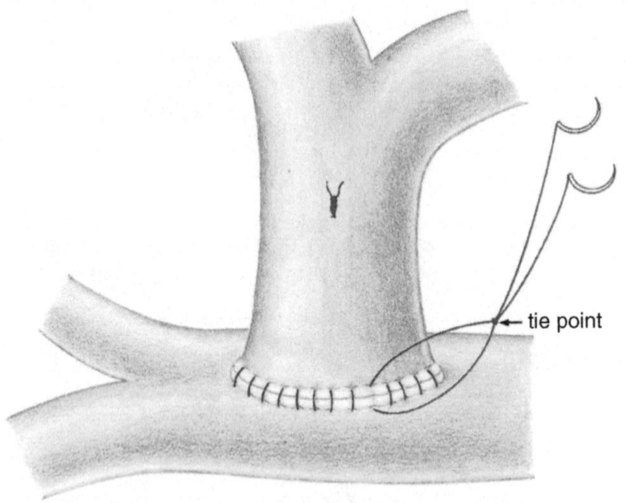

Fig. II-30-6. Completion of the superior vena cava–right pulmonary artery anastomosis. An air knot is demonstrated

In patients with bilateral superior vena cavae, after BCPA, the central pulmonary artery occasionally becomes hypoplastic or thrombosed because the respective cavopulmonary blood flows compete with each other [3]. In such cases, the central pulmonary artery is reconstructed at the time of Fontan completion. In the presence of unfavorable hemodynamic factors for Fontan circulation, such as atrioventricular valve regurgitation, restrictive interatrial communication, subaortic stenosis, or pulmonary vein stenosis, these defects should be addressed at the time of BCPA; this will minimize risk at the time of Fontan completion.

The benefit of additional pulmonary blood flow such as forward flow through the pulmonary valve or residual systemic-to-pulmonary shunt flow at the time of BCPA is still controversial. Potential advantages of additional pulmonary blood flow include higher oxygen saturation, improved growth of the pulmonary artery, and the inclusion of hepatic factors in the pulmonary circulation that may prevent formation of pulmonary arteriovenous fistula [4]. Disadvantages include persistence of volume load to the ventricle and increased pulmonary artery pressure. In the presence of ventricular dysfunction and atrioventricular valve regurgitation, additional pulmonary blood flow should be avoided. The application of banding of the main pulmonary artery, if antegrade flow is to be retained, is determined by the pulmonary artery pressure, degree of pulsatility, and arterial saturation. There are no established criteria for pulmonary artery banding at the time of BCPA, so each case is handled on its merits. When forward flow is completely eliminated, division and closure of the main pulmonary artery should be accomplished so as to avoid distortion. When the main pulmonary artery is ligated or divided, the pulmonary valve tissue should be imbricated or resected to avoid thrombus formation, which may cause systemic embolism.

References

1. Tanoue Y, Sese A, Ueno Y, et al (2001) Bidirectional Glenn procedure improves the mechanical efficiency of a total cavopulmonary connection in high-risk Fontan candidates. Circulation 103:2176–2180

2. Knott-Craig CJ, Fryar-Dragg T, Overholt ED (1995) Modified hemi-Fontan operation: an alternative definitive palliation for high-risk patients. Ann Thorac Surg 60:s554–s557
3. Iyer GKT, van Arsdell GS, Dick FP, et al (2000) Are bilateral superior vena cavae a risk factor for single ventricle palliation. Ann Thorac Surg 70:711–716
4. Uemura H, Yagihara T, Kawashima Y, et al (1995) Use of the bidirectional Glenn procedure in the presence of forward flow from the ventricles to the pulmonary arteries. Circulation 92(suppl 9):II-228–II-232

II-31. Single Ventricle: Total Cavopulmonary Connection (TCPC)

Fontan Procedure

The Fontan procedure was reported in 1971 as a functional repair for a patient with tricuspid atresia [1]. Several modifications have been introduced over the ensuing 35 years. This type of surgery is now applied to patients with all types of functional single ventricles, and those patients with two ventricles but with an anomaly that precludes biventricular repair. Initially, the atriopulmonary connection (APC) was introduced, and there is therefore the longest experience with this type of Fontan. After demonstration of improved hemodynamics, with a total cavopulmonary connection (TCPC) [2], by either lateral tunnel creation or an extracardiac conduit [3], these two versions of the Fontan procedure have been the most commonly performed. There seems to be a preference in the majority of centers for the extracardiac conduit TCPC procedure [4–6]. Advantages of the extracardiac conduit TCPC procedure include possible hemodynamic superiority [7]; avoidance of aortic cross-clamping, which may decrease ventricular function; elimination of the atrial suture lines that may predispose to late atrial arrhythmias [4]; and the ability to perform the Fontan operation in the presence of complex venous anatomy. Other factors contributing to the improvement of surgical results are a staged approach, that is, placement of a bidirectional cavopulmonary shunt between the initial operation and the final Fontan procedure [8], limitation of cardiopulmonary bypass or aortic cross-clamping, usage of ultrafiltration, and early weaning from ventilatory support. Current focus areas of research are directed toward ways to avoid or prevent ventricular dysfunction, atrial arrhythmias, protein-losing enteropathy, thrombus formation in the Fontan pathway, and pulmonary vein compression by the Fontan pathway. Because a dilated atrium late after APC often causes these complications [9], APC is increasingly converted to an extracardiac conduit TCPC in the patient with Fontan failure [10]. We routinely apply a staged approach and perform the extracardiac conduit TCPC procedure.

Ideally, the Fontan completion is performed between the ages of 2 and 4 years, although it may be performed at an even younger age. In such cases, however, it may not be possible to use a large conduit. If ventricular function is compromised, the indication of surgery must be carefully evaluated because completion of the Fontan will not improve ventricular function. If the Nakata's pulmonary artery index [11] is between 100 and 150, without significant stenosis and with low pulmonary resistance, the Fontan conversion may be accomplished at low pulmonary resistance (<2 Wood units·m^2). Even if the preoperative pulmonary artery pressure is relatively high, so long as the resistance is low, the Fontan procedure is likely to be successful. It is especially in this situation that a staged approach is of greatest value.

Extracardiac Conduit TCPC

In many cases, bidirectional cavopulmonary anastomosis (BCPA) has been performed previously, and extensive dissection may be required. It is important to fully dissect the inferior vena cava (IVC) low at the junction of the hepatic veins. To avoid compression of the right pulmonary vein by the conduit, the right pulmonary veins and right pulmonary artery (PA) are fully dissected, to keep the pulmonary veins posterior (Fig. II-31-1). When pulmonary arterioplasty is required, extensive preliminary dissection is accomplished. Otherwise, minimal dissection over the PA is preferable to shorten the time of surgery. Care is taken to avoid damaging the phrenic nerve at the time of dissection. When aortic cross-clamping is necessary for atrioventricular valve repair or atrial septal defect (ASD) enlargement, the ascending aorta is dissected.

Cardiopulmonary bypass is instituted with ascending aortic and bicaval cannulation. The IVC cannula should be placed sufficiently inferior to leave an adequate IVC cuff. Surgery is continued with mild hypothermia and the heart beating.

An expanded polytetrafluoroethylene (ePTFE) tube is used for the conduit. Graft sizes between 16 and 24 mm are determined according to the weight of the patient. In a patient less than 8 kg, a 16-mm tube is used; if weighing 8 to 20 kg, an 18-mm tube; if 20–40 kg, a 20-mm size; and in patients over 40 kg, a 24-mm tube is used. In concordant atrioventricular connection, the conduit faces the right atrium (RA), bulging to the right side and staying inside the pericardium (Fig. II-31-2). The distal end of the conduit is cut obliquely, long medially and short laterally (Fig. II-31-3). The lower end is cut straight. An incision on the right pulmonary artery (PA) is made along the inferior surface. To avoid fluid dynamic energy loss, it is believed that this anastomosis should be created slightly leftward [7]. The anastomosis can be initiated from either side. We prefer to start anastomosis from the PA end, because the visualization of the IVC is generally adequate. When forward flow through

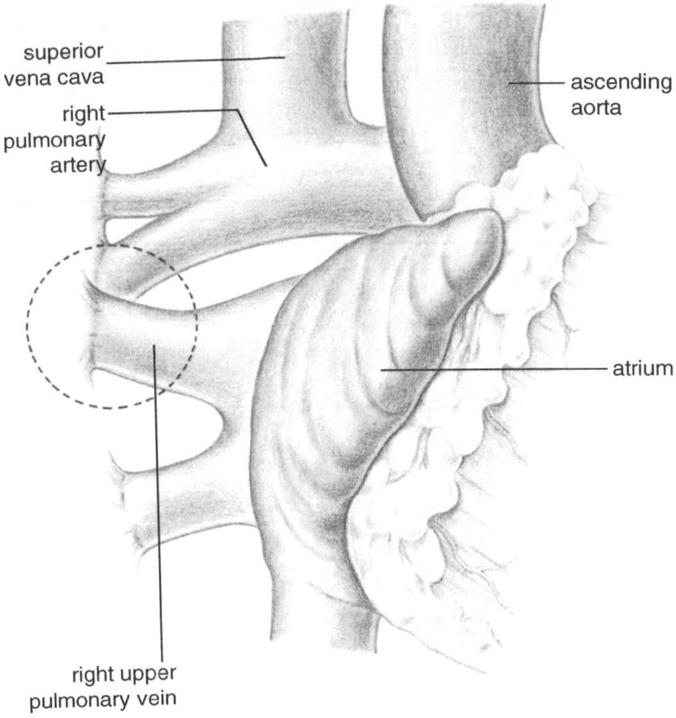

Fig. II-31-1. Dissection around the right upper pulmonary vein. To avoid right upper pulmonary vein compression by a conduit, mobilization of the right upper pulmonary vein is improved by dissection of the pulmonary vein–pericardial reflection and the space between the right lower pulmonary artery (PA) and right upper pulmonary vein

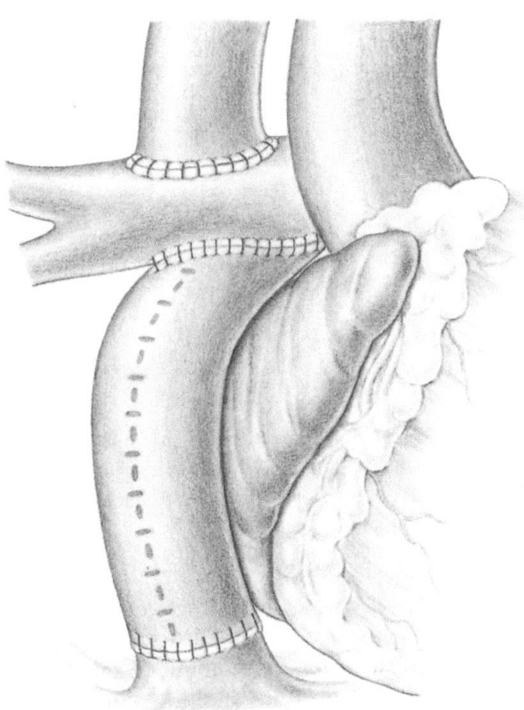

Fig. II-31-2. Completion of conduit placement. A tube graft is placed in the right side of the right atrium to create a gentle curve

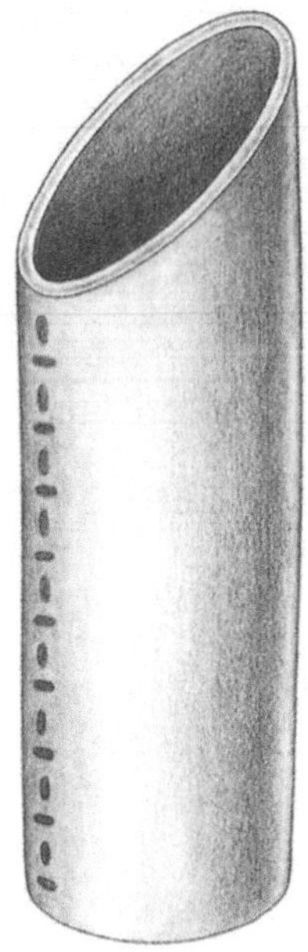

Fig. II-31-3. An expanded polytetrafluoroethylene (ePTFE) graft for the extracardiac conduit. The left superior end of the graft is cut longer and the right superior end is cut shorter, to create an oblique end. The inferior end is cut straight

the main PA is present, the main PA is divided and the proximal side is closed with running suture after the pulmonary valve tissue is oversewn to avoid thrombus formation in the main PA stump. The incision is advanced from a stump of the distal main PA to the right PA. A stay suture is placed to the anterior edge of the pulmonary arteriotomy site to keep open this arteriotomy. The anastomosis is started from the midpoint of the posterior suture line and advanced to the right (Fig. II-31-4). After the suture line comes to the right-side edge, the other suture line is carried to the left. When this suture line comes to the left side of the edge, the anterior suture line is accomplished.

A vascular clamp is applied to the IVC–atrial junction with care taken to avoid distorting the coronary sinus, and the IVC is transected (Fig. II-31-5). Before this takes place, a mattress suture is placed to the clamping site to avoid clamp slippage. To avoid IVC cuff slippage through the tourniquet, a traction suture is placed on the inferior edge of the cuff. When an aortic cross-clamp is required, the IVC transection and closure of the atrial side of IVC stump can be performed during the cross-clamp interval. The valve tissue at the IVC is excised to avoid stenosis. Suturing is initiated from the midposterior point of anastomosis using 5-0 monofilament suture (Fig. II-31-6). When the hepatic vein and the IVC return separately, venous cannulae are inserted into both vessels. The two vessels are joined at their facing edges to create one orifice for the conduit (Fig. II-31-7).

In patients with apicocaval juxtaposition, two types of surgical procedures are applied. (1) When the conduit is placed on the side opposite the apex, the IVC cuff is left long to bring the anastomosis between the IVC and conduit

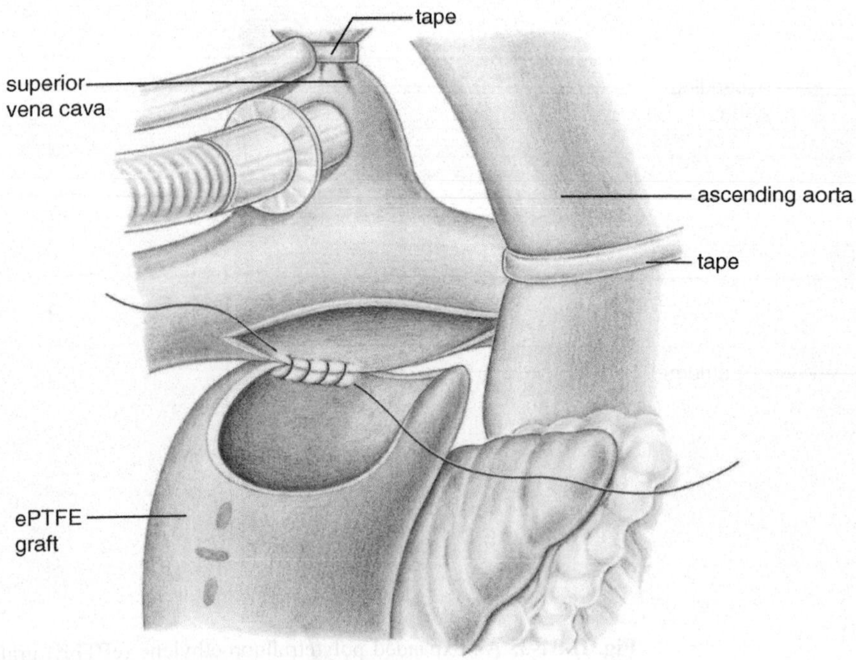

Fig. II-31-4. Anastomosis between the right PA and a graft. The ascending aorta is retracted to improve visualization

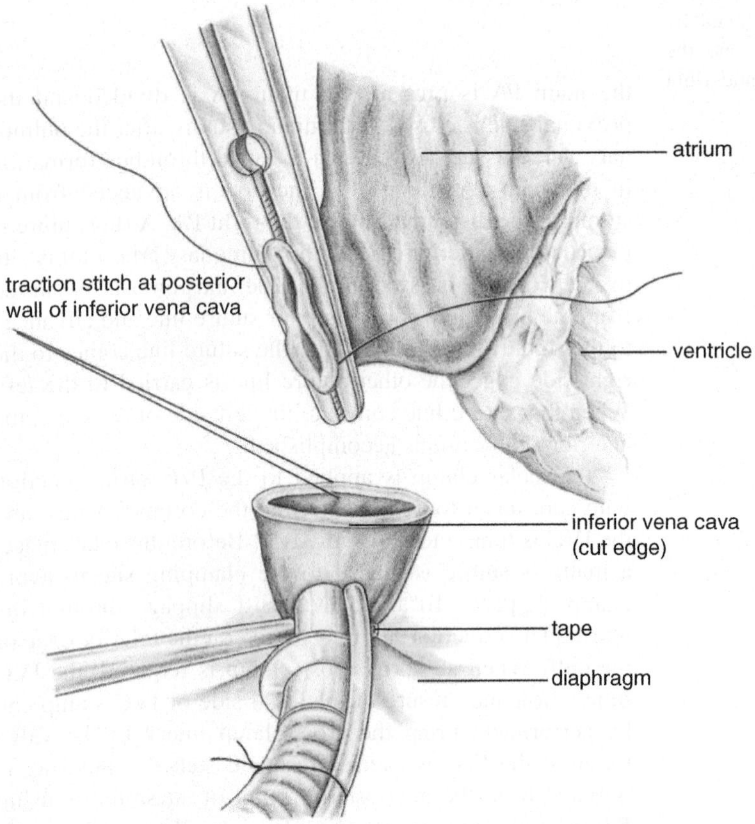

Fig. II-31-5. Transection of the inferior vena cava (IVC)–atrial junction and closure of cardiac end. The cardiac end is closed in a clamp placement using two layers of suture

to the side opposite to the apex, which avoids compression of the conduit by the spine. (2) When the conduit is placed on the same side as the apex, a longer conduit is used, creating a laterally curved pathway that prevents pulmonary vein compression by the conduit or conduit stenosis caused by compression by the apex of the heart (Fig. II-31-8).

A benefit of the extracardiac conduit TCPC procedure is the ability to create a fenestration after cardiopulmonary bypass. Side-biting clamps are applied to the conduit and atrium, and side-to-side anastomosis is performed over a 4-mm hole or a PTFE tube is interposed between the atrium and the conduit.

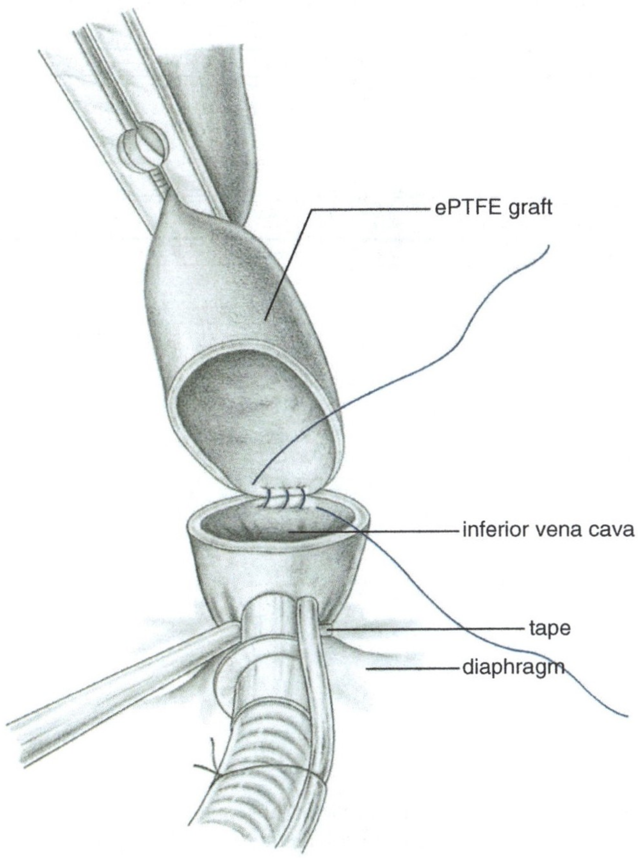

Fig. II-31-6. Anastomosis between the IVC end and a PTFE graft

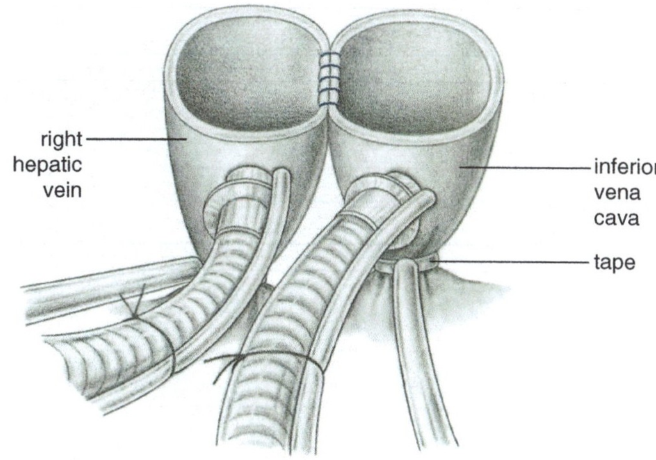

Fig. II-31-7. Separate return of the IVC and the hepatic veins. Venous cannulae are inserted to both the IVC and hepatic vein; these are combined by suturing the facing venous walls to create a double-barreled vessel. This combined orifice is anastomosed to a graft

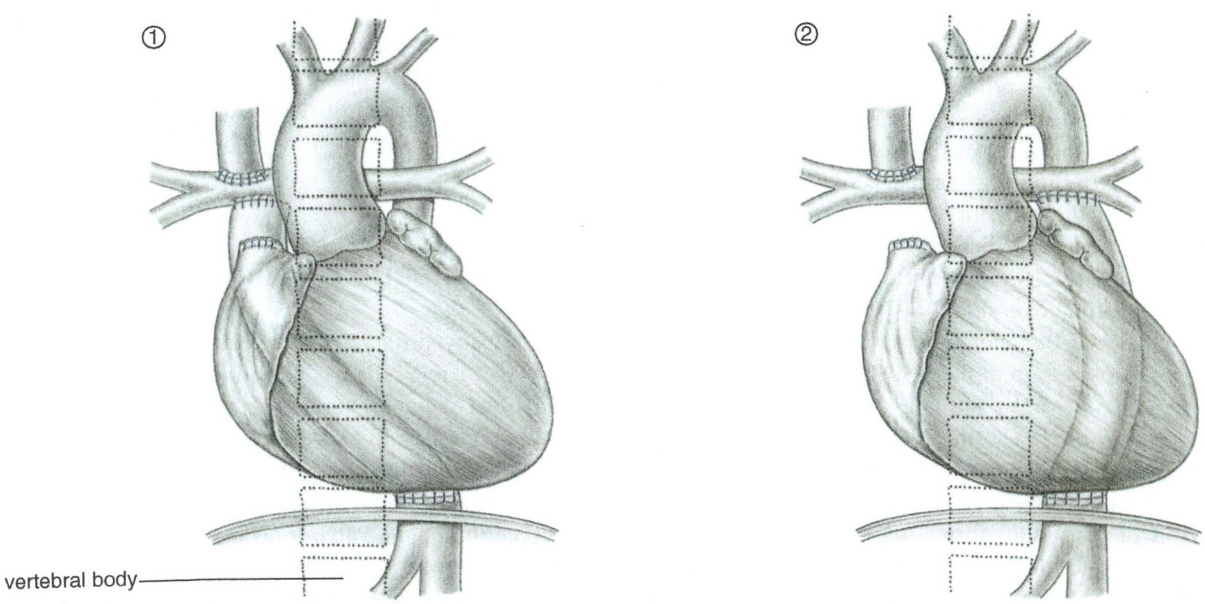

Fig. II-31-8. In the presence of apiocaval juxtaposition: ① contralateral apex conduit; ② ipsilateral apex conduit

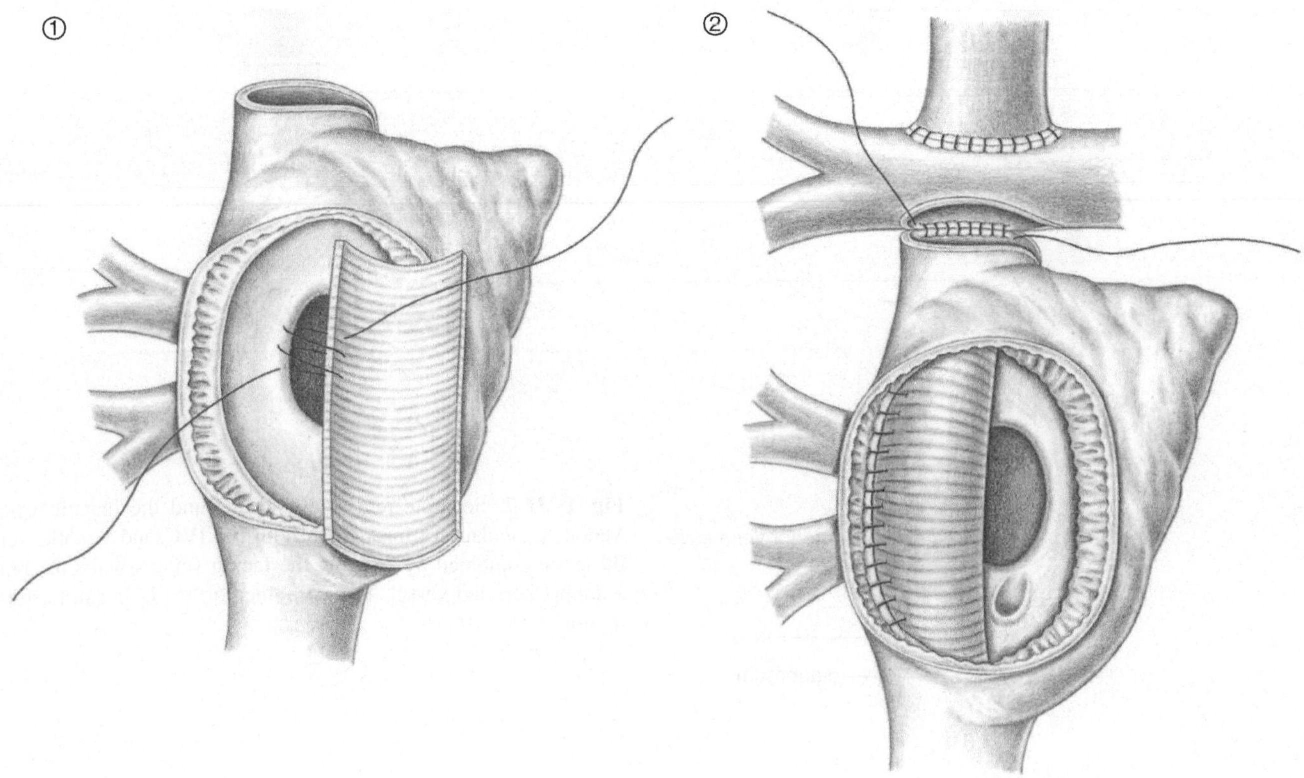

Fig. II-31-9. Lateral tunnel TCPC procedure. ① Anastomosis is started at the posterior margin of the atrial septal defect. ② The suture line of the lateral tunnel should be kept straight. The superior vena cava (SVC) site is opened and enlarged leftward before anastomosis to the right PA

Lateral Tunnel TCPC

In 1988, de Leval and colleagues [2] reported hemodynamic superiority of a lateral tunnel-type Fontan over APC-type Fontan, and many centers continue to utilize the lateral tunnel version. This procedure requires cardiopulmonary bypass and aortic cross-clamping. A right atriotomy is performed parallel to the atrioventricular groove, and the atrial septum, crista terminalis, coronary sinus, Thebesian vein, and orifices of the superior vena cava (SVC) and IVC are carefully inspected. When the ASD is restrictive, it is enlarged. A 14- to 18-mm PTFE tube is cut longitudinally to create a baffle covering 50%–70% of the circumference of the tunnel. A 5-0 monofilament running suture is initiated at the posterior margin of the ASD (Fig. II-31-9). The patch is designed to create a straight tunnel. The suture line is carried toward the IVC orifice. The coronary sinus is left to the left atrial side. When an ASD is present, the suture line is kept a distance from the orifices of the right pulmonary vein to avoid thrombus formation in the LA. The anterior suture line arrives at the crista terminalis with care to avoid leaving the space between the crista terminalis and atrial trabeculation so as not to damage the conduction system. The superior end of the crista terminalis area should be avoided while suturing as this area is trabeculated and may result in baffle leakage. When this area needs to be used for the suture line, stitches are placed to imbricate the trabeculation. The SVC end is usually enlarged leftward, because the SVC end is retracted after BCPA (Fig. II-31-9). An autologous pericardial patch may be used to enlarge this anastomosis. An incision is made on the inferior aspect of the right PA (when BCPA was performed previously, care is taken to avoid creating this anastomosis just beneath the BCPA site), and the anastomosis of the atriotomy to the PA completes the Fontan pathway.

Atrioventricular Valve Repair

When atrioventricular valve regurgitation is present at an early age, valve repair is performed at the time of BCPA to reduce the volume overload on the ventricle and minimize cardiopulmonary bypass time at the time of Fontan operation. Occasionally, the volume load reduction by BCPA alone may reduce valve regurgitation, although usually intervention on the valve is necessary if preoperative regurgitation is moderate or worse. In mitral valve regurgitation, a cleft at the anterior leaflet is often observed. In this case, cleft closure may reduce regurgitation. If the atrioventricular valve is a common valve type, as in heterotaxy syndrome, successful repair is difficult because of leaflet dysplasia and abnormality of the subvalvular apparatus (shortening of the chorda and annular dilation).

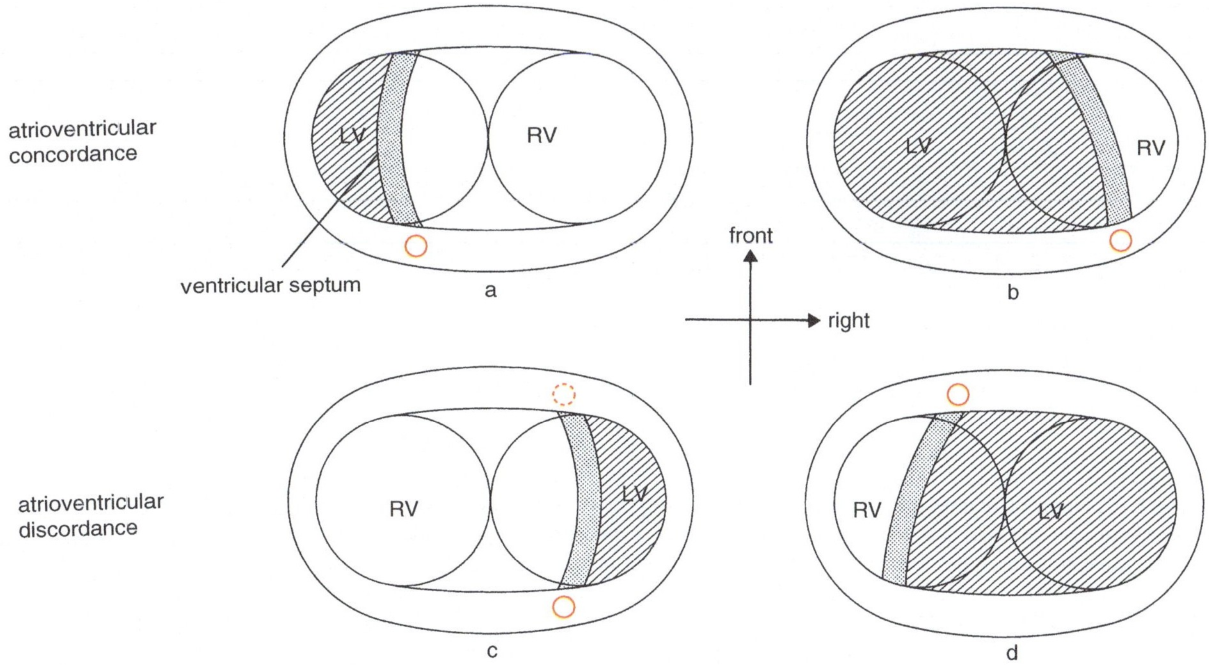

Fig. II-31-10. Possible position of the atrioventricular (AV) node in a single ventricle. *Red circle* shows possible position of the AV node. In patients with AV concordance (*a*, *b*), the AV node is located posteriorly and laterally in mitral (*a*) and tricuspid (*b*) overriding, respectively. In patients with AV discordance (*c*, *d*), the AV node is located posteriorly or both anteriorly and posteriorly in mitral overriding (*c*) and anteriorly in tricuspid (*d*) overriding. *LV*, left ventricle; *RV*, right ventricle

Circular Annuloplasty or Partial Circular Annuloplasty

Avoiding damage to the conduction system is challenging with this surgical procedure (Fig. II-31-10). After identification of the ventricular septum, one avoids placing sutures to the annulus above the septum, and sutures are placed to the leaflet itself to protect the conduction system. In right ventricle (RV) type and concordant atrioventricular (AV) connection single ventricle, the AV node is located at the posterior portion of the ventricular septum. In left ventricle (LV) type, the AV node is situated at the posterolateral portion of the ventricular septum. In RV type and discordant AV connection single ventricle, the AV node is located at the posterior node or both anterior and posterior nodes. In LV type and discordant AV connection single ventricle, the AV node is located at the anterior node [12]. When the ventricular septum is not identified, the area around the posterior node is not used to protect the conduction system during annuloplasty.

Double-layer 3-0 braided sutures are utilized for annuloplasty. These sutures are attached to felt pledgets at each end. At the area where the conduction system is thought to be located, sutures are placed in the valve itself. The size of the annuloplasty is limited to 80% or more of the diameter of the normal mitral valve annulus by Rowlatt (see Supplement, Fig. 1). In pediatric patients, total circumferential annuloplasty is avoided to maintain growth potential.

Creation of a Double Orifice in the Common Atrioventricular Valve

This surgical procedure is effective for the patient with two relatively equal-sized ventricles. The anterior and posterior bridging leaflets are sutured to each other with pledgetted mattress sutures, and double orifices are created (Fig. II-31-11). In the patient with the common AV valve and AV discordance, as both anterior and posterior AV nodes are considered to be present, an annuloplasty suture is placed, thus avoiding the annulus at the ventricular septum (Fig. II-31-11). When valve regurgitation is predominantly through one orifice, that orifice is closed completely and an annuloplasty is performed on the other orifice to create 80% of the normal valve annulus.

Valvuloplasty for Subvalvular Apparatus

When valve prolapse with chordal elongation or rupture is present, an artificial chord constructed of PTFE suture can be placed. In a tricuspid valve or common AV valve, valvuloplasty with an artificial chord has limited effect. When the coaptation site is shifted to the apex of the heart by shortening of the chord, valvuloplasty is fairly difficult, and valve replacement may be necessary.

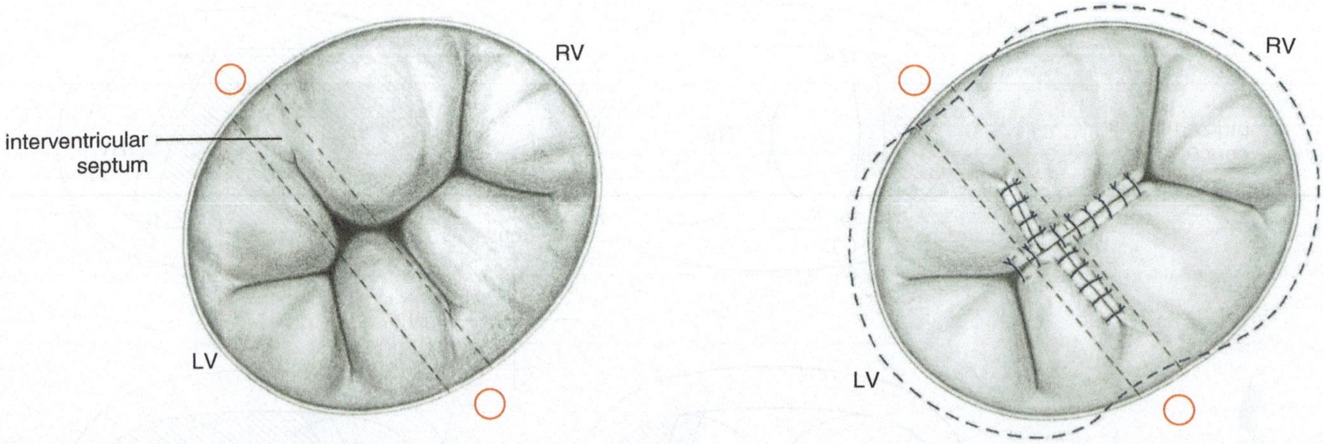

Fig. II-31-11. Creation of double-orifice valve. *Left:* in patients with a common AV valve and functional single ventricle, when the ventricular septum is identified, possible positions of the anterior and posterior AV nodes can be recognized. *Right:* when annuloplasty is performed, the sutures are placed to avoid these possible locations of the AV nodes

References

1. Fontan F, Baudet E (1971) Surgical repair of tricuspid atresia. Thorax 26:240–248
2. de Leval MR, Kilner P, Gewillig M, et al (1988) Total cavopulmonary connection: a logical alternative to atriopulmonary connection for complex Fontan operations. Experimental studies and early clinical experience. J Thorac Cardiovasc Surg 96:682–695
3. Marcelletti C, Corno A, Giannico S, et al (1990) Inferior vena cava-pulmonary artery extracardac conduit. A new form of right heart bypass. J Thorac Cardiovasc Surg 100:228–232
4. Azakie A, McCrindle BW, Arsdell GV, et al (2001) Extracardiac conduit versus lateral tunnel cavopulmonary connections at a single institution: impact on outcomes. J Thorac Cardiovasc Surg 122:1219–1228
5. Haas GS, Hess H, Black M, et al (2000) Extracardiac conduit Fontan procedure: early and intermediate results. Eur J Cardiothorac Surg 17:648–654
6. Petrossian E, Reddy VM, McElhinney DB, et al (1999) Early results of the extracardiac conduit operation. J Thorac Cardiovasc Surg 117:688–696
7. Lardo AC, Webber SA, Friehs I, et al (1999) Fluid dynamic comparison of intra-atrial and extracardiac cavopulmonary connections. J Thorac Cardiovasc Surg 117:697–704
8. Masuda M, Kado H, Shiokawa Y, et al (1998) Clinical results of the staged Fontan procedure in high-risk patients. Ann Thorac Surg 65:1721–1725
9. Van Son JAM, Mohr FW, Hambsch J, et al (1999) Conversion of atriopulmonary or lateral tunnel cavopulmonary anastomosis to extracardiac conduit Fontan modification. Eur J Cardiothorac Surg 15:150–158
10. Mavroudis C, Backer CL, Deal BJ, et al (2001) Total cavopulmonary conversion and maze procedure for patients with failure of the Fontan operation. J Thorac Cardiovasc Surg 122:863–871
11. Nakata S, Imai Y, Takanashi Y, et al (1984) A new method for the quantitative standardization of cross-sectional areas of the pulmonary arteries in congenital heart diseases with decreased pulmonary blood flow. J Thorac Cardiovasc Surg 88:610–619
12. Kurosawa H, Becker AE (1987) Congenitally corrected transposition and double inlet ventricle. In: Kurosawa H, Becker AE (eds) Atrioventricular conduction in congenital heart disease. Springer-Verlag, Tokyo, pp 225–253

II-32. Hypoplastic Left Heart Syndrome: Norwood Procedure

A staged approach is utilized in this disease, resulting ultimately in the Fontan circulation. The first stage is the Norwood procedure, performed in the neonatal period. The key points of this procedure are the following: (1) unobstructed systemic circulation, (2) adequate pulmonary blood flow, (3) unrestrictive atrial communication, (4) preserved coronary circulation, and (5) preserved right ventricular function. Before surgery, a meticulous survey should be made of the following anatomic factors: the presence of aortic coarctation, the size and shape of the aortic arch, the size and shape of the ascending aorta, size and function of the aortic and pulmonary valves, adequacy of the atrial communication, and the degree of tricuspid valve regurgitation.

Operative Procedure

There are several alternative surgical procedures applied for aortic arch reconstruction and creation of pulmonary blood flow. In the United States, a homograft patch is most commonly used for arch reconstruction. In Japan, a xenograft patch has been used, and recently arch reconstruction without a patch has been performed [1]. Three general approaches to the ascending aorta and arch have been taken, with consistent focus on preservation of coronary perfusion. (1) The ascending aorta is not cut but is kept intact in its entire length, and arch repair is performed. (2) The entire length of the ascending aorta is opened longitudinally and used for neo-aortic reconstruction. (3) The ascending aorta is transected, longitudinal incisions are made into the facing sinuses of Valsalva, and side-by-side anastomosis is made to the main pulmonary artery.

To provide pulmonary blood flow, a central shunt was originally used. Currently, a modified Blalock–Taussig (BT) shunt between the brachiocephalic artery and right pulmonary artery is more commonly used if the source of pulmonary blood flow is the systemic artery-to-pulmonary artery shunt. In Japan, at the majority of centers, a right ventricle-to-pulmonary artery (RV–PA) conduit has gained popularity, and with this modification better surgical results seems to have been obtained [2,3]. Deep hypothermic circulatory arrest (DHCA) has been used traditionally in many centers during aortic reconstruction, although recently regional cerebral perfusion, via the brachiocephalic artery, has been preferred because it is believed to provide superior central nervous system protection. Perfusion through the descending aorta is also combined in some institutions to maintain lower body circulation and eliminate the need for deep hypothermia, thus possibly preventing coagulopathy [4,5]. In this chapter, cardiopulmonary bypass without circulatory arrest, arch reconstruction with and without a patch, and both alternatives for pulmonary blood flow are discussed and demonstrated.

Establishment of Cardiopulmonary Bypass

Via standard median sternotomy, the ascending aorta, aortic arch, arch branches, branch pulmonary arteries, and both vena cavae are dissected and tapes are placed. If necessary, the ascending aorta may be dissected during cardiopulmonary bypass to avoid coronary insufficiency. After heparin is administered, a C-shaped clamp is applied to the brachiocephalic artery, and a polytetrafluoroethylene (PTFE) tube is anastomosed. For patients under 3.0 kg, a 3-mm tube is used; for those over 3.0 kg, a 3.5-mm tube is chosen. A Y-shaped connector is placed in the arterial side of the bypass circuit. An aortic cannula is inserted into the PTFE tube and connected to the Y-connector (Fig. II-32-1). Because this PTFE tube may later be used as the modified Blalock–Taussig shunt, the PTFE tube is anastomosed to the lateral aspect of the brachiocephalic artery to avoid kinking of the shunt. One venous cannula is inserted into the inferior vena cava through the right atrium, and bypass is initiated. Tapes around the branch pulmonary arteries are fastened. After initiation of bypass, a right-angled arterial cannula is inserted into the descending aorta at the level of the diaphragm via an incision in the posterior pericardium (see Figs. II-4-5 and II-4-6) [6].

A second venous cannula is inserted into the superior vena cava from the right atrial appendage. In a small neonate, a venous cannula is not inserted into the superior vena cava, and a pump sucker is used during the atrial septectomy, which is performed in all cases. In patients with aortic atresia, the intracardiac procedure can be performed while the heart is beating. The ductus is subsequently ligated.

Aortic Arch Reconstruction

The arch branches are mobilized completely and a vascular clamp is applied between the brachiocephalic and left carotid

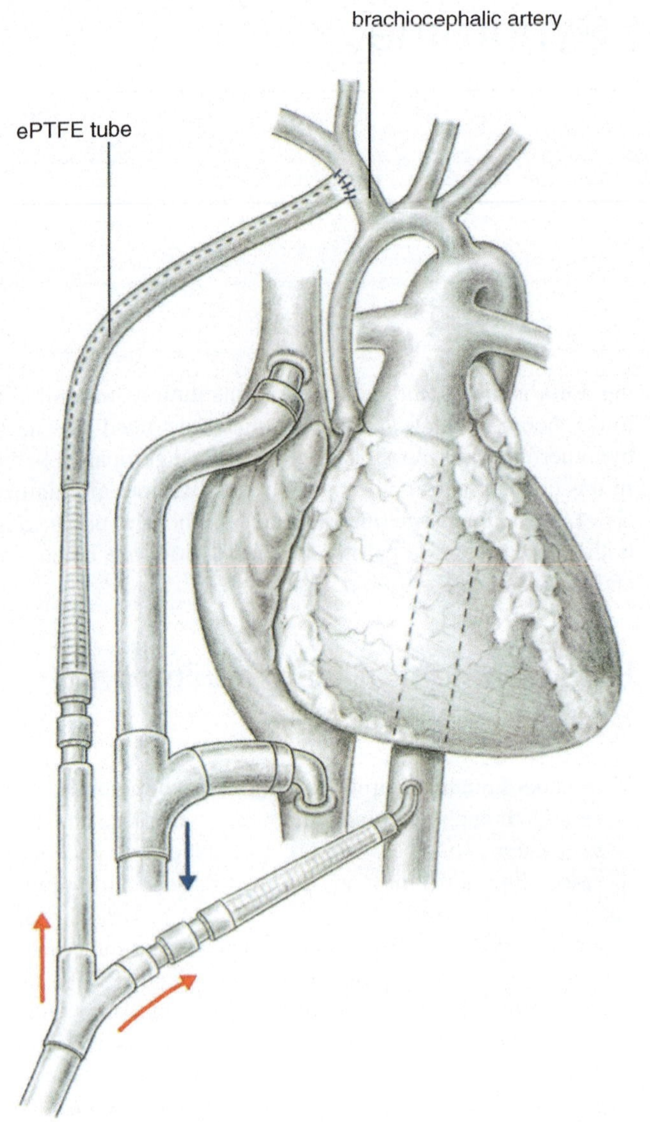

Fig. II-32-1. Cardiopulmonary bypass without circulatory arrest with arterial perfusion through the brachiocephalic artery and the descending aorta

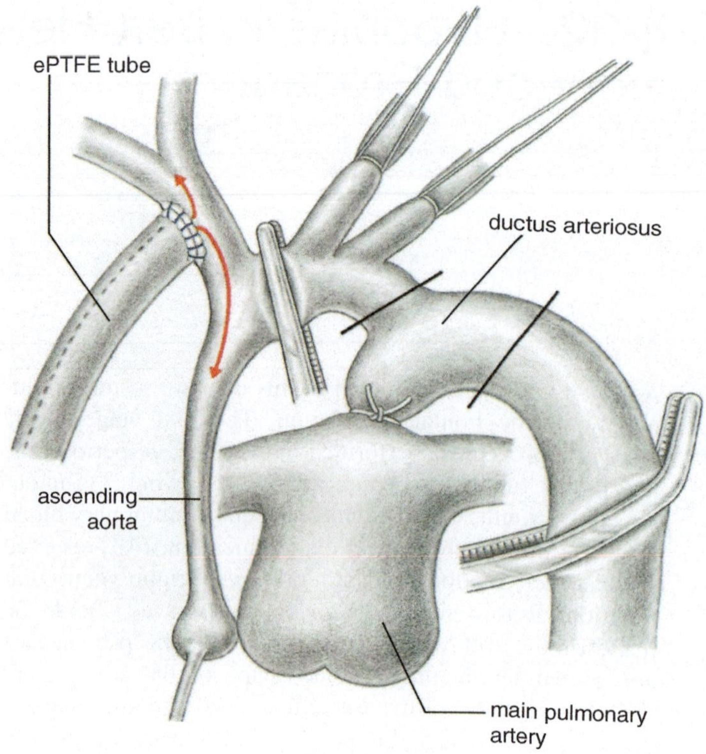

Fig. II-32-2. Ligation of ductus arteriosus and excision of ductal tissue. All ductal tissue is removed from the aorta. The *two straight lines* indicate division lines

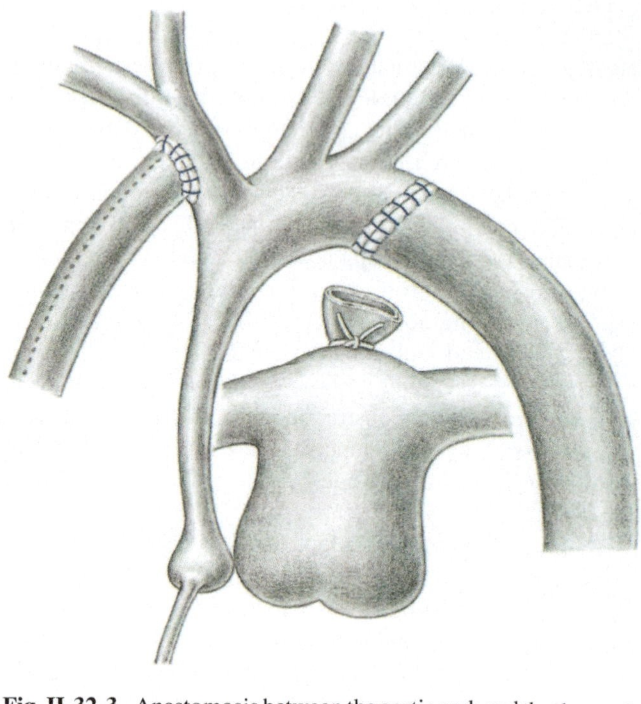

Fig. II-32-3. Anastomosis between the aortic arch and the descending aorta with 7-0 polydioxanone (PDS) running suture

arteries. The left carotid and subclavian arteries are controlled with encircling heavy silk string or vessel loops. A vascular clamp is applied to the descending aorta. The duct is divided distal to the ligation site. Ductal tissue should be completely removed, even if the coarctation seems mild, to avoid recurrent coarctation in the late postoperative period (Fig. II-32-2). Further caudal dissection of the descending aorta is easily performed after ductal tissue resection. With division of the first one or two sets of intercostal arteries, when necessary, mobilization of the descending aorta is enhanced. During this period, perfusion of the head, heart, and lower body is maintained. The aortic arch and the descending aorta are anastomosed with running suture (Fig. II-32-3).

The main pulmonary artery is transected proximal to its bifurcation. The left branch pulmonary artery typically originates distal to the right branch pulmonary artery, and so the main pulmonary artery is transected obliquely (Fig. II-32-4). A key technical point is that the anterior portion of the main pulmonary artery is opened 1 cm proximal to the duct ligation site. The orifices of the branch pulmonary arteries are identified from the inside, and the main pulmonary artery is transected. The distal main pulmonary artery is repaired with an autologous pericardial patch.

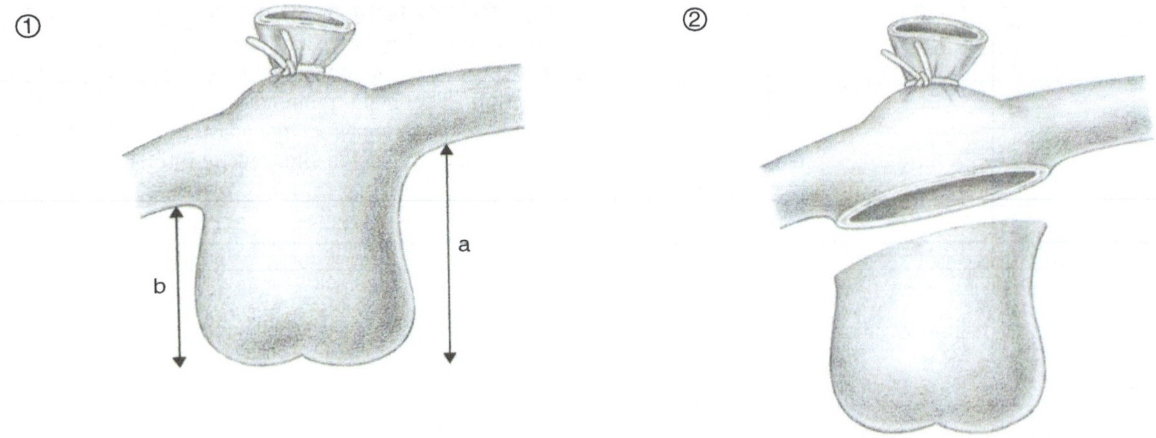

Fig. II-32-4. The shape and transection line of the main pulmonary artery. ① The left branch pulmonary artery typically originates distal to the right branch pulmonary artery. *a* is significantly longer than *b*. ② Transection of the main pulmonary artery is proximal to the take-off of the branch pulmonary arteries

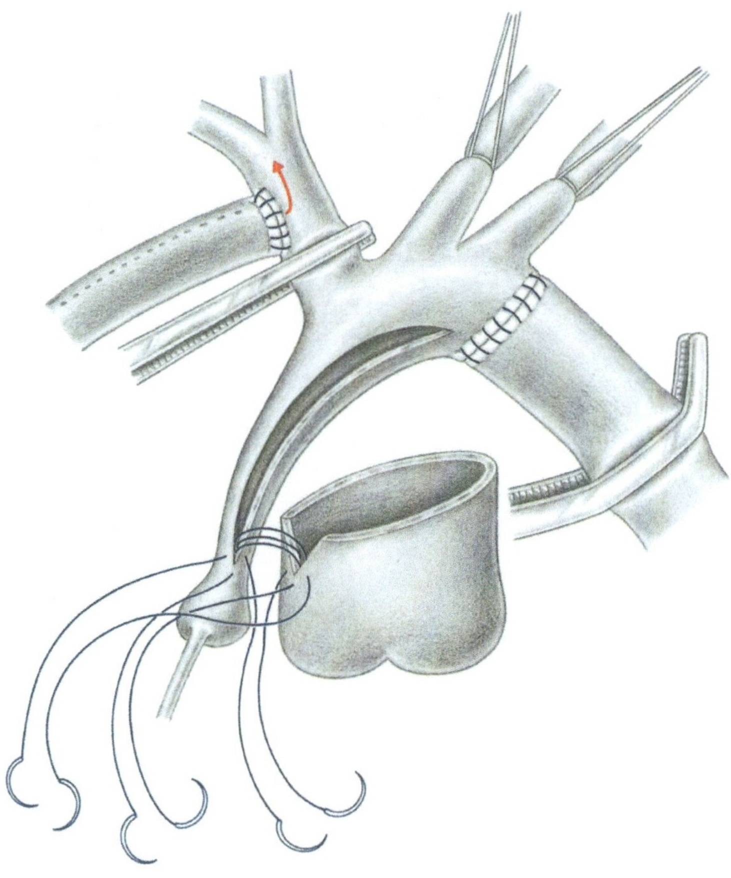

Fig. II-32-5. Anastomosis of the ascending aorta and the main pulmonary artery with PDS sutures

The ascending aorta is opened longitudinally, and cardioplegic solution is injected through this opening. This aortotomy is brought down to the base of the ascending aorta. The main pulmonary artery and the ascending aorta are directly anastomosed, taking care to avoid stenosis of the coronary source (Fig. II-32-5). The incision on the ascending aorta terminates above the sinotubular junction to avoid coronary injury. A wedge incision is made to the main pulmonary artery opposite the incision in the ascending aorta. This relationship of the aortic incision to the pulmonary artery incision is shown in Fig. II-32-6. To avoid coronary stenosis, interrupted sutures are used at the lowest part of the anastomosis, which is then completed between the obliquely transected pulmonary artery and the aortotomy. After neo-aortic reconstruction, de-airing is accomplished and coronary perfusion is resumed by releasing the clamp on the brachiocephalic artery. The snares on the arch branches are removed.

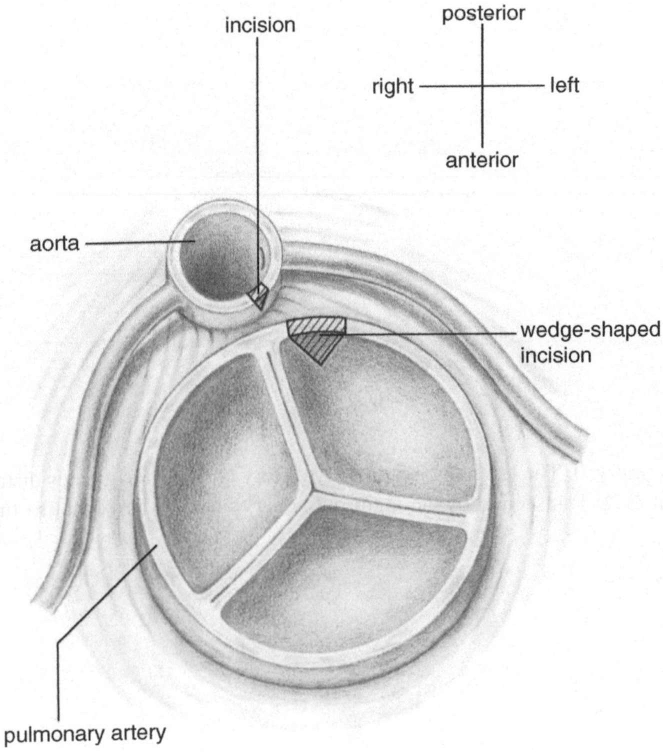

Fig. II-32-6. Incisions in the ascending aorta and the main pulmonary artery. Incisions are made at the *shaded positions*. The incision in the ascending aorta is kept above the sinotubular junction. The main pulmonary arterial wall is excised in a wedge shape to create a large anastomosis. At the bottom of this wedge-shaped incision site, several interrupted sutures are used

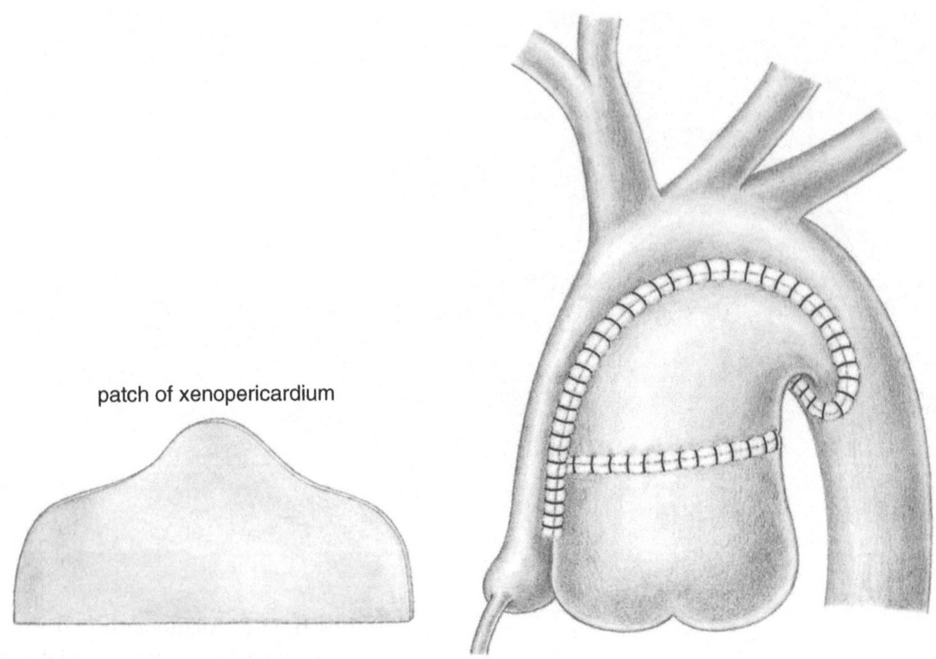

Fig. II-32-7. Neo-aortic arch reconstruction: 1. The aortic arch is reconstructed using a xenopericardial patch

Other Arch Reconstruction Techniques

If the aortic arch is hypoplastic, a homograft or xenograft patch maybe used to augment the arch. A tube graft should not be created, and continuity with autologous tissue must be maintained to allow for growth even if using a foreign material for arch reconstruction (Fig. II-32-7). When hypoplastic arch reconstruction is pursued without patch material, half the descending aorta is anastomosed to the distal part of the aortic arch, before aortic cross-clamp (Fig. II-32-8), and a tube graft should be avoided. After aortic cross-clamp, the main pulmonary artery is anastomosed to the arch. Another technique is shown in Fig. II-32-9. In this technique, the entire arch is reconstructed

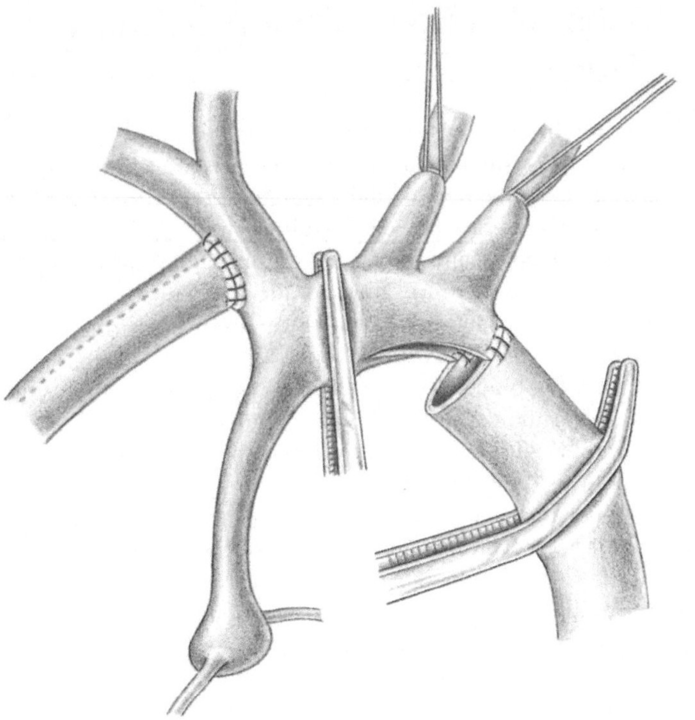

Fig. II-32-8. Neo-aortic arch reconstruction: 2. When the aortic arch is small, the distal aortic arch and part of the descending aorta (about half the circumference) are anastomosed

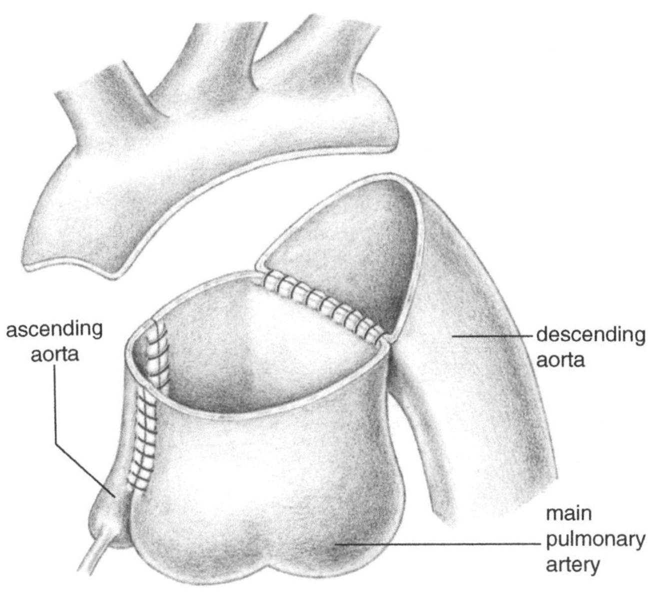

Fig. II-32-9. Neo-aortic arch reconstruction: 3. After aortic cross-clamping, the base of the neo-aorta is reconstructed, and then the left side of the main pulmonary artery and one-third of the right side of the descending aorta are anastomosed. Finally, the isolated aortic arch is sutured to the confluence

after aortic cross-clamping. The ascending aorta is transected and anastomosed to the facing main pulmonary artery in a side-to-side fashion. One-third of the circumference of the descending aorta and main pulmonary artery is anastomosed. The inferior side of the arch is cut open, and the arch is prepared as a flap which contains the arch vessels. This flap is anastomosed to the confluence of the main pulmonary artery and descending aorta.

Construction of the Pulmonary Blood Source

When a modified Blalock–Taussig shunt is used for pulmonary blood flow, the PTFE tube at the brachiocephalic artery is cut to the appropriate length for anastomosis to the right pulmonary artery, and this tube is anastomosed in an end-to-side fashion (Fig. II-32-10). During anastomosis of the Blalock–Taussig shunt (BT shunt) to the right pulmonary artery, systemic perfusion is maintained through an arterial cannula placed on the descending aorta. The tube is anastomosed to the pulmonary artery as centrally as possible to obtain equal pulmonary blood flow to both lungs. The Blalock–Taussig shunt is temporarily occluded until separation from bypass.

When a right ventricle-to-pulmonary-artery conduit (RV–PA conduit) is used as the source of pulmonary blood flow, a 5-mm PTFE tube is used if the patient is less than 3 kg, and a 6-mm tube is chosen if the patient is over 3 kg. An autologous pericardial patch is sutured to the one end of the PTFE tube before bypass is initiated. Before pericardial patch removal, a small hole is made to the pericardium, and the PTFE tube is sutured in with the pericardium in situ. The pericardium is then cut to create a large patch, which is ultimately a patch anastomosed to the distal pulmonary artery site. Although this procedure may be performed after arch reconstruction, it is more easily accomplished before. The right ventriculotomy is placed to the left side of the right ventricular outflow tract, 1 cm from the pulmonary annulus. Trabeculations of the free wall should be excised through the ventriculotomy site to prevent anastomosis stenosis. The PTFE tube is cut obliquely and anastomosed with a running suture (Fig. II-32-11). The RV–PA conduit is temporarily clamped with a bulldog clamp until separation from bypass.

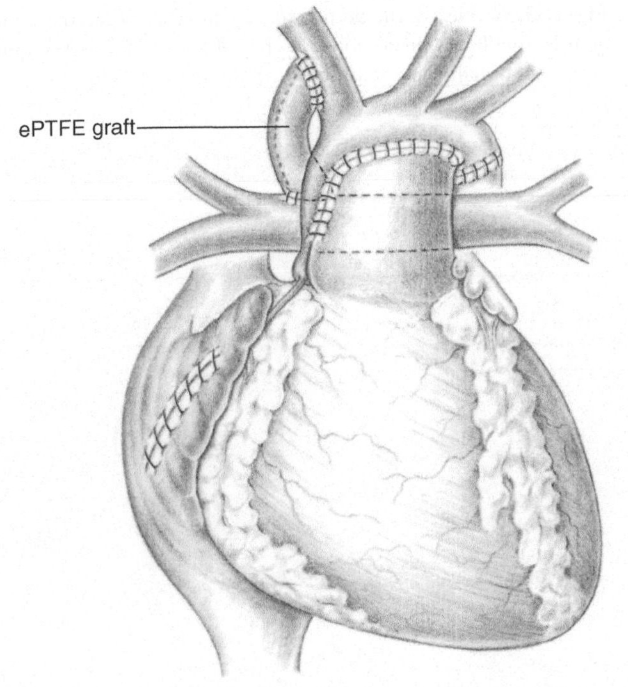

Fig. II-32-10. Norwood procedure with Blalock–Taussig (BT) shunt. An expanded polytetrafluoroethylene (ePTFE) tube originally used for cerebral perfusion is anastomosed to the proximal right pulmonary artery with 6-0 monofilament running suture

Separation from Cardiopulmonary Bypass

During the early postoperative period, patients are managed with low systemic and pulmonary vascular resistance to avoid acute hemodynamic changes [7]. Nitroglycerin is administered into the cardiopulmonary bypass circuit as a 250-μg bolus and is given by continuous infusion after bypass (2 μg/kg/min). Nitric oxide (20 ppm), an inspired FiO_2 of 100%, and hyperventilation are instituted as bypass flow is weaned. Bypass flow is gradually decreased as guided by blood pressure and oxygen saturation. While assessing the cardiac motion and pulse pressure, inotropic support is adjusted and the clamp on the BT shunt or RV–PA conduit is removed slowly.

When the balance between systemic and pulmonary perfusion is acceptable, evidenced by an arterial oxygen saturation of 75%–80% and systolic blood pressure greater than 60 mmHg with atrial pressure less than 10 mmHg, then bypass is discontinued. If the systemic saturation is higher and the systemic pressure is lower, hemoclips are applied to partially occlude the RV–PA conduit tube (Fig. II-32-12). If a BT shunt is used for the pulmonary blood source, the adventitia of the brachiocephalic artery proximal to the shunt placement is plicated to decrease pulmonary blood flow.

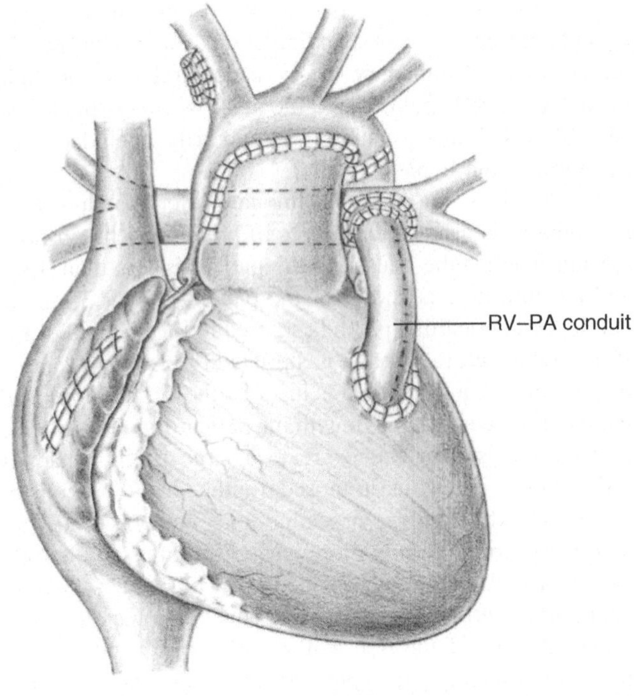

Fig. II-32-11. Norwood procedure with the right ventricle–pulmonary artery conduit (*RV–PA conduit*)

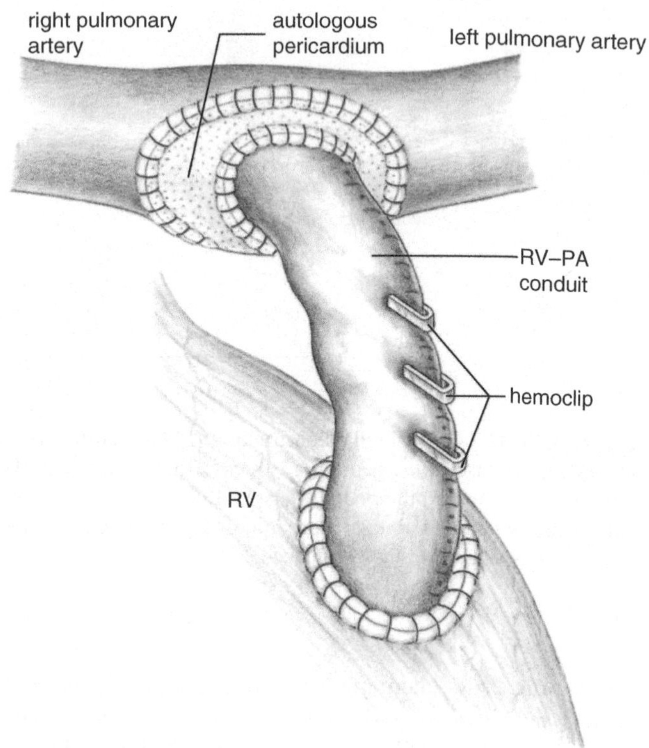

Fig. II-32-12. Banding of the RV–PA conduit. Several hemoclips are applied to the RV–PA conduit obliquely to adjust the pulmonary blood flow. If the patient develops hypoxia, these clips are easily removed

Insufficient pulmonary blood flow resulting from increased pulmonary vascular resistance is considered if desaturation and hypotension are observed after separation from bypass. The clips on the RV–PA conduit or plication sutures on the brachiocephalic artery are removed, and hyperventilation or inhaled nitric oxide is started to reduce pulmonary vascular resistance. On rare occasions, an additional BT shunt is required. A peritoneal dialysis catheter is inserted in all cases. The chest is left open in all cases, and delayed sternal closure is instituted several days after surgery when stabilization of hemodynamics is obtained.

References

1. Fraser CD, Mee RBB (1995) Modified Norwood procedure for hypoplastic left heart syndrome. Ann Thorac Surg 60: S546–S549
2. Kishimoto H, Kawahira Y, Kawata H, et al (1999) The modified Norwood palliation on a beating heart. J Thorac Cardiovasc Surg 118:1130–1132
3. Sano S, Ishino K, Kado H, et al (2004) Outcome of right ventricle-to-pulmonary artery shunt in first-stage palliation of hypoplastic left heart syndrome: a multi-institutional study. Ann Thorac Surg 78:1951–1957; discussion 1957–1958
4. Asou T, Kado H, Imoto Y, et al (1996) Selective cerebral perfusion technique during aortic arch repair in neonates. Ann Thorac Surg 61:1546–1548
5. Imoto Y, Kado H, Shiokawa Y, et al (2001) Experience with Norwood procedure without circulatory arrest. J Thorac Cardiovasc Surg 122:879–882
6. Imoto Y, Kado H, Shiokawa Y, et al (1999) Norwood procedure without circulatory arrest. Ann Thorac Surg 68: 559–561
7. Nakano T, Kado H, Shiokawa Y, et al (2004) The low resistance strategy for the perioperative management of the Norwood procedure. Ann Thorac Surg 77:908–912

II-33. Coronary Fistula

A coronary fistula is defined as the presence of a communication between the coronary artery and a cardiac chamber, the coronary sinus, the superior vena cava, the pulmonary artery, or a pulmonary vein. The communication may originate in the main coronary artery or a more peripheral segment of a coronary artery. Coronary fistulae may involve either the right or left coronary artery, although the incidence of right coronary involvement is greater than left. The fistula communicates with the right side of the heart in 90% of cases [1].

Surgical Indication

Surgical treatment is indicated in the presence of (1) symptoms of congestive heart failure such as fatigue during exercise or dyspnea on exertion, (2) symptoms of coronary ischemia, (3) aneurysm formation, and (4) significant shunt. If the patient is asymptomatic, and the shunt is small, there is no surgical indication, although if the patient requires cardiac surgery for another reason, the anomaly should be repaired simultaneously.

Preoperative Evaluation

Multiplane coronary angiography is performed to confirm the position of the fistula and the coronary arteries, as well as the entry and exit sites of the fistula. Treatment options for coronary fistulae include coil embolization, fistula ligation, fistula division, and surgical occlusion of the fistula orifice from inside the cardiac chamber. When coil embolization can be performed with low risk, this interventional treatment has become the treatment of choice [2]. If surgical intervention is chosen for fistula at the distal coronary artery, ligation or division can be used. For fistula at the proximal coronary artery, occlusion at the entry or exit site of the fistula is performed with cardiopulmonary bypass. Anticoagulation is used postoperatively after intervention to avoid thrombosis.

Ligation/Division

The coronary fistula is dissected, and ligatures are applied around the fistula. Test occlusion is instituted. When the thrill on the fistula disappears, without alteration in the electrocardiogram and hemodynamics, the fistula is doubly ligated (Fig. II-33-1). If division is chosen, both ends of the fistula are closed using monofilament sutures. In the case of a fistula originating from a main coronary artery, the orifice is closed with a pledgetted mattress suture, and absence of a palpable thrill is confirmed after closure (Fig. II-33-2).

Fistula Occlusion from Inside the Heart and the Coronary Artery

If the fistula is not identified outside the heart, the exit orifice of the fistula may be closed from inside the heart (Figs. II-33-3–II-33-5). The patient is placed on cardiopulmonary bypass with ascending aortic and bicaval cannulation. Under cardioplegic arrest or fibrillation, the target cardiac chamber is opened. When cardioplegic arrest is used, to obtain adequate cardiac protection, the fistula is compressed to avoid steal of cardioplegic solution. The exit orifice of the fistula is closed with simple sutures, and a mattress pledgetted suture is additionally applied. When cardioplegic arrest is used, completeness of the fistula occlusion is checked with cardioplegic solution injection. If the coronary artery becomes aneurysmal, the coronary artery is opened, and the fistula is closed from inside the coronary artery (the Symbas procedure [3]) (Fig. II-33-5). Under cardioplegic arrest, the aneurysmal coronary artery is opened longitudinally and the opening of the fistula is closed directly with a fine monofilament running suture. The excessive coronary arterial wall is excised and closed with monofilament running suture. When the aneurysm is located at the distal coronary artery or small branch, the coronary orifices to the aneurysm as well as fistula are closed from the inside and outside, then the aneurysm is completely isolated.

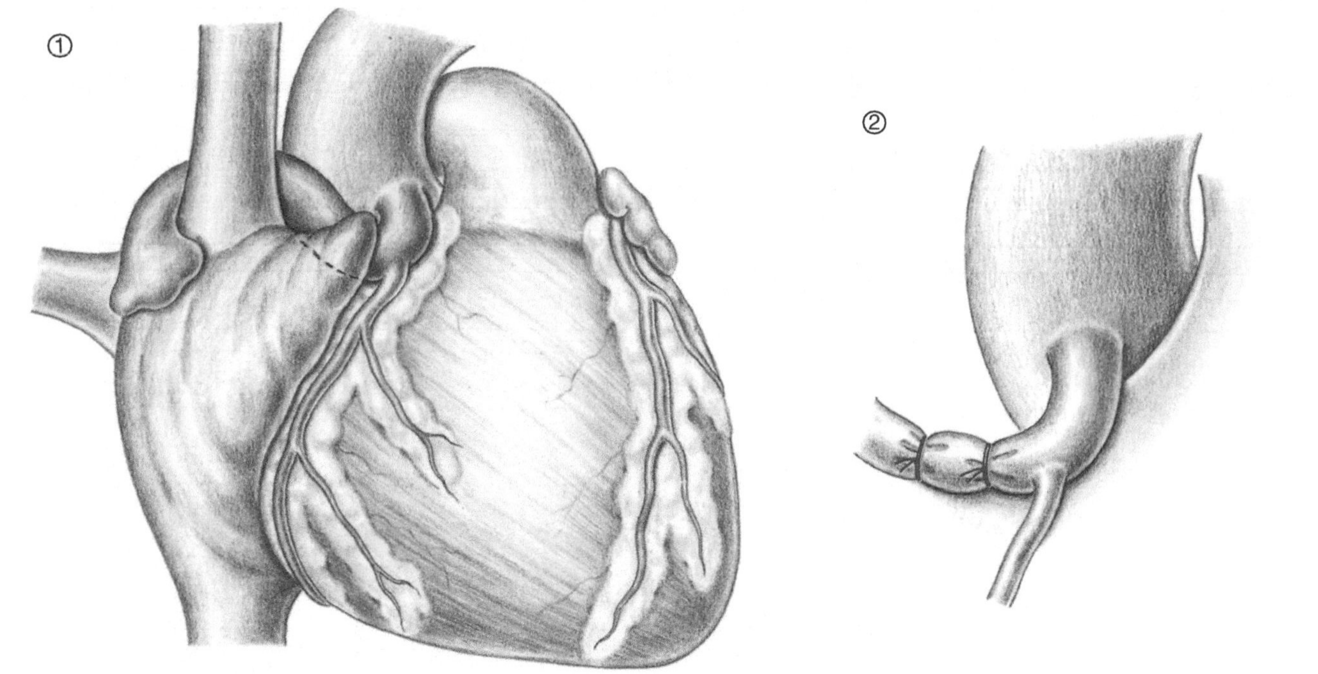

Fig. II-33-1. Fistula from the sinus node artery to the right atrium. The entry of the fistula is the sinus node artery. The fistula is ligated after test clamping as closure may cause rhythm disturbance.

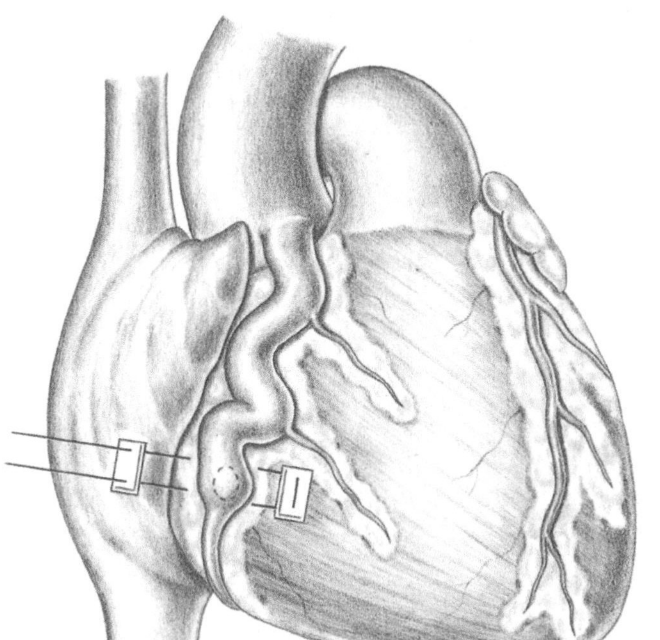

Fig. II-33-2. Fistula from the right coronary artery to the right ventricle. The fistula is closed with a monofilament pledgetted horizontal mattress suture

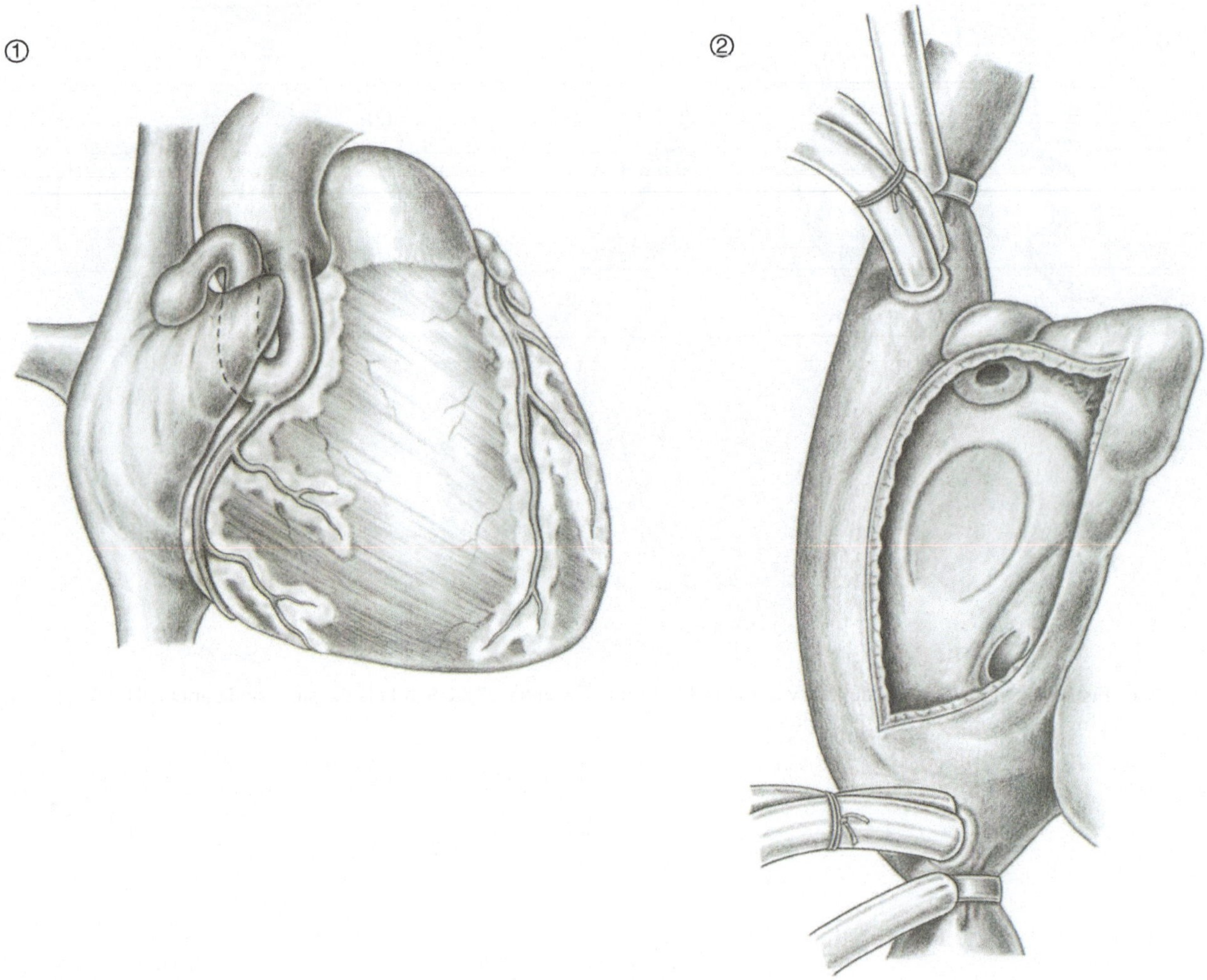

Fig. II-33-3. Fistula from the sinus node artery to the right atrium. The exit site is located anterolateral in the right atrium. Preservation of the sinus node artery is expected by closure of exit site from the inside. On cardiopulmonary bypass, an aortic cross-clamp is placed, and cardioplegic solution is infused with temporary obstruction of the fistula. After right atriotomy, the exit of the fistula can be easily identified during cardioplegic injection

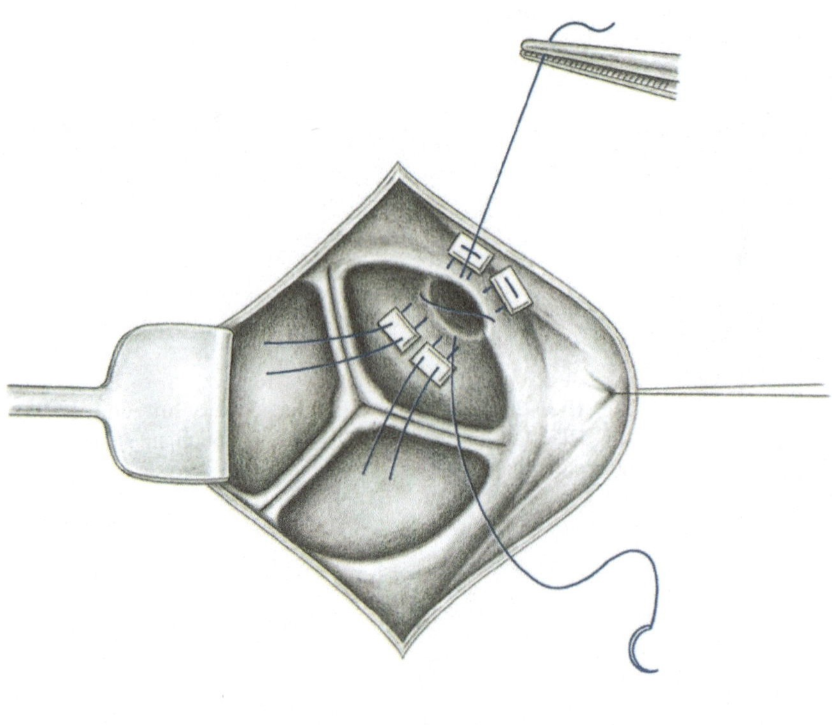

Fig. II-33-4. Fistula from both the right and left coronary arteries to the main pulmonary artery. The enlarged and torturous fistula formed an aneurysm. In this case, the course was not discernible on external inspection. Under cardioplegic arrest, the exit of the fistula is closed with direct sutures which was reinforced with pledgetted horizontal mattress sutures

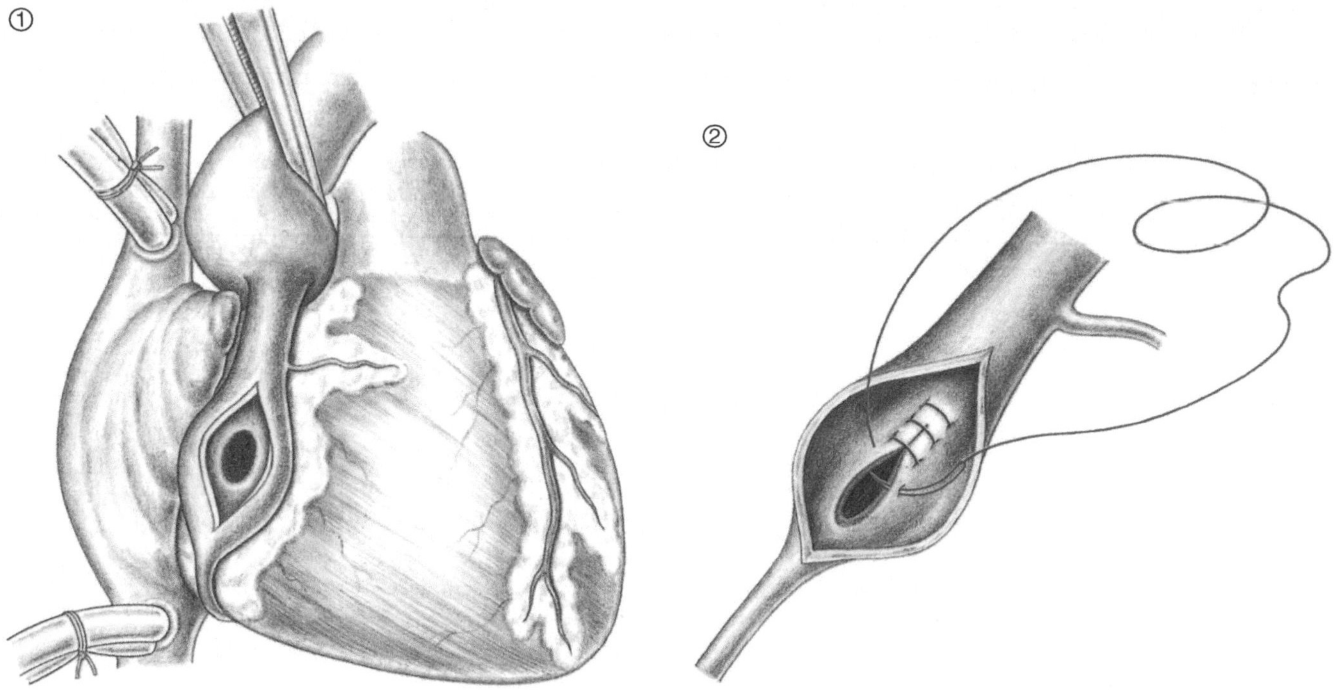

Fig. II-33-5. Aneurysmal formation of the fistula between the right coronary artery and the right ventricle. After cardioplegic arrest, the aneurysmal portion of the coronary artery is opened longitudinally, and the orifice of the fistula is closed directly. Excess aneurysmal tissue is excised and closed, taking care not to compromise the resultant lumen of the coronary artery

References

1. Lowe JE, Oldham HN Jr., Sabiston DC Jr (1981) Surgical management of congenital coronary artery fistulas. Ann Surg 194:373–380
2. Mavroudis C, Backer CL, Rocchini AP, et al (1997) Coronary artery fistulas in infants and children: a surgical review and discussion of coil embolisation. Ann Thorac Surg 63:1235–1242
3. Symbas PN, Schlant RC, Hatcher CR Jr, et al (1967) Congenital fistula of right coronary artery to right ventricle complicated by *Actinobacillus actinomycetemcomitans* endarteritis. J Thorac Cardiovasc Surg 53:379–384

II-34. Anomalous Origin of the Left Coronary Artery from the Pulmonary Artery

In patients with Bland–White–Garland syndrome, the left coronary artery arises from the pulmonary artery (Fig. II-34-1). In the neonatal period, patients are usually asymptomatic because of the neonatal elevation in pulmonary vascular resistance. As the pulmonary vascular resistance decreases, a left-to-right shunt develops in the anomalous coronary, resulting in a coronary "steal" phenomenon. Myocardial ischemia and heart failure ensue, and as many as 80% of patients die within 1 year without surgery. If collateral vessels develop to an adequate extent, the patient may survive. The aim of the surgical procedure is the establishment of a two-coronary artery system [1]. In the majority of cases, the left coronary artery arises from the posterior wall of the main pulmonary artery [2], allowing for direct translocation of the left coronary artery to the aorta. Occasionally direct transfer is impossible, and thus several other techniques have been reported [1,3–5]. In the presence of severe mitral regurgitation caused by myocardial ischemia [5,6] mitral valve repair may be necessary at the time of coronary reconstruction.

Direct Anastomosis

A standard median sternotomy is performed. The ascending aorta, vena cavae, and branch pulmonary arteries (PAs) are dissected. Tapes are placed around the branch PAs. After cardiopulmonary bypass (CPB), cardioplegic catheters are placed in both the ascending aorta and the main PA. Following aortic cross-clamping, the tapes on the branch PAs are tightened, and cardioplegic solution is injected into both the aorta and the PA. When significant mitral regurgitation is present, the left atrium is opened, and mitral valve repair is performed. Repair of the valve may be accomplished by Wooler or Reed annuloplasty at the commissures or a posterior suture annuloplasty. The incision site on the main PA is determined. When the coronary artery arises from the posterior wall of the main PA, an anterior pulmonary arteriotomy is created just proximal to the bifurcation. Through the arteriotomy, the orifice of the coronary artery is identified. The main PA is transected, and the coronary button is resected with a 5-mm cuff of PA, if transfer of the coronary button is considered feasible.

Initially, only the pulmonary arterial wall is cut using fine scissors; then the connective tissue around the coronary artery is carefully dissected using diathermy, protecting the collateral vessels. The coronary artery is mobilized at least 1 cm in length from the orifice to facilitate transfer to the aorta (Fig. II-34-2). A small aortotomy is created on the left aspect of the ascending aorta for implantation. The aortotomy is enlarged with a 4-mm punch (Fig. II-34-3). The coronary button is anastomosed using a running suture. After anastomosis, the aortic cross-clamp is released and hemostasis is checked. Given the difficulty of hemostasis after PA reconstruction, complete hemostasis must be achieved at this stage. The defect in the main PA is reconstructed using an autologous pericardial patch (Fig. II-34-4), and PA anastomosis is completed with a running suture. The aortic cross-clamp is released, and separation from cardiopulmonary bypass is accomplished.

Takeuchi Procedure

When direct implantation is not feasible, a Takeuchi procedure can be used [3] (Fig. II-34-5). A transverse incision is made in the anterior surface of the distal main PA, and the orifice of the coronary artery is identified. This incision is advanced to create a flap with a width of about 8 mm. Holes 4 mm in diameter are made at the base of the flap and the left side of the ascending aortic wall with a punch. These two holes are anastomosed in a side-to-side fashion. The previously created flap is anastomosed to the posterior wall of the main PA to generate a tunnel from the left coronary orifice to the ascending aorta. This suture line must be intact to prevent left-to-right shunting. The anterior wall of the main PA is reconstructed with a generous autologous pericardial patch to prevent supravalvar pulmonary stenosis.

Spiral-Cuff Procedure [4]

A portion of the main PA wall with a width of 5 mm is excised in a ring shape. This ring is opened at the right to the coronary orifice. The pulmonary arterial wall is anastomosed to coronary orifice at the proximal side. When this suture line is advanced, a funnel-shaped extension of the main coronary artery is created (Fig. II-34-6). At the new

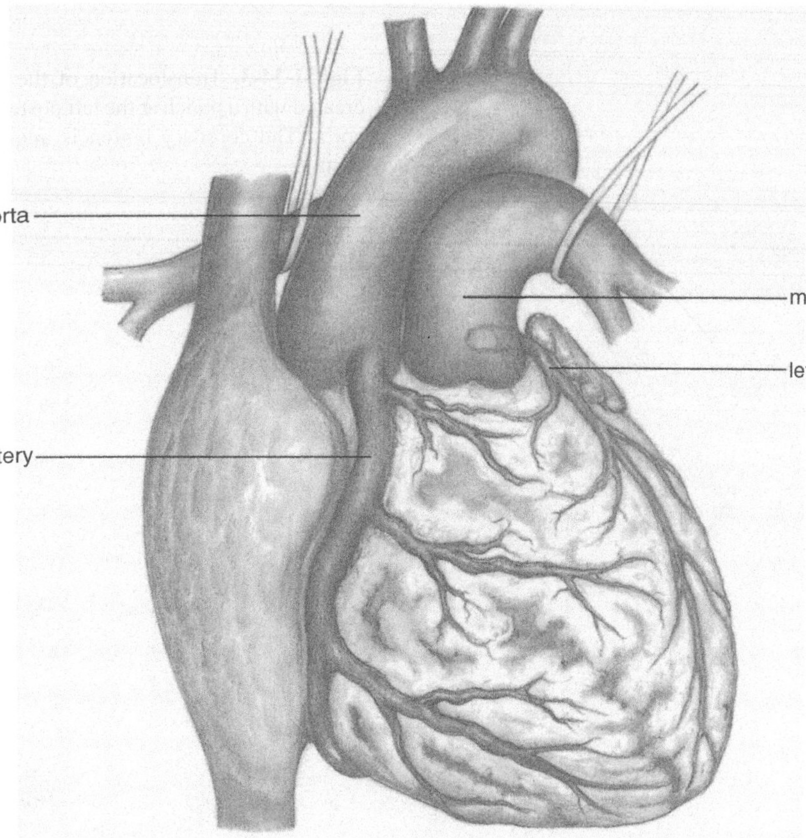

Fig. II-34-1. Anomalous origin of the left coronary artery from the pulmonary artery. The right coronary artery is enlarged and tortuous. The left coronary artery arises from the posterior aspect of the main pulmonary artery in the majority of cases

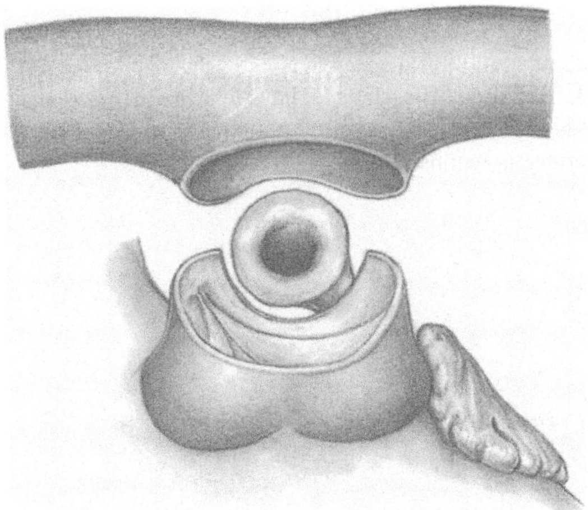

Fig. II-34-2. Excision of the coronary button. The main pulmonary artery is transected distal to the coronary orifice. The coronary artery is excised as a button with a generous cuff of main pulmonary wall tissue

origin of the coronary artery, redundant tissue is excised, and the coronary is anastomosed to the ascending aorta. The proximal and distal main PAs are directly anastomosed to each other after pericardial patch repair of the sinus defect (Fig. II-34-7).

Pulmonary Artery Flap Procedure [5]

When the left coronary artery arises from the left and anterior aspect of the main pulmonary artery, the distance between the orifice of the anomalous coronary artery and ascending aorta is greatest. A coronary button is created with a long segment of flap from the anterior main PA. Another large flap, hinged posteriorly, is created from the ascending aorta to receive the coronary button (Fig. II-34-8). After the main PA defect is repaired with an autologous pericardial patch, the aortic wall and coronary flap are anastomosed (Fig. II-34-9).

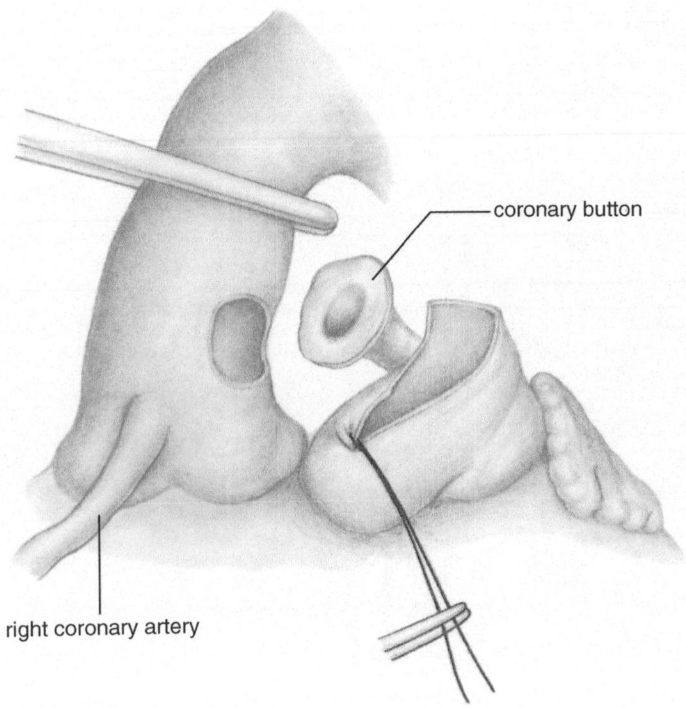

Fig. II-34-3. Translocation of the coronary artery. A hole is created with a punch at the left posterior aspect of the ascending aorta. The coronary button is anastomosed to the ascending aorta

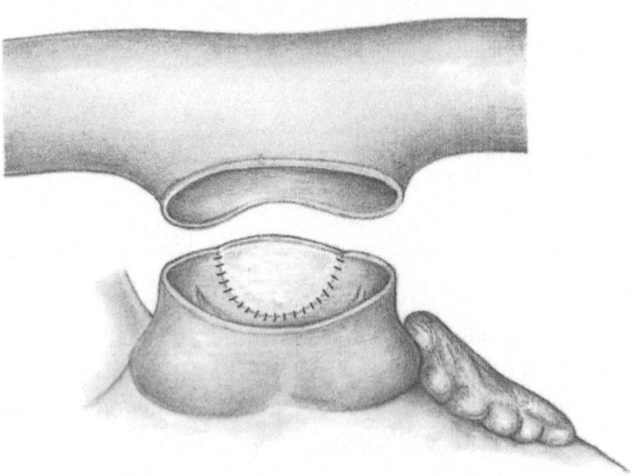

Fig. II-34-4. Repair of the sinus defect. The main pulmonary artery sinus defect is repaired with an autologous pericardial patch. The main pulmonary artery is reconstructed by direct anastomosis

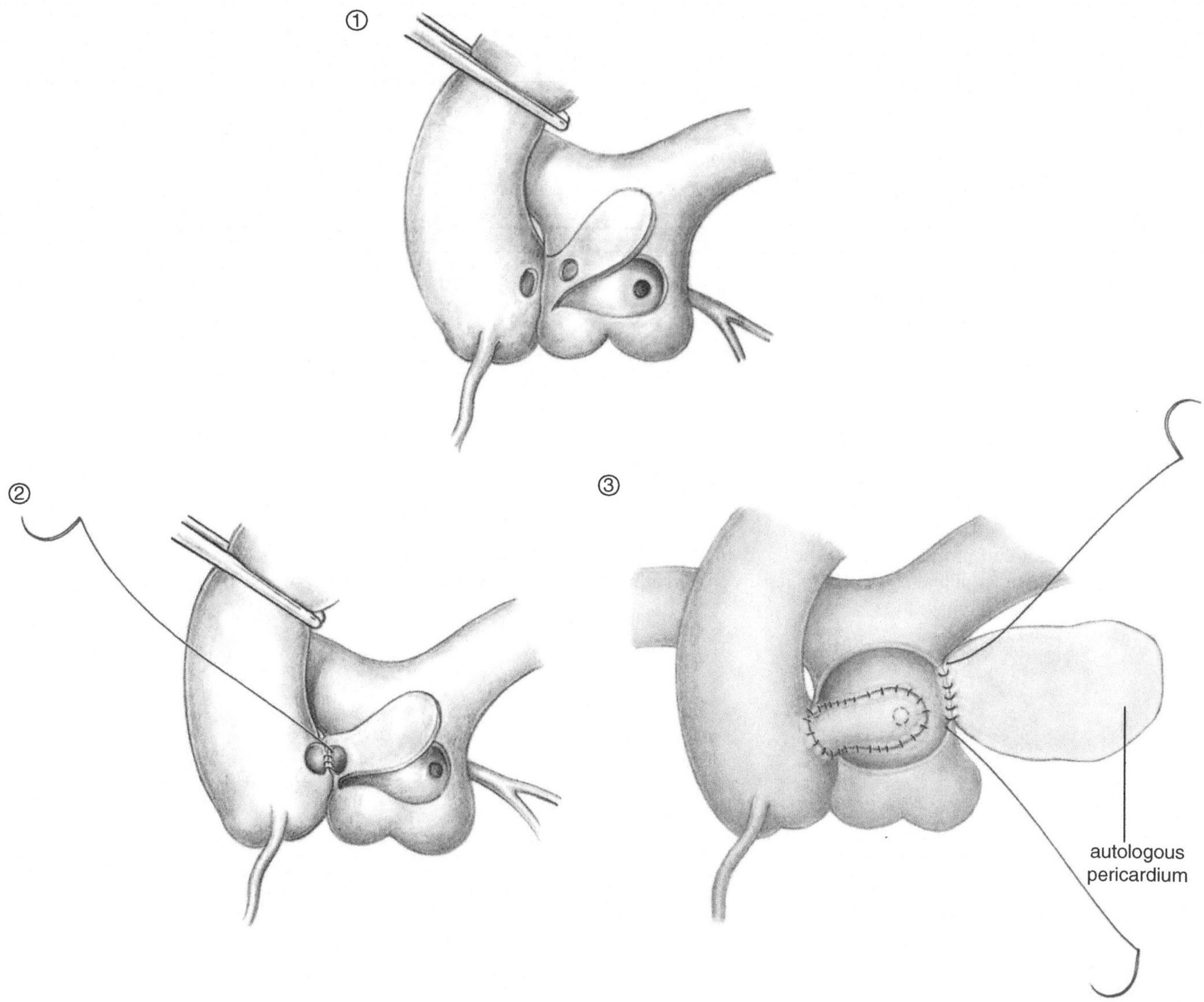

Fig. II-34-5. Takeuchi procedure. (See text for description)

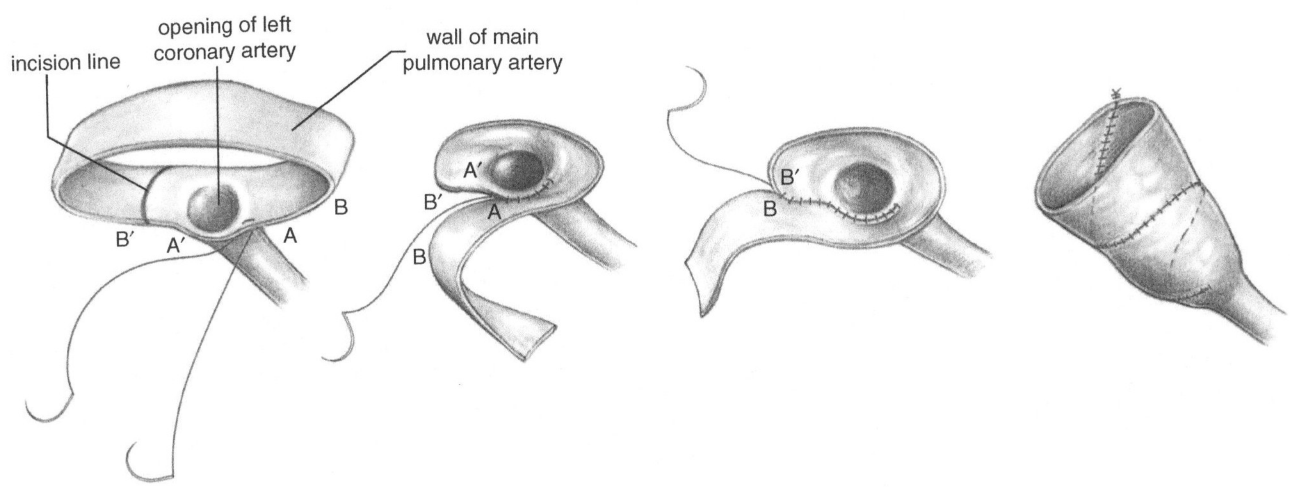

Fig. II-34-6. Spiral-cuff procedure: 1. The proximal side of the main pulmonary arterial wall is anastomosed to the coronary orifice portion of the pulmonary arterial wall. A funnel-shaped proximal portion of the coronary artery is created

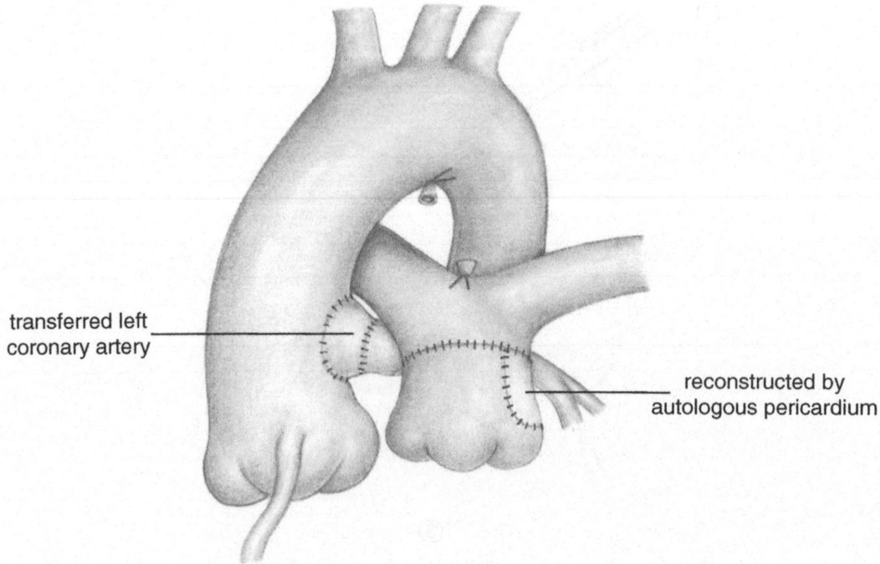

Fig. II-34-7. Spiral-cuff procedure: 2. The new proximal portion of the left coronary artery is anastomosed to the ascending aorta. The sinus defect of the main pulmonary artery is repaired with an autologous pericardial patch. The distal and proximal main pulmonary arteries are directly anastomosed

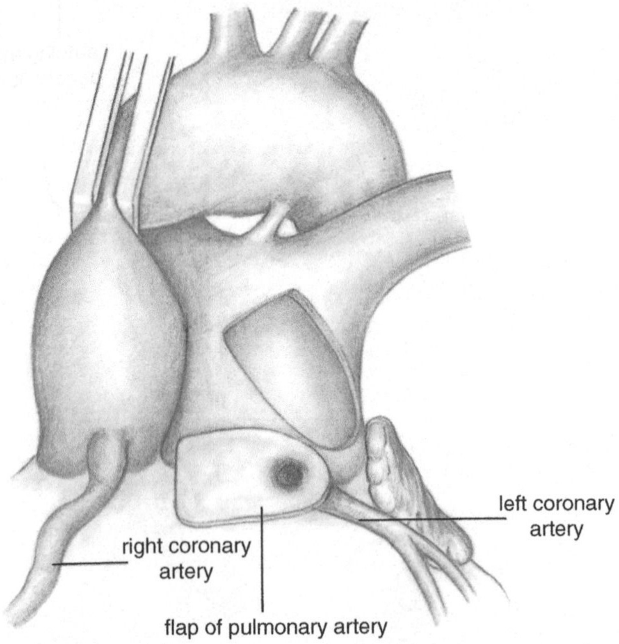

Fig. II-34-8. Pulmonary artery flap procedure: 1. A pulmonary artery flap is excised with a long flap of anterior pulmonary artery wall

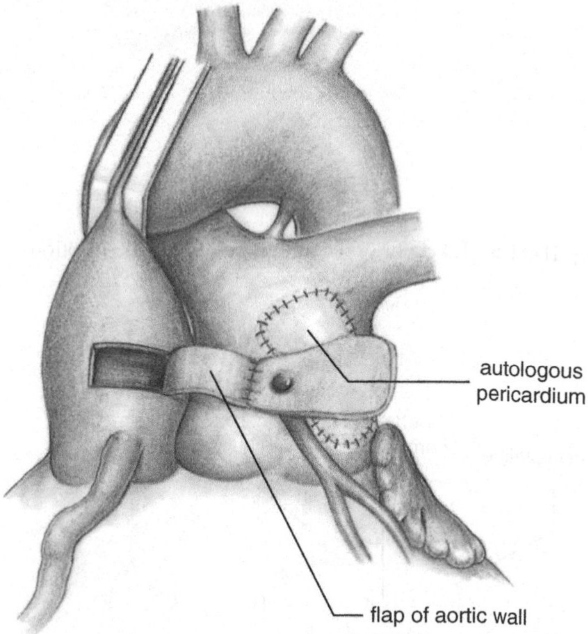

Fig. II-34-9. Pulmonary artery flap procedure: 2. A posteriorly based flap of the ascending aorta is created, and an overlapping long anastomosis of the two flaps is accomplished. The pulmonary artery defect is closed with a patch of autologous pericardium

References

1. Backer CL, Stout MJ, Zales VR, et al (1992) Anomalous origin of the left coronary artery. A twenty-year review of surgical management. J Thorac Cardiovasc Surg 103:1049–1058
2. Smith A, Arnold R, Anderson RH, et al (1989) Anomalous origin of the left coronary artery from the pulmonary trunk. Anatomic findings in relation to pathophysiology and surgical repair. J Thorac Cardiovasc Surg 98:16–24
3. Takeuchi S, Imamura H, Katsumoto K, et al (1979) New surgical method for repair of anomalous left coronary artery from pulmonary artery. J Thorac Cardiovasc Surg 78:7–11
4. Ando Y, Kado H, Masuda M, et al (2008) "Spiral-cuff" technique for repair of anomalous left coronary artery from the pulmonary artery. Ann Thorac Surg 86:667–668
5. Sese A, Imoto Y (1992) New technique in the transfer of an anomalously originated left coronary artery to the aorta. Ann Thorac Surg 53:527–529
6. Burchell HB, Brown AL (1962) Anomalous origin of coronary artery from pulmonary artery masquerading as mitral insufficiency. Am Heart J 63:388–393

II-35. Systemic to Pulmonary Artery Shunt, Pulmonary Artery Banding, and Blalock–Hanlon Procedure

Systemic–Pulmonary Artery Shunt, Takedown of Shunt

A systemic–pulmonary artery shunt increases pulmonary blood flow, ameliorates desaturation, and promotes pulmonary arterial growth. After the original technique for systemic–pulmonary artery shunt creation was described by Blalock and Taussig [1], other techniques were developed by Potts et al. [2] and Waterston [3]. Currently, systemic–pulmonary shunting is most commonly performed by interposing a synthetic tube graft, typically a polytetrafluoroethylene (PTFE) graft, between a systemic artery and a branch pulmonary artery (PA), the so-called modified Blalock–Taussig shunt [4]. In the presence of small PAs, a central shunt is performed by placement of an interposition graft between the ascending aorta and the main PA [5].

Surgical Indication

A systemic–pulmonary shunt is indicated in a patient with decreased pulmonary blood flow who is not a candidate for complete repair, typically in neonates or young infants, and in children with a single ventricle as a first staging procedure. For patients who cannot undergo complete repair or cavopulmonary anastomosis, this procedure is performed as a final palliative procedure.

Preoperative Evaluation

A systemic–pulmonary shunt increases the volume load to the ventricle as well as increasing pulmonary blood flow. Acute volume overload with systemic–pulmonary shunt placement may cause acute heart failure and acute deterioration, which is especially likely in cases of single ventricle anatomy, with significant atrioventricular valve regurgitation, decreased ventricular function, and anemia. The physiology is also worsened by the low diastolic pressure that accompanies systemic–pulmonary shunts and which may diminish coronary perfusion pressure. Inotropic support and transfusion are often required during the acute postoperative course. Partial or complete anomalies of pulmonary venous return should be sought before surgery, because in the presence of this condition pulmonary congestion often worsens after shunt placement.

Side of the Shunt

The following points are taken into consideration.

1. The shunt is placed to the pulmonary artery, which is more hypoplastic.
2. The right PA is chosen in patients with single ventricle anatomy who will later undergo right-sided bidirectional cavopulmonary anastomosis.
3. If the ductus arteriosus requires intervention, the left PA is selected.
4. When a classic Blalock–Taussig shunt is chosen, the contralateral side to the aortic arch is utilized.

Classic Shunt or Modified Shunt

For systemic–pulmonary shunting, the modified shunt (interposition graft) is the surgical treatment of choice. Advantages of the modified shunt include preservation of the subclavian artery, availability of either side of the aortic arch for use, and simplified take-down of the shunt. Advantages of the classic shunt are less intimal hyperplasia, probable better long-term patency, and growth potential.

The optimal material for a tube graft is a PTFE tube; Dacron should be avoided because of the high incidence of occlusion.

Size of Tube Graft

The following points are taken into consideration.

1. In neonates, infants, and toddlers, or all other children, 3.5- to 4-mm tubes, 4- to 5-mm tubes, and 6-mm tubes are used, respectively.
2. The size of the subclavian artery: in infants, a graft size more than twice as large as the subclavian artery size should be avoided.
3. When atrioventicular (AV) valve regurgitation or ventricular dysfunction is present, especially in the case of a single ventricle, a tube graft one size smaller than the normal is utilized.

Operative Procedure

Right Modified BT Shunt

The patient is placed in left lateral decubitus position. The chest is entered through the third or fourth intercostal space. The lung is retracted inferiorly, and the visceral pleura over the superior surface of the hilum is opened. The right PA is located most superiorly, posterior to the right pulmonary veins, and anterior to the right bronchus. When collateral vessels are present, they are divided after double ligation or cauterized with a diathermy, and dissection is advanced. Care is taken to avoid injury to the phrenic nerve, which courses anterior to the hilum (Fig. II-35-1 ①). When the PA is small, identification may be difficult. To confirm identification and avoid shunt placement to the pulmonary vein, blood is drawn from the vessel for blood gas analysis, and the vessel is dissected. A vessel loop is placed around the right PA using a right-angle clamp. Care is necessary not to mistake the right upper lobe branch for the main right pulmonary artery. The azygous vein is doubly ligated and divided, and connective tissue around it is removed. Traction stitches are placed on the pericardium, and exposure of the operative field behind the superior vena cava is facilitated. The right PA is dissected as proximal as possible behind the vena cava to obtain enough space for graft placement. Vessel loops are encircled around the upper and lower branch of the right PA to control blood flow. The right subclavian artery is dissected. Generally, the subclavian artery is visible. When the subclavian artery is not visible, the area posterior to the subclavian vein is palpated. The pleura is opened over the pulse, and the subclavian artery is dissected and encircled with a vessel loop. This dissection is advanced proximally, and the brachiocephalic and the right carotid arteries are identified. Care is taken to avoid damage to the vagus and phrenic nerves, which are located at the base of the subclavian artery (Fig. II-35-1 ②).

For the anastomosis site, the proximal subclavian artery is chosen. Adjacent peribronchial lymph nodes are ligated and divided. When more shunt flow is necessary, the proximal anastomosis is performed on the brachiocephalic artery. Before constructing the anastomosis, 100 units/kg heparin is administered. The proximal end of a PTFE tube is beveled to fit to the subclavian artery, and the distal end is cut to the appropriate length. A C-shaped vascular clamp is applied to the subclavian artery, and the inferior aspect of this vessel is opened longitudinally with a scalpel. Care is taken to avoid damage to the posterior wall of the vessel. This opening is enlarged with Potts' scissors. The anastomosis is performed with a fine monofilament running suture, with the assistant only holding the suture because of the small operative field. The tube graft is placed on the left side of the subclavian artery. The suture is carried from the distal end of the arteriotomy from inside to outside of the subclavian artery, then from outside to inside of the graft (Fig. II-35-1 ③). After two or three stitches are placed at the heel, the other end of the double-armed suture is used to complete the anastomosis (Fig. II-35-1 ④).

The suture is tied, and the graft is clamped. The clamp on the subclavian artery is released. The suture line is checked for bleeding, and a sponge is placed at the anastomosis site for hemostasis. If bleeding is excessive, the clamp is replaced on the subclavian artery and hemostatic fibrin glue is applied.

Next, a clamp is applied to the proximal right PA, taking care to avoid placing the clamp on the main PA or ductus arteriosus. The distal PA flow is controlled with vessel loops. The superior surface of the right PA is longitudinally opened to a length two-thirds to three-fourths of the graft diameter. Three or four suture bites are placed through the graft and the proximal PA, after which the graft is lowered into place (Fig. II-35-1 ⑤). The suture is placed from outside-in on the graft, and a subsequent stitch is placed from the inside of the PA along the posterior wall of the anastomosis. After the first suture line arrives at the distal PA, the other arm of the suture is started. All stitches are placed forehand except at the proximal end. After the suture is tied, the vessel loops and the clamp are released, and de-airing occurs through the suture line. Finally, the clamp on the tube graft is released (Fig. II-35-1 ⑥). A thrill on the graft and increase in systemic saturation confirm graft patency. Protamine is usually not administered. After hemostasis is confirmed by minimal chest tube output, a low-dose heparin infusion is started in the intensive care unit.

Left Modified BT Shunt

The patient is placed in a right lateral decubitus position, and the chest is entered through the third or fourth intercostal space. The lung is retracted inferiorly, and the left PA is located as the most superior structure in the hilum (Fig. II-35-2 ①). The left PA is dissected in a similar fashion for a right-sided shunt. The left PA is dissected as far proximally as possible. If excessive pericardial fluid is hampering visualization, pericardial fluid is drained by opening the pericardium. The upper and lower left PA branches are encircled with vessel loops for subsequent distal control. In the presence of a patent ductus arteriosus, dissection is accomplished with care to protect the vagus and recurrent nerves, and a heavy silk string is placed around the ductus. When ductus ligation is necessary, this is performed after shunt placement. If pulmonary blood flow is ductal dependent, care is taken not to compromise blood flow through the duct with the clamp on the PA. The left subclavian artery is usually visible through the pleura. The pleura overlying the subclavian artery is opened, and a tape is placed around the subclavian artery. The subclavian artery is dissected for enough distance to allow placement of a vascular clamp (Fig. II-35-2 ②), and heparin (100 units/kg) is administered intravenously. A PTFE tube graft is cut to appropriate length, and one end is trimmed obliquely to fit to the subclavian artery. A C-shaped vascular clamp is applied to the subclavian artery. The vessel is opened longitudinally with a scalpel. The suture is placed from inside-out on the graft, and a subsequent stitch is placed from the outside of the subclavian artery (Fig. II-35-2 ③, ④). The suture is advanced with running technique to the heel, and the other suture is

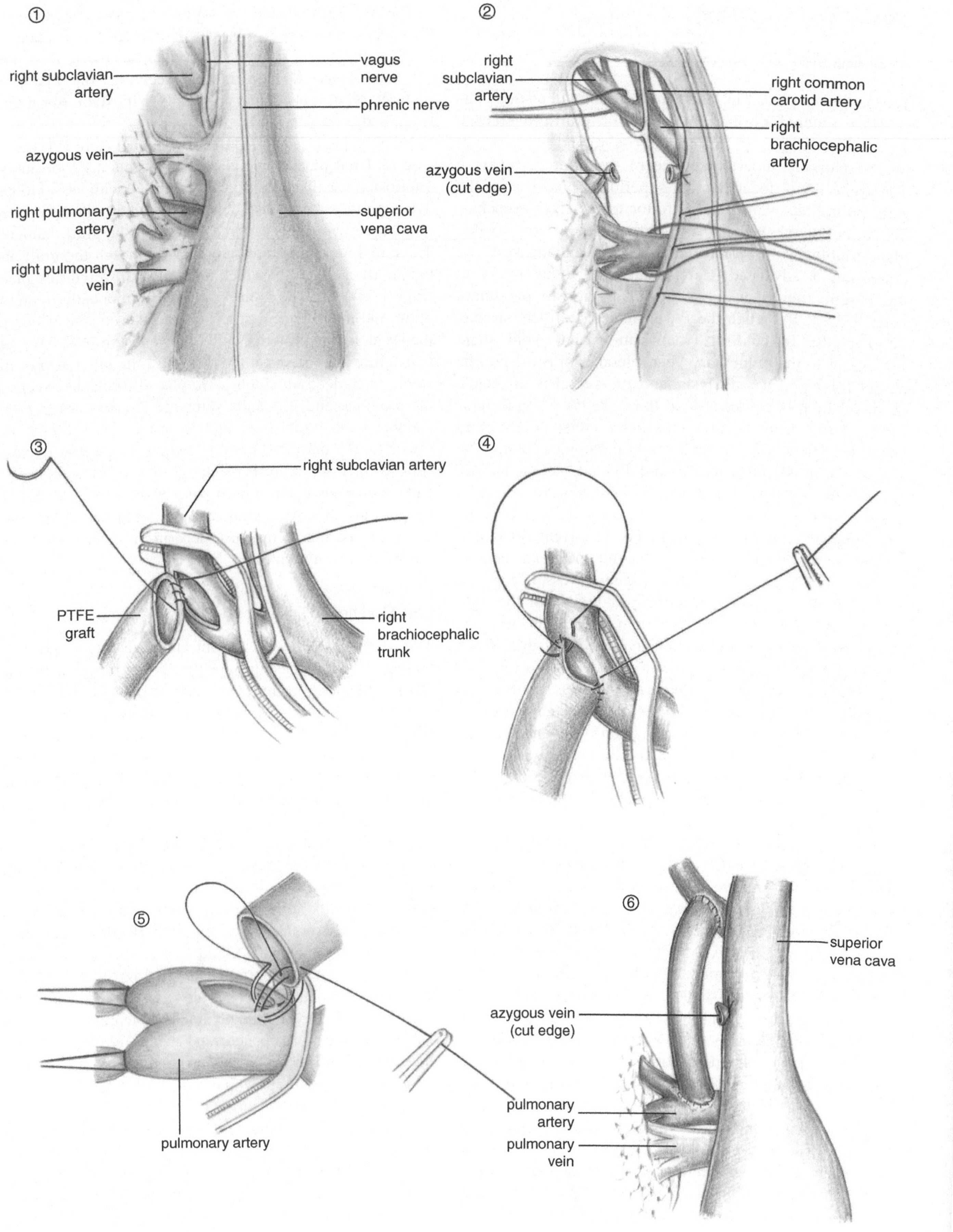

Fig. II-35-1. Right modified Blalock–Taussig (BT) shunt

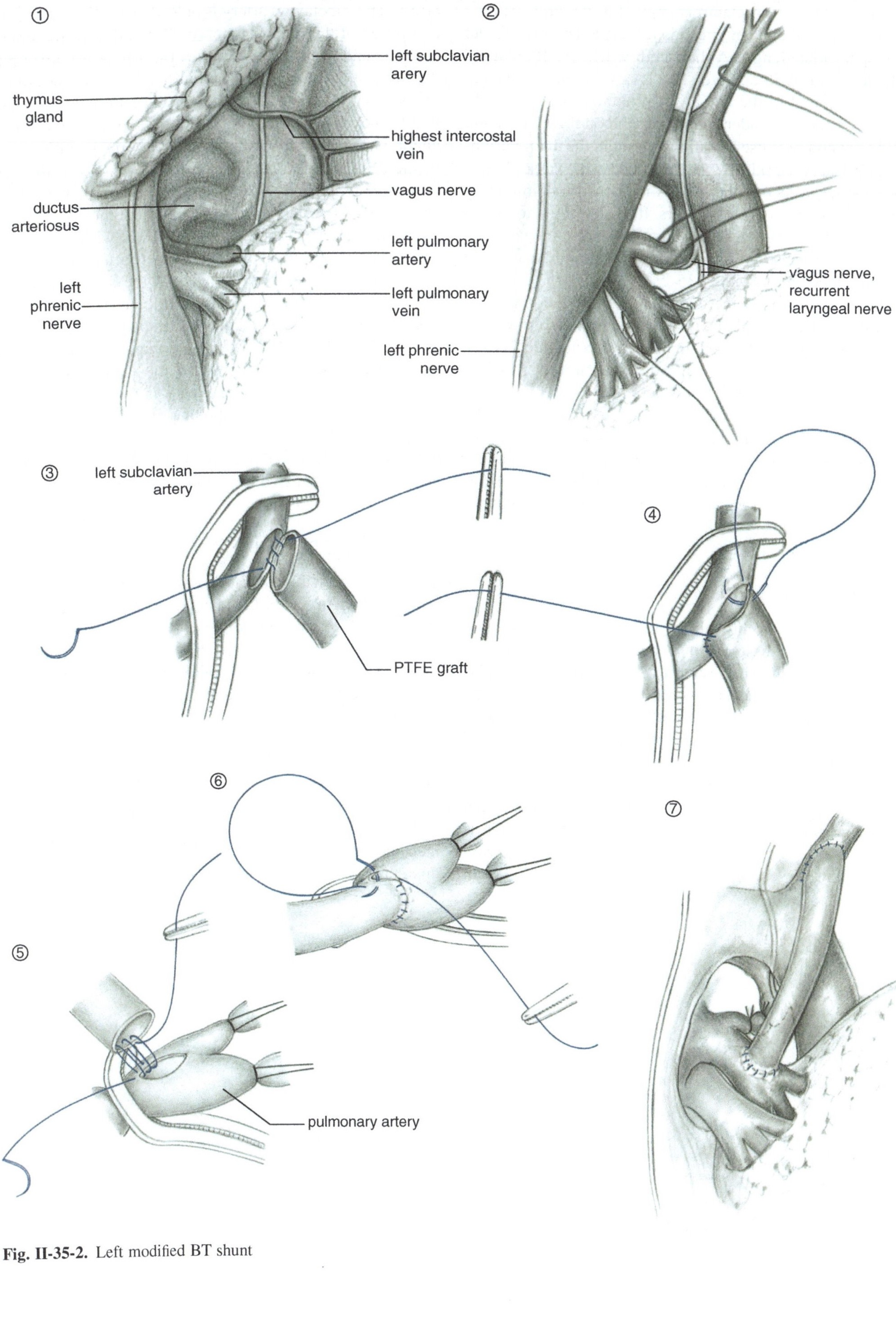

Fig. II-35-2. Left modified BT shunt

brought to the heel. A clamp is applied to the graft and the clamp on the subclavian artery is released. The graft is cut to an appropriate length. A short graft will cause PA tenting, and a long graft will compress the PA. A C-shaped vascular clamp is applied to the left PA as proximal as possible. In the case of duct-dependent pulmonary blood flow, the clamp should not compromise blood flow through the duct. Peripheral pulmonary blood flow is controlled with vessel loops. The superior aspect of the left PA is opened longitudinally and enlarged with a Potts' scissors. If the left PA is too short for an appropriately long incision, a transverse incision can be used. The anastomosis is performed similarly as for a right modified shunt (Fig. II-35-2 ⑤, ⑥).

After completion of the distal suture line, the clamp on the graft is released, and the thrill on the graft and improvement of saturation is checked. In the patient with duct dependent pulmonary circulation, the duct is carefully ligated. Before double ligation of the duct, stable saturation and hemodynamics are checked with temporary occlusion of the duct (Fig. II-35-2 ⑦). In the event of unstable saturation and hemodynamics, the duct is left open with discontinuation of prostaglandin infusion. If the discontinuation of prostaglandin infusion compromises hemodynamics, prostaglandin infusion is continued, with attention to the possibility of pulmonary overcirculation.

Right Classic BT Shunt

The chest is entered through the third or fourth intercostal space. The PA is dissected in a similar fashion as for the modified BT shunt. The azygous vein is divided, and adjacent connective tissue is dissected. The right subclavian artery is dissected and encircled with a tape. This dissection is advanced proximally to the right carotid and brachiocephalic arteries. Distally, the vertebral, internal thoracic, and thyroid arteries are doubly ligated and divided to obtain enough length of the subclavian artery. The subclavian artery is clamped proximally then ligated and divided as distally as possible. A right-angle clamp is placed beneath the recurrent nerve, holding the distal end of the subclavian artery. The subclavian artery is pulled down through the loop composed of the recurrent nerve. Dissection of the brachiocephalic and right carotid arteries facilitates mobilization of the subclavian artery and obtaining a larger anastomosis. Division of the azygous vein and dissection of the connective tissue around it facilitates a direct route to the PA. The clamp is placed to the subclavian artery proximally, and the inside of the vessel lumen is flushed. The end of the vessel is trimmed. Heparin (100 units/kg) is administered before application of a clamp to the proximal right PA. The distal pulmonary artery branches are controlled with vessel loops. The superior aspect of the pulmonary artery is opened to an extent determined by the size of the subclavian artery. The posterior and anterior suture lines are completed with running and interrupted technique, respectively (Fig. II-35-3 ①, ②). After the anastomosis is completed, air is flushed by releasing the vessel loops and the clamp from the PA. The clamp on the subclavian artery is removed. A thrill on the subclavian artery or Doppler probe is used to confirm the patency of the shunt. Protamine is not used so long as excessive bleeding is not encountered. After the patient arrives in the intensive care unit, continuous heparin infusion is started.

Left Classic BT Shunt

For the patient with a left aortic arch, a left classic BT shunt is performed in a similar fashion as the right classic BT shunt. Thoracotomy and dissection and preparation of the subclavian artery are the same as for the right classic BT shunt. The anastomosis is performed in a similar way, with posterior continuous and anterior interrupted sutures (Fig. II-35-4 ①, ②).

When the length of the artery is not adequate, stenosis can occur at the origin of the left subclavian artery as a result of kinking. To avoid this complication, a Laks–Castaneda procedure [6] is performed. A partial clamp is placed on the aortic arch at the base of the left subclavian artery. A longitudinal incision is placed to the base of the left subclavian artery, and this opening is enlarged toward proximally to the aorta and

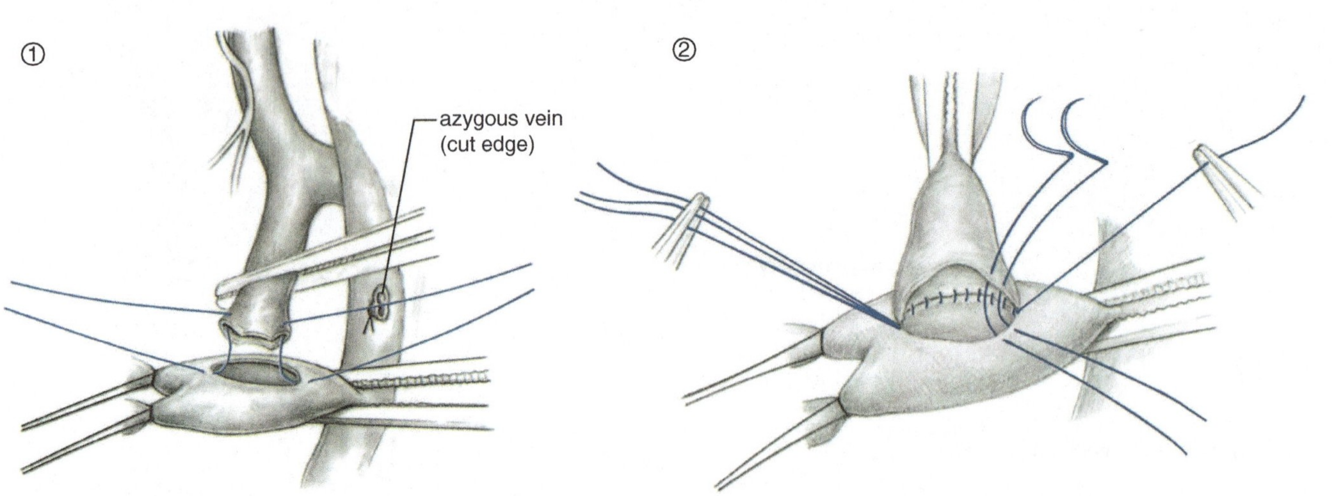

Fig. II-35-3. Right classic BT shunt

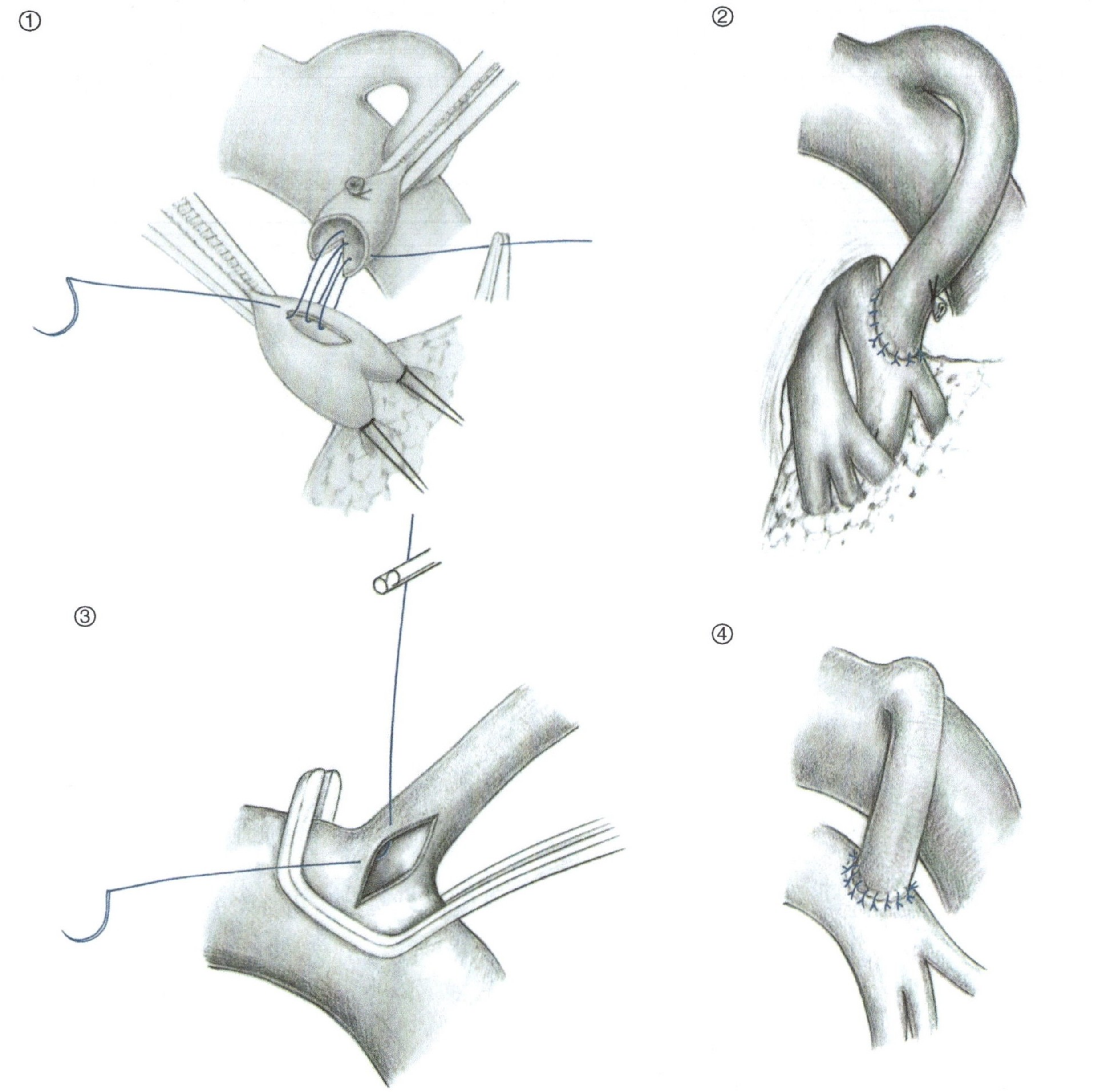

Fig. II-35-4. Left classic BT shunt

distally. The opening is closed transversely with fine monofilament sutures. This maneuver may prevent stenosis at the origin of the left subclavian artery (Fig. II-35-4 ③, ④).

Central Shunt

The benefits of a central shunt include greater shunt flow and less distortion of the branch PAs. Disadvantages include the potential for "overshunting" and consequent heart failure, and the requirement of redoing a median sternotomy at the time of complete repair, so this procedure is not often used. Central shunting is most often performed when the distal branch PAs are hypoplastic or a modified BT shunt has failed. If desaturation or hemodynamic instability occurs after clamping the main PA or a vascular clamp cannot be applied to a small ascending aorta, cardiopulmonary bypass is required. Thus, bypass standby is required for this surgery. A median sternotomy is performed, and the ascending aorta and main PA are dissected. One end of a 3.5- or 4-mm PTFE tube is obliquely trimmed. The graft should be cut short at this stage because an excessively long graft may cause kinking and occlusion of the graft. Heparin (100 units/kg) is administered. The main pulmonary artery is clamped with a C-shaped vascular clamp and opened with a scalpel and Potts' scissors. The graft is anastomosed to the arteriotomy with a fine monofilament suture (Fig. II-35-5 ①). The suture is initially placed from outside to in on the graft, and subsequently from the inside to out on the pulmonary artery. This suture line is brought to one end of the graft, and then the other arm is used to complete the anastomosis. Another clamp is applied to the graft, and the clamp on the main PA is slowly released.

A partial clamp is applied to the left side of the ascending aorta, which is then longitudinally opened

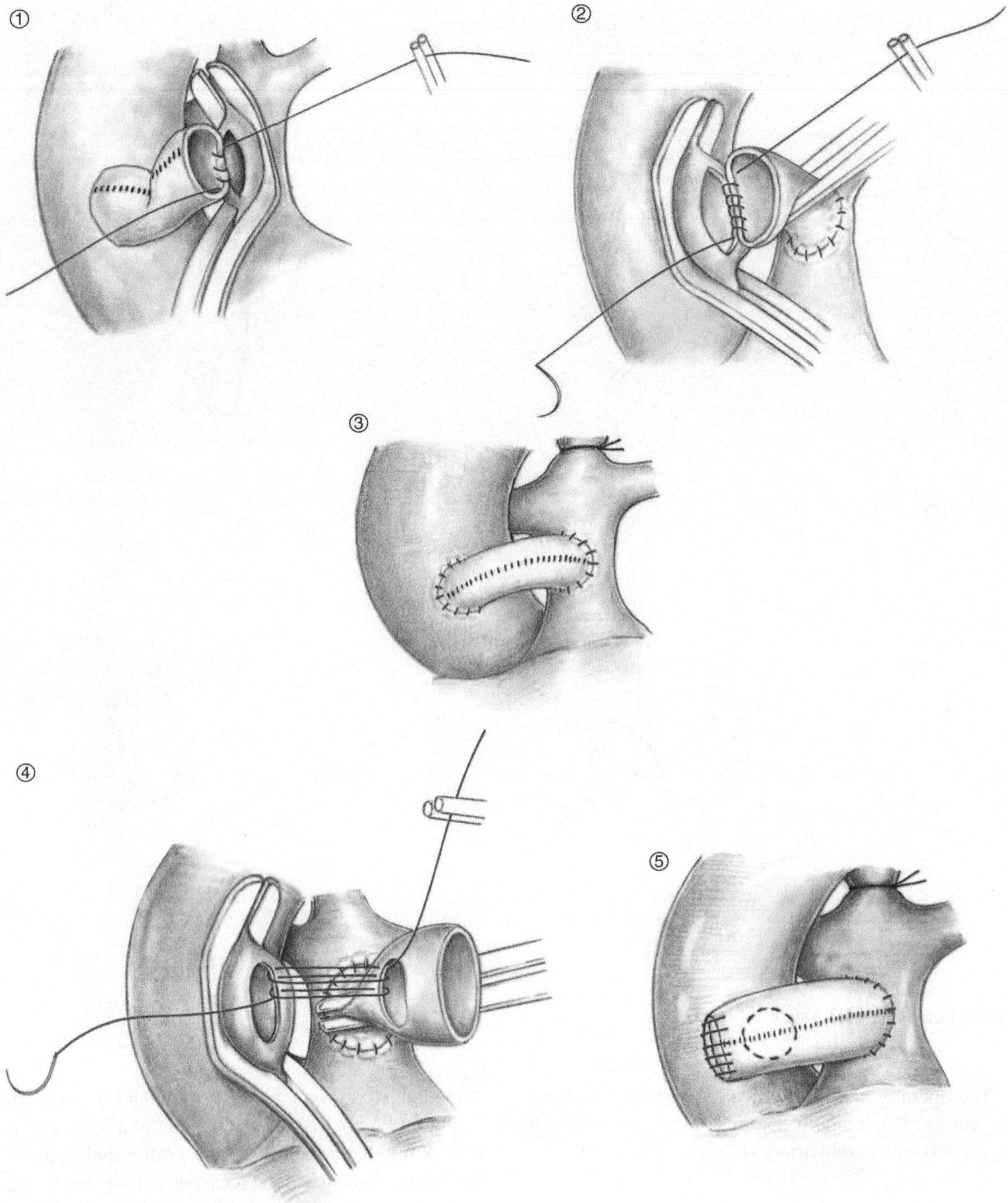

Fig. II-35-5. Central shunt

with a knife. The graft is trimmed and anastomosed with a fine monofilament suture in an end-to-side fashion (Fig. II-35-5 ②). The clamp on the graft is released for de-airing and the partial clamp on the ascending aorta is released (Fig. II-35-5 ③).

An alternative approach is a side-to-side anastomosis between the graft and the ascending aorta to avoid kinking of the graft. A side hole is made in the graft facing the ascending aorta. Using this side hole, a side-to-side anastomosis is completed with a fine monofilament suture (Fig. II-35-5 ④). The open end of the graft is clamped. The partial clamp on the ascending aorta and clamp on the graft are released. The end of the tube graft is then closed with a running suture (Fig. II-35-5 ⑤).

Takedown of BT Shunt

At the time of complete repair, the native vessel in a classic BT shunt is ligated and the PTFE tube in a modified BT shunt is divided to avoid distortion of the branch PA with growth of the patient.

Takedown of the right shunt is straightforward. Graft position is confirmed by palpation behind the superior vena cava. The posterior pericardium is opened longitudinally above the right PA. The vena cava is pushed laterally, and the connective tissue 1 cm superior to the pulmonary artery is dissected because of potential difficulty in dissecting the anastomosis site. A heavy silk ligature is passed around the graft using a right-angle clamp. After initiation of cardiopulmonary bypass, the graft is doubly ligated and divided. Each end is closed with a running suture.

Takedown of the left side shunt is more difficult than on the right side. The graft may be identified by tracing the left PA. The left side of the pericardium adjacent to the ascending aorta is longitudinally opened, and the left pulmonary artery is dissected. Dissection is advanced to the peripheral PA, and the anastomosis site is identified. If intervention on the branch PA is required, this approach is utilized (Fig. II-35-6). An alternative approach is to trace from the left subclavian artery. In the patient with a classic BT shunt, this approach is often utilized. The innominate vein is brought anteriorly, and dissection is advanced to the left subclavian artery along the brachiocephalic artery in right arch and along the aortic arch in case of left arch. The subclavian artery is ligated with a heavy silk ligature after initiation of cardiopulmonary bypass.

Pulmonary Artery Banding

Pulmonary artery banding (PAB) was invented by Muller and associates in 1952 [7]. It has been widely used to treat heart failure and to prevent pulmonary vascular disease in the infant [8]. Since results for neonatal complete repair have improved, the indications for PAB are relatively limited. However, it is still applied in small neonates with certain complex congenital heart diseases, especially those with univentricular hearts.

Surgical Indication

PAB is performed in patients with congestive heart failure caused by increased pulmonary blood flow who are thought to be at high risk for complete repair. In patients with d-transposition of the great arteries with decreased left ventricular pressure, PAB is performed in conjunction with systemic-to-pulmonary shunt before the arterial switch operation [9].

Preoperative Evaluation

The following points are evaluated before the surgery.

1. Based on the relationship of the great arteries, the surgical approach is decided.
2. Based on the length of the main PA, the width of the band is decided.

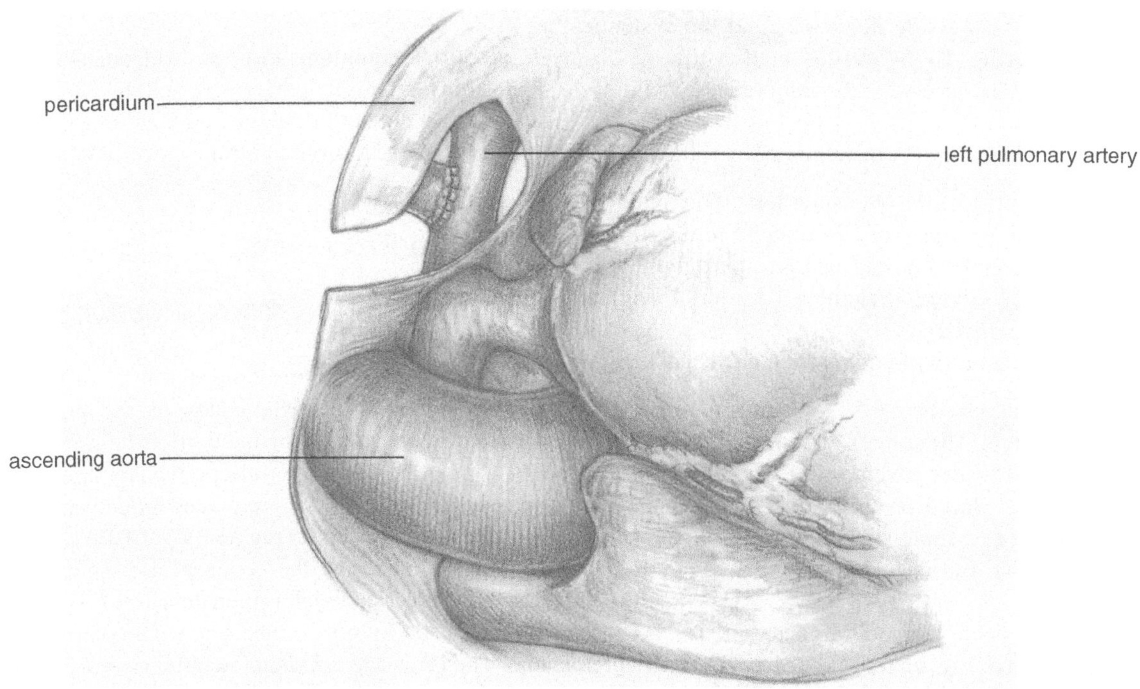

Fig. II-35-6. Takedown of modified BT shunt

3. Presence of left ventricular outflow tract (LVOT) obstruction [10].
4. Presence of patent ductus arteriosus.

Operative Procedure

A lateral thoracotomy, a median sternotomy, or an anterolateral thoracotomy may be used. Exposure via a left anterolateral thoracotomy approach is shown. The chest is entered through the third or fourth intercostal space. The lung is retracted posteriorly, and the pericardium, thymus, and phrenic nerve are identified. The left lobe of thymus is dissected from the pericardium with care to protect the phrenic nerve. The thymus may be partially excised. The pericardium is opened longitudinally anterior to the phrenic nerve, proximal enough to visualize the main PA. Traction sutures are placed on the edges of the pericardium to facilitate visualization of the operative field (Fig. II-35-7 ①). The ascending aorta and the main PA are separated, and a tape is placed around the main PA. Care is taken to avoid damage to the right PA and not to place the band distally, which may cause right PA stenosis.

Silicon-coated Teflon tape that is 3 mm wide is used as a band. Silicon coating facilitates smooth removal of the band at the time of PA debanding. At the middle of the tape, marking stitches are placed. At the distance of (18 + body weight in kg) mm in single ventricle anatomy and (20 + body weight in kg) mm in other than single ventricle anatomy, two sutures are placed on the band tape. The band is attached to the tape, which was placed previously around the main PA. The tape is pulled from behind the PA, drawing the band around the main PA (Fig. II-35-7 ②). A catheter is placed in the main PA, distal to the band site, to measure the pressure continuously. One stitch of the band is put to the marking spot and this string is temporarily tied. The PA pressure decreases, and the systemic pressure increases (Fig. II-35-7 ③). If bradycardia or distention of the heart is observed, the temporary banding is loosened.

The target parameters of PA banding are as follows.

1. Pulmonary artery systolic pressure less than half the systemic systolic pressure (or less than 30 mmHg).
2. In patients with single ventricle anatomy, partial pressure of oxygen (Pao_2) above 35 mmHg or arterial oxygen saturation above 75%.
3. Stable hemodynamics without ventricular distension.

Band tightness is adjusted by 0.5- to 1-mm increments to meet these parameters. The sutures on the band are tied, and the band is sutured to the adventitia of the main PA. The adventitial suture is placed on the main PA to avoid compromising the right PA. Care is taken to avoid distortion of the pulmonary valve by placing the band too proximally (Fig. II-35-7 ④).

The pericardium is closed, and the chest tube is left in the left hemithorax. The key to this procedure is the degree of tightening of the banding, guided by the ratio of systemic to pulmonary blood flow. Because there is no reasonable modality to measure this parameter, pressure is used as a surrogate to assess the adequacy of band tightness.

Management of PA Banding

Debanding is performed at the time of complete repair via median sternotomy. Because the tissue around the band is usually tightly adherent, scissors are used to dissect the band. The site of tightening the band is the landmark for dissection. From this point, dissection of the band is advanced along the middle of the band (Fig. II-35-8 ①). After the sutures securing the band are removed, the band is pulled out smoothly (Fig. II-35-8 ②). When the interval between the band placement and debanding is less than 3 months, growth of the main PA without stenosis is expected. At the time of repair, a Hegar dilator is put through the main PA from the right ventricle to assess size. If stenosis is present, the main PA is opened longitudinally and augmented with an autologous pericardial patch, or reconstructed after resection of the stenotic area (Fig. II-35-8 ③, ④).

Blalock–Hanlon Procedure

This operation was devised and successfully performed by Blalock and Hanlon for the treatment of transposition of the great arteries [11]. It is designed to provide mixing of systemic and pulmonary venous blood. Nowadays, balloon atrial septostomy [12] is usually done for this purpose; in addition, an atrial septal defect can be enlarged through the atrial appendage using a special instrument, so that the Blalock–Hanlon procedure is performed relatively rarely.

Surgical Indication

If interatrial communication is inadequate, balloon atrial septostomy cannot be performed, and the patient is not considered to be a candidate for complete repair or cardiopulmonary bypass, a surgical atrial septectomy is done.

Operative Procedure

The chest is opened via right anterolateral thoracotomy, using the fourth intercostal space. The lung is retracted posteriorly. The pericardium is opened in front of the phrenic nerve longitudinally. The edges of the pericardium are retracted to improve visualization of the operative field. A tape is placed around the right pulmonary artery. Heavy silk ligatures or vessel loops are placed around each pulmonary vein for desired control (Fig. II-35-9 ①). Fine monofilament sutures are placed at the cephalad and caudal ends of the interatrial groove, which is then developed. Two stay sutures are placed on both right and left atrium along this incision line. The PA is snared, then the pulmonary veins are snared. A C-shaped clamp is applied to the left atrium behind the pulmonary veins and anterior to the right atrium. During this

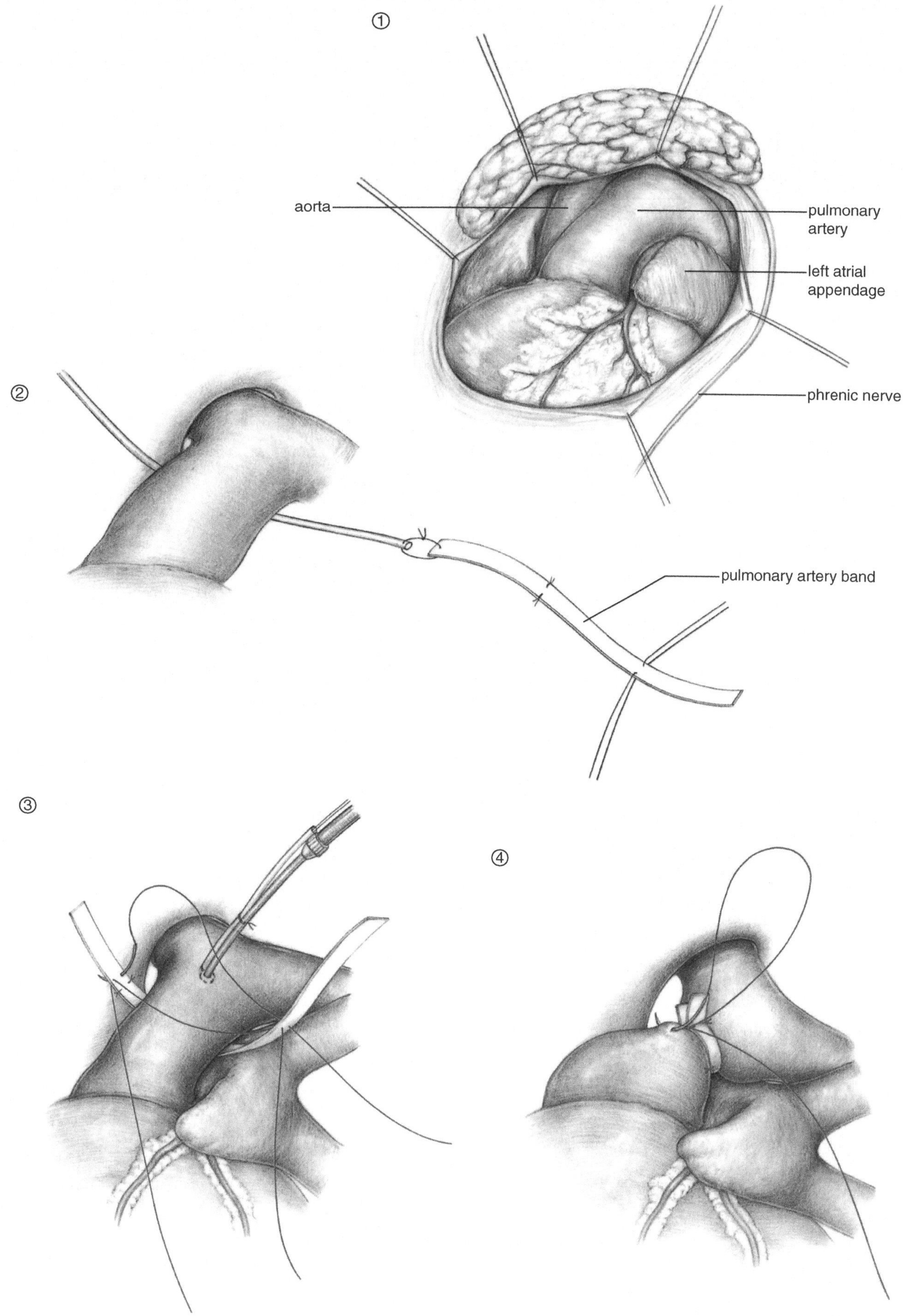

Fig. II-35-7. Pulmonary artery banding: 1

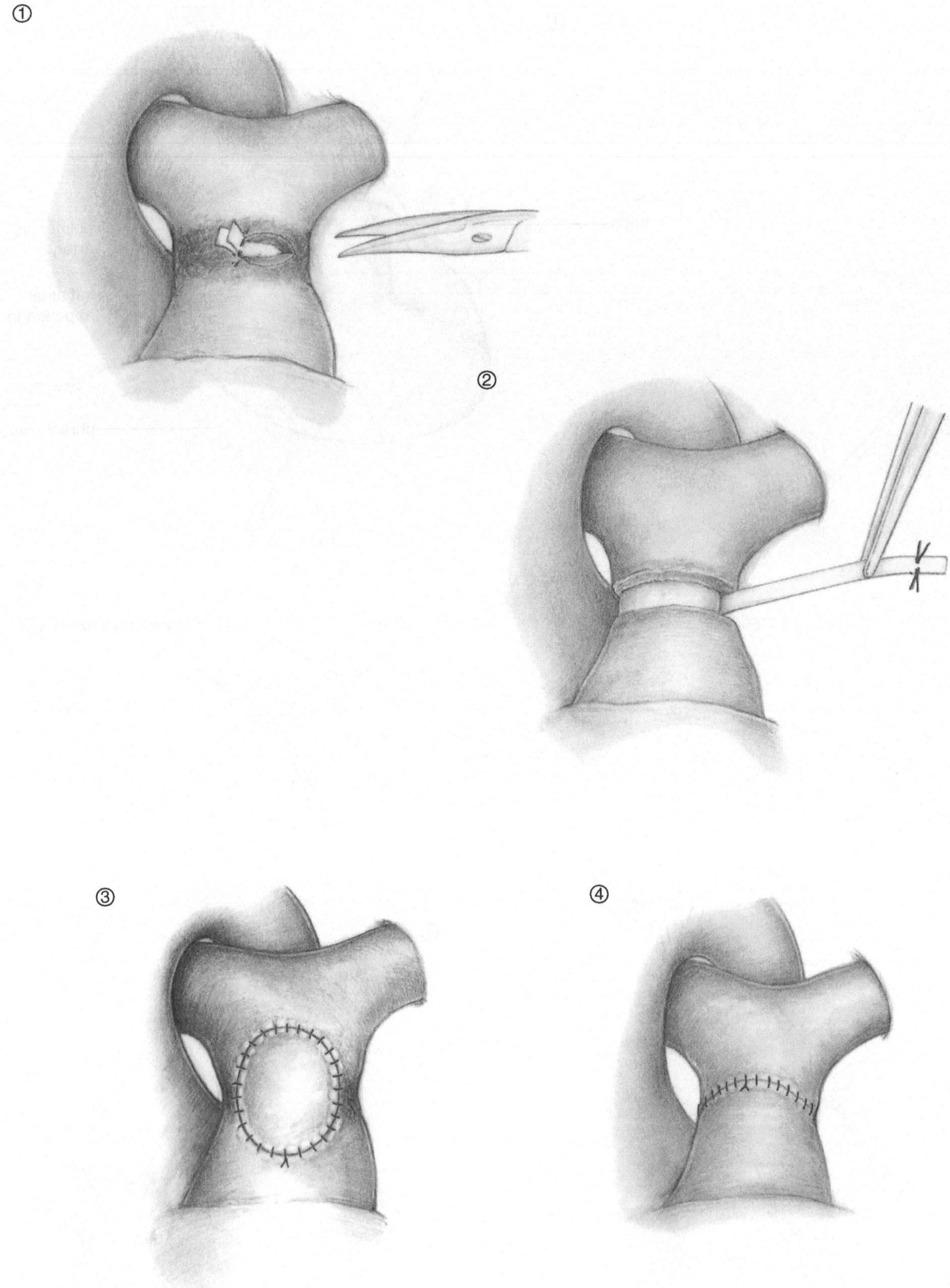

Fig. II-35-8. Pulmonary artery banding: 2. Debanding

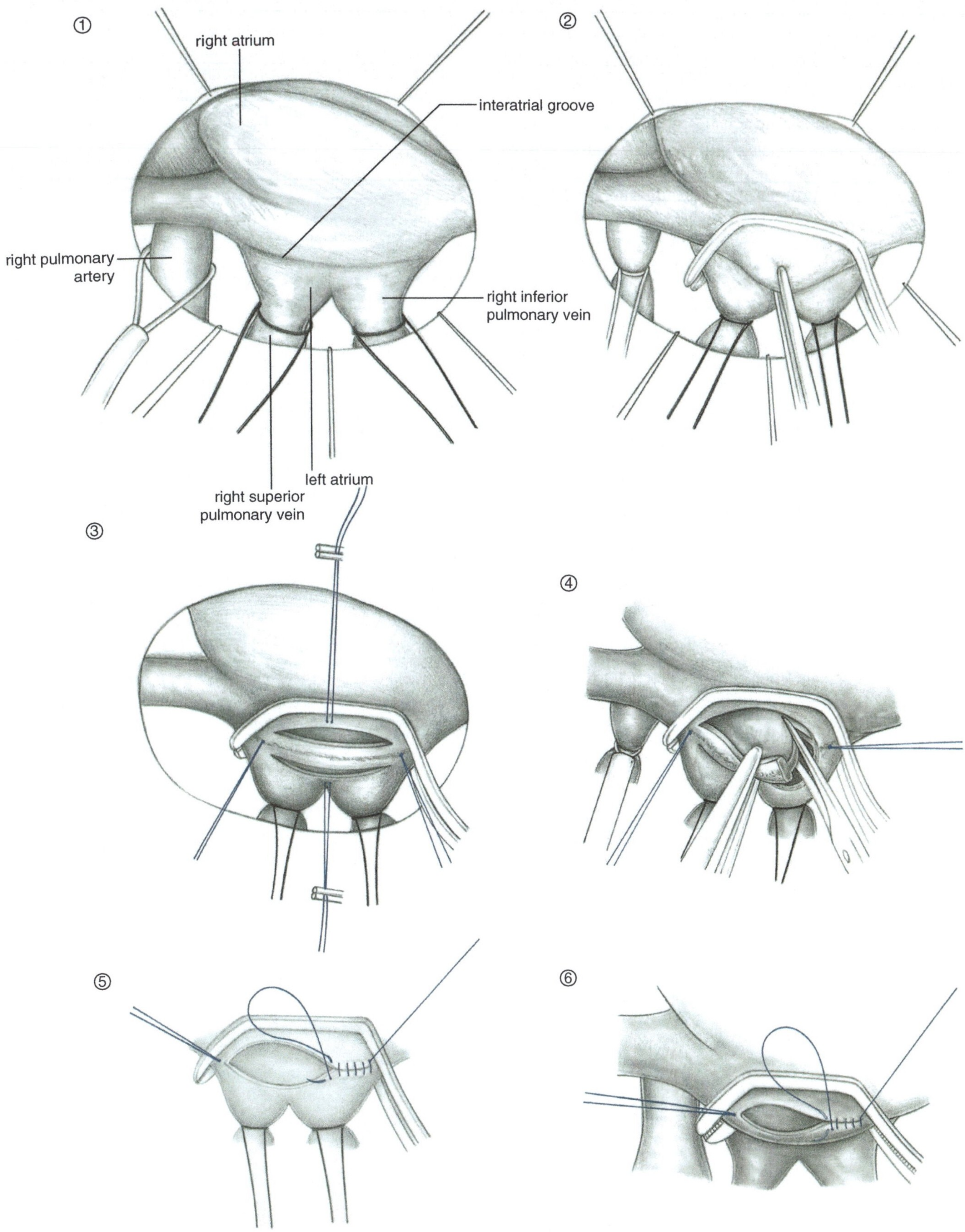

Fig. II-35-9. Blalock–Hanlon Procedure

clamp application the interatrial groove is held firmly and care is taken to protect the sinus node (Fig. II-35-9 ②). The right and left atria are opened longitudinally parallel to the interatrial groove. Because this incision can be placed into the atrial septum, the endocardium of the atria should be carefully identified (Fig. II-35-9 ③). If an inadequate atrial septum is present in the jaws of the clamp, the atrial septum is grasped, the clamp is slightly loosened, and the septum is pulled, with reapplication of the clamp. The atrial septum and the interatrial groove are excised with scissors (Fig. II-35-9 ④). To avoid suturing the atrial septum with free walls, the clamp is loosened, and the septum is released, again with reapplication of the clamp. Using monofilament sutures placed previously, the atrial free wall is closed with running suture (Fig. II-35-9 ⑤). After one layer is sutured, de-airing is accomplished, and the clamp is released. The snares are released from the pulmonary vein and then from the PA. The second layer of closure is then accomplished.

If the free wall of the atrial wall is large enough, another clamp is applied after septum excision, shallower than the previously placed clamp (anterior to the pulmonary veins). Then, the snare to the pulmonary veins and the C-shaped clamp are released. The snare on the PA is also released, and the closure is performed with the right lung reperfused (Fig. II-35-9 ⑥).

References

1. Blalock A, Taussig HB (1945) The surgical treatment of malformations of the heart in which there is pulmonary stenosis or pulmonary atresia. JAMA 128:189–192
2. Potts WJ, Smith S, Gibson S (1946) Anastomosis of the aorta to a pulmonary artery for certain types of congenital heart disease. JAMA 132:627–631
3. Waterston D (1962) Treatment of Fallot's tetralogy in children under one year of age. Rozhl Chir 41:181–183
4. de Leval MR, McKay R, Jones M, et al (1981) Modified Blalock–Taussig shunt. Use of subclavian artery orifice as flow regulator in prosthetic systemic-pulmonary artery shunts. J Thorac Cardiovasc Surg 81:112–119
5. Amato JJ, Marbey ML, Bush C, et al (1988) Systemic-pulmonary polytetrafluoroethylene shunts in palliative operations for congenital heart disease. Revival of the central shunt. J Thorac Cardiovasc Surg 95:62–69
6. Laks H, Castaneda AR (1975) Subclavian arterioplasty for the ipsilateral Blalock–Taussig shunt. Ann Thorac Surg 19:319–321
7. Muller WH Jr, Dammann JF Jr (1952) The treatment of certain congenital malformations of the heart by the creation of pulmonic stenosis to reduce pulmonary hypertension and excessive pulmonary blood flow, a preliminary report. Surg Gynecol Obstet 95:213–219
8. Trusler GA, Mustard WT (1972) A method of banding the pulmonary artery for large isolated ventricular septal defect with and without transposition of the great arteries. Ann Thorac Surg 13:351–355
9. Yacoub MH, Radley-Smith R, Maclaurin R (1977) Two-stage operation for anatomical correction of transposition of the great arteries with intact ventricular septum. Lancet 1:1275–1278
10. Freed MD, Rosenthal A, Plauth WH, et al (1973) Development of subaortic stenosis after pulmonary artery banding. Circulation 48(suppl III):III-7–III-10
11. Blalock A, Hanlon CR (1950) The surgical treatment of complete transposition of the aorta and the pulmonary artery. Surg Gynecol Obstet 90:1–15
12. Rashkind WJ, Miller WW (1966) Creation of an atrial septal defect without thoracotomy. A palliative approach to complete transposition of the great arteries. JAMA 196:991–992

II-36. Minimum Access Cardiac Surgery

Currently, less invasive cardiac surgery is performed in many situations. Less invasive cardiac surgery means cardiac surgery with a partial sternotomy or even avoidance of sternotomy altogether. However, the option to avoid using cardiopulmonary bypass as in off-pump coronary bypass grafting in adult surgery is virtually never available in congenital heart operations.

For limited skin incision pediatric cardiac surgery, approaches are generally either anterior (partial or complete sternotomy, or parasternal) or lateral. Anterior skin incisions for trans-sternal access may be (1) T-shaped [1], (2) inverted T-shape [2], (3) inverse L-shape [3,4], (4) inverted reverse L-shape (J-shape) [5], or (5) transverse sternotomy [6]. An anterior parasternal approach is also possible [6–8] (Fig. II-36-1). For lateral access anterolateral [9], lateral, and posterolateral thoracotomies, axial approaches are applied.

Surgery via Sternotomy

Atrial septal defect, ventricular septal defect, atrioventricular septal defect, and simple repair of tetralogy of Fallot are good indications for this procedure. The sternum of young children is very flexible, and a partial median sternotomy is sufficient to obtain good visualization to perform many types of cardiac operations. Although it has been suggested that the skin incision should begin at the level of the areola and extend to the tip of the xiphoid, we recommend that the incision begin 1 cm above the nipple line. With this incision, a standard aortic cross-clamp can be applied. The sternum is cut from the xiphoid to the body of the sternum, but the manubrium is not divided. This preservation of the manubrium enhances stability of the sternum after surgery. With application of a Kent retractor to the superior edge of the skin incision and retraction cephalad, good visualization of the operating field is obtained.

The pericardium is opened in reverse T shape. The inferior margin of the pericardium is retracted to the inferior margin of the skin incision. The cephalad pericardial edges are retracted caudally. The ascending aorta is pulled caudally and anteriorly. To avoid excessive traction of the superior vena cava (SVC), the pericardial refection of the SVC is dissected. If the thymus impedes visualization, a traction suture is placed to the pericardial reflection above the ascending aorta, and this stitch is fixed to the edge of the skin incision to keep the thymus out of the operative field.

After the ascending aorta is pulled down with delicate hemostatic forceps, purse-string sutures are easily placed on the ascending aorta. A flexible straight aortic cannula is used. Purse-string sutures are placed on the SVC and inferior vena cava (IVC). Right-angle venous cannulae are inserted into both cavae directly. The IVC cannula is inserted first to provide better visualization and avoid hemodynamic compromise. After initiation of cardiopulmonary bypass (CPB), the SVC cannula is inserted. Tapes are snared around both cavae. A cardioplegic needle is inserted into the root of the ascending aorta, and the aortic cross-clamp is applied.

Surgery via Thoracotomy

Atrial septal defect and anomalous drainage of right pulmonary vein to the right atrium are good indications for this procedure. From a cosmetic point of view, a median sternotomy incision is far more visible than a thoracotomy scar. Because the standard vertical incision is made at right angles to the lines of Langer, the scar widens with time. Additionally, keloids tend to develop at the sternum. On the other hand, because a thoracotomy incision can be parallel to the Langer's lines, the scar will not widen and may be less likely to develop keloids. This approach is especially applicable in female patients as the incision can be hidden by a swimsuit.

Although the anterolateral thoracotomy gives an excellent surgical view in infants, it is very difficult to predict the lower margin of the mammary tissue in prepubescent girls. Because an anterolateral thoracotomy incision may thus impair breast development, we prefer the lateral thoracotomy. The skin incision is started 1 cm beneath the inferior margin of the scapula and carried toward the midpoint between the nipple and costal arch. This incision should not be extended anterior to the anterior axial line. The latissimus dorsi and serratus anterior muscles are partially divided. The fourth intercostal space is entered. Exposure is gained by extending the incision medially to the internal mammary artery and laterally to the iliocostalis muscles.

The pericardium is opened longitudinally 1.5 cm anterior to the phrenic nerve. At the level of the diaphragm, the pericardial incision is carried anteriorly. After the thymus is dissected from the pericardium, the incision is extended cephalad. Traction sutures are applied to the edges of the pericardial opening. To elevate the operative field, cephalad and caudad traction sutures are retracted inferiorly and superiorly, respectively.

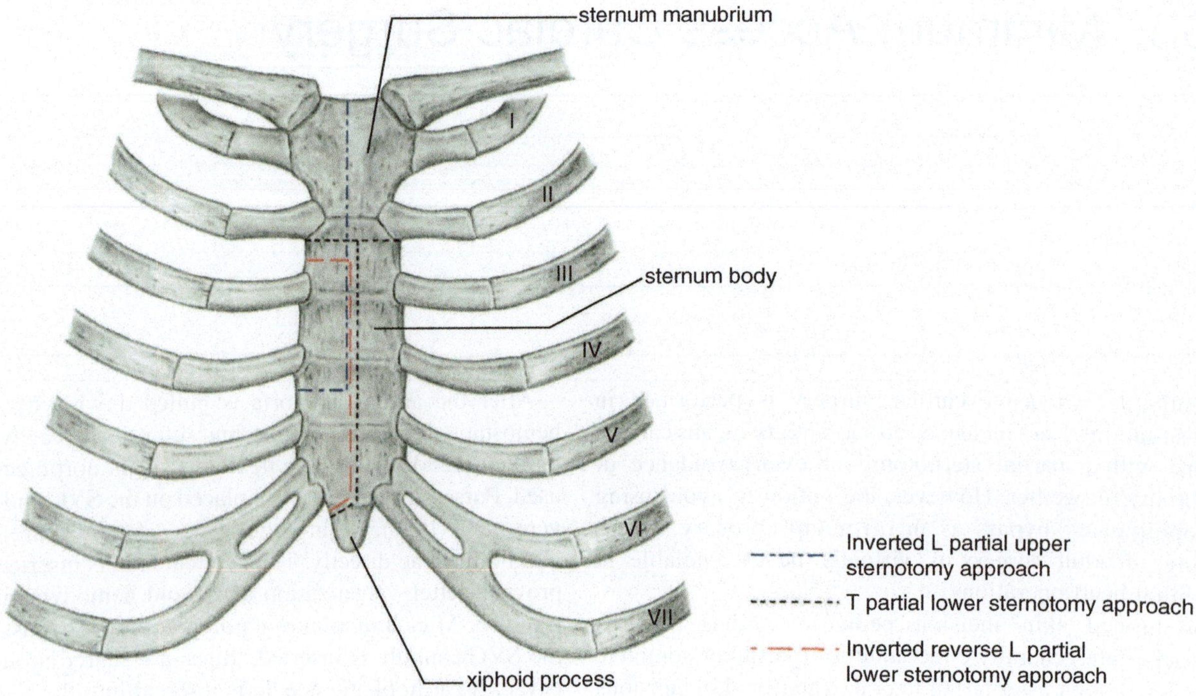

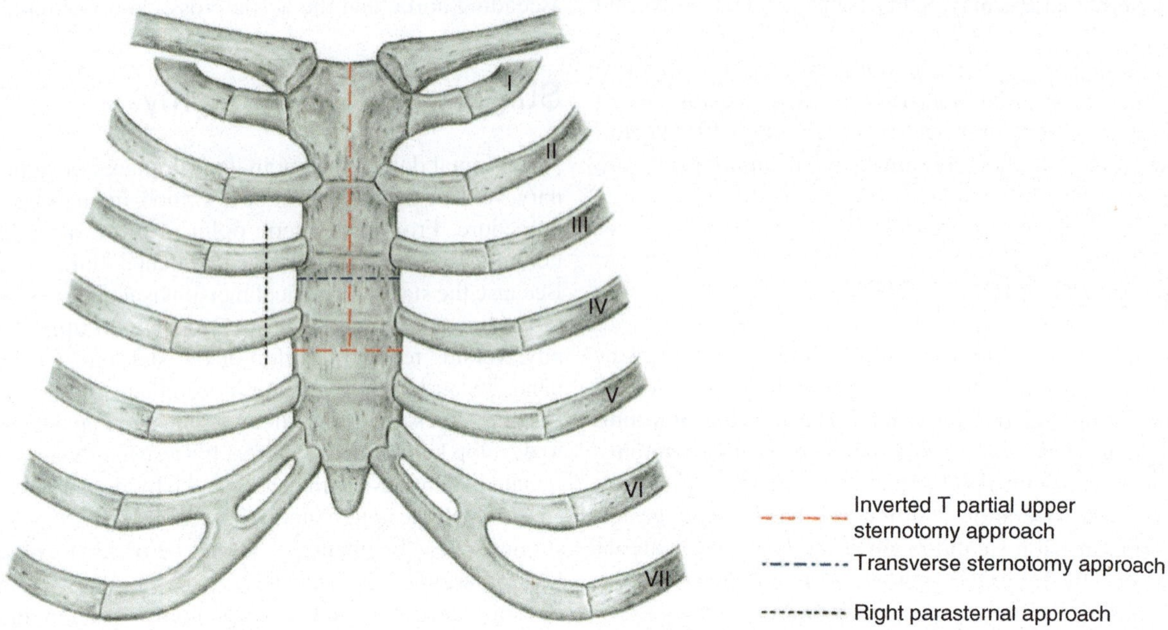

Fig. II-36-1. Access to heart via minimal skin incision

Two purse-string sutures are always placed in the ascending aorta, and a straight aortic cannula is used. Care is taken not to exceed the line pressure on the arterial cannulation side. Purse-string sutures are placed in the SVC and IVC, and right-angle venous cannulae are directly inserted. The IVC is cannulated first, because access is easier than for the SVC. The cardioplegic cannula is inserted into the ascending aorta. The SVC cannula is placed last. Tapes are applied to both cavae. The ascending aorta is cross-clamped, and then a standard operation is performed as would be accomplished via a full sternotomy. The following surgical procedures should be referred to each cardiac defect and surgical procedure chapter.

References

1. Doty DB, DiRusso GB, Doty JR (1998) Full-spectrum cardiac surgery through a minimal incision. Mini-sternotomy (lower half) technique. Ann Thorac Surg 65:573–577
2. Gundry SR, Shattuck OH, Razzouk AJ (1998) Facile minimally invasive cardiac surgery via ministernotomy. Ann Thorac Surg 65:1100–1104

3. Nair RU, Sharpe DAC (1998) Limited lower sternotomy for minimally invasive mitral valve replacement. Ann Thorac Surg 65:273–274
4. Rodriguez JE, Cortina J, Sota EP, et al (1998) A new approach to cardiac valve replacement through a small midline incision and inverted L shape partial sternotomy. Eur J Cardiothorac Surg 14:S115–S116
5. Svensson LG, D'Agostino RS (1998) "J" incision minimal-access valve operations. Ann Thorac Surg 66:1110–1112
6. Cosgrove DM, Sabik JF (1996) Minimally invasive approach for aortic valve operations. Ann Thorac Surg 62:596–597
7. Frazier BL, Derrick MJ, Purewal SS, et al (1998) Minimally invasive aortic valve replacement. Eur J Cardiothorac Surg 14:S122–S125
8. Matsuda H (1998) Minimally invasive cardiac surgery: Principle and prospects. Surg Today 28:775–779
9. Giamberti A, Mazzera E, Di Chiara L, et al (2000) Right submammary minithoracotomy for repair of congenital heart defects. Eur J Cardiothorac Surg 18:678–682

II-37. Pediatric Cardiac Transplantation

Cardiac transplantation is performed for pediatric patients with severe heart failure that results from cardiomyopathy, myocarditis, congenital heart disease, or cardiac tumor. Although any type of congenital heart defect may lead to end-stage heart failure, patients with a simple congenital heart defect usually do not develop severe heart failure. As an exception to the rule, some patients with a partial atrioventricular canal, however, may develop end-stage heart failure as a consequence of atrioventricular valve regurgitation, subaortic stenosis, and complete atrioventricular block. Cardiac transplantation is often required in patients with hypoplastic left heart syndrome, single ventricle, congenitally corrected transposition of great arteries, and anomalous origin of the left coronary artery from the pulmonary artery. Before transplantation, some children require mechanical circulatory support such as extracorporeal membrane oxygenation (ECMO) or ventricular assist device (VAD).

In this chapter, we discuss cardiac transplantation for patients with cardiomyopathy, hypoplastic left heart syndrome, ECMO support, and VAD support (Berlin Heart EXCOR).

Donor Heart Selection and Recovery

At the time of donor selection, the following should be taken into consideration: blood type, weight difference, sex difference, heart function, amount of inotropic support, cause of death, and expected ischemic time.

The cardiac procurement is generally performed as part of a multi-organ procurement. Before recovery, the surgeon should check whether he or she needs to recover additional parts of the great vessels such as distal ascending aorta, aortic arch, branch pulmonary artery, superior vena cava, or innominate vein. During organ retrieval, the recovery team must continuously update the recipient team. A standard median sternotomy is performed. The pericardium is opened longitudinally and the heart is inspected for external signs of ventricular function or major damage caused by trauma or cardiac resuscitation.

The aorta and pulmonary artery are dissected superiorly, and a tape is placed around the ascending aorta. The superior vena cava is also dissected superiorly. When the abdominal organ recovery team finishes preparation for explantation and cannulation, intravenous heparin at a dose of 300 units/kg body weight is administered. Three minutes after heparin administration, a purse-string suture is placed in the root of the ascending aorta and a cardioplegic needle is inserted. The ascending aorta is clamped, and cardioplegic solution is administered. After aortic clamping, the inferior vena cava is incised above the diaphragm to vent the preservation solutions from the abdominal organs. To decompress the left heart, the base of the right upper pulmonary vein is cut. When the lungs are recovered simultaneously, the tip of the left atrial appendage is cut to obtain better venting of the left side of the heart. Topical iced saline is applied to achieve rapid cardiac cooling. After completion of cardioplegic solution administration, the cardioplegic needle is removed and the purse-string suture tied. The cardiectomy is begun by transection of the inferior vena cava. Next, the apex of the heart is elevated, and the pulmonary veins are divided, or the left atrium is opened between the pulmonary vein orifices and coronary sinus if the lungs are to be recovered simultaneously. Then, the ascending aorta and main pulmonary artery are divided at the necessary levels.

For recipients with an aortic arch anomaly such as hypoplastic left heart syndrome, the entire aortic arch and proximal descending aorta are recovered en bloc with the heart. Similarly, if the recipient has hypoplasia or stenosis of the branch pulmonary arteries, the branch pulmonary arteries are taken with the heart if the lungs are not being recovered. Last, the superior vena cava is divided with or without the innominate vein. The heart is brought to a back table, where the donor heart is placed into a bag with cold solution. This bag is placed into a larger bag, which is put into a plastic container with cold saline. This plastic container is placed in the transport cooler box. Lymph nodes, which are recovered from the abdominal organ recovery team, are placed in an appropriate container and brought back to the recipient hospital for a retrospective cross-match.

Implantation

Transplantation is usually accomplished by either a right atrial or bicaval technique. In many pediatric patients, high pulmonary vascular resistance is often observed. Therefore, we primarily use the bicaval insertion technique, because this technique seems to be associated with less tricuspid valve regurgitation after transplant.

A standard median sternotomy and ascending aortic with bicaval cannulation are utilized. A left atrial vent is inserted

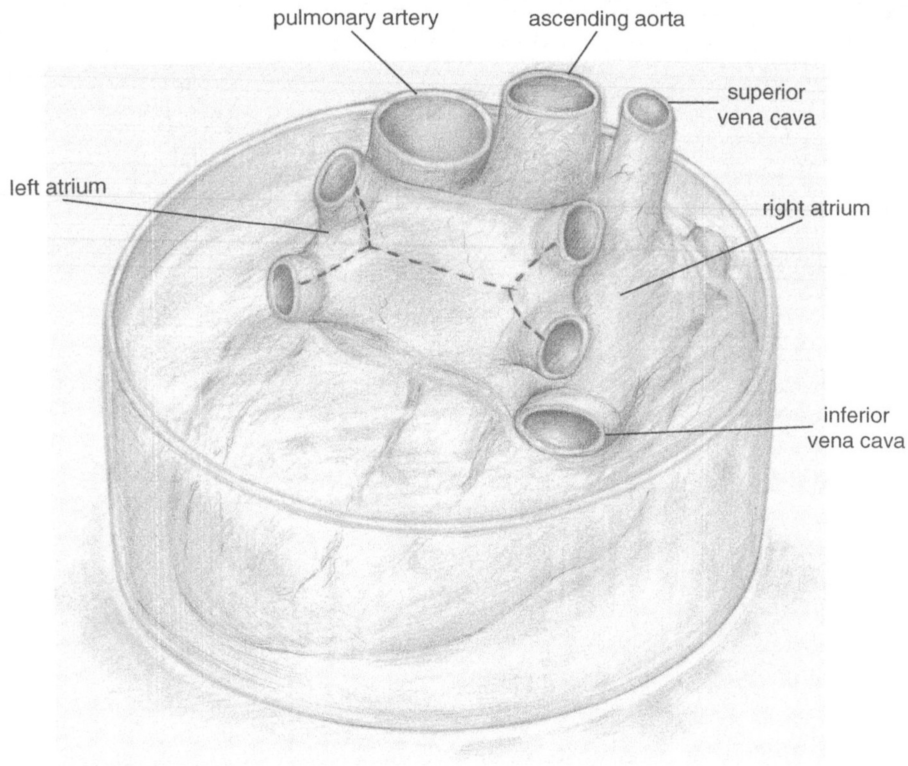

Fig. II-37-1. Preparation of donor heart. Preparation of the donor heart is performed in a bowl with cold saline. The left atrium is opened by connecting the orifices of the pulmonary veins. Excess left atrial tissue is removed to create a cuff sized to fit the recipient left atrial cuff

from the base of the right upper pulmonary vein. After both the superior and inferior vena cavae are snared with tapes, the aorta is cross-clamped. The heart is excised beginning with division of the inferior vena cava. The left atrium is opened between the left pulmonary veins and coronary sinus, and the left atrial cuff is created. The ascending aorta and main pulmonary artery are transected at the level of the sinotubular junction. The superior vena cava is transected at its junction with the right atrium. If additional repair is required for the pulmonary arteries, this repair is accomplished before donor heart implantation to reduce ischemic time.

When the recipient operating field is ready for implantation, the donor heart is removed from the transport cooler box, and the donor heart is placed in a bowl of cold saline. (The preparation of the donor heart is performed in this bowl to reduce warm ischemic time.) The left atrium is opened by incisions connecting the orifices of the pulmonary veins (Fig. II-37-1). Excess left atrial tissue is removed to optimize the size match to the recipient left atrial cuff. The atrial septum should be inspected for a patent foramen ovale, which, if present, should be closed with a running suture. The posterior aspect of the pulmonary artery is dissected from the roof of the left atrium.

Here, bicaval anastomosis technique is discussed [1]. Implantation consists of a series of five sequential anastomoses: the left atrium, the inferior vena cava, the pulmonary artery, the ascending aorta, and finally the superior vena cava. A cold saline-soaked sponge is placed on the left side of the sternal retractor. The donor heart is placed on this sponge to keep the left atrium up and the ascending aorta superior (Fig. II-37-2). A running suture is started at the base of the donor left atrial appendage and the recipient left atrium anterior to the left pulmonary vein orifice. After the first few stitches are placed, the donor heart is lowered into the pericardium. The suture line is advanced toward the inferior vena cava. The anterior and superior portion of the left atrial anastomosis is completed using the second arm of the suture. Before finishing this suture line, the tip of the left atrial vent tube is relocated to the left ventricle through the mitral valve (Fig. II-37-3). Next, the inferior vena cava is anastomosed. The pulmonary artery is then shortened appropriately and anastomosed. Next, the aorta is trimmed and anastomosed. After completion of the aortic suture line, a steroid bolus is given and the heart is de-aired. De-airing is accomplished by clamping the ventricular vent while aspirating a catheter in the root of the ascending aorta. Alternatively, a tiny aortotomy may be created for de-airing. To minimize the possibility of air embolism, the operating field is flooded with carbon dioxide until all the anastomoses are completed. The superior vena cava is anastomosed after the cross-clamp is removed. Care is taken to avoid twisting or narrowing the anastomosis. To reduce the chance of a purse-string effect, we tie an "air-knot," purposely leaving 1–2 mm of looseness in the knot (shown in Fig. II-30-6). As an alternative, the superior vena cava may be distended while tying the knot, by temporarily occluding the donor superior vena cava with a clamp while simultaneously clamping the superior vena caval cannula. Before separation from bypass, hemostasis at the left atrial suture line should be checked because it is difficult to expose this suture line after weaning from bypass.

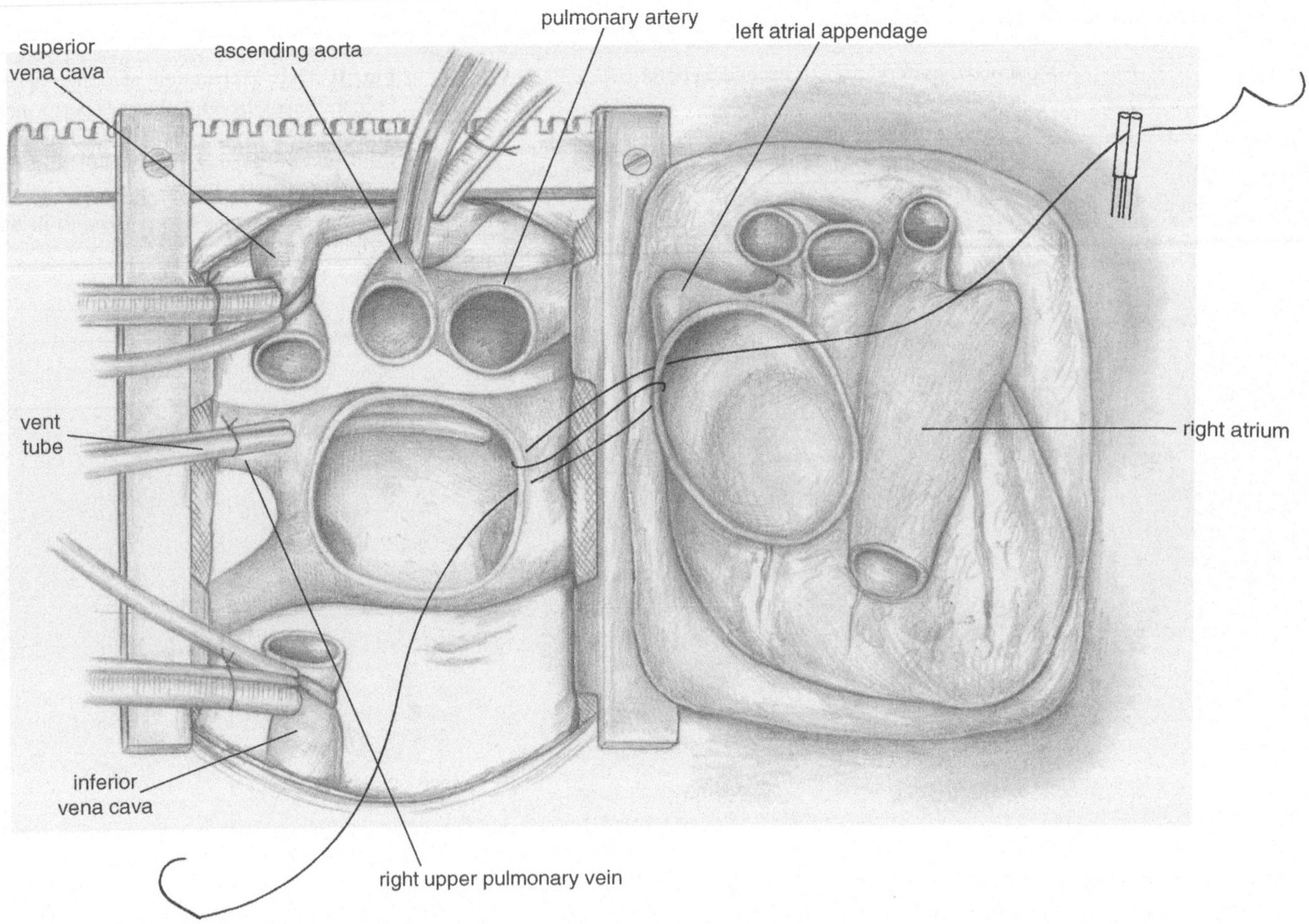

Fig. II-37-2. Bypass is started with ascending aortic and bicaval cannulation. A left atrial vent is inserted via the base of the right upper pulmonary vein. After tapes on the cavae are snugged down, cardiectomy is performed. The donor heart is placed on a cold saline-soaked sponge, on the left side of the chest retractor. Anastomosis is begun at the base of the left atrial appendage. This running suture line is advanced in a clockwise direction

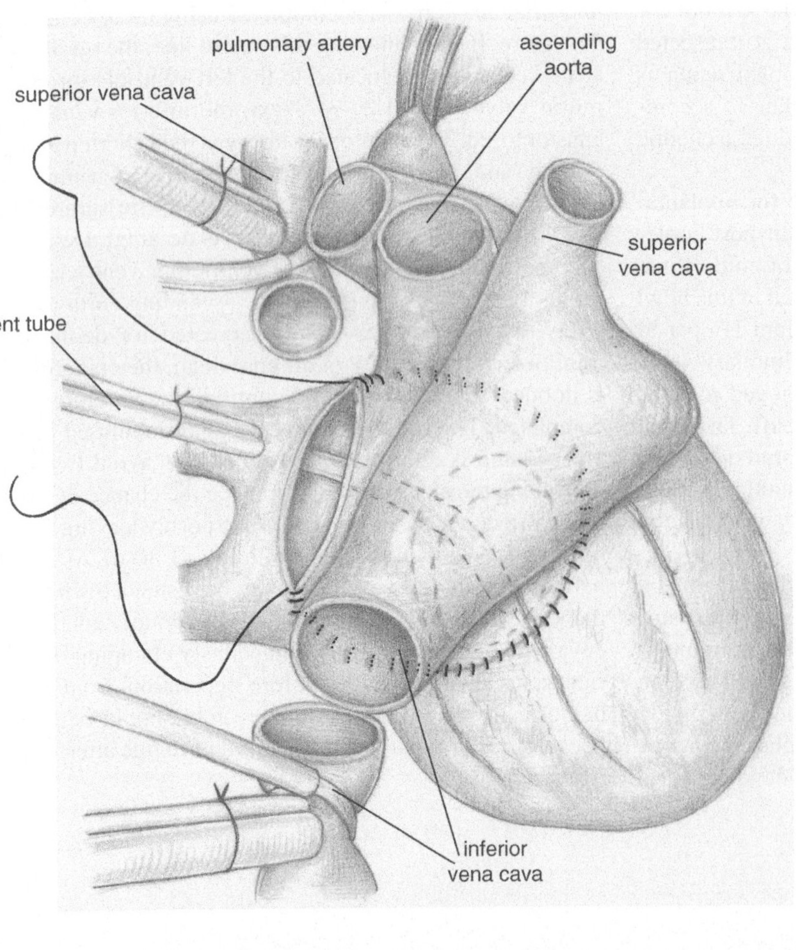

Fig. II-37-3. When the first arm suture line comes past the inferior vena cava, the other arm is used to complete the superior suture line. Before finishing this suture line, the tip of the left atrial vent is passed into the left ventricle

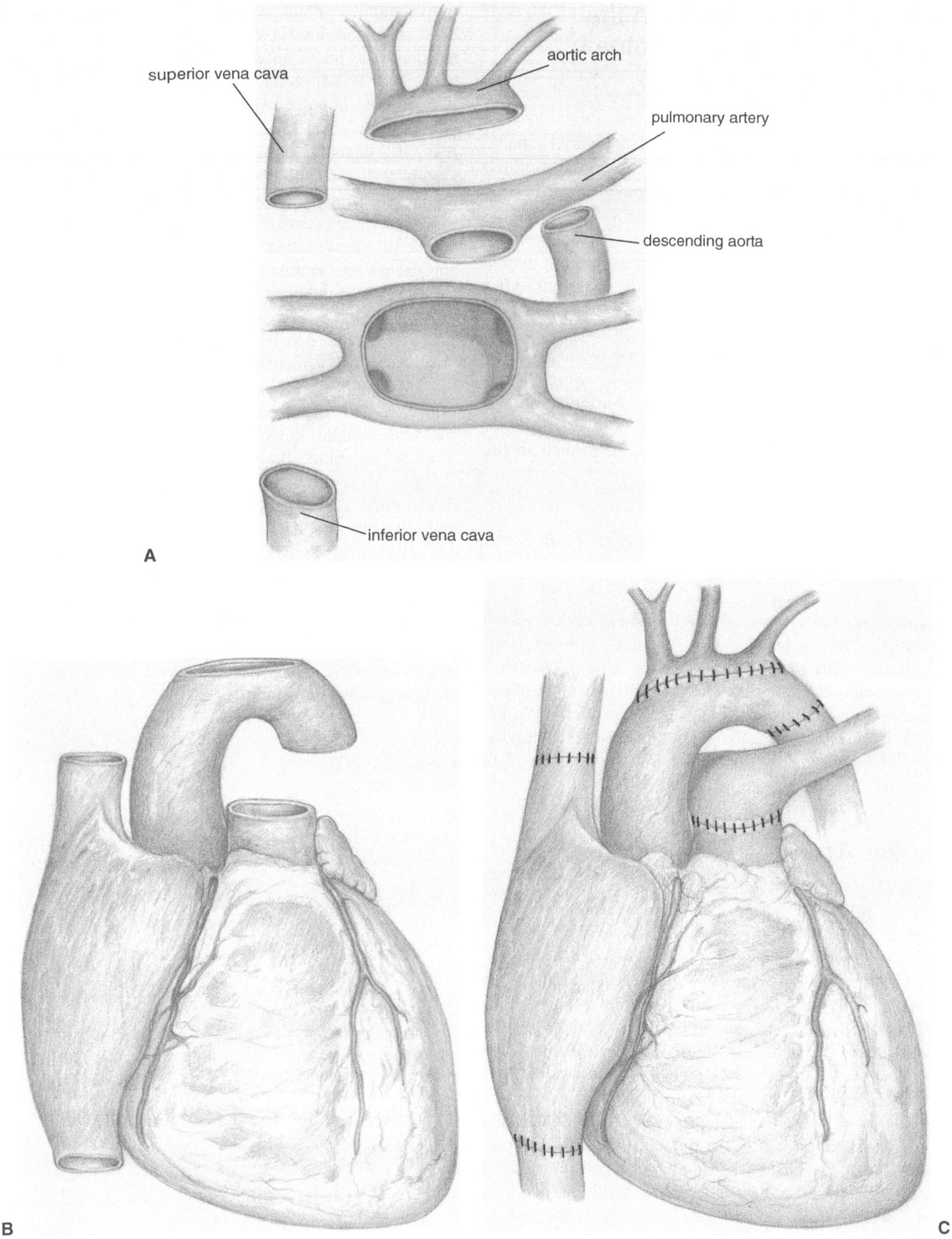

Fig. II-37-4. Transplantation for hypoplastic left heart syndrome. **A** Cardiectomy. Preparation for a bicaval approach is shown here. **B** Donor heart recovery. A donor heart is recovered with the aortic arch and proximal descending aorta. **C** Implantation. The donor descending aorta is anastomosed to the recipient descending aorta with end-to-end technique, and the island patch of recipient brachiocephalic vessels is anastomosed to the donor arch

Cardiac Transplantation in the Presence of Complex Anatomy

Hypoplastic Left Heart Syndrome [2]

Cardiopulmonary bypass is initiated with an arterial cannula through a polytetrafluoroethylene (PTFE) tube anastomosed to the base of the brachiocephalic artery and regular bicaval cannula. The ductus arteriosus is dissected and ligated. Dissection is advanced to the aortic arch, arch branches, and descending aorta. The bases of the arch branches are snared, and regional cerebral low flow perfusion is started. After tapes are snared on the superior and inferior vena cavae, and a clamp is applied to the descending aorta, cardiectomy is started. The aortic arch is kept as a patch with the three arch branches (Fig. II-37-4). The donor descending aorta is anastomosed to the recipient descending aorta distal to the ductus. The recipient arch patch is anastomosed to the donor aortic arch. The other anastomoses are performed in the usual fashion.

Transplantation in the Presence of Left Superior Vena Cava [3]

When a recipient has a persistent left superior vena cava, the innominate vein is recovered at the time of donor heart procurement. The recipient left superior vena cava is then anastomosed to the donor innominate vein. Other anastomoses are performed in the usual fashion. As an alternative, the right atrial anastomosis technique may be used, leaving the native left superior vena cava draining to the recipient right atrial cuff.

Cardiac Transplantation for the Patient on ECMO or VAD

When a patient is supported with ECMO, there are two surgical approaches. One is to employ standard cannulation, and the other is to use the ECMO arterial cannula as an arterial cannula for bypass. With both techniques, superior and inferior vena cavae are ultimately cannulated in the usual fashion. For initiation of bypass, right atrial or inferior vena cava cannulation is used. Then, the venous ECMO cannula is removed from the right jugular vein, and the superior vena cava is cannulated. Repair of the jugular vein should be accomplished. If the duration of ECMO support has been short, repair of the carotid artery is recommended. If cannulae have been in place for more than 2 weeks, repair of the artery is not recommended because of the risk of pseudoaneurysm formation. Cardiac implantation technique after cardiectomy is otherwise the same as regular cardiac transplantation. Patients who have been on ECMO before heart transplant are typically very edematous, and the time required for post-implant hemostasis is often prolonged because of ECMO-related coagulopathy.

Currently, in North America and Europe, the most commonly used ventricular assist device is the Berlin Heart EXCOR, which is a paracorporeal, pneumatically driven system with pulsatile flow. Cardiac transplantation under this device support is discussed here [4].

If the available ascending aorta is short because of previous aortic cannulation for the assist device, alternative approaches are cannulation in the aortic arch, cannulation of a graft sewn on the brachiocephalic artery or the artery itself, or right carotid artery cannulation via a right cervical incision as with ECMO cannulation.

When a left ventricular assist device (LVAD) is used, venous cannulae are inserted into the superior and inferior vena cava. However, if adhesions are severe, bypass is initiated with a single right atrial cannula, and further dissection is accomplished to allow direct caval cannulation.

When Bi-VAD is used, dissection can be particularly challenging. For initiation of bypass, the right ventricular assist device (RVAD) venous cannula can be used, after discontinuation of VAD support. The RVAD inflow cannula is doubly clamped and divided, and the venous tubing for bypass is connected.

At the time of cardiac transplantation after VAD support, the old tunnels used for VAD cannulae may be the site of profuse bleeding, and it is mandatory to be sure these areas are completely hemostatic.

References

1. el Gamel A, Yonan NA, Grant S, et al (1995) Orthotopic cardiac transplantation: a comparison of standard and bicaval Wythenshawe techniques. J Thorac Cardiovasc Surg 109:721–729
2. Bailey L, Concepcion W, Shattuck H, et al (1986) Method of heart transplantation for treatment of hypoplastic left heart syndrome. J Thorac Cardiovasc Surg 92:1–5
3. Chartrand C, Guerin R, Kangah M, et al (1990) Pediatric heart transplantation: surgical considerations for congenital heart diseases. J Heart Transplant 9:608–616
4. Hetzer R, Loebe M, Potapov EV, et al (1998) Circulatory support with pneumatic paracorporeal ventricular assist device in infants and children. Ann Thorac Surg 66:1498–1506

Suggested Readings

Franco KL (ed) (1997) Pediatric Cardiopulmonary Transplantation. Futura, Armok, NY, pp 97–114

Gardner TJ, Spray TL (eds) (2004) Operative Cardiac Surgery. Arnold, London, pp 351–361

Supplement

For right ventricular volume measurement, Simpson's rule was used, and for left ventricular volume measurement, the area–length method was used.

References

Rowlatt normal valve diameter

Rowlatt UF, Rimoldi HJA, Lev M (1963) The quantitative anatomy of the normal child's heart. Pediatr Clin N Am 10:499–588

Kishimoto normal valve diameter, Kishimoto normal ventricular volume

Kishimoto H, Hirose H, et al (1985) Normal left and right ventricle volume and normal atrioventricular and semilunar valve size measured by the cardiac angiogram. Shinzou 17:711–716

Tokyo Women's Medical College normal ventricular volume

Nakazawa M, Marks RA, et al (1976) Right and left ventricular volume characteristics in children with pulmonary stenosis and intact ventricular septum. Circulation 53:884–890

PA index (Nakata index)

{[the cross-sectional area of the right pulmonary artery immediately proximal to the origin of the first branches (mm^2)] + [the cross-sectional area of the left pulmonary artery immediately proximal to the origin of the first branches (mm^2)]} / body surface area (M^2)

Nakata S, Imai Y, et al (1984) A new method for the quantitative standardization of cross-sectional areas of the pulmonary arteries in congenital heart disease with decreased pulmonary blood flow. J Thorac Cardiovasc Surg 88:610–619

● Rowlatt normal valve diameter

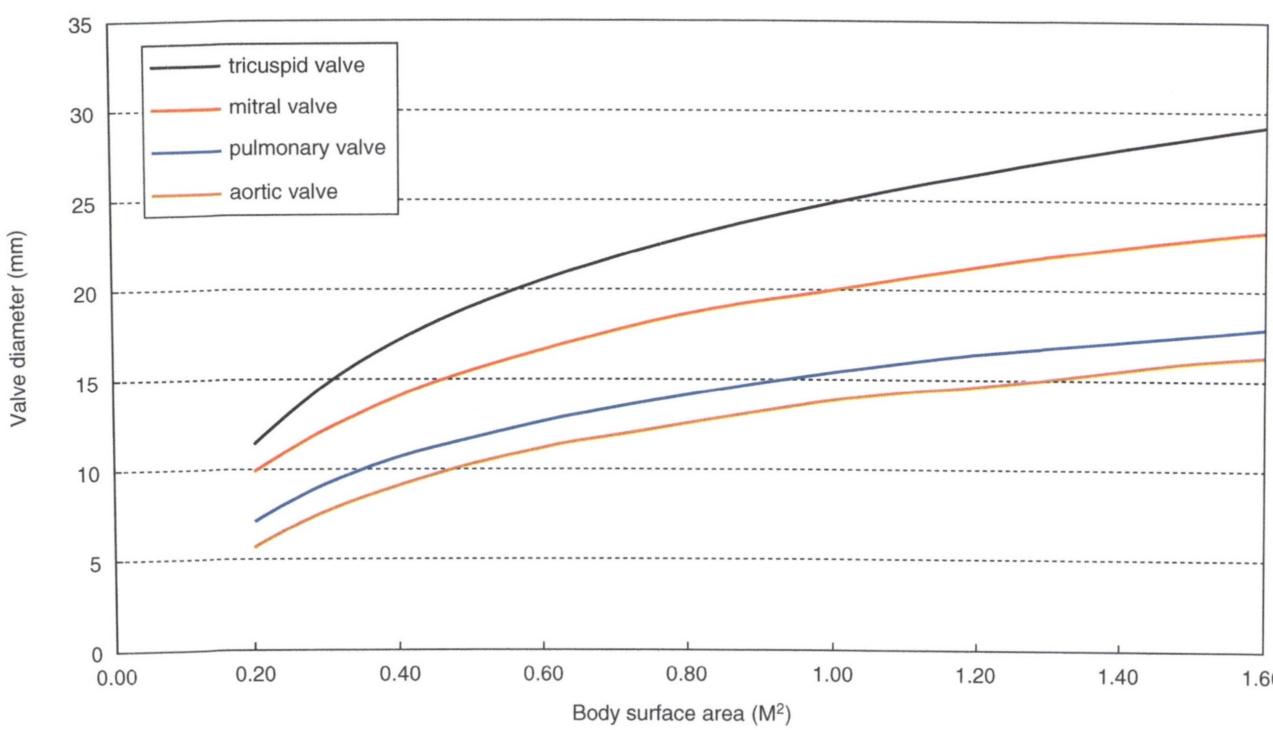

● Kishimoto normal valve diameter

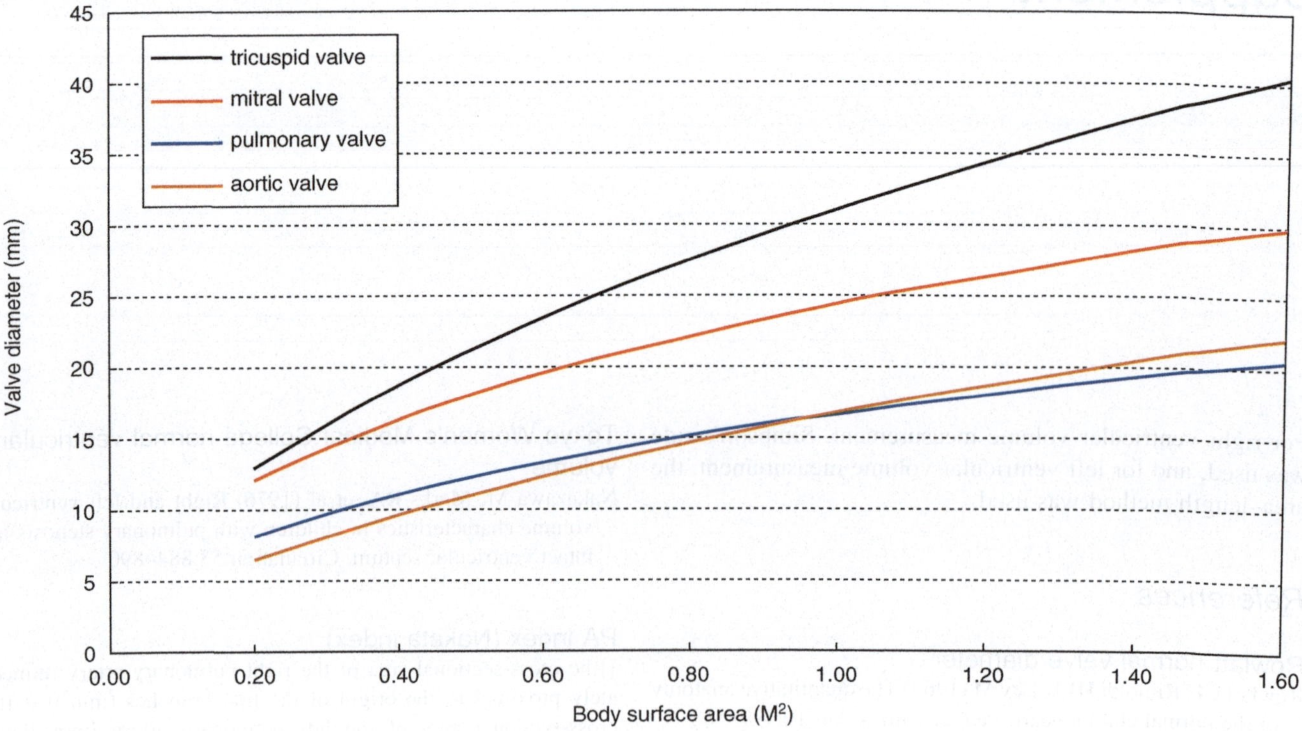

● Kishimoto normal ventricular volume

For right ventricular volume measurement, Simpson's rule was used and for left ventricular volume measurement, the area–length method was used.

Ventricular volume measured by an angiogram was corrected by the formula below.

Relation between ventricular volume and body surface area is shown in the figure.

Right ventricle: 0.76 × measured value +1.5

Left ventricle: 0.974 × measured value −3.05 (measured value >15)

0.733 × measured value +0.03 (measured value ≤15)

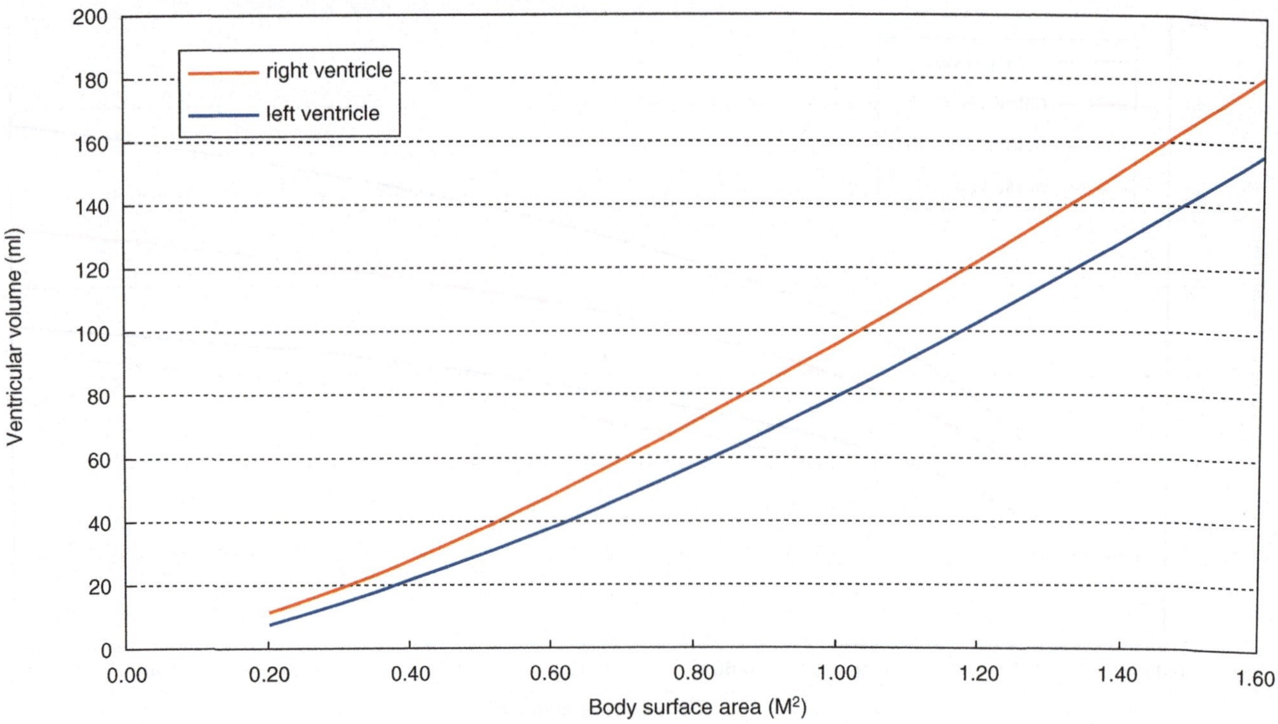

● Tokyo Women's Medical College normal ventricular volume

For right ventricular volume measurement, Simpson's rule was used and for left ventricular volume measurement, the area–length method was used.
Ventricular volume measured by an angiogram was corrected by the formula below.
Relation between ventricular volume and body surface area is shown in the figure.
Right ventricle: 0.649 × measured value
Left ventricle: 0.974 × measured value −3.05

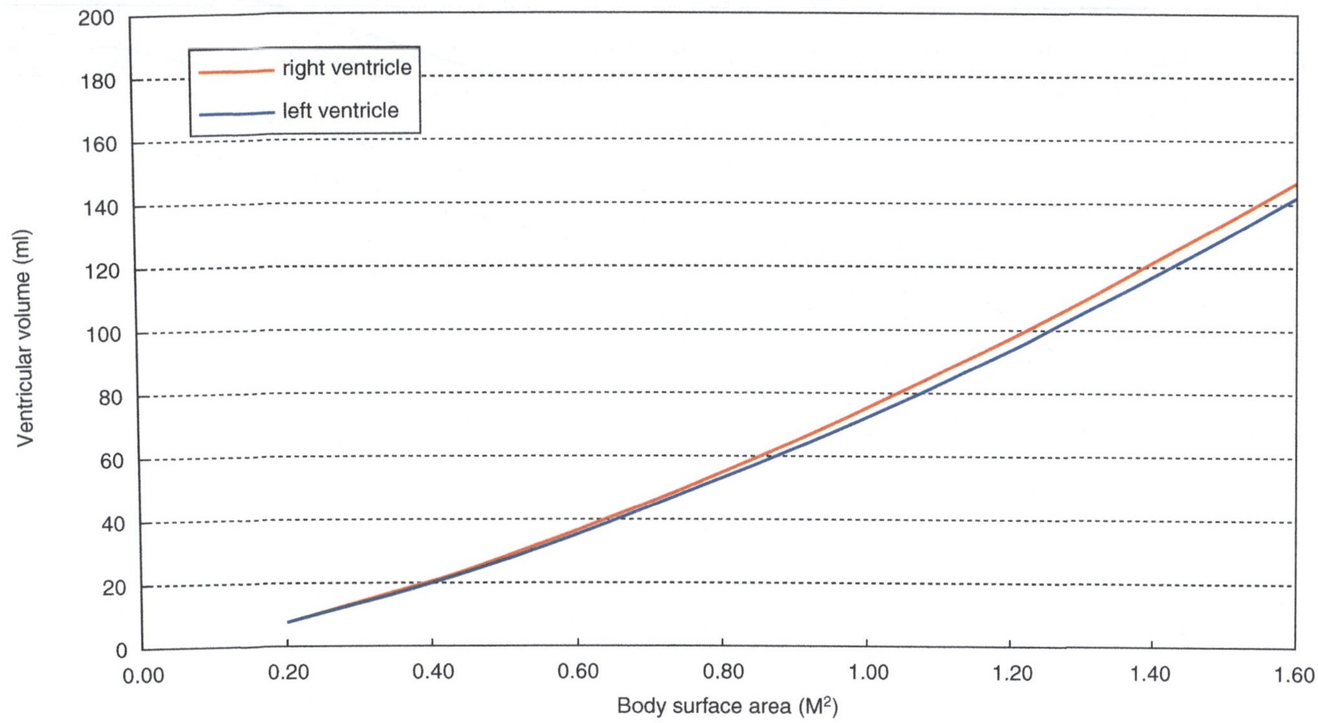

● Pulmonary valve area index (valve area cm²/BSA M²)

Relations between pulmonary annulus diameter (mm) and body surface area (M²) are shown in those cases where the pulmonary valve area index is 1.2, 1.4, 1.6, 1.8, and 2.0.

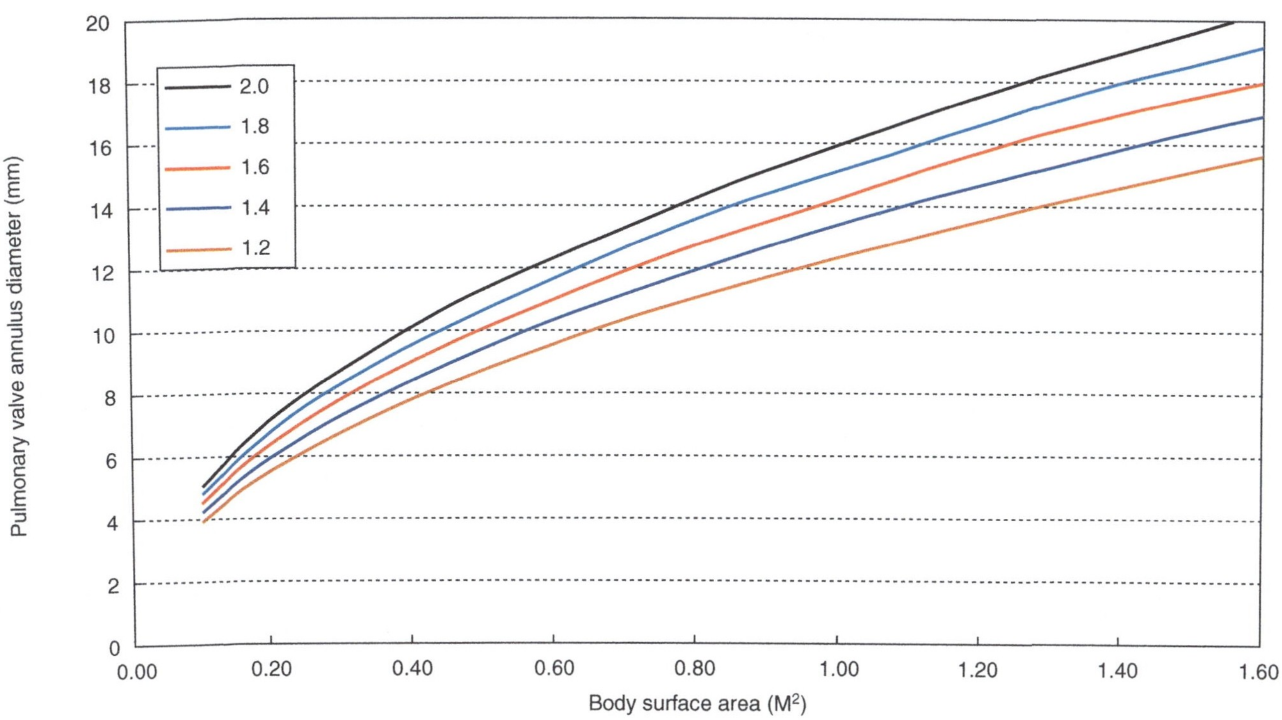

● Unilateral pulmonary artery index (mm^2/M^2)

Relations between either right or left pulmonary artery diameter (mm) and body surface area (M^2) are shown in those cases where the unilateral pulmonary artery index is 200, 150, 125, 100, 75, and 50.

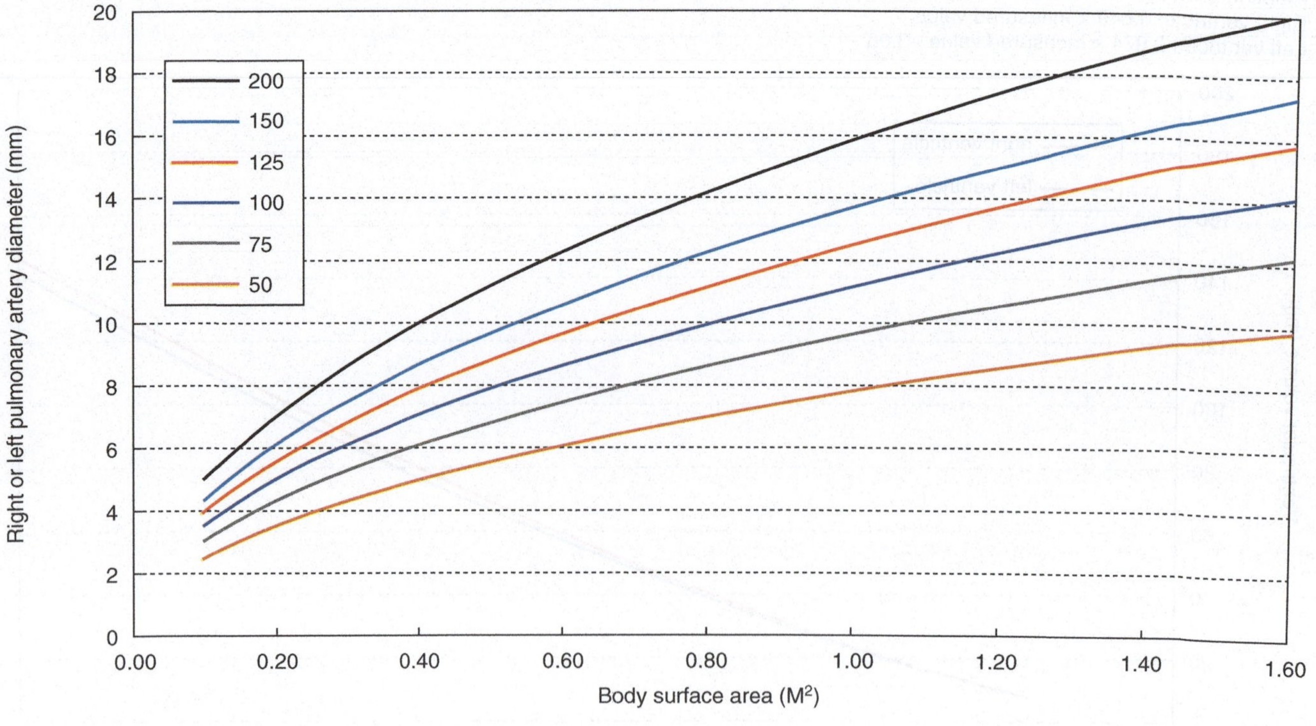

Subject Index

The manufacturer's authorised representative in the EU is Springer Nature Customer Service Centre GmbH, Europaplatz 3, 69115 Heidelberg, Germany. If you have any concerns regarding our products, please contact ProductSafety@springernature.com

Printed and bound by CPI Group (UK) Ltd, Croydon, CR0 4YY
22/09/2026
02221075-0001